The Spectrum of Mineral and Bone Disorders in Chronic Kidney Disease

The Spectrum of Mineral and Bone Disorders in Chronic Kidney Disease

SECOND EDITION

Edited by

Klaus Olgaard

Isidro B. Salusky

Justin Silver

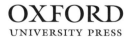

OXFORD
UNIVERSITY PRESS

OXFORD
UNIVERSITY PRESS

Great Clarendon Street, Oxford OX2 6DP

Oxford University Press is a department of the University of Oxford.
It furthers the University's objective of excellence in research, scholarship,
and education by publishing worldwide in

Oxford New York

Auckland Cape Town Dar es Salaam Hong Kong Karachi
Kuala Lumpur Madrid Melbourne Mexico City Nairobi
New Delhi Shanghai Taipei Toronto

With offices in

Argentina Austria Brazil Chile Czech Republic France Greece
Guatemala Hungary Italy Japan Poland Portugal Singapore
South Korea Switzerland Thailand Turkey Ukraine Vietnam

Oxford is a registered trade mark of Oxford University Press
in the UK and in certain other countries

Published in the United States
by Oxford University Press Inc., New York

British Library Cataloguing in Publication Data
Data available

Library of Congress Cataloging in Publication Data
Data available

Typeset by Glyph International, Bangalore, India
Printed by Ashford Colour Press

ISBN 978–0–19–955917–6

10 9 8 7 6 5 4 3 2 1

Whilst every effort has been made to ensure that the contents of this book are as complete, accurate and
up-to-date as possible at the date of writing, Oxford University Press is not able to give any guarantee or
assurance that such is the case. Readers are urged to take appropriately qualified medical advice in all cases.
The information in this book is intended to be useful to the general reader, but should not be used as a
means of self-diagnosis or for the prescription of medication.

Contents

Contributors

Judith Adams
Diagnostic Radiology School of
Medicine,
University of Manchester,
Manchester, UK.

Yaakov H. Applbaum
Department of Radiology,
Hadassah-Hebrew University Medical
Center, Jerusalem, Israel.

Sevcan A. Bakkaloglu
Gazi University, Department of
Paediatric Nephrology,
Besevler, Ankara,
Turkey.

T. Bardin
Université Paris VII and
Rheumatology Department,
Hôpital Laridoisière,
Paris, France.

Ezequiel Bellorin-Font
Division of Nephrology,
University Hospital of Caracas and
Universidad Central de Venezuela,
Venezuela.

Ishir Bhan
Nephrology Division, Massachusetts
General Hospital,
Boston, MA, USA.

Geoffrey A. Block
Denver Nephrologists,
Denver, CO, USA.

Alex J. Brown
Renal Division, Washington University
School of Medicine,
St. Louis, MO, USA.

Edward M. Brown
Division of Endocrinology, Diabetes
and Hypertension,
Department of Medicine, Brigham
and Women's Hospital and Harvard
Medical School,
Boston, MA, USA.

Marc Bürzle
Institute of Biochemistry and
Molecular Medicine,
University of Bern,
Bern, Switzerland.

David A. Bushinsky
University of Rochester School of
Medicine and Dentistry, and
University of Rochester Medical Center,
Rochester, NY, USA.

Jorge B. Cannata-Andia
Andia, Bone and Mineral Research
Unit, Instituto "Reina Sofía"
de Investigación. REDinREN—ISCIII,
Hospital Universitario Central de
Asturias, Universidad de Oviedo,
Oviedo, Spain.

John Cunningham
The Centre for Nephrology,
The Royal Free and University
College Medical School,
London, UK.

Tilman B. Drüeke
Division of Nephrology,
Necker Hospital,
Paris, France.

Adriana Dusso
Department of Internal Medicine/Renal,
Washington University School
of Medicine,
St. Louis, MO, USA.

Ogo I. Egbuna
Division of Endocrinology,
Diabetes and Hypertension,
Department of Medicine, Brigham
and Women's Hospital and Harvard
Medical School, and Division of
Nephrology Department of Medicine,
Beth Israel Deaconess Medical Center
and Harvard Medical School
Boston, MA, USA.

Yifu Fang
Division of Pediatric Nephrology,
Washington University,
St. Louis, MO, USA.

Arnold J. Felsenfeld
University of California, Los Angeles,
and Department of Medicine,
Greater Los Angeles VA Healthcare
System,
Los Angeles, CA, USA.

Jian Q. Feng
Department of Biomedical Sciences,
Texas A&M Health Science Center,
Baylor College of Dentistry,
Dallas, Texas, USA.

Jürgen Floege
Renal Division, University Hospital
RWTH Aachen, Germany.

Masafumi Fukagawa
Division of Nephrology and
Metabolism,
Tokai University School of Medicine,
Isehara, Japan.

David Goldsmith
Consultant Nephrologist,
Clinical Director of NIHR,
London (South) Comprehensive
Local Research Network,
Member of the Faculty of Translational
Medicine, Guy's and St Thomas'
NHS Foundation Trust,
King's Health Partners ASHC,
London, UK.

David Goltzman
Calcium Research Laboratory and
Department of Medicine,
McGill University and Royal Victoria
Hospital of the McGill University
Health Centre,
Montreal, Quebec, Canada.

Esther A. González
Division of Nephrology, Saint Louis
University School of Medicine,
St. Louis, MO, USA.

Alain P. Guerin
Service d'Hémodialyse,
Hôpital F.H. Manhès,
Fleury-Mérogis Cedex, France.

Matthias A. Hediger
Institute of Biochemistry and
Molecular Medicine,
University of Bern,
Bern, Switzerland.

Keith A. Hruska
Division of Pediatric Nephrology,
Washington University,
St. Louis, MO, USA.

T. Keefe Davis
Division of Pediatric Nephrology,
Washington University,
St. Louis, MO, USA.

Markus Ketteler
Nephrology Division,
Klinikum Coburg,
Coburg, Germany.

Hirotaka Komaba
Division of Nephrology and Kidney
Center,
Kobe University School of Medicine,
Kobe, Japan.

Rajiv Kumar
Mayo Clinic,
Rochester, MN, USA.

Makoto Kuro-o
Department of Pathology,
The University of Texas Southwestern
Medical Center,
Dallas, TX, USA.

Ewa Lewin
Department of Nephrology,
Herlev Hospital,
Herlev, Denmark.

Gérard M. London
Service d'Hémodialyse,
Hôpital F.H. Manhès,
Fleury-Mérogis Cedex, France.

Sylvain J. Marchais
Service d'Hémodialyse,
Hôpital F.H. Manhès,
Fleury-Mérogis Cedex, France.

Kevin J. Martin
Division of Nephrology,
Saint Louis University,
Saint Louis, MO, USA.

Suresh Mathew
Division of Pediatric Nephrology,
Washington University,
St. Louis, MO, USA.

Imran Memon
Division of Pediatric Nephrology,
Washington University,
St. Louis, MO, USA.

Sharon M. Moe
Indiana University School of Medicine
and Roudebush VAMC,
Indianapolis, IN, USA.

Tally Naveh-Many
Minerva Center for Calcium and Bone
Metabolism,
Nephrology Services,
Hadassah Hebrew University Medical
Center,
Jerusalem, Israel.

Edward F. Nemeth
MetisMedica,
Toronto, Canada.

Klaus Olgaard
Department of Nephrology,
Righospitalet, University of
Copenhagen,
Copenhagen, Denmark.

Susan M. Ott
University of Washington,
Seattle, WA, USA.

Bruno Pannier
Service d'Hémodialyse, Hôpital F.H.
Manhès,
Fleury-Mérogis Cedex, France.

Paulo Raggi
Emory University School of Medicine,
Division of Cardiology and Department
of Radiology,
Atlanta, GA, USA.

Mariano Rodriguez
Unidad de Investigacion y Servicio
de Nefrologia,
Hospital Universitario Reina Sofia,
Cordoba, Spain.

Isidro B. Salusky
University of California,
Los Angeles, CA, USA.

Emile Sarfati
Centre Hospitalier Universitaire
Saint-Louis,
Paris, France.

Susan C. Schiavi
Endocrine and Renal Sciences,
Genzyme Corporation,
Framingham, MA, USA.

Catherine M. Shanahan
British Heart Foundation Centre,
Cardiovascular Division,
Kings College London,
London, UK.

Rukshana C. Shroff
British Heart Foundation Centre,
Cardiovascular Division,
Kings College London,
London, UK.

Justin Silver
Minerva Center for Calcium
and Bone Metabolism,
Nephrology Services, Hadassah
Hebrew University Medical Center,
Jerusalem, Israel.

Mukesh Sinha
Mayo Clinic,
Rochester, MN, USA.

Eduardo Slatopolsky
Renal Division,
Washington University School of
Medicine,
St. Louis, MO, USA.

Stuart M. Sprague
Division of Nephrology and Hypertension,
NorthShore University
HealthSystem-University of Chicago
Pritzker School of Medicine,
Chicago, IL, USA.

Yoshiro Suzuki
Institute of Biochemistry and
Molecular Medicine,
University of Bern,
Bern, Switzerland.

Motoko Tanaka
Department of Nephrology,
Akebono Clinic,
Kumamoto, Japan.

Ravi Thadhani
Nephrology Division,
Massachusetts General Hospital,
Boston, MA, USA.

Leslie Thomas
Mayo Clinic,
Rochester, MN, USA.

Masanori Tokumoto
Renal Division, Department of Internal
Medicine,
Washington University School of
Medicine,
St. Louis, MO, USA.

Armando Torres
Nephrology Section,
University of La Laguna, Tenerife,
Canary Islands, Spain.

Pablo Ureña
Clinique du Landy. Service de
Néphrologie et Dialyse,
Saint Ouen; Hôpital
Necker-Enfants Malades,
Service d'Explorations Fonctionnelles,
Paris; and Centre de Recherche
Croissance et Signalisation.
Université Paris Descartes,
Faculté de Médecine,
Paris, France.

Katherine Wesseling-Perry
David Geffen School of Medicine at
University of California,
Los Angeles, CA, USA.

Myles Wolf
University of Miami,
Miami, FL, USA.

Acknowledgements

The colour printing of this book was made possible by an unrestricted grant from Genzyme.
The cover painting was kindly provided by the artist Pamela Silver, Jerusalem, Israel.

Abbreviations

2HPT	secondary hyperparathyroidism	BMD	bone mineral density
AA	arachidonic acid	BMI	body mass index
ABD	adynamic bone disease	BMP	bone morphogenetic protein
AC	arterial calcification	BMU	bone metabolic units
ACE	angiotensin converting enzyme	BSAP	bone-specific alkaline phosphatase
Acf	activation frequency	BSP	bone sialoprotein
ACTH	adrenocorticotropin hormone	BUA	broadband ultrasound attenuation
AD	adynamic		
ADH	autosomal dominant hypoparathyroidism	CAC	coronary artery calcification
AGE	advanced glycation end products	CAD	coronary artery disease
AHSG	α2-Schmid Heremans glycoprotein	CAP	carbonated apatite
		CAPD	continuous ambulatory peritoneal dialysis
AoCS	aortic calcification score	CaR	calcium receptor
AP	alkaline phosphatase	CARE2	Calcium Acetate Renagel Evaluation-2 Study
ApoE	apolipoprotein E		
ARB	angiotensin receptor blocker	CaSR	calcium-sensing receptor
ARE	AU-rich elements	CAT	chloramphenicol acetyl transferase
ARHR	autosomal recessive hypophosphatemic rickets	cdk	cyclin-dependent kinases
ARIC	Atherosclerosis Risk in Communities Study	CgA	chromogranin A
		CHO	Chinese hamster ovary fibroblasts
ASBMR	American Society for Bone and Mineral Research	CIMT	carotid intima-media thickness
AT	autotransplantation	CKD	chronic kidney disease
ATP	adenosine triphosphate	CN	carbon:nitrogen
AUC	area under the plasma concentration–time curve	COX	cyclo-oxygenase
		CPPD	calcium pyrophosphate dehydrate
AVN	avascular necrosis		
baPWV	brachial-ankle pulse wave velocity	CPPDD	calcium pyrophosphate dihydrate deposition disease
bFGF	basic fibroblast growth factor	CRE	cyclic AMP response element
BFR	bone formation rate	CREB	cyclic AMP response element binding protein
BGP	bone Gla protein		
BLC	Blomstrand lethal chondrodysplasia	CRP	C-reactive protein
		CSF	colony-stimulating factors
BMAD	bone mineral apparent density	CT	computed tomography
BMC	bone mineral content	CTAL	cortical thick ascending limb

CTS	carpal tunnel syndrome	FEPi	fractional excretion of Pi
CUA	calcific uremic arteriolopathy	FGF	fibroblast growth factor
CV	cardiovascular	FHH	familial hypocalciuric hypercalcemia
CVC	calcifying vascular cell		
DAPI	death associated protein 1	FRAX	fracture risk assessment
DBP	diastolic blood pressure	GABA	gamma-aminobutyric acid
DCOR	Dialysis Clinical Outcomes Revisited Study	GFP	green fluorescent protein
		GFR	glomerular filtration rate
DCT	distal convoluted tubule	GH	growth hormone
DEXA	dual energy X-ray absorptiometry	GHRH	growth hormone-releasing hormone
DMP1	dentin matrix protein 1		
DNA	deoxyribonucleic acid	GI	gastrointestinal
DOPPS	Dialysis Outcomes and Practice Patterns Study	GM-CSF	granulocyte macrophage colony–stimulating factor
DPD	deoxypyridinoline	GPCR	G protein-coupled receptors
DRI	daily recommended intake	GTP	guanosine-5'-triphosphate
DXA	dual energy X-ray absorptiometry	HD	hemodialysis
		HETE	hydroxyeicosatetranoic acid
DXA	dual X-ray absorptiometry	HHRH	hypophosphatemic rickets with hypercalciuria
EBCT	electron beam computed tomography		
ECD	extracellular C-terminal domain	HNF1B	hepatocyte nuclear factor 1B
ECF	extracellular fluids	HPETE	hydroxyperoxyeicosatetranoic acid
EDTA	European Dialysis and Transplant Association	HPT	hyperparathyroidism
		HR	hazard ratio
EGF	epidermal growth factor	HRCT	high resolution computed tomography
EGFR	epidermal growth factor receptor		
ELISA	enzyme-linked immunoabsorbent assay	HRMRI	high resolution magnetic resonance imaging
		HSC	hematopoietic stem cell
EMG	electromyogram	HSH	hypomagnesemia with secondary hypocalcemia
EMT	epithelial-to-mesenchymal transition		
		HTBD	high bone remodeling
ENPP1	ecto-nucleotide pyrophosphatase/phosphodiesterase 1	HTLV-I	human T-cell leukemia virus type I
		HVDRR	hereditary vitamin D-resistant rickets
ENS	epidermal nevus syndromes		
ER	endoplasmic reticulum	ICD	intracellular C-terminal domain
ESKD	end-stage kidney disease	ICTP	type I cross-linked carboxy-terminal telopeptide
ESRD	end-stage renal disease		
ET-1	Endothelin-1	IDBP	intracellular vitamin D binding protein
EVOLVE	evaluation of cinacalcet HCl therapy to lower cardiovascular events study		
		IGF	insulin-like growth factors
		IHC	immunohistochemistry
FBHH	familial benign hypocalciuric hypercalcemia	IMCD	inner medullary collecting duct
		IP	inositol phosphate
FD	fibrous dysplasia	IP$_3$	inositol-tri-phosphate

iPTH	intact parathyroid hormone	MUO	mixed uremic osteodystrophy
IRMA	radio-immunometric assays	NBR	natural background radiation
IRS	insulin receptor substrates	NHANES III	Third National Health and Nutrition Examination Survey
ISCD	International Society of Clinical Densitometry	NHERF	Na^+/H^+ exchanger regulatory factor
ITAM	immunoreceptor tyrosine-based activation motifs	NLS	nuclear localization signal
IV	intravenous	NSHPT	neonatal severe primary hyperparathyroidism
JG	juxtaglomerular		
JNK	c-Jun N-terminal kinases	NTBD	normal bone remodeling
K/DOQI	Kidney Dialysis Outcomes Quality Initiative	NTX	N-terminal crosslink telopeptide
		OC	osteocalcin
KDIGO	Kidney Disease: Improving Global Outcomes	OCT	22-oxacalcitriol
		OD	osteoglophonic dysplasia
KI	knock-in	OF	osteitis fibrosa
KSRP	KH-type splicing regulatory protein	OGR1	ovarian G-protein coupled receptor 1
LDL	low density lipoprotein	OM	osteomalacia
LH	luteinizing hormone	ON	osteonectin
LRP	low-density-lipoprotein-receptor-related protein	OPG	osteoprotegerin
		OPN	osteopontin
LTBD	low bone remodeling	OVX	ovariectomized
LV	left ventricular	PA	postero-anterior
LVH	left ventricular hypertropy	PBM	peak bone mass
MAC	medial artery calcification	PC	perichondrium
MAP	mean arterial pressures	PCNA	proliferating cell nuclear antigen
MAPK	mitogen-activated protein kinases	PCPE-1	procollagen C-proteinase enhancer 1
MAS	McCune–Albright syndrome	PDDR	Pseudovitamin D-deficiency rickets
MBD	mineral and bone disorder		
MCP-1	macrophage chemoattractant protein 1	PDGF	platelet-derived growth factor
M-CSF	macrophage colony stimulating factor	PDIT	percutaneous vitamin D injection therapy
MEPE	matrix extracellular phosphoglycoprotein	PEIT	percutaneous ethanol injection therapy
mGluRs	metabotropic receptors for glutamate	PHEX	phosphate regulating protein with homology to endopeptidases on the X-chromosome
MGP	matrix Gla protein		
MIBI	^{99m}Tc-methoxyisobutyl isonitrile		
MLT	mineralization lag time	PICP	procollagen type I C-terminal propeptide
MMP	matrix metalloproteinase		
MRI	magnetic resonance imaging	PII	inferior parathyroid
MSCT	multi-slice computed tomography	PINP	procollagen type I N-terminal propeptide
MTAL	medullary thick ascending limb	PIV	superior parathyroid

PKA	protein kinase A
PKC	protein kinase C
PLA_2	phospholipase A_2
PLC	phospholipase C
PLD	phospholipase D
PMCA	plasma membrane calcium ATPase
pQCT	peripheral quantitative computed tomography
PRIMO	paricalcitol benefits in renal failure induced cardiac morbidity
PT	proximal tubule
PTH	parathyroid hormone
PTHrP	parathyroid hormone related peptide
PTX	parathyroidectomy
PWV	pulse wave velocity
PYD	pyridinoline
QCT	quantitative computed tomography
QMR	quantitative magnetic resonance
QUS	quantitative ultrasound
RAS	renin-angiotensin system
rhGH	recombinant human GH
RIA	radioimmunoassay
RIND	Renagel in New Dialysis Patients
RNA	ribonucleic acid
ROI	regions of interest
ROS	reactive oxygen species
RR	relative risk
RTK	receptor tyrosine kinase
RT-PCR	reverse transcriptase-polymerase chain reaction
RXR	retinoic X receptor
SBP	systolic blood pressure
SC	subcutaneous
SDS	1 standard deviation
SEM	scanning electron microscopy
SERM	selective estrogen receptor modulator
sFRP	secreted frizzled-related protein
SIBLING	small integrin-binding ligand, N-linked glycoprotein
SLC	solute carrier series
SMA	smooth muscle actin
SNP	single nucleotide polymorphisms
SNX	subtotal nephrectomy
SOS	speed of sound
SPECT	single-photon emission computed tomography
TEM	transmission electron microscopy
TGF	transforming growth factor
TLR	toll-like receptor
TMD	transmembrane domain
TMV	turnover, mineralization, and volume
TNF	tumor necrosis factor
TRAP	tartrate-resistant acid phosphatase
TRL	carboxyl terminal residues
TRP	tubular reabsorption of phosphate
TRPV6	transient receptor potential vanilloid 6
TSH	thyroid-stimulating hormone
TTG	Treat-to-Goal
TTP	tristetraprolin
US	ultrasound
UTR	untranslated regions
VC	vascular calcification
VDBP	vitamin D binding protein
VDDR	vitamin D-resistant rickets
VDIR	VDR interacting repressor
VDR	vitamin D-receptor
VDRE	vitamin D response element
VEGF	vascular endothelial growth factor
VFTM	Venus fly trap motif
VSMC	vascular smooth muscle cell
WTh	wall thickness
XLH	X-linked hypophosphatemic

Introduction

Chronic kidney disease (CKD) is a global public health problem, affecting up to 10% of the world's population and increasing in prevalence and adverse outcomes. The progressive loss of kidney function is invariably complicated by disorders of bone and mineral metabolism and cardiovascular disease, resulting in premature death.

The disturbances in mineral metabolism begin early in the course of progressive CKD with a reduced capacity to fully excrete a phosphate load and to convert vitamin D into the biological active 1,25-dihydroxy-vitamin-D, resulting in a compensatory secondary hyperparathyroidism. A number of factors appear to be involved in or affected in this abnormal regulation. Recently, elevated FGF23 and disturbed klotho levels have been found in early CKD in addition to hyperparathyroidism, hyperphosphatemia, vitamin D deficiency, bone disease, and extraskeletal calcifications. This complex pathophysiology has led to the development of a number of new drugs and therapeutic approaches, and it motivated the publication in 2003 of "The Clinical Practice Guidelines" by the Kidney/Dialysis Outcomes Quality Initiative (K/DOQI).

In 2006, the term Chronic Kidney Disease-Mineral and Bone Disorder (CKD-MBD) was introduced and defined at the Kidney Disease: Improving Global Outcome (KDIGO) conference as the clinical syndrome combining the mineral, bone, and cardiovascular abnormalities that develop as complications to CKD. Conferees further decided that the term renal osteodystrophy should be used to refer only to the bone pathology associated with CKD. In follow-up, KDIGO published in 2006 the "Clinical Guide to Bone and Mineral Metabolism in CKD" in collaboration with the National Kidney Foundation. Subsequently, in August 2009, KDIGO published the "Clinical Practice Guideline for the Diagnosis, Evaluation, Prevention, and Treatment of Chronic Kidney Disease-Mineral and Bone Disorder (CKD-MBD)" in *Kidney International*.

This book is the second edition of the textbook *The Spectrum of Renal Osteodystrophy*, originally published 2000. In 32 new and completely updated chapters, written by the best experts in the field, the book deals with the physiology and pathophysiology of the whole spectrum of CKD-MBD. The chapter authors describe and evaluate the latest knowledge in bone biology, calcium and related receptors, parathyroid hormone and vitamin D regulation, disturbances in other hormone regulation, pathogenesis of vascular calcifications and their relation to bone disease, klotho and the different phosphatonins in health and disease, diagnosis and treatment of bone disease, secondary hyperparathyroidism, and vascular calcification in uremic adult patients, children, and kidney-transplanted patients. There is also a chapter on the morbidity and mortality related to disturbances in mineral metabolism in CKD.

Fascinating breakthroughs are presented in nearly all of the chapters. Examples include advances in our understanding of the "bone-vascular-kidney" axis and the new hormones and factors involved in phosphate homeostasis.

The purpose of this book is to provide a state-of-the-art overview of both the basic and the clinical aspects of all the various disturbances of CKD-MBD. Our aim is to bring to the attention of adult and pediatric nephrologists, as well as other specialists and practitioners, the new diagnostic and therapeutic developments in the pathogenesis and treatment of the many different and challenging aspects of CKD-MBD.

We offer sincere thanks and great appreciation to all of the book's contributors for their outstanding chapters. We hope that this book will have an impact on the quality of care provided to children and adults affected with complications of CKD.

March 2010
Editors
Klaus Olgaard, Isidro B. Salusky, Justin Silver

Chapter 1

Definition and classification of renal osteodystrophy and chronic kidney disease–mineral bone disorder (CKD–MBD)

Sharon M. Moe

Chronic kidney disease (CKD) is a worldwide public health problem affecting 5–10% of the world's population with increasing prevalence and adverse outcomes, including progressive loss of kidney function, cardiovascular disease, disorders of bone and mineral metabolism, and premature death.[1] In people with healthy kidneys, normal serum levels of phosphorus and calcium are maintained through the combined effects of three hormones: parathyroid hormone (PTH), $1,25(OH)_2D$ (calcitriol), and phosphatonins. These hormones act on three target organs: the kidney, bone, and intestine. The kidneys serve to regulate PTH mediated calcium reabsorption and phosphate excretion, convert vitamin D to its metabolite calcitriol, and increase phosphate excretion in response to changes in serum phosphorus mediated by fibroblast growth factor 23 (FGF23) and PTH. Thus, the kidneys play a critical role in the regulation of normal serum calcium and phosphorus concentrations, leading to abnormal homeostasis in the setting of CKD.

Disturbances in mineral metabolism are common complications of CKD, beginning early in the course of progressive CKD. Beginning in stage 3 CKD, the damaged kidney is unable to fully excrete a phosphorus load nor convert vitamin D into its metabolite calcitriol, leading to a compensatory secondary hyperparathyroidism. Elevated PTH and decreased calcitriol levels are found in 40% of patients with a glomerular filtration rate (GFR) between 40 and 50ml/min, and 80% of patients with GFR below 20ml/min.[2] Elevated FGF23 is also observed beginning in CKD stage 4.[3] The progression of kidney disease is eventually associated with the inability to completely compensate for the loss of GFR ultimately resulting in hyperphosphatemia, bone disease, and extra-skeletal calcification. This complex pathophysiology has led to an evolution of new drugs and therapeutic approaches over the last 30 years. In 2003, the clinical practice guidelines from K/DOQI (Kidney Dialysis Outcomes Quality Initiative) were published.[4] The publication of these guidelines led to a more uniform approach to the care and management of patients by general nephrologists, but also pointed out the lack of high quality evidence-based data for such treatment and a need for research.

To stimulate collaborative research, the National Kidney Foundation held an international conference of basic and clinical researchers in Washington DC in 2003. Three work groups focused on the assessment of bone turnover, osteoporosis, and vascular calcification.[5] To briefly summarize the conclusions, the bone turnover work group determined that parathyroid hormone and other bone biomarker assays, and interpretation of bone biopsy by histomorphometry require international standardization.[6] The osteoporosis work group determined that the assessment of bone fragility in CKD patients was complicated and that the use of dual energy X-ray absorptiometry (DEXA) assessments must be interpreted simultaneously with bone turnover prior to initiating anti-resorptive therapies. Because of this, the group recommended that the term osteoporosis be avoided in patients with advanced CKD.[7] The third work group concluded that arterial calcification was common in CKD, in part because of the increased prevalence of medial calcification in addition to intimal/atherosclerotic calcification. The group recommended that there be increased education to nephrologists and cardiologists about the differences and similarities of these types of vascular calcification, and that simple screening methods be developed and validated.[8] The conclusion of this consensus conference was that all three of these processes (abnormal mineral metabolism, abnormal bone, and extra-skeletal calcification) are closely interrelated and, together, make a major contribution to the morbidity and mortality of patients with CKD.

This meeting was followed in 2005 by another international conference sponsored by KDIGO (Kidney Disease: Improving Global Outcomes). The purpose of this meeting was to better define renal osteodystrophy. The conclusions of this expert panel of over 80 individuals from around the world was that the term 'CKD-mineral and bone disorder (CKD-MBD)' should be used to describe the broader clinical syndrome encompassing mineral, bone and cardiovascular abnormalities that develop as a complication of CKD. The term 'renal osteodystrophy' should be restricted to describing the bone pathology associated with CKD (Table 1.1).[9] Renal osteodystrophy is

Table 1.1 Kidney disease improving global outcomes (KDIGO) classification of CKD-MBD and renal osteodystrophy

---

Definition of CKD-MBD

A systemic disorder of mineral and bone metabolism due to CKD manifested by either one or a combination of the following:

◆ Abnormalities of calcium, phosphorus, PTH, or vitamin D metabolism

◆ Abnormalities in bone turnover, mineralization, volume, linear growth, or strength

◆ Vascular or other soft tissue calcification

Definition of Renal Osteodystrophy

◆ Renal osteodystrophy is an alteration of bone morphology in patients with CKD.

◆ It is one measure of the skeletal component of the systemic disorder of CKD-MBD that is quantifiable by histomorphometry of bone biopsy.

Adapted from Moe et al. (2006)[9] with permission.

defined as an alteration of bone morphology in patients with CKD. It is one measure of the skeletal component of the systemic disorder of CKD-MBD that is quantifiable by histomorphometry of bone biopsy. In this chapter we will discuss both disorders: renal osteodystrophy and CKD-MBD.

Renal osteodystrophy

The spectrum of bone abnormalities in CKD

The mineral and endocrine functions disrupted in CKD are critically important in the regulation of bone remodelling. As a result, bone abnormalities are found almost universally in patients with CKD requiring dialysis and in the majority of patients with CKD Stages 3–5.[10–12] In 1966, Pendras et al.[13] reported the experience with the first 22 patients to receive long-term hemodialysis, stating 'the bone disease of chronic renal failure has been most troublesome'. Thus, it became clear that dialysis does not cure bone and mineral disorders of kidney disease. Unfortunately, over 40 years later, there is still increased prevalence of hip fracture compared with the general population across the entire range of CKD stages 3–5 and in dialysis patients.[14–24] Dialysis patients in their 40s have a relative risk of hip fracture 80-fold that of age- and sex-matched controls.[16] In patients with stage 4 CKD, the risk of hip fracture was nearly 4-fold that of the general population without CKD.[20] Furthermore, a hip fracture in patients with a GFR <45ml/min or on dialysis is associated with a doubling of the mortality observed in non-dialysis patients with a hip fracture.[17,23,25]

In the general population the factors associated with fragility fractures are called osteoporosis. Studies in patients without CKD have demonstrated that low bone mineral density is associated with increased fracture risk, even when adjusted for age.[26] This led to an emphasis on bone mass, generally assessed by DEXA. However, there was recognition of an apparent discrepancy between the small increase in bone mineral density by DEXA and much larger decrease in fracture risk in various therapeutic trials.[27] These data and advances in other imaging modalities, led to a National Institutes of Health consensus conference to redefine osteoporosis as 'a skeletal disorder characterized by compromised bone strength that results in an increased risk of fracture. Bone strength reflects the integration of two main features: bone density and bone quality'. These 'quality' factors include abnormal bone turnover or remodelling, and other indices of bone architecture, such as geometry, connectivity, mineralization, and collagen cross-linking. These factors appear additive to bone mineral density as determinants of bone strength.[28] Abnormal bone quality may be especially prominent in dialysis patients due to the co-existence of disordered bone remodelling and this abnormal quality may be the cause of the increased fractures observed in CKD.

Early in the course of CKD, secondary hyperparathyroidism leads to the development of osteitis fibrosa cystica. However, many patients with CKD (both pre dialysis and on dialysis) also have low-turnover bone disease, primarily adynamic bone where there is a paucity of both osteoblasts and osteoclasts.[29–31] In bone biopsies series in patients with CKD, only 5% of patients have normal bone formation rate. In addition to abnormalities in turnover, patients with CKD may have abnormal bone mineralization or bone volume.[12] Clinically, there is also a high prevalence of low bone mineral density by DXA in both CKD and dialysis patients.[14,19,32–34] Thus, both histomorphometry and bone mineral density are frequently abnormal in patients with CKD, and thus both bone quality and bone mass are impaired. It is therefore not surprising that patients with CKD suffer fragility fractures. However, bone quality is likely the primary determinant of increased fracture risk with progressive CKD, additive to the effects of low bone mass. Low bone mass may be from pre-existing loss of bone prior to the onset of kidney disease, concomitant therapies such as corticosteroids, or abnormal bone remodelling from CKD resulting in net loss of bone (Fig. 1.1). The complicated pathogenesis of abnormal bone fragility in CKD was the rationale to not use the term 'osteoporosis' in patients with CKD,[7] and for recent international guidelines to not recommend routine use of DXA as a screening tool.[35]

Classification of renal osteodystrophy

Of all the factors that result in abnormal bone quality, bone turnover, or remodelling is the best characterized in CKD, and can be assessed by bone biopsy. Sherrard and others proposed a classification system for renal osteodystrophy that utilized the parameters of osteoid (unmineralized bone) area as a percentage of total bone area, and fibrosis. These two static parameters, together with the dynamic bone turnover assessed by bone formation rate or activation frequency have been used to distinguish the various forms of renal osteodystrophy over the past 20 years (Table 1.2).[31] The histological features of high turnover disease (predominant hyperparathyroidism or osteitis fibrosa) are characterized by increased rate of bone formation, increased bone resorption, extensive osteoclastic and osteoblastic activity, and progressive increase in endosteal peritrabecular fibrosis. High osteoblast activity is manifested by an increase in unmineralized bone matrix. In osteitis fibrosa, the alignment of strands of collagen

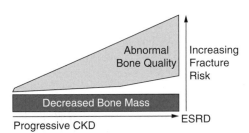

Fig. 1.1 Contribution of bone quality and bone mass to fractures in chronic kidney disease (CKD). As patients have progressively deteriorating kidney function (left to right, x axis) there is an increasing risk of fracture. This comes from two components—decreased bone mass and abnormal bone quality. The decreased bone mass may be due to pre-existing conditions and likely worsens with progression of CKD due to net bone resorption over bone formation in patients with secondary hyperparathyroidism. Abnormal bone quality increases more substantially due to abnormal turnover and mineralization with progressive CKD due to associated mineral metabolism derangements. As a result, by the time a patient requires dialysis, the contribution of abnormal bone quality to fracture risk is greater than that from decreased bone mass.

Table 1.2 1993 Histological classification of renal osteodystrophy

Lesion	Area of fibrosis % of tissue area	Area of osteoid % of total bone area	Bone formation rate μm²/ mm² tissue area day
Mild	<0.5%	<15%	>108
Osteitis fibrosa	>0.5%	<15%	X
Mixed	>0.5%	>15%	X
Osteomalacia	<0.5%	>15%	X
Adynamic	<0.5%	<15%	<108
Normal range	0	1–7%	108–500

X is not a diagnostic criterion. Adapted with permission from Sherrard et al. (1993).[31]

in the bone matrix has an irregular woven pattern that contrasts with the normal lamellar (parallel) alignment of strands of collagen in normal bone.

Although low turnover disease is common in the absence of aluminium, it was initially described as a result of aluminium toxicity. Osteomalacia is characterized by an excess of unmineralized osteoid as a percentage of bone volume, manifested as wide osteoid seams and a markedly decreased mineralization rate. The presence of increased unmineralized osteoid *per se* does not necessarily indicate a mineralizing defect, because increased quantities of osteoid appear in conditions associated with high rates of bone formation when mineralization lags behind the increased synthesis of matrix. The histological features of adynamic bone disease are characterized histologically by absence of cellular (osteoblast and osteoclast) activity, osteoid formation, and endosteal fibrosis. Mixed uremic osteodystrophy is the term that has been used to describe bone biopsies that have features of secondary hyperparathyroidism together with evidence of a mineralization defect. There is extensive osteoclastic and osteoblastic activity coupled with increased osteoid as a percentage of bone volume, than expected. Unfortunately, mixed uremic osteodystrophy been inconsistently defined by different laboratories.

Utilizing this classification system, the prevalence of different forms of renal osteodystrophy has changed over the past decade (Fig. 1.2). Whereas osteitis fibrosa cystica due to severe hyperparathyroidism had previously been the predominant lesion, the prevalence of mixed uremic osteodystrophy and adynamic bone disease has recently increased. However, the overall percentage of patients with high bone formation compared with low bone formation has not changed dramatically over the last 20–30 years, but osteomalacia has been essentially replaced with adynamic bone disease. Importantly, the series of bone biopsies yield widely different results depending on the level of GFR, and the country in which the study was done.[36,37]

New classification of renal osteodystrophy: the 'Turnover, Mineralization and Volume' system

Historically, renal osteodystrophy has been defined as a spectrum of disorders ranging from low turnover (adynamic) to high turnover disease (osteitis fibrosa) as detailed

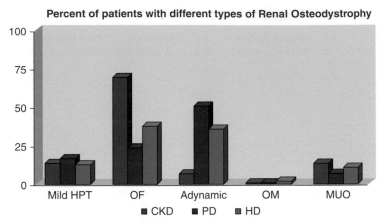

Fig. 1.2 The spectrum of histological types of renal osteodystrophy in patients with chronic kidney stages 3–5. This graph represents the distribution of various pathologic forms of renal osteodystrophy in three recent studies with a total *n* of 319 subjects.[67–69] HPT = hyperparathyroidism; OF = osteitis fibrosa or severe HPT; Adynamic = adynamic bone disease; OM = osteomalacia; MUO = mixed uremic osteodystrophy. Reproduced with permission from Moe SM & Sprague S, *Brenner and Rector's The Kidney*, 8th edn, p. 1800.

above. As our understanding of bone biology progresses, there is increased appreciation of diverse physiological processes leading to similar bone biopsy findings. In addition, there has been new information on bone volume as an independent parameter.[12] In order to clarify the interpretation of bone biopsy results and develop international standardization in the evaluation of renal osteodystrophy, the biopsy working group at the KDIGO International Consensus Conference in 2005 agreed to use three key histological descriptors—bone turnover, mineralization, and volume (TMV) system, with any combination of each of the descriptors possible in a given specimen (Table 1.3). The TMV classification scheme provides a clinically relevant description of the underlying bone pathology as assessed by histomorphometry, which in turn helps define the pathophysiology and thereby guide therapy.

Turnover reflects the rate of skeletal remodelling that is normally the coupled process of bone resorption and bone formation. It is assessed with histomorphometry by dynamic measurements of osteoblast function using double-tetracycline labeling. Bone formation rates (BFR) and activation frequency (Acf) represent acceptable parameters for assessing bone turnover. Bone turnover is affected mainly by hormones, cytokines, mechanical stimuli, and growth factors that influence the recruitment, differentiation, and activity of osteoclasts and osteoblasts. It is important to clarify that although bone formation rate is frequently similar to bone resorption rate, which cannot be measured directly, this is not always true. Imbalance in these processes can affect bone volume. For example, excess resorption over formation will lead to negative bone balance and decreased bone volume. *Mineralization* reflects how well bone

Table 1.3 2005 TMV classification system for renal osteodystrophy

Turnover	Mineralization	Volume
Low		Low
	Normal	
Normal		Normal
	Abnormal	
High		High

Adapted from Moe et al. (2006)[9] with permission.

collagen becomes calcified during the formation phase of skeletal remodelling. It is assessed with histomorphometry by static measurements of osteoid volume and osteoid thickness, and by dynamic, tetracycline-based measurements of mineralization lag time and osteoid maturation time. Causes of impaired mineralization include inadequate vitamin D nutrition, mineral (calcium or phosphorus) deficiency, acidosis, or bone aluminium toxicity. *Volume* indicates the amount of bone per unit volume of tissue. It is assessed with histomorphometry by static measurements of bone volume in cancellous bone. Determinants of bone volume include age, gender, race, genetic factors, nutrition, endocrine disorders, physical activity, toxicities, neurological function, vascular supply, growth factors, and cytokines.

This new TMV classification is consistent with the 1993 used classification system (Table 1.2),[31] but provides more information on parameters other than turnover. A comparison of the new system to the old system is shown in Fig. 1.3.

Chronic kidney disease–mineral bone disorder

Renal osteodystrophy beyond bone

Renal ostedystrophy, literally translated to bone pathology from renal impairment was introduced by Liu and Chu in 1943.[38,39] However, the term has also been used to describe mineral related abnormalities in CKD and even arterial calcification, both of which may be associated with cardiovascular disease and all cause mortality.[40] Cardiovascular disease accounts for 70% of all deaths in patients with CKD, with an overall mortality of 20% per year in patients on dialysis.[41] In individuals with stage 5 CKD on dialysis, cardiovascular mortality rates are 10–500 times higher than in the general population, even after adjustment for gender, race, and presence of diabetes.[15] Importantly, individuals at earlier stages of CKD not yet on dialysis (stages 3–5), are up to 17 times more likely to die of cardiovascular disease than they are of progressing to dialysis.[42] Multiple cross-sectional studies in dialysis patients have found that disordered mineral metabolism, especially hyperphosphatemia, increase the risk of cardiovascular and all cause mortality.[43–45]

One mechanism by which abnormal mineral metabolism may increase cardiovascular risk is by inducing or accelerating arterial and valvular calcification. Patients on dialysis have 2–5-fold more coronary artery calcification than age matched individuals

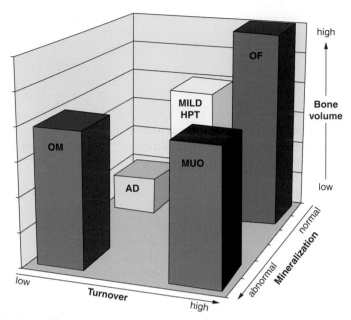

Fig. 1.3 TMV classification system for bone histomorphometry. The figure is a graphical example of how the TMV system provides more information than the present, commonly used classification scheme. Each axis represents one of the descriptors in the TMV classification: turnover (from low to high), mineralization (from normal to abnormal), and bone volume (from low to high). Individual patient parameters could be plotted on the graph, or means and ranges of grouped data could be shown. For example, many patients with renal osteodystrophy cluster in areas shown by the bars. The red bar (OM, osteomalacia) is currently described as low-turnover bone with abnormal mineralization. The bone volume may be low to medium, depending on the severity and duration of the process and other factors that affect bone. The green bar (AD, adynamic bone disease) is currently described as low-turnover bone with normal mineralization, and the bone volume in this example is at the lower end of the spectrum, but other patients with normal mineralization and low turnover will have normal bone volume. The yellow bar (mild HPT, mild hyperparathyroid-related bone disease) and purple bar (OF, osteitis fibrosa or advanced hyperparathyroid-related bone disease) are currently used distinct categories, but in actuality represent a range of abnormalities along a continuum of medium to high turnover, and any bone volume depending on the duration of the disease process. Finally, the blue bar (MUO, mixed uremic osteodystrophy) is variably defined internationally. In the present graph, it is depicted as high-turnover, normal bone volume, with abnormal mineralization. In summary, the TMV classification system more precisely describes the range of pathologic abnormalities that can occur in patients with CKD. Taken from Moe et al. (2006).[9]

with angiographically proven coronary artery disease.[46] In patient not yet on dialysis, there is also increased coronary artery calcification.[47,48] Peripheral artery calcification can lead to claudication and systolic hypertension, and this in turn can lead to increased cardiac afterload resistance and left ventricular hypertrophy. Coronary artery calcification can lead to cardiac ischemia and sudden death, and the latter is the leading cause of cardiovascular death in patients on dialysis.[49]

Epidemiological studies on both post-menopausal women and the general aging population have demonstrated that patients with osteoporosis have increased atherosclerosis and increased coronary artery calcification.[50–54] Drake et al. recently found genetic evidence linking atherosclerosis with osteoporosis in mice with diet-induced atherosclerotic disease,[55] and several knockout mice models demonstrate a linkage between bone demineralization and vascular calcification including the osteoprotegerin and matrix Gla protein deficient animals.[56,57] This same inverse relationship has been found in humans with CKD, as Braun et al. also found a significant inverse correlation between coronary artery calcification and bone mineral density by computed tomography (CT) in a cross-sectional analysis.[46] London and colleagues demonstrated that indices of impaired bone remodelling on biopsy was associated with increased vascular calcification by ultrasound.[58] Supporting this relationship are studies in which agents given to improve bone have been found helpful in preventing vascular calcification in animal models.[59–65]

Defining CKD-MBD

Patients with CKD develop abnormalities in the serum levels of phosphorus, calcium, PTH, vitamin D, and FGF23 leading to abnormal bone. Both the laboratory changes and bone abnormalities contribute to vascular calcification, and all three of these processes are closely interrelated and may account for the significant morbidity and mortality of patients with CKD. The increased mortality is due not only to the magnitude of risk but also the high prevalence of disorders of mineral metabolism, together assessed by determining the population attributable risk. Disorders of calcium, phosphorous and PTH have lead to a population attributable risk of mortality of 17.5%. This is substantially greater than the risk of anemia (6%), or low urea reduction ratio (5.5%).[66] Unfortunately, the traditional definition of renal osteodystrophy does not reflect all of these manifestations associated with mineral and bone disorders. Thus, providing the rationale for linking the many clinical, biochemical, and imaging abnormalities as a clinical syndrome called chronic kidney disease-mineral and bone disorder (CKD-MBD) (Table 1.1).[9]

The initial evaluation of CKD-MBD should include: PTH, calcium (either ionized or total corrected for albumin), phosphorus, alkaline phosphatases (total or bone-specific), bicarbonate, and imaging for soft tissue calcification. If there are inconsistencies in the biochemical markers (e.g. high PTH, but low alkaline phosphatases), unexplained bone pain, or unexplained fractures, a bone biopsy would be indicated. In children with CKD, additional tests to assess linear growth rate are also needed. A proposed framework was put forth for CKD-MBD, which divides patients into groups based on the presence or absence of abnormalities in the three primary components used in the definition of the disorder: laboratory abnormalities (L), bone disease (B), and calcification of extra-skeletal tissue (C). This framework is only a working model, and should be modified and improved in the future as new data becomes available.[9]

Co-existence of CKD-MBD with other causes of bone and vascular disease

The use of CKD-MBD should be as specific as possible and limited to disturbances caused by advanced CKD, stages 3–5D, as this is the level of GFR below which abnormalities in calcium, phosphorus, PTH, and vitamin D metabolism are detectable.[2] However, in pediatric patients the level of GFR at which CKD-MBD abnormalities are detectable is higher (GFR $< 89ml/min/1.73m^2$). On the other hand, disease states such as osteoporosis (increased bone fragility observed with aging or menopause) and atherosclerotic disease with calcified intimal plaques may be present in patients with CKD who have normal or only slightly reduced kidney function, may be present for reasons other than CKD and can co-exist with CKD-MBD after its onset. Thus, CKD may alter the diagnosis, treatment, and prognosis of osteoporosis and atherosclerosis. Bone is likely to be more severely affected by CKD than might be expected from normal aging, either due to the extremes of turnover or remodelling that occur in CKD in adults and children, or from abnormalities of modeling that occur in growing children. Thus, while CKD-MBD should refer to conditions that are caused by CKD, the contribution of CKD-related changes to diseases commonly found in the general population will require additional research.

Conclusion

Mineral and bone disorders are complex abnormalities that cause morbidity and mortality in patients with CKD. In order to raise awareness of the systematic manifestations of mineral and bone disorders, KDIGO established a new term 'chronic kidney disease–mineral and bone disorder' (CKD–MBD) to describe the syndrome of biochemical, bone, and extra-skeletal calcification abnormalities that occur in patients with CKD. The term *renal osteodystrophy* should be used exclusively to define alterations in bone morphology associated with CKD, assessed by bone biopsy with or without histomorphometry. The results of the biopsies should be reported based on a classification system that includes parameters of turnover, mineralization, and volume. These updated definitions, and classification schemes of these two disorders due to CKD reflect new scientific advances, and the adoption of this terminology should further enhance research and improve patient care.

References

1. Eknoyan G, Lameire N, Barsoum R, et al. The burden of kidney disease: improving global outcomes. *Kidney Int* 2004;**66**:1310–14.
2. Levin A, Bakris GL, Molitch M, et al. Prevalence of abnormal serum vitamin D, PTH, calcium, and phosphorus in patients with chronic kidney disease: results of the study to evaluate early kidney disease. *Kidney Int* 2007;**71**:31–8.

3. Tomida K, Hamano T, Mikami S, et al. Serum 25-hydroxyvitamin D as an independent determinant of 1–84 PTH and bone mineral density in non-diabetic predialysis CKD patients. *Bone* 2009;**44**:678–83.

4. K/DOQI NKF. Clinical practice guidelines for bone metabolism and disease in chronic kidney disease. *Am J Kidney Dis* 2003;**42**:S1–201.

5. Moe S, Drueke T. Controversies in mineral metabolism in chronic kidney disease: a bridge to improving healthcare outcomes an quality of life in patients with CKD. *Am J Kidney Dis* 2004;**43**:552–7.

6. Martin KJ, Olgaard K, Coburn JW, et al. Diagnosis, assessment, and treatment of bone turnover abnormalities in renal osteodystrophy. *Am J Kidney Dis* 2004;**43**:558–65.

7. Cunningham J, Sprague SM, Cannata-Andia J, et al. Osteoporosis in chronic kidney disease. *Am J Kidney Dis* 2004;**43**:566–71.

8. Goodman WG, London G, Amann K, et al. Vascular calcification in chronic kidney disease. *Am J Kidney Dis* 2004;**43**:572–9.

9. Moe S, Drueke T, Cunningham J, et al. Definition, evaluation, and classification of renal osteodystrophy: a position statement from kidney disease: improving global outcomes (KDIGO). *Kidney Int* 2006;**69**:1945–53.

10. Sprague SM. The role of the bone biopsy in the diagnosis of renal osteodystrophy. *Semin Dial* 2000;**13**:152–5.

11. Malluche HH, Monier-Faugere MC. Renal osteodystrophy: what's in a name? Presentation of a clinically useful new model to interpret bone histologic findings. *Clin Nephrol* 2006;**65**:235–42.

12. Barreto FC, Barreto DV, Moyses RM, et al. Osteoporosis in hemodialysis patients revisited by bone histomorphometry: a new insight into an old problem. *Kidney Int* 2006;**69**: 1852–7.

13. Pendras JP, Erickson RV. Hemodialysis: a successful therapy for chronic uremia. *Ann Intern Med* 1966;**64**:293–311.

14. Stehman-Breen CO, Sherrard D, Walker A, et al. Racial differences in bone mineral density and bone loss among end-stage renal disease patients. *Am J Kidney Dis* 1999;**33**:941–6.

15. Foley RN, Parfrey PS, Sarnak MJ. Clinical epidemiology of cardiovascular disease in chronic renal disease. *Am J Kidney Dis* 1998;**32**:S112–19.

16. Alem AM, Sherrard DJ, Gillen DL, et al. Increased risk of hip fracture among patients with end-stage renal disease. *Kidney Int* 2000;**58**:396–9.

17. Coco M, Rush H. Increased incidence of hip fractures in dialysis patients with low serum parathyroid hormone. *Am J Kidney Dis* 2000;**36**:1115–21.

18. Atsumi K, Kushida K, Yamazaki K, et al. Risk factors for vertebral fractures in renal osteodystrophy. *Am J Kidney Dis* 1999;**33**:287–93.

19. Jamal SA, Hayden JA, Beyene J. Low bone mineral density and fractures in long-term hemodialysis patients: a meta-analysis. *Am J Kidney Dis* 2007;**49**:674–81.

20. Dooley AC, Weiss NS, Kestenbaum B. Increased risk of hip fracture among men with CKD. *Am J Kidney Dis* 2008;**51**:38–44.

21. Fried LF, Biggs ML, Shlipak MG, et al. Association of kidney function with incident hip fracture in older adults. *J Am Soc Nephrol* 2007;**18**:282–6.

22. Nickolas TL, McMahon DJ, Shane E. Relationship between moderate to severe kidney disease and hip fracture in the United States. *J Am Soc Nephrol* 2006;**17**:3223–32.

23. Nitsch D, Mylne A, Roderick PJ, et al. Chronic kidney disease and hip-fracture-related mortality in older people in the UK. *Nephrol Dial Transplant* 2009;**24**:1539–44.

24. Ball AM, Gillen DL, Sherrard D, et al. Risk of hip fracture among dialysis and renal transplant recipients. *J Am Med Ass* 2002;**288**:3014–18.

25. Mittalhenkle A, Gillen DL, Stehman-Breen CO. Increased risk of mortality associated with hip fracture in the dialysis population. *Am J Kidney Dis* 2004;**44**:672–9.

26. Hui SL, Slemenda CW, Johnston CC, Jr. Age and bone mass as predictors of fracture in a prospective study. *J Clin Invest* 1988;**81**:1804–9.

27. Chesnut CH, 3rd, Rose CJ. Reconsidering the effects of antiresorptive therapies in reducing osteoporotic fracture. *J Bone Mineral Res* 2001;**16**:2163–72.

28. Watts NB. Bone quality: getting closer to a definition. *J Bone Miner Res* 2002;**17**:1148–50.

29. Monier-Faugere MC, Malluche HH. Trends in renal osteodystrophy: a survey from (1983) to (1995) in a total of 2248 patients. *Nephrology, Dialysis, Transplantation* 1996;**11** (Suppl. 3):111–20.

30. Torres A, Lorenzo V, Hernandez D, et al. Bone disease in predialysis, hemodialysis, and CAPD patients: evidence of a better bone response to PTH. *Kidney Int* 1995;**47**:1434–42.

31. Sherrard DJ, Hercz G, Pei Y, et al. The spectrum of bone disease in end-stage renal failure—an evolving disorder. *Kidney Int* 1993;**43**:436–42.

32. Lobao R, Carvalho AB, Cuppari L, et al. High prevalence of low bone mineral density in pre-dialysis chronic kidney disease patients: bone histomorphometric analysis. *Clin Nephrol* 2004;**62**:432–9.

33. Stehman-Breen C, Walker A, Sadler R, et al. Bone loss among end stage renal disease (ESRD) patients treated with calcitonin. *Dialysis: Complicat Haemodialysis* A1378.

34. Moe SM, Yu BO, Sprague SM. Maintenance of bone mass in patients receiving dialytic therapy. *Am J Kidney Dis* 1993;**22**:300–7.

35. KDIGO. Clinical practice guidelines for the management of CKD-MBD. *Kidney International Supp.* 2009;**113**:51–130.

36. Moe SM. Calcium, phosphorus, and vitamin D metabolism in renal disease and chronic renal failure. In: Kopple JD, Massry SG (eds) Nutritional Management of Renal Disease, 2nd edn. Lippincott Williams & Wilkins: Philadelphia, 2004, pp 261–85.

37. Sprague SM, Ho LT. Oral doxercalciferol therapy for secondary hyperparathyroidism in a peritoneal dialysis patient. *Clin Nephrol* 2002;**58**:155–60.

38. Liu SH, Chu HI. Treatment of renal osteodystrophy with dihydrotachysterol (A.T.10) and Iron. *Science* 1942;**95**:388–9.

39. Stanbury SW. Azotaemic renal osteodystrophy. *Br Med Bull* 1957;**13**:57–60.

40. Block GA, Raggi P, Bellasi A, et al. Mortality effect of coronary calcification and phosphate binder choice in incident hemodialysis patients. *Kidney Int* 2007;**71**:438–41.

41. USRDS. (2003) *Annual Data Report: Atlas of End-Stage Renal Disease in the United States. Bethesda, USRDS*, 2003.

42. Go AS, Chertow GM, Fan D, et al. Chronic kidney disease and the risks of death, cardiovascular events, and hospitalisation. *N Engl J Med* 2004;**351**:1296–305.

43. Block GA, Klassen PS, Lazarus JM, et al. Mineral metabolism, mortality, and morbidity in maintenance hemodialysis. *J Am Soc Nephrol* 2004;**15**:2208–18.

44. Kalantar-Zadeh K, Kuwae N, Regidor DL, et al. Survival predictability of time-varying indicators of bone disease in maintenance hemodialysis patients. *Kidney Int* 2006;**70**: 771–80.

45. Kestenbaum B, Sampson JN, Rudser KD, et al. Serum phosphate levels and mortality risk among people with chronic kidney disease. *J Am Soc Nephrol* 2005;**16**:520–8.

46. Braun J, Oldendorf M, Moshage W, et al. Electron beam computed tomography in the evaluation of cardiac calcification in chronic dialysis patients. *Am J Kidney Dis* 1996;**27**:394–401.

47. Mehrotra R, Adler S. Coronary artery calcification in nondialyzed patients with chronic kidney diseases. *Am J Kidney Dis* 2005;**45**:963.

48. Mehrotra R, Budoff M, Christenson P, et al. Determinants of coronary artery calcification in diabetics with and without nephropathy. *Kidney Int* 2004;**66**:2022–31.

49. Moe SM, Chen NX. Pathophysiology of vascular calcification in chronic kidney disease. *Circ Res* 2004;**95**:560–7.

50. Banks LM, Lees B, MacSweeney JE, Stevenson JC. Effect of degenerative spinal and aortic calcification on bone density measurements in post-menopausal women: links between osteoporosis and cardiovascular disease? *Eur J Clin Invest* 1994;**24**:813–17.

51. Kiel DP, Hannan MT, Cupple LA, et al. Low bone mineral density (BMD) is associated with coronary artery calcification. *J Br Med Rev* 2000;**15**:S160.

52. Boukhris R, Becker KL. Calcification of the aorta and osteoporosis. A roentgenographic study. *J Am Med Ass* 1972;**219**:1307–11.

53. Kiel DP, Kauppila LI, Cupples LA, et al. Bone loss and the progression of abdominal aortic calcification over a 25 year period: the Framingham Heart Study. *Calcif Tissue Int* 2001;**68**:271–6.

54. Hak AE, Pols HA, van Hemert AM, et al. Progression of aortic calcification is associated with metacarpal bone loss during menopause: a population-based longitudinal study. *Arterioscler Thromb Vasc Biol* 2000;**20**:1926–31.

55. Drake TA, Schadt E, Hannani K, et al. Genetic loci determining bone density in mice with diet-induced atherosclerosis. *Physiol Genomics* 2001;**5**:205–15.

56. Wallin R, Wajih N, Greenwood GT, Sane DC. Arterial calcification: a review of mechanisms, animal models, and the prospects for therapy. *Med Res Rev* 2001;**21**:274–301.

57. Giachelli CM. Inducers and inhibitors of biomineralization: lessons from pathological calcification. *Orthod Craniofac Res* 2005;**8**:229–31.

58. London GM, Marty C, Marchais SJ, et al. Arterial calcifications and bone histomorphometry in end-stage renal disease. *J Am Soc Nephrol* 2004;**15**:1943–51.

59. Price PA, June HH, Buckley JR, Williamson MK. Osteoprotegerin inhibits artery calcification induced by warfarin and by vitamin D. *Arterioscler Thromb Vasc Biol* 2001;**21**:1610–16.

60. Price PA, Buckley JR, Williamson MK. The amino bisphosphonate ibandronate prevents vitamin D toxicity and inhibits vitamin D-induced calcification of arteries, cartilage, lungs and kidneys in rats. *J Nutr* 2001;**131**:2910–15.

61. Price PA, Faus SA, Williamson MK. Bisphosphonates alendronate and ibandronate inhibit artery calcification at doses comparable to those that inhibit bone resorption. *Arterioscler Thromb Vasc Biol* 2001;**21**:817–24.

62. Price PA, June HH, Buckley JR, Williamson MK. SB 242784, a selective inhibitor of the osteoclastic V-H+ATPase, inhibits arterial calcification in the rat. *Circ Res* 2002;**91**: 547–52.

63. Lomashvili KA, Monier-Faugere MC, Wang X, et al. Effect of bisphosphonates on vascular calcification and bone metabolism in experimental renal failure. *Kidney Int* 2009.

64. Gonzalez EA, Lund RJ, Martin KJ, et al. Treatment of a murine model of high-turnover renal osteodystrophy by exogenous BMP-7. *Kidney Int* 2002;**61**:1322–31.

65. Lund RJ, Davies MR, Brown AJ, Hruska KA. Successful treatment of an adynamic bone disorder with bone morphogenetic protein-7 in a renal ablation model. *J Am Soc Nephrol* 2004;**15**:359–69.

66. Block GA, Klassen P, Danese M, et al. Association between proposed NKF-K/DOQI bone metabolism and disease guidelines and mortality risk in hemodialysis patients. *J Am Soc Nephrol* 2003;**14**:474A.

67. Ho LT, Sprague SM. Renal osteodystrophy in chronic renal failure. *Semin Nephrol* 2002;**22**:488–93.

68. Coen G, Bonucci E, Ballanti P, et al. PTH 1-84 and PTH '7–84' in the noninvasive diagnosis of renal bone disease. *Am J Kidney Dis* 2002;**40**:348–54.

69. Wang M, Hercz G, Sherrard DJ, et al. Relationship between intact 1–84 parathyroid hormone and bone histomorphometric parameters in dialysis patients without aluminium toxicity. *Am J Kidney Dis* 1995;**26**:836–44.

Chapter 2

New aspects of normal bone biology

Susan M. Ott

Introduction

Bone as a structural material must be strong enough to support the body weight and light enough for efficient movement. Some of the most important new developments in bone biology help explain the mechanisms of sensing and responding to mechanical loading. New genetic approaches combined with clinical observations have led to discoveries of signaling pathways that may eventually lead to new therapies to treat or prevent bone diseases. This chapter will focus on some recently defined factors that influence bone remodelling, with an emphasis on those that could potentially be modified to improve the bone strength.

Basic multicellular units

Before discussing new developments, I will briefly review bone remodelling. Turnover of bone is different from dermal turnover, where the entire surface is continuously forming new skin while shedding old skin. Healthy bone is a dynamic tissue, continually resorbing bone and replacing it with new bone in discrete areas know as basic multicellular units, also called bone metabolic units (BMU). A BMU is not a permanent structure. It forms in response to a signal, performs its function, and disbands, leaving residual lining cells and osteocytes. Each BMU undergoes its functions in the same sequence: origination and organization of the BMU, activation of osteoclasts, resorption of old bone, recruitment of osteoblasts, formation of new bone matrix, and mineralization. On the cancellous surfaces, a BMU does not just dissolve a pit on the surface, but it spreads across the surface leaving behind an area filled with new bone. In the cortex the osteoclasts form a cutting edge and bore through the solid bone, and osteoblasts follow, filling in the tunnels and leaving behind a small vascular channel.

Some BMUs originate when the bone has been damaged; others may originate at random surfaces on the bone. The osteocytes can initiate a BMU in response to microdamage and perhaps after mechanical loading. It is not clear if systemic hormones or local cytokines initiate new BMUs, or if they work by increasing activity or lifespan of existing BMUs. The first sign of activity seen by standard microscopy is bone resorption, so early histologists thought that the first step in a remodelling cycle was performed by the osteoclasts. Now, however, it is known that osteoclasts must be activated by cells in the osteoblast lineage, a process that occurs on the molecular level. After activation of pre-osteoclasts, which fuse and form mature osteoclasts, the second step is bone resorption. At a given spot on the bone surface, resorption is rapid for the first 10 days, and continues for about a month. The osteoclasts undergo apoptosis; the lifespan and activity of the osteoclasts determine the depth of the resorption cavity. Meanwhile, the pre-osteoblasts that were generated by the marrow stem cells have proliferated, and when the osteoclasts retire a team of osteoblasts line the cavity. The osteoblasts form a matrix and after about 14 days directs mineralization of the matrix. The osteoblasts continue to form and to mineralize osteoid until the cavity is filled or nearly filled. The time to fill in the cavity at any given place on the surface is 124–168 days in normal individuals. After formation is concluded, that spot on the surface is quiescent for about 2–5 years, during which time the newly formed bone gradually accumulates mineral and become denser.[1] A dynamic review of bone remodelling is available online (Fig. 2.1).[2]

Recently, more attention has been paid to structures within the marrow spaces that accompany the BMU. At the initiation of a BMU, the lining cells separate from the bone matrix and merge with the marrow vasculature, forming a canopy that provides a protected space for bone resorption and formation, and provide a mechanism for the correct spacial and temporal organisation. It is likely that the stem and marrow stromal cells reside close to these vascular structures. The marrow stromal cells secrete local factors that begin to assemble the osteoclasts and the osteoblasts and the canopy restricts the action to the correct location.[3]

The bone cells

Two major families of cells control bone remodelling: the osteoclasts and the osteoblasts.

Osteoclasts originate from cells in the hematopoetic line from precursors of macrophages. Osteoblasts are derived from stem cells in the marrow stromal that are also precursors to adipocytes and chondrocytes. The cells differentiated into pre-osteoblasts,

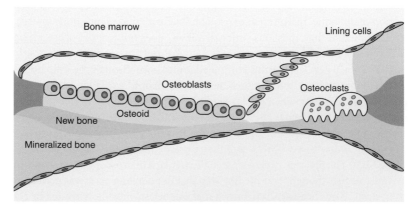

Fig. 2.1 A BMU travelling along the surface of cancellous bone.

then mature osteoblasts that secrete collagen and form bone. The osteoblasts which do not undergo apoptosis further differentiate into lining cells or osteocytes (Fig. 2.2).

Osteoclasts

The osteoclast precursors circulate in the bloodstream. They proliferate in response to several growth factors, particularly macrocyte colony-stimulating factor that is expressed by cells in the osteoblast line. The pre-osteoclasts express surface receptor activator of nuclear factor κB (RANK). When RANK-ligand occupies these receptors the cells become active and merge with other pre-osteoclasts to form large, mature, multinucleated osteoclasts. The RANK-RANK-ligand signaling is the key regulator of bone resorption; many systemic hormones increase bone resorption indirectly by acting on cells in the osteoblast line, which then express the RANK-ligand. TNFα and IL-1 enhance activity of RANK-ligand. Other signaling pathways between the osteoblast and osteoclast include newly described immunoreceptor tyrosine-based activation motifs (ITAM) which are similar to systems found in immune cells and which modulate osteoclast fusion (Fig. 2.3).[4,5] After RANK activation, the intracellular pathway is mediated by calcineurin. Thus, inhibitors such as FK506 and cyclosporin A inhibit osteoclastogenesis. The activated mature osteoclast generates a complex of RANK, TRAF6, and c-Src. This leads to polarization of the cell and cytoskeletal changes.

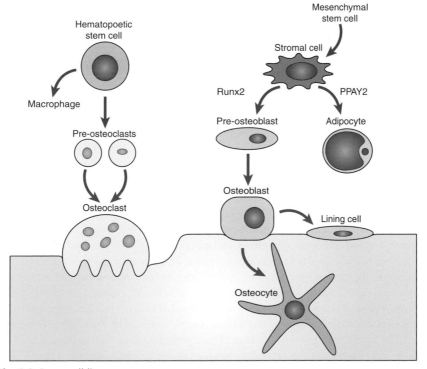

Fig. 2.2 Bone cell lineage.

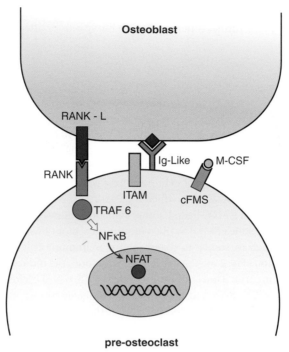

Fig. 2.3 Osteoblast signals to pre-osteoclasts. TRAF 6 = receptor-associated factor 6. ITAM = immunoreceptor tynosine-based activation motif. M-CSF = macrophage colony-stimulating factor CFMS is the receptor for M-CSF. NFκB = nuclear factor. κB NFAT = nuclear factor of activated T-cells. Figure modified from figures in Takayengi[5] and Novack and Teitelbaum.[4]

The small GTPase Rab3D is necessary for formation of the ruffled border and integrins, particularly αvβ3, are expressed on the surface. Integrins convey signals from the bone matrix to the osteoclast interior. The integrins are adherins that act with actin to form tight circular junctions attached to the bone mineral, creating a space between the bone and the osteoclast's ruffled border, which is separated from the rest of the marrow space (Fig. 2.4). Into this space, the osteoclast secretes cathepsin, which degrades collagen. The osteoclasts also pump hydrogen ions that dissolve the mineral. To maintain electroneutrality, a chloride channel coupled to H^+ATP-ase secretes chloride into the resorption space. The hydrogen pump and carbonic anhydrase are similar to those in the nephron, and a Cl^-/HCO_3^- exchanger on the anti-resorbing surface maintains the cellular pH. In the acid environment, growth factors that were embedded within the bone matrix are released. These include TGFß, insulin-like growth factor (IGF), and fibroblast growth factor (FGF), which were deposited into the matrix by the previous generation of osteoblasts. Some, like TGFß, may be activated by the acid environment caused by osteoclastic proton secretion. These growth factors (delayed autocrine factors) might contribute to the coupling between resorption and formation that is seen in normal situations, but direct evidence for this theory is lacking. The osteoclast can

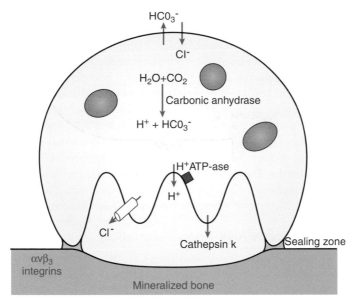

Fig. 2.4 Mature osteoclast resorbing bone. Modified from Novack and Teitelbaum.[4]

also engulf material through endocytosis, similar to the macrophages (which are the cells most closely related to the osteoclasts). Osteoclasts thus resorb the bone, moving deeper into the bone and also spreading along the surface. Eventually, they undergo apoptosis, under the influence of factors such as oestrogen (which promotes the apoptosis and thereby limits the amount of bone which is resorbed).

Although the primary function of the osteoclast is to resorb bone, there is emerging evidence that they also are necessary for the functioning of osteoblasts, which will form new bone to fill the resorbed cavities.[4] It appears that bone resorption *per se* is not necessary for bone formation.[6] Osteoclasts have been shown to excrete interleukin-6 and annexin-II, both of which could signal the osteoblasts. Osteoclasts secrete sphingosine-1 phosphate and WNT10b which stimulate production of pre-osteoblasts[7]. Patients with osteopetrosis have non-functioning osteoclasts due to mutation in the chloride channel, so bone resorption is decreased, but formation is normal. Animal studies suggest that the number of osteoclasts, and not the bone resorption, signals osteoblasts.

Excess bone resorption causes bone loss and osteoporosis. Many medications have been developed to inhibit bone resorption in order to improve the fracture risk of patients with osteoporosis. On the other hand, when osteoclasts are unable to resorb bone, patients develop osteopetrosis. The thickened bone, unfortunately, is not strong and these patients suffer from chalk-stick fractures.

Bisphosphonate mechanism of action

Bisphosphonates are stable analogs of inorganic pyrophosphate, which is one of the body's defenses against metastatic calcification. All bisphosphonates can, therefore, inhibit mineralization if used at high enough concentrations. The bisphosphonates bind tightly to minerals. The affinity for the hydroxyaptite crystals, the major mineral form in the bone, determines their duration of action. They enter the osteoclasts via endocytosis. The amino-bisphosphonates inhibit farnesyl pyrophosphate synthase, an enzyme within the mevalonate pathway. They bind to an aspartic acid-rich region of the enzyme and the potency of bone resorption is related to the closeness of the fit. The downstream enzymes are necessary for prenylation of small GTP-ases, including Rho, Rab, and Rac. Therefore, the osteoclasts are not able to form a cytoskeleton.[7] Recent reports have documented very large multinucleated osteoclasts in patients who have used long-term bisphosphonate; the cells are not as close to the bone like normal osteoclasts and they do not have a ruffled border. The long-term effects of pronounced inhibition of both bone resorption and, secondarily, of bone formation remain unknown. There is one case of osteopetrosis in a boy who received excessive doses of a bisphosphonate.[9]

Inhibition of RANK-RANK-ligand signaling

RANK-RANK-L signaling is an obvious target for pharmaceutical intervention. Denosumab, a human monoclonal antibody to RANK-L, has been extensively studied in patients with osteoporosis, rheumatoid arthritis, and metastatic bone lesions. This antibody causes rapid and marked decrease in bone resorption, lasting for about 6 months. The bone density increases. In a recent large randomized clinical trial of postmenopausal osteoporosis the fracture rates were significantly decreased (S. R. Cummings, ASBMR Annual Meeting, 2008).[10] The RANK, RANK-L signaling pathway is not unique to the bone cells. These receptors are in the tumor necrosis factor family and are also expressed in immune cells, but to date no increase in side effects related to the immune system has been reported.

Inhibition of integrins

In mice deletion of the β3 intergrin subunit causes high bone mass and one case of osteopetrosis has been reported in a patient with thrombathenia, which is caused by a mutation in the β3 intergrin. A study in women with osteoporosis given a small molecule inhibitor of αvβ3 integrin has shown evidence of decreased bone resorption, with decreases in serum and urine markers of bone resorption (collagen cross-linking molecules) and increases in the bone density.[11]

Inhibition of cathepsin or hydrogen pump

Pycnodysostosis is a disease caused by a mutation in cathepsin. These patients have increased bone density, but the bone is fragile and, on biopsy, they have layers of unmineralized osteoid under the osteoclasts. The osteoclasts are able to form normal ruffled borders and actin rings to bind to the bone matrix and are able to secrete the hydrogen ions which dissolve the mineral from the bone, but the lack of cathepsin means the collagen matrix is not degraded.[12] Small molecules that inhibit cathepsin have been developed and tested in early clinical trials of patients with osteoporosis. The patients show improved bone density and reduced bone resorption. More studies about safety and efficacy are in progress.

The most common genetic form of osteopetrosis is carbonic anhydrase deficiency. This demonstrated the importance of the hydrogen pump for bone resorption. This has not been a target for drug therapy because inhibition could cause systemic acidosis. It is interesting to note that thiazide diuretics, which cause a mild metabolic alkalosis, also cause a mild reduction of bone resorption, and this is possibly related to osteoclast function.

Osteoblasts

Stem cells

Stem cells near the vasculature within the bone marrow give rise to pre-osteoblasts,[13] which can proliferate under the influence of local and systemic growth factors. Two transcription factors control the fate of the cells. RUNX2 (formerly known as CBFA1), the earliest marker of an osteoblast lineage cell, promotes maturation into osteoblasts, but PPAR-γ causes the stem cells to become adiopocytes. The lipids in the environment partly determine which of these transcription factors is prominent. Treatment of diabetic patients with roziglitazone, a PPAR-γ agonist, increased the incidence of fractures in a large randomized clinical trial. Animal studies show that this drug increases the number of marrow adipocytes, but decreases the number of osteoblasts. On the other hand, bortezomib, a proteasome inhibitor used in treatment of multiple myeloma, induces the mesenchymal stem cells to differentiate into the osteoblastic pathway, and this improves the bone mass in mice with osteoporosis.[14]

Both osteoblasts and fat cells are involved in a complex regulation of body fat and energy metabolism.[15] Fat cells convert androgens to estrogens, which are beneficial to the bones. Also they secrete the adipocyte hormones leptin and adiponectin. Epidemiological observations find a strong correlation between serum leptin levels and bone density within populations; in addition, body fat mass is closely linked to bone density. The precise role of leptin is still not clear;[16] some investigators found no local activity of leptin and hypothesized that the effects were all central, because intra-cerebroventricular injections of leptin caused bone loss that could be reversed by blockade of the sympathetic nervous system. Others have found leptin receptors on osteoblasts, and leptin directly supports osteoblastic activity, while reducing the levels of RANK-ligand.[17] Osteoblasts also increase osteocalcin production after exposure to leptin; new research suggests that the osteocalcin is associated with lower fasting glucose levels, providing a feedback loop related to energy metabolism.[18]

Pre-osteoblasts

Growth factors such as TGF-β, fibroblast growth factor, bone morphogenic proteins, platelet-derived growth factors and colony-stimulating factors (CSF) can increase proliferation of pre-osteoblasts. More details about these factors are discussed in other chapters of this book. Bone morphogenic protein 7 is of particular interest to nephrologists because it is made in the kidney and deficiency will retard the differentiation of pre-osteoblasts into osteoblasts.[19] The spindle-shaped pre-osteoblasts accumulate near the bone surface and have been mis-named 'peri-trabecular fibrosis' for years because early histologists thought they looked like fibroblasts.

The pre-osteoblasts have receptors for many of the hormones and cytokines that were classically felt to increase bone resorption (such as PTH, interleukins, and calcitriol). Pre-osteoblasts express RANK-ligand on their surface, which stimulates the pre-osteoclasts. The gene profiles of the cells in the osteoblast lineage change in a complicated way during differentiation. The cells have decreasing proliferative capacity as they become more differentiated, under the influence of transcription factors such as RUNX2 and OSTERIX.[20] There are different developmental routes to the same endpoint and mature osteoblasts have heterogeneous gene profiles.

Mature osteoblasts

The mature osteoblasts secrete collagen and bone matrix proteins, as well as several growth factors. Osteocalcin and osteopontin are expressed in these mature cells, as well as osteoprotegerin (OPG), a decoy receptor for RANK-ligand that will block osteoclast formation. When a team of osteoblasts first starts forming matrix, the cells are cuboidal and plump, and have many mitochondria. As they fill in the resorption cavity, they become flatter and less metabolically active. Some of them stop making matrix, and are left behind the other cells and surrounded by matrix. These cells differentiate into the osteocytes. Some of the osteoblasts undergo apoptosis. When the cells have finished making osteoid they differentiate into lining cells. These cells are flat, pancake-like cells that form tight junctions with each other and essentially separate the bone from the rest of the body. The osteocytes remain in contact with the lining cells. The lining cells make alkaline phosphatase, which prevents pyrophosphate from entering the bone and dissolving the mineral. Patients with hypophosphatasia have mutations in the alkaline phosphatase gene and develop severe fatal osteomalacia.

The osteoblasts and the vascular sinusoids in the marrow function as a niche for the hematopoetic stem cells. Recent studies using real-time imaging have shown that these cells home to the endosteum surface in irradiated mice, near preosteoblasts that are positive for N-cadherin. This special zone normally maintains the stem cells, but promotes their expansion in response to bone marrow damage.[21]

The Wnt-signaling pathway

In 1997 clinical investigators from Creighton University reported a kindred with high bone mass.[22] The proband was an 18-year-old girl who had back pain after an automobile accident. Radiographs showed dense, but otherwise normal bones and the bone mineral density was 5.6 SD above average for age. Her mother had similarly dense bones. This led to an extended survey of this family whose members carried the 'high bone mass' gene. Using linkage analysis, they demonstrated that the family members with high bone mass had a single point mutation in the *LRP-5* gene (low-density-lipoprotein-receptor-related protein 5). This was not on any list of candidate genes involved in bone metabolism. Shortly afterwards, an unrelated kindred was reported that carried the identical mutation. In both studies, the inheritance was autosomal dominant. Meanwhile, another group of investigators discovered that a different mutation in the *LRP-5* gene caused the osteoporosis-pseudoglioma syndrome, a devastating disease manifested by multiple fractures and blindness which was inherited as an autosomal recessive disorder. *LRP-5* is a member of the Wnt-signaling

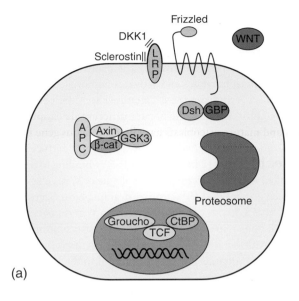

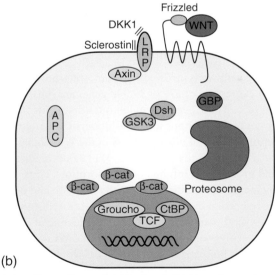

Fig. 2.5 The Wnt signaling pathway. (a) No signal. (b) Ligand occupies receptor and pathway is activated. Modified from Moon, R.[30]

pathway (Fig. 2.5). The Wnt genes are homologous to segment-polarity genes that are critical in embryonic development.

Several of the Wnt-related proteins have been shown to be important in the regulation of bone metabolism. The signal is Wnt, a protein secreted by many cell types (the name is a combination of the *Drosophila* gene *wingless* and the mouse gene *int*), which occupies Frizzled, a 7-transmembrane domain receptor, and *LRP-5* is a co-factor necessary for signal transduction. Intracellular proteins include Dishevelled, Axin, GSK3, and ß-catenin. When there is no signal, the intracellular GSK phosphorylates ß-catenin, so it is ubiquitinated and broken down by the proteosome. When Wnt binds the Frizzled receptor, it phosphorylates and activates Dishevelled, which represses GSK3, which in turn releases Axin from the ß-catenin. The Axin is then restrained by the intracellular part of LRP-5, and so the ß-catenin accumulates, and enters the nucleus and binds TCF transcription factors. This pathway, that involves Wnt and ß-catenin, is called the canonical Wnt-signaling pathway. Several extracellular proteins can inhibit this process. Dickkopf (Dkk) ties up LRP-5 by binding to it and another membrane protein called Kremen. Sclerostin, homologue of Wise, also binds to the LRP-5 protein. These each prevent the LRP-5 from restraining Axin. Secreted Frizzled-related protein (sFRP) acts as a decoy receptor and binds to Wnt. In patients with the G171V mutation and high bone mass, the mutated LRP-5 resists binding to Dkk. Therefore, the Wnt-signaling pathway is more active. In the patients with osteoporosis pseudoglioma syndrome, the protein is non-functional and so the Wnt-signaling pathway is inhibited.[23]

Gene array analysis on bone marrow cells from patients with myeloma compared those who had bone lesions on MRI scans with those without lesions found that those with bone lesions expressed Dkk1, which is one of the extracellular proteins that inhibits Wnt signaling. Animal models of myeloma show response to pharmacological inhibition of Dkk1 and transgenic mice without the *Dkk1* gene have high bone density.

The Wnt-signaling pathway is involved in pleomorphic processes. Gene array technology shows that expression of 879 of 39,000 genes are statistically different after treatment with Wnt3a. These genes included ones that control cell differentiation (promotion of osteoblastic as opposed to adiopocytic phenotypes), inhibition of apoptosis (longer lifespan), and other proteins in the Wnt-signaling pathway (feedback). Of particular interest is the finding that Wnt 3a up-regulates osteoprotegerin (OPG), a secreted protein that inhibits bone resorption. Thus, the Wnt-signaling pathway not only increases osteoblastic cell differentiation and bone formation, but also inhibits bone resorption by blocking the RANK-L/RANK interaction.[24]

During the last several years there has been an epidemic of transgenic mice with knock-outs or over-expression of proteins within the Wnt-signaling pathway, and they all have either high bone mass or osteopenia as would be predicted by whether the pathway was activated or inhibited, respectively. Drugs that enhance this pathway, however, could have side effects because many other systems also use the same pathway. Malignancies could occur with over-stimulation of the pathway; recently it was demonstrated that osteosarcomas silence one of the inhibitors of Wnt.

Treatment with intermittent parathyroid hormone

There is nothing new about the fact that PTH increases the bone formation rate and that the osteoblasts have PTH receptors. When PTH is consistently elevated, the bone resorption rate exceeds the bone formation rate and thus bone is lost, especially on the endocortical surfaces. However, when given intermittently (once a day) a different set of genes is expressed by the bone cells, and the net effect is a net increase in bone volume because bone formation is greater than bone resorption. There are more osteoblasts, they are more active, and the mineral apposition rate is faster. Teriparatide (1–34 human PTH) is now used to treat serious osteoporosis. The mechanisms for the differential effects of continuous versus intermittent PTH are still not known.

Osteocytes

The osteocytes, once thought to be 'trapped' in the bone mineral, are actually quite active within their lacunae and canaliculae.[6] They have multiple long cell processes that extend within the bone and form junctions with other osteocytes. The resulting network resembles a neuronal network and the osteocytes could be considered the brains of the bones. A special cell process like a cilia can be found on these extensions, which is firmly attached to the mineral of the canalicular wall. When mechanical loads are applied to the bone, the cilia can detect the fluid movement, and thus the osteocytes can sense mechanical strains. The osteocytes can secrete several stimulatory factors into the marrow, including prostaglandins, nitric oxide, and IGF. When there is more serious micro-damage, the osteocytes undergo apoptosis. This signals the surface cells to originate a new BMU, most likely because the osteocytes tonically secrete sclerostin, which inhibits bone formation.

Sclerostin

Within the group of bone diseases with high bone mass are Van Buchem's disease and sclerosteosis. Patients with Van Buchem's disease have abnormally thick skulls, square jaws, and may have abnormalities in fingers. The bones can be painful. Some of the patients were found to have mutations in the *LRP-5* gene, but others did not. Sclerosteosis is a serious, autosomal recessive disease. Patients have very thick bones, especially in the skull, with entrapment of cranial nerves leading to deafness and facial nerve palsy, increased intracranial pressure and greater risk of stroke. Bones in the rest of the skeleton are also thick and dense, and frequently syndactyly is present. Most of the patients are Afrikaans from South Africa, and bone fractures are not seen. Patients with sclerosteosis were found to have homozygous mutations in the *SOST* gene and those with Van Buchem's disease had mutations in an area on the same chromosome as *SOST*, which is upstream and is involved in regulation of the gene transcription.

Relatives of patients with sclerosteosis were tested to see if they were heterozygous for the mutation in the *SOST* gene. The bone densities of these heterozygous persons were high and they did not have fractures. The carriers were healthy and had no symptoms of skeletal dysfunction. Sclerosteosis is, therefore, a human model of a gene knock-out showing a beneficial effect in heterozygotic carriers, but serious disease in homozygote knock-outs.

Sclerostin, the *SOST* gene product, was initially thought to function as a BMP (bone morphogenetic protein) antagonist. This antagonistic function, however, is weak and does not really explain the disease. Now we know that sclerostin is a circulating inhibitor of the Wnt-signaling pathway, which acts to inhibit LRP-5 function. Sclerostin is expressed almost exclusively in the osteocytes. In fact, the sclerostin is not present in osteocytes near the bone surface, but only in the more mature osteocytes that are deeper in the bone. The osteocytes tonically suppress the lining cells via sclerostin, and then stop secreting it when the need arises to form new bone. While the exact mechanism is not known, it now seems likely that sclerostin plays an important role in skeletal adaptation to mechanical forces.

An elegant study by Robling and colleagues[25] established the importance of sclerostin as a mechanisms to link biomechanical forces to bone formation. They studied mice and rats whose forearms were loaded by mild bending. The opposite limbs were used as controls. In the control limb, the osteocytes diffusely expressed sclerostin. This was seen by immunohistochemistry and also documented by *in situ* hybridization. In the loaded forearm, the osteocytes appeared normal on routine staining, proving that they were still alive, but on the third day, the sclerostin secretion was inhibited. Furthermore, the suppression of sclerostin secretion was very specifically located to the area of the bone that was most stressed. The mRNA for sclerostin was decreased in locations corresponding to the decreased immunohistochemistry, so the mechanical loading response of the *SOST* gene was partly at the transcriptional level. The animals were labeled with fluorochrome, and the bone formation rates 10 days later were increased in proportion to the decrease in the sclerostin.

Antibodies against sclerostin have been given to normal mice and rats, and their bone density increases. One small study of 45 post-menopausal women showed that an antibody against human sclerostin increased the biochemical markers of bone formation. Sclerostin inhibition has potential for becoming a useful anabolic agent because it is targeted to the bone, and because there is a genetic model of partial suppression in which bones are strong, but otherwise the people are healthy.

Mechanical loading

One of the most novel new aspects of bone biology is the ability of bone to show an anabolic response to mechanical loading at precise loading stress and frequency. This response is seen at a variety of vibration frequencies and mechanical loads, but always with a particular ratio between the frequency and the load. Thus, low-frequency-high load and high-frequency-low loads can both give anabolic responses. This led to the development of low-level, high-frequency platforms (30Hz, 0.3g), which have been shown in pilot studies to increase the bone density of the legs and spine. These loads are similar to those caused by muscle contractibility during postural control. Further studies are in progress, and to date there are not enough subjects to tell if this approach will reduce the risk of fractures.[26]

Systemic hormones

It seems that every systemic hormone influences bone biology, but the response depends on the context. Factors such as age, stage of development, level of the hormone, whether the level is changing or not, levels of other hormones and minerals, and degree of mechanical loading all can play a role. Bone cells have receptors for a long list of hormones, including the traditional mineral-regulating hormones (PTH, PTHrp, calcitonin, and its gene-related product, and calcitriol), the gonadal hormones, IGF1, energy-related hormones (thyroid, insulin, leptin, ghrelin), gluco-corticoids, and serotonin. They even have receptors for calcium, and probably for phosphate, although that has not yet been definitely identified. Details about all of these are beyond the scope of this chapter, but a few new findings deserve mention.

Estrogen

New studies have not tarnished the important role of estrogen in maintaining bone health. Even in males, estrogens are important regulators of bone resorption, and testosterone is converted into estrogen by aromatases. Several mechanisms are involved:

- estrogen increases osteoclast apoptosis;
- by suppressing interleukins and pro-inflammatory cytokine expression in bone marrow cells, estrogen decreases the number of osteoclasts;
- by inhibiting the production of RANK-ligand, estrogen reduces the number and activity of osteoclasts;
- by increasing stromal cell/osteoblast cell expression of TGFβ, estrogen inhibits osteoclast activity.

Estrogen also has some positive effects on bone formation by acting as a mitogen to cells early in the osteoblast line, reducing apoptosis of osteoblasts, and increasing expression of TGFβ, bone morphogenetic proteins, and IGF-I.[27]

Glucocorticoids

These hormones cause devastating loss of bone mineral and increase in fracture rates, and in the past it was taught that they increased bone resorption rates. Now it has been shown that the major physiological action of these steroids is to inhibit bone formation—this effect is so strong that decreased markers of bone formation can be detected in healthy people after 1 week of treatment with prednisone. Contrary to popular opinion, the direct effect of glucocorticoids on osteoclasts is actually an inhibition of resorption.[4]

Serotonin

A recent series of genetic studies in mice has suggested a role of gut-derived serotonin in the control of bone formation.[28] Mice with knock-out of the *LRP-5* gene developed serious osteoporosis. The protein profile of these mice, compared with normal litter-mates, showed high levels of tryptophan hydroxylase, the enzyme that converts tryptophan to serotonin. The serum levels of serotonin were markedly elevated in the LRP-5 knock-out animals. Of interest, the serotonin levels were also elevated in humans with the osteoporosis pseudoglioma syndrome, who have an inactivating mutation in *LRP-5* gene. Furthermore, in the knock-out animals, either a tryptophan-reduced diet or an inhibitor of serotonin reduced serotonin serum levels normalized the bone density. Serotonin receptors were identified in the osteoblasts, and when activated they inhibited osteoblast activity. All of these findings suggest that serum serotonin plays a role in osteoblast function. In the LRP-5 knock-out mice, the origin of the excess serotonin was the gut. Selected knock-out in the gut reproduced the osteopenia, but selected knock-out in osteoblast cells had no effect. The authors felt this meant that the Wnt-signaling pathway in the osteoblasts was not responsible for the disease in the LRP-knockout, and that the gut serotonin was inhibiting the bone.[28]

Other laboratories have found that mice with selective knock-out of various steps within the Wnt-signaling pathway do have osteoporosis. Results from genetically modified animal models must be interpreted with some caution, because deleting one gene could activate alternate pathways.

Also, the osteoblast family is heterogeneous, and it is not yet clear which of the cells are most involved with either Wnt or serotonin signaling. Although it is plausible that a gut-derived hormone could modulate bone formation, it makes heuristic sense that the major regulators would be factors derived from the local osteocytes. Physiological bone formation should be targeted to the part of the skeleton which is bearing the most mechanical load. Further research will help to clarify the exact role of the LRP-5, and serotonin in both normal and pathological conditions.

Serotonin also is an important neuro-transmitter. This small molecule does not pass through the blood–brain barrier, so medications that increase brain serotonin levels may not necessarily increase the systematic serum serotonin levels. There is, however, an increasing body of evidence that patients treated with selective serotonin reuptake inhibitors have increased fracture rates and/or decreased bone density. The mechanisms are still unclear.[29]

Summary

This chapter has briefly reviewed the normal sequence of bone remodelling, and discussed new findings about the differentiation, function, and interactions of the bone cells. The importance of mechanical loading was stressed. Some mechanisms of medications used for osteoporosis, as well as potential new targets for influencing the bone strength are particularly interesting to clinicians and to the millions of patients with metabolic bone diseases.

References

1. Ott S. Histomorphometric analysis of bone remodelling. In: J Bilezikian, L Raisz, Ga R (eds) *Principles of Bone Biology*. San Diego: Academic Press; 2002:303–20.

2. Ott SM. *Osteoporosis and Bone Physiology*. Available at: http://courses.washington.edu/ bonephys (accessed 29/01/2010).

3. Eriksen EF, Eghbali-Fatourechi GZ, Khosla S. Remodelling and vascular spaces in bone. *J Bone Miner Res* 2007;**22**:1–6.

4. Novack DV, Teitelbaum SL. The osteoclast: friend or foe? *Ann Rev Pathol* 2008;**3**:457–84.

5. Takayanagi H. Osteoimmunology: shared mechanisms and crosstalk between the immune and bone systems. *Nat Rev Immunol* 2007;**7**(4):292–304.

6. Henriksen K, Neutzsky-Wulff AV, Bonewald LF, Karsdal MA. Local communication on and within bone controls bone remodelling. *Bone* 2009;**44**(6):1026–33.

7. Pederson L, Ruan M, Westerndorf JJ, Oursler JM. Regulation of bone formation by osteoclasts involves Wnt/BNP signaling and the chemokin sphingosin-1-phosphate. *PNAS* 2008;**105**:20761–9.

8. Russell RG, Xia Z, Dunford JE, et al. Bisphosphonates: an update on mechanisms of action and how these relate to clinical efficacy. *Ann N Y Acad Sci* 2007;**1117**:209–57.

9. Whyte MP, McAlister WH, Novack DV, Clements KL, Schoenecker PL, Wenkert D. Bisphosphonate-induced osteopetrosis: novel bone modeling defects, metaphyseal osteopenia, and osteosclerosis fractures after drug exposure ceases. *J Bone Miner Res* 2008;**23**:1698–707.

10. Cummings SR, San Martin J, McClung MR, et al. FREEDOM Trial. Denosumab for prevention of fractures in postmenopausal women with osteoporosis. *N Engl J Med.* 2009;**20**;361(8):756–65.

11. Murphy MG, Cerchio K, Stoch SA, Gottesdiener K, Wu M, Recker R. Effect of L-000845704, an alphaVbeta3 integrin antagonist, on markers of bone turnover and bone mineral density in postmenopausal osteoporotic women. *J Clin Endocrinol Metab* 2005;**90**:2022–8.

12. Fratzl-Zelman N, Valenta A, Roschger P, et al. Decreased bone turnover and deterioration of bone structure in two cases of pycnodysostosis. *J Clin Endocrinol Metab* 2004;**89**: 1538–47.

13. Sacchetti B, Funari A, Michienzi S, et al. Self-renewing osteoprogenitors in bone marrow sinusoids can organise a hematopoietic microenvironment. *Cell* 2007;**131**:324–36.

14. Mukherjee S, Raje N, Schoonmaker JA, et al. Pharmacologic targeting of a stem/progenitor population *in vivo* is associated with enhanced bone regeneration in mice. *J Clin Invest* 2008;**118**:491–504.

15. Rosen CJ, Klibanski A. Bone, fat, and body composition: evolving concepts in the pathogenesis of osteoporosis. *Am J Med* 2009;**122**(5):409–14.

16. Hamrick MW, Ferrari SL. Leptin and the sympathetic connection of fat to bone. *Osteoporos Int* 2008;**19**:905–12.

17. Reid IR. Relationships between fat and bone. *Osteoporos Int* 2008;**19**:595–606.

18. Pittas AG, Harris SS, Eliades M, Stark P, Dawson-Hughes B. Association between serum osteocalcin and markers of metabolic phenotype. *J Clin Endocrinol Metab* 2009;**94**: 827–32.

19. Gonzalez EA, Lund RJ, Martin KJ, et al. Treatment of a murine model of high-turnover renal osteodystrophy by exogenous BMP-7. *Kidney Int* 2002;**61**:1322–31.

20. Aubin JE. Advances in the osteoblast lineage. *Biochem Cell Biol* 1998;**76**:899–910.

21. Yin T, Li L. The stem cell niches in bone. *J Clin Invest* 2006;**116**:1195–201.

22. Johnson ML, Gong G, Kimberling W, Recker SM, Kimmel DB, Recker RB. Linkage of a gene causing high bone mass to human chromosome 11 (11q12-13). *Am J Hum Genet* 1997;**60**:1326–32.

23. Krishnan V, Bryant HU, Macdougald OA. Regulation of bone mass by Wnt signaling. *J Clin Invest* 2006;**116**:1202–9.

24. Jackson A, Vayssiere B, Garcia T, et al. Gene array analysis of Wnt-regulated genes in C3H10T1/2 cells. *Bone* 2005;**36**:585–98.

25. Robling AG, Niziolek PJ, Baldridge LA, et al. Mechanical stimulation of bone in vivo reduces osteocyte expression of SOST/sclerostin. *J Biol Chem* 2008;**283**:5866–75.

26. Gilsanz V, Wren TA, Sanchez M, Dorey F, Judex S, Rubin C. Low-level, high-frequency mechanical signals enhance musculoskeletal development of young women with low BMD. *J Bone Miner Res* 2006;**21**:1464–74.

27. Riggs BL, Khosla S, Melton LJ, 3rd. Sex steroids and the construction and conservation of the adult skeleton. *Endocr Rev* 2002;**23**:279–302.

28. Yadav VK, Ryu JH, Suda N, et al. LRP-5 controls bone formation by inhibiting serotonin synthesis in the duodenum. *Cell* 2008;**135:**825–37.

29. Ziere G, Dieleman JP, van der Cammen TJ, Hofman A, Pols HA, Stricker BH. Selective serotonin reuptake inhibiting antidepressants are associated with an increased risk of nonvertebral fractures. *J Clin Psychopharmacol* 2008;**28:**411–17.

30. Moon, R. *Labratory of Randall Moon*. Available at: http://faculty.washington.edu/rtmoon (accessed 29/1/2010).

Chapter 3

Osteocytes and mineral metabolism

Susan C. Schiavi and Jian Q. Feng

Introduction

Osteocytes, the terminally differentiated cell of the osteoblast lineage, reside within the mineralized matrix of bone and account for over 90% of all bone cells. Recently, genetically-based studies in both humans and mice have unveiled a previously unknown osteocyte function in the systemic regulation of mineral. It is now recognized that osteocytes and late stage osteoblasts are the primary site for production of a recently identified phosphaturic hormone, fibroblast growth factor 23 (FGF23) and several associated proteins involved in bone mineralization including dentin matrix protein 1 (DMP1), matrix extracellular phosphoglycoprotein (MEPE), and phosphate regulating protein with homology to endopeptidases on the X-chromosome (PHEX). FGF23 is elevated in chronic kidney disease and expression of each of these genes is altered in genetic and/or acquired diseases associated with hypophosphatemia. Additionally, DMP1, a non-collagenase matrix protein that serves as a scaffold for calcium phosphate deposition also appears to be involved in the regulation of systemic phosphate homeostasis through its direct or indirect effects on FGF23 expression. Cumulatively, these findings have led to the speculation that cells of the osteoblast/ osteocyte lineage may play a prominent role in maintenance of systemic phosphate homeostasis through the local control of bone mineral, the major reservoir for calcium and phosphate.

The osteoblast/osteocyte lineage

More than 90% of total calcium and phosphate content within the body resides within mineralized bone. It is therefore not surprising that changes in bone remodelling can contribute to the systemic mineral dysregulation associated with pathological conditions, such as chronic kidney disease–mineral bone disorder (CKD-MBD) by altering the bone's capacity to buffer excess calcium and phosphate. It is well understood that bone remodelling typically occurs on bone surfaces through the concerted actions of osteoclasts and osteoblasts. New evidence now suggests that the third bone cell type, the osteocyte, may also play an active role in bone remodelling and mineral maintenance in addition to its known role as a transducer of mechanical load. To understand how the osteocyte is linked to bone remodelling, it is useful to consider that it is a highly differentiated cell within the osteoblast lineage.

Osteoblasts are cuboidal-shaped cells with well-developed Golgi complexes. They reside adjacently on surfaces of existing bone tissue or calcified cartilage where they play a critical role in the formation and growth of new bone through their sequential deposition of osteoid followed by calcium and phosphorus. The life span of a typical osteoblast is 3 months in humans,[1] and less than 20 days in mice.[2] The osteoblast then undergoes one of three potential fates: cell death, transition to a bone lining cell, or further differentiation into an osteocyte.[3]

A complete understanding of how osteocytes are formed and specifically influence the remodeling process has been limited by the difficulties associated with isolating live cells from mineralized matrix coupled to the inability to recapitulate the environment necessary to fully maintain differentiated osteocytes *in vitro*. Nonetheless, microscopy studies suggest that there are several phenotypically distinct stages representing cell transitions between the mature osteoblast and osteocyte, including osteoblast, osteoblastic osteocyte, osteoid osteocyte, and mature osteocyte.[3–5] These studies suggest that osteoblasts are actively differentiating toward a mature osteocyte as they are engulfed within mineralizing matrix. During these concurrent processes, cell organelles, and cytoplasm are reduced, and the cell acquires exceptionally long dendritic cell processes. The slender branched dendritic processes of the differentiated osteocyte occupy the many minute canals, named canaliculi, which radiate in all directions from the cell body encased within the core spaces referred to as lacunae. Within the bone, individual osteocyte lacunocanalicular units form a large network allowing osteocytes to communicate with each other, surface osteoblast cells, and blood vessels (Figs 3.1 and 3.2). This system of osteocyte-filled caves and channels provide osteocytes the flexible environment required to coordinate adaptive bone remodeling in response to mechanical strain.[6] It also provides a route in which released paracrine and endocrine factors may reach their local or systemic destination including osteoblast and osteocyte targets.

Osteocyte role in mineralization

The limited understanding of the osteocyte's role in matrix production and mineralization has been based on static pictures from transmission electron microscopy (TEM).[3] More recently, live imaging techniques have been used to correlate differentiation with the mineralization process. A pivotal study by the Dallas laboratory examined *in vitro* differentiation of primary rat calvarial cells (a rich source of pre-osteoblasts and osteoblasts) which have been isolated from transgenic mice expressing green fluorescent protein (GFP) under control of an 8kb *DMP1* osteocyte selective promoter. Mineralization was observed using the vital calcium stain, alizarin red. Time-lapsed photography demonstrated that the mineral process started from small focal areas within clusters of GFP-positive cells and radiated outwards. The entire mineralization was complete within 10 h. These studies demonstrate that osteocytes may play an active role in the mineralization process, rather than passively being buried alive by neighboring osteoblasts.[7] The relevance of this finding is that it suggests the same cell type regulates mineralization and systemic phosphate homeostasis.

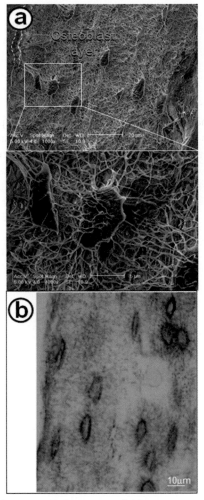

Fig. 3.1 Complexity of the osteocyte lacunocanalicular system and DMP1 expression in osteocytes. Resin embedded 3-month-old mouse alveolar bone was polished and acid-etched to remove mineral leaving behind the plastic for visualization of the osteocyte lacunocanalicular system using scanning electron microscopy. (a) This image displays the connections between osteocytes and the osteoblast layer on bone surfaces, as well as connections between osteocytes. The insert shows an enlargement of the area outlined in the top panel. The figure is adapted from Feng et al. in *Nature Genetics* (2006).[14] (b) An immunohistochemistry stain shows that DMP1 is highly expressed in osteocytes in a wild-type 4-week-old tibia mid-shaft.

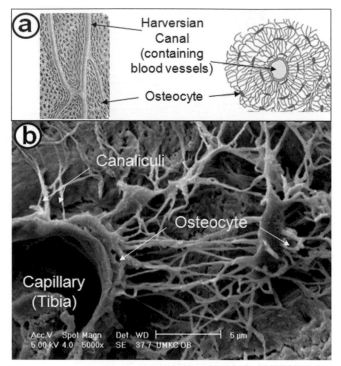

Fig. 3.2 Connections between blood vessels and osteocyte-lacunocanaliculi (a). Parallel (×100, left panel) and transverse (×250, right panel) sections of the cortical bone (decalcified). Osteocyte-lacunocanaliculi are arranged concentrically around the Haversian canal, which contains blood vessels and nerves, suggesting that there might be connections between blood vessels and osteocytes. (Adapted from *Gray's Anatomy of the Human Body* from the classic 1918 publication, http://www.bartleby.com/107/18.html). (b) The image is an acid-etched resin embedded rabbit tibia and visualized by scanning electron microscopy, documenting that there are direct connections of a capillary and osteocyte-lacunocanaliculi either by cell bodies or by canaliculi (adapted from Feng et al. 2009[58]).

Osteocyte function has also been studied in genetic mouse models in which genes associated with human genetic or acquired disorders of phosphate dysregulation are either over-expressed transgenically or deleted through homologous recombination techniques. The group of proteins associated with hypophosphatemic diseases include:

+ the secreted phosphaturic hormone, FGF23;

+ the Wnt inhibitor, sFRP4;

+ bone matrix proteins of the small integrin-binding ligand, N-linked glycoprotein (SIBLING) family, DMP1 and MEPE;

+ the membrane bound endopeptidase, PHEX.[8–10]

In addition to being linked to changes in serum phosphate, each of these molecules has been shown to be directly or indirectly associated with changes in bone mineral content and with the exception of sFRP4, each of these proteins is expressed in osteocytes. sFRP4 is a secreted protein that attenuates bone formation at least partially through inhibition of the canonical Wnt signaling pathway in osteoblasts.[11]

The *DMP1* null mouse model provides a good example of how genetic approaches have increased our understanding of genes associated with the mineralization process. DMP1 is a secreted serine-rich acidic protein in the SIBLING family that has numerous potential phosphorylation sites to promote mineral formation at the perilacunar surfaces of osteocytes (Fig. 3.1b).[12,13] While full length DMP1 is susceptible to proteolytic cleavage resulting in the generation of specific N- and C-terminal fragments, the biological functions of intact versus these fragments are not clear. Although these mice clearly show that DMP1 is not essential for mineralization in early development,[7] they display striking defects in osteocyte morphology, bone remodelling, and mineralization during postnatal development when the skeleton bears mechanical loading.[12–15] A combination of sensitive microscopy techniques revealed changes in osteocyte cell morphology and mineral deposition in the *DMP1* null relative to wild-type mice. The co-ordinate use of fluorescent dyes provided a strategy to examine the relationship of osteocytes (DAPI nuclear stain), active mineralization (calcein), total mineral content (alizarin red), and lacunocanalicular space (procian red).[14] Backscattered scanning electron microscopy (SEM) was also used to view the lacunae and density of the surrounding mineral. These studies confirmed that loss of DMP1 resulted in profound changes in both osteocyte structure and total bone mineralization[14–18] and are in agreement with previous studies in adult wild-type animals, where DMP1 osteocyte expression is dramatically up-regulated in response to mechanical loading induced bone remodeling.[19,20]

Two additional SIBLINGs proteins, MEPE and osteopontin, have also been shown to play a role in the regulation of bone mineral content. Similar to DMP1, both osteopontin and MEPE are expressed by late stage osteoblasts and osteocytes, and are also localized to the extracellular matrix adjacent to the canaliculi and lacunae walls. It is now well established that osteopontin is a negative regulator of bone mineralization.[21] Osteopontin inhibits mineralization *in vitro* and knockout mice have increased mineral content.[22] MEPE also appears to be a negative regulator of mineralization as MEPE null mice have increased bone density.[23] The ASARM peptide, a cleavage product of MEPE can directly block mineralization both *in vitro*[24] and *in vivo*.[25] Current data support a hypothesis that these molecules may be transducers of strain and participate in local mineral content of the perilacunar space. One model proposes that the function of osteopontin and ASARM is to reduce local mineral content in lacunae, whereas DMP1 has been proposed to be a positive regulator of mineralization at the same site.[26–28]

The emerging data suggests that the phosphate regulated SIBLING proteins control the degree of mineralization at the interface of bone surfaces lining the lacunocanalicular space. It is further hypothesized that the degree of mineralization dictates the flexibility of the osteocyte, thereby altering how it responds to mechanical induction and how it transmits signals that regulate active remodelling on the bone surface.

Roles of osteocytes in the control of Pi homeostasis

Pi is essential not only for skeletal health and integrity, but also required for a diverse array of biological processes, including numerous cellular mechanisms involved in energy metabolism, cell signaling, nucleic acid synthesis, and membrane function.[29] As mentioned above, 90% of total body phosphorus is stored in bone, with only 1% in circulation. The relationship between control of phosphorus homeostasis by the kidney and bone mineralization is clearly illustrated by the known functions of parathyroid hormone (PTH). PTH directly induces phosphorus release from bone via activation of osteoclast-induced resorption and simultaneously promotes renal phosphate excretion, thereby providing a mechanism by which the body can handle excess phosphorus during net catabolic states of bone remodeling.

FGF23 also promotes phosphorus excretion, but its local actions at its main site of expression within bone are not entirely understood.[14,30,31] Despite earlier reports failing to identify FGF23 expression in bone, it is now fully recognized that depending on the mouse model, FGF23 can be expressed in late stage osteoblasts and/or osteocytes.[30,32] Liu and colleagues[30,33] crossed a *FGF23*-deficient GFP reporter mouse (where GFP is used to reflect the endogenous *FGF23* expression) with the PHEX-deficient *Hyp* mouse model of the human disease, XLH (X-linked hypophosphatemic rickets) and demonstrated that FGF23 was expressed in osteocytes, but not in PHEX-deficient osteoblast cells. Furthermore, in bone marrow stromal cells derived from *FGF23*-null/*Hyp* mice, GFP expression was selectively increased in osteocyte-like cells within mineralization nodules consistent with osteocyte-specific expression.[34] In contrast, a separate group reported that FGF23 expression was localized to osteoblasts in calvaria sections of *FGF23*-lacZ knock-in mice (where the LacZ reporter was used to reflect the endogenous *FGF23* expression).[32] There are a variety of explanations that may explain discrepancies in the identified FGF23 expression sites including differential sensitivity of detection methods, abnormal expression of related pathway genes in individual genetic models, variable age-dependent expression, and/or differential expression in specific bone regions. As discussed below, detection using the more sensitive method of *in situ* hybridization suggests FGF23 is expressed in both osteoblasts and osteocytes.

A recent study visually examined the relationship between FGF23 and DMP1 protein expression and the physical characteristics of the osteocyte lacunocanicular system in long bones of 12-week-old wild-type mice to assess the potential role of these proteins in bone remodelling.[35] The physical arrangement of the osteocyte lacunocanicular system is thought to reflect the relative speed of bone formation and/or osteocyte maturation in a given bone area. Disorganized osteocyte lacunocanicular patterns are found in bone areas undergoing more rapid bone formation, such as the metaphyseal regions of cortical bone and the primary trabeculae, whereas linearly well-spaced osteocyte lacunocanicular are found in areas with slower bone formation rates, such as the secondary trabeculae and the cortical endosteal region of the diaphysis. Importantly, DMP1 expression was observed throughout the epiphysis, metaphysis, and diaphysis in both cortical and trabecular bone. This relatively ubiquitous expression of DMP1 supports its role as a local regulator of mineralization. In contrast, FGF23 immunostaining was significantly greater in areas known to have reduced bone formation and organized osteocytes. Thus, strong FGF23 expression was observed in secondary trabeculae and in the endosteal region of the cortical epiphysis, where osteocytes were regularly organized. The authors speculated that well arranged canaliculi and osteocyte connectivity would promote more efficient transport of FGF23 and other small molecules. DMP1 positive osteocytes did not express FGF23, supporting earlier studies suggesting DMP1 is a negative regulator of FGF23.[14] Taken together, these data suggest that FGF23 expression is correlated with areas of reduced mineralization.

FGF23 expression can impact mineralization simply by removing the critical substrate, phosphate. Consequentially, hypophosphatemia induced by high levels of circulating FGF23 leads to rickets and osteomalacia in both humans and mice with fully functioning kidneys. However, recent studies also support specific FGF23 effects on mineralization that appear independent of its renal actions on systemic phosphate levels. Although FGF23 null mice are hyperphosphatemic and have a general increase in bone mineral density, there is a localized increase in osteoid with corresponding decrease in mineralization. Furthermore, mice deficient in both FGF23 and its main target protein, the renal phosphate co-transporter, Npt2a, exhibit reversal of hyperphosphatemia while retaining skeletal defects suggesting that FGF23 may also control bone mineralization independently of its roles on regulation of systemic phosphate homeostasis.[36] Finally, physiological concentrations of FGF23 can inhibit nodule formation and mineralization of an osteoblast cell line, as well as bone formation in the parietal bone organ culture model, supporting a direct role of FGF23 on bone *in vitro*.[37] Despite these lines of evidence, the apparent absence in bone of the FGF23 co-receptor, KLOTHO raises mechanistic questions regarding how FGF23 may direct specific effects on bone mineralization.

Additional data supporting the concept that osteocytes control Pi homeostasis in association with the anabolic mineralization process are mainly from studies of two hypophosphatemic animal models: *DMP1*-null mice and *Hyp* mice, in which the membrane bound endopeptidase *PHEX* is deleted. PHEX is predominately located in osteoblasts and osteocytes. Inactive *PHEX* mutations lead to increased FGF23 production in osteocytes by an unknown matrix-derived FGF23 stimulatory factor.[30,33,34] These two animal models share essentially the same phenotype: hypophosphatemia rickets/osteomalacia and high FGF23 levels.[14,30,38] Humans harboring lose of function mutations in either the *PHEX* or *DMP1* genes also have elevated FGF23 levels.[14,39–41] While the similarities between these phenotypes suggest that DMP1 and PHEX might function in the same pathway, current evidence suggests that intact DMP1 is not a substrate for PHEX.[42]

In situ hybridization and immunohistochemistry have demonstrated that in young wild-type mice, FGF23 is mainly expressed in osteoblasts with relatively low expression in osteocytes.[14] In contrast, relative to WT mice, young *DMP1* null mice had a dramatic FGF23 increase in osteocytes with expression unchanged in osteoblast cells.[14] These observations suggested that DMP1, a protein highly expressed in osteocytes and associated with mineralization negatively regulates FGF23 expression, a protein associated with reduced mineralization. This hypothesis is consistent with the fact that expression of multiple genes is typically repressed during osteocyte differentiation and the mineralization process. Many markers of osteoblasts, such as alkaline phosphatase activity and collagen type 1 mRNA, as well as osteoid-osteocyte markers, such as E11/ gp38 protein16, are greatly elevated in *DMP1*-null osteocytes regardless of whether they are newly formed or deeply embedded.[14] These observations not only explain the abnormal skeletal phenotype of *DMP1*-null mice, but also reveal a failure to repress osteoblastic gene expression in the *DMP1*-null osteocytes. Interestingly, recent staining in wild-type mice demonstrates that DMP1 and FGF23 do not co-localize to the same osteocytes.[35]

The most striking change in the *DMP1*-null osteocyte is the dramatically increased production and secretion of FGF23 causing hypophosphatemia.[14] By definition, an endocrine cell should release hormones into the bloodstream easily and quickly. Unlike the osteoblast lining cells, which are directly exposed to the blood circulation, osteocytes are embedded in the mineralized matrix. Based on the molecule weight of FGF23, it is too large to pass through the gap junctions connecting osteocytes and osteoblasts. However, the lacunocanalicular transportation system containing proteoglycans and extravascular fluid surrounding the osteocyte[43] provides an environment for transportation of fluid and signals. It is also known that there is a close connection between large blood vessels and osteocytes (Fig. 3.2a). The relationship between a capillary blood vessel (10μm diameter) and neighboring osteocytes was examined using a resin-casted SEM method with acid etching of the sample surface. Figure 3.2b depicts direct contacts between an osteocyte cell body or dendrites, and the capillary wall. Thus, physical evidence is consistent with the osteocyte's endocrine function.

While the above studies clearly demonstrate a role for FGF23 in pathological conditions, evidence also demonstrates that it has a physiological role in normal Pi homeostasis. Yamazaki and colleagues showed that a single injection of neutralizing FGF23 antibodies into wild-type mice nearly doubled the serum phosphate level, supporting a PTH-independent function in regulation of Pi homeostasis.[44] Furthermore, increases in serum phosphate or vitamin D leads to elevations in serum FGF23 levels within hours. FGF23 also inhibits 1α-hydroxylase, the rate limiting enzyme for $1,25(OH)_2D_3$ production and inhibits PTH synthesis via KLOTHO/FGFR1 complexes on the parathyroid system.[45,46] These findings suggest that FGF23 is an important component of a hormonal feedback system and demonstrate how FGF23 can indirectly influence bone remodelling through regulation of PTH and $1,25(OH)_2D_3$. Evidence suggests that the role of FGF23 in this potential feedback system is to manage phosphate changes over hours since changes in FGF23 serum levels respond more slowly to challenges relative to PTH. Recently, Tatsumi and colleagues showed that mice with ablated osteocytes do not have changes in Pi homeostasis or serum FGF23 levels[47] suggesting that FGF23 actions might be redundant or secondary to the actions of PTH. However, caution in the over-interpretation of these experiments is warranted as increased FGF23 from osteoblasts or residual osteocytes may account for the apparent lack of affects on systemic phosphate levels.

Cumulatively, these data suggest that FGF23 and its associated osteocyte SIBLING proteins may co-ordinate mineralization with systemic regulation of phosphorus levels. One possibility is that these proteins directly regulate the differentiation of osteoblasts into mature osteocytes with either direct or indirect regulation of mineral deposition within active remodelling units. Another scenario is that these molecules regulate the mineral density along the perilacunar surfaces adjacent to embedded osteocytes. Released mineral from these sites could be a potential source of serum calcium and phosphorus. It is also proposed that changes in perilacunar mineralization might alter the ability of the osteocyte to respond to mechanical load with resulting changes in released signals such as sclerostin that regulate normal bone remodelling at the bone surface. Regardless of the mechanism, the release of FGF23 appears to be correlated with decreased mineralization states in the presence of a functional kidney.

Osteocytes' role in phosphate dysregulation associated with CKD

In addition to the hypophosphatemic diseases associated with normal renal function, FGF23 levels are progressively increased during CKD-MBD. These elevations occur early in CKD before increases in PTH or serum phosphate, and correlate strongly with cardiovascular calcification and mortality.[48–50] Serum phosphate elevations even in the normal range have been linked to increased mortality within both the general and the CKD population.[51] It is currently unclear whether FGF23 has direct effects on disease progression or whether the dramatic progressive increases in FGF23 are simply a consequence of uncontrolled increases in serum phosphate. Given the evidence described above, it is appealing to consider that FGF23 may be an important molecule signaling early changes in bone health. This possibility is consistent with new histological evidence demonstrating that renal osteodystrophy[52,53] and vascular calcification can be found early in CKD and are not limited to ESKD. In a pivotal radiolabel study performed in the early 1990s, it became clear that different forms of renal osteodystrophy with reduced or enhanced turnover can alter the ability of bones to 'buffer' excess calcium[54] and presumably, by extension, phosphorus. This study demonstrated how alterations in bone remodelling can dramatically impact systemic calcium and phosphorus load. By extension, it is conceivable that alterations in proteins such as FGF23 that either directly regulate or sense changes in bone mineralization could contribute to the early and progressive dysregulation in mineral metabolism.

The above concept was explored in a study utilizing a gene delivery technique to introduce elevated FGF23 levels early in a progressive rat CKD model. Despite the attenuation of glomerulosclerosis and improved renal function by the early introduction of the phosphaturic hormone FGF23, renal osteodystrophy developed more aggressively as noted by increased bone fibrosis and enhanced bone formation.[55] These FGF23 effects on bone could be attributed at least in part to decreased $1,25(OH)_2D_3$ production and subsequent increased PTH production. Results of this study highlight the difficulties in defining the direct effects of individual components within a hormonal feedback loop and the need for additional studies to determine whether FGF23 has direct bone effects that contribute to the progression of renal osteodystrophy.

A recent cross-sectional study in pediatric ESKD patients with high turnover disease revealed a positive correlation between serum FGF23 levels and improved indices of mineralization with no significant correlation between FGF23 and bone formation rates.[56] These results are not entirely inconsistent with the results from immunostaining cited above which demonstrate that FGF23 is expressed in localized regions of organized osteocyte lacunocanalicular systems. These regions are also likely to be regions with more densely packed crystals as mineralization continues for some time after osteocytes are embedded.[57] Thus, FGF23 may be most prominently expressed by osteocytes that have matured beyond the stage of rapid mineralization and are structurally equipped for efficient secretion into the bloodstream. Additional studies examining the organization of osteocyte lacunocanalicular systems and osteocyte morphology in other forms of renal osteodystrophy, with and without mineralization defects, is necessary to fully understand the relationship of FGF23, mineralization, and osteocyte maturation.

The influence of CKD on osteocyte function

In addition to delineating the mechanisms by which osteocytes may contribute to dysregulation of mineral homeostasis, it is also relevant to understand how other pathological parameters of CKD may influence osteocyte health. It is known that apoptotic osteocytes may also support osteoclast activation and formation at the site of micro-damage by the release of specific signals.[47] Co-morbidities in CKD such as inflammation could contribute to declining bone health by promoting osteocyte apoptosis. For example, TNFα and interleukin-1 have been shown to promote osteocyte apoptosis in parallel with estrogen deficiency and could conceivably contribute to increased osteoclast activity observed in high turnover diseases of CKD.[59] It will be important to characterize how various metabolic factors influence osteocyte health to understand how underlying causes and co-morbidities can impact overall bone health in CKD.

Summary

Emerging data incorporating genetic models and specialized microscopy techniques have established a new paradigm in which the osteocyte plays an active, rather than passive role in the mineralization process. Additionally, it is now recognized that the osteocyte also co-ordinates mineralization with systemic phosphate regulation through its expression of multi-functional proteins that simultaneously regulate mineralization and production of the phosphaturic hormone, FGF23. Thus, DMP1, a matrix protein that has a positive influence on mineralization, is a negative regulator of FGF23, whereas MEPE, a protein that is associated with reduced mineralization, appears to enhance FGF23 expression. It is currently unclear whether FGF23 expression is more tightly controlled by the extent of mineralization or the stage of osteocyte maturation. Furthermore, conflicting information exists regarding potential local effects of FGF23 during normal and abnormal states of bone remodelling. FGF23 elevations in CKD have illuminated the potential contributions of the osteocyte in renal osteodystrophy and raised new questions regarding the role of FGF23 in the mineralization process. Analysis of the physical attributes of osteocyte lacunocanalicular systems in conjunction with the parameters outlined by KDIGO will assist in defining the extent in which variations of osteocyte functions may contribute to the spectrum of renal osteodystrophy.

Acknowledgments

The osteocyte work is partly supported by NIH AR-46798, AR051587, and Genzyme Renal Innovations Program.

References

1. Manolagas SC. Birth and death of bone cells: basic regulatory mechanisms and implications for the pathogenesis and treatment of osteoporosis. *Endocr Rev* 2000;**21**:115–37.

2. McCulloch CA, Heersche JN. Lifetime of the osteoblast in mouse periodontium. *Anat Rec* 1988;**222**:128–35.

3. Franz-Odendaal TA, Hall BK, Witten PE. Buried alive: how osteoblasts become osteocytes. *Dev Dyn* 2006;**235**:176–90.

4. Knothe Tate ML, Adamson JR, Tami AE, Bauer TW. The osteocyte. *Int J Biochem Cell Biol* 2004;**36**:1–8.

5. Palumbo C, Palazzini S, Zaffe D, Marotti G. Osteocyte differentiation in the tibia of newborn rabbit: an ultrastructural study of the formation of cytoplasmic processes. *Acta anatomica* 1990;**137**:350–8.

6. Bonewald LF. Mechanosensation and Transduction in Osteocytes. *Bonekey* 2006;**3**:7–15.

7. Dallas SL, Veno PA, Rosser JL *et al.* Time lapse imaging techniques for comparison of mineralization dynamics in primary murine osteoblasts and the late osteoblast/early osteocyte-like cell line MLO-A5. *Cells, tissues, organs* 2009;**189**:6–11.

8. Shimada T, Mizutani S, Muto T *et al.* Cloning and characterization of FGF23 as a causative factor of tumor-induced osteomalacia. *Proc Natl Acad Sci U S A* 2001;**98**:6500–5.

9. Strom TM, Juppner H. PHEX, FGF23, DMP1 and beyond. *Curr Opin Nephrol Hypertens* 2008;**17**:357–62.

10. De Beur SM, Finnegan RB, Vassiliadis J *et al.* Tumors associated with oncogenic osteomalacia express genes important in bone and mineral metabolism. *J Bone Miner Res* 2002;**17**:1102–10.

11. Nakanishi R, Akiyama H, Kimura H *et al.* Osteoblast-targeted expression of Sfrp4 in mice results in low bone mass. *J Bone Miner Res* 2008;**23**:271–7.

12. Qin C, Brunn JC, Cook RG *et al.* Evidence for the proteolytic processing of dentin matrix protein 1. Identification and characterization of processed fragments and cleavage sites. *J Biol Chem* 2003;**278**:34700–8.

13. Qin C, D'Souza R, Feng JQ. Dentin matrix protein 1 (DMP1): new and important roles for biomineralization and phosphate homeostasis. *J Dent Res* 2007;**86**:1134–41.

14. Feng JQ, Ward LM, Liu S *et al.* Loss of DMP1 causes rickets and osteomalacia and identifies a role for osteocytes in mineral metabolism. *Nature genetics* 2006;**38**:1310–5.

15. Rios HF, Ye L, Dusevich V, Eick D, Bonewald LF, Feng JQ. DMP1 is essential for osteocyte formation and function. *J Musculoskelet Neuronal Interact* 2005;**5**:325–7.

16. Ling Y, Rios HF, Myers ER, Lu Y, Feng JQ, Boskey AL. DMP1 depletion decreases bone mineralization in vivo: an FTIR imaging analysis. *J Bone Miner Res* 2005;**20**:2169–77.

17. Ye L, Mishina Y, Chen D *et al.* Dmp1-deficient mice display severe defects in cartilage formation responsible for a chondrodysplasia-like phenotype. *J Biol Chem* 2005;**280**: 6197–203.

18. Ye L, Zhang S, Ke H, Bonewald LF, Feng JQ. Periodontal breakdown in the Dmp1 null mouse model of hypophosphatemic rickets. *J Dent Res* 2008;**87**:624–9.

19. Yang W, Kalajzic I, Lu Y *et al.* In vitro and in vivo study on osteocyte-specific mechanical signaling pathways. *J Musculoskelet Neuronal Interact* 2004;**4**:386–7.

20. Yang W, Lu Y, Kalajzic I *et al.* Dentin matrix protein 1 gene cis-regulation: Use In osteocytes to characterize local responses to mechanical loading in vitro and In vivo. *J Biol Chem* 2005;**280**:20680–90.

21. McKee MD, Nanci A. Osteopontin at mineralized tissue interfaces in bone, teeth, and osseointegrated implants: ultrastructural distribution and implications for mineralized tissue formation, turnover, and repair. *Microsc Res Tech* 1996;**33**:141–64.

22. Giachelli CM, Steitz S. Osteopontin: a versatile regulator of inflammation and biomineralization. *Matrix Biol* 2000;**19**:615–22.

23. Gowen LC, Petersen DN, Mansolf AL *et al.* Targeted disruption of the osteoblast/osteocyte factor 45 gene (OF45) results in increased bone formation and bone mass. *J Biol Chem* 2003;**278**:1998–2007.

24. Addison WN, Nakano Y, Loisel T, Crine P, McKee MD. MEPE-ASARM peptides control extracellular matrix mineralization by binding to hydroxyapatite: an inhibition regulated by PHEX cleavage of ASARM. *J Bone Miner Res* 2008;**23**:1638–49.

25. Rowe PS, Garrett IR, Schwarz PM *et al.* Surface plasmon resonance (SPR) confirms that MEPE binds to PHEX via the MEPE-ASARM motif: a model for impaired mineralization in X-linked rickets (HYP). *Bone* 2005;**36**:33–46.

26. Robling AG, Niziolek PJ, Baldridge LA *et al.* Mechanical stimulation of bone in vivo reduces osteocyte expression of Sost/sclerostin. *J Biol Chem* 2008;**283**:5866–75.

27. Yang W, Lu Y, Kalajzic I *et al.* Dentin matrix protein 1 gene cis-regulation: use in osteocytes to characterize local responses to mechanical loading in vitro and in vivo. *J Biol Chem* 2005;**280**:20680–90.

28. Harris SE, Gluhak-Heinrich J, Harris MA *et al.* DMP1 and MEPE expression are elevated in osteocytes after mechanical loading in vivo: theoretical role in controlling mineral quality in the perilacunar matrix. *J Musculoskelet Neuronal Interact* 2007;**7**:313–5.

29. Foster BL, Tompkins KA, Rutherford RB *et al.* Phosphate: known and potential roles during development and regeneration of teeth and supporting structures. *Birth Defects Res C Embryo Today* 2008;**84**:281–314.

30. Liu S, Zhou J, Tang W, Jiang X, Rowe DW, Quarles LD. Pathogenic role of Fgf23 in Hyp mice. *Am J Physiol Endocrinol Metab* 2006;**291**:E38–49.

31. Schiavi SC. Bone talk. *Nat Genet* 2006;**38**:1230–1.

32. Sitara D, Razzaque MS, Hesse M *et al.* Homozygous ablation of fibroblast growth factor-23 results in hyperphosphatemia and impaired skeletogenesis, and reverses hypophosphatemia in Phex-deficient mice. *Matrix Biol* 2004;**23**:421–32.

33. Quarles LD. Endocrine functions of bone in mineral metabolism regulation. *J Clin Invest* 2008;**118**:3820–8.

34. Liu S, Gupta A, Quarles LD. Emerging role of fibroblast growth factor 23 in a bone-kidney axis regulating systemic phosphate homeostasis and extracellular matrix mineralization. *Curr Opin Nephrol Hypertens* 2007;**16**:329–35.

35. Ubaidus S, Li M, Sultana S *et al.* FGF23 is mainly synthesized by osteocytes in the regularly distributed osteocytic lacunar canalicular system established after physiological bone remodeling. *J Electron Microsc (Tokyo)* 2009;**58**:381–92.

36. Sitara D, Kim S, Razzaque MS *et al.* Genetic evidence of serum phosphate-independent functions of FGF23 on bone. *PLoS genetics* 2008;**4**:e1000154.

37. Wang H, Yoshiko Y, Yamamoto R *et al.* Overexpression of Fibroblast Growth Factor 23 Suppresses Osteoblast Differentiation and Matrix Mineralization in vitro. *J Bone Miner Res* 2008; **23**:939–48.

38. Liu S, Guo R, Simpson LG, Xiao ZS, Burnham CE, Quarles LD. Regulation of fibroblastic growth factor 23 expression but not degradation by PHEX. *J Biol Chem* 2003;**278**: 37419–26.

39. Lorenz-Depiereux B, Bastepe M, Benet-Pages A *et al.* DMP1 mutations in autosomal recessive hypophosphatemia implicate a bone matrix protein in the regulation of phosphate homeostasis. *Nature genetics* 2006;**38**:1248–50.

40. Yamazaki Y, Okazaki R, Shibata M *et al.* Increased circulatory level of biologically active full-length FGF23 in patients with hypophosphatemic rickets/osteomalacia. *The Journal of clinical endocrinology and metabolism* 2002;**87**:4957–60.

41. Jonsson KB, Zahradnik R, Larsson T *et al.* Fibroblast growth factor 23 in oncogenic osteomalacia and X-linked hypophosphatemia. *The New England journal of medicine* 2003;**348**:1656–63.

42. Lu Y, Qin C, Xie Y, Bonewald LF, Feng JQ. Studies of the DMP1 57-kDa functional domain both in vivo and in vitro. *Cells Tissues Organs* 2009;**189**:175–85.

43. Knothe Tate ML. "Whither flows the fluid in bone?" An osteocyte's perspective. *Journal of biomechanics* 2003;**36**:1409–24.

44. Yamazaki Y, Tamada T, Kasai N *et al.* Anti-FGF23 neutralizing antibodies show the physiological role and structural features of FGF23. *J Bone Miner Res* 2008;**23**:1509–18.

45. Shimada T, Hasegawa H, Yamazaki Y *et al.* FGF23 is a potent regulator of vitamin D metabolism and phosphate homeostasis. *J Bone Miner Res* 2004;**19**:429–35.

46. Ben-Dov IZ, Galitzer H, Lavi-Moshayoff V *et al.* The parathyroid is a target organ for FGF23 in rats. *J Clin Invest* 2007;**117**:4003–8.

47. Tatsumi S, Ishii K, Amizuka N *et al.* Targeted ablation of osteocytes induces osteoporosis with defective mechanotransduction. *Cell metabolism* 2007;**5**:464–75.

48. Gutierrez OM, Mannstadt M, Isakova T *et al.* Fibroblast growth factor 23 and mortality among patients undergoing hemodialysis. *The New England journal of medicine* 2008;**359**:584–92.

49. Gutierrez O, Isakova T, Rhee E *et al.* Fibroblast growth factor-23 mitigates hyperphosphatemia but accentuates calcitriol deficiency in chronic kidney disease. *J Am Soc Nephrol* 2005;**16**:2205–15.

50. Fliser D, Kollerits B, Neyer U *et al.* Fibroblast growth factor 23 (FGF23) predicts progression of chronic kidney disease: the Mild to Moderate Kidney Disease (MMKD) Study. *J Am Soc Nephrol* 2007;**18**:2600–8.

51. Kestenbaum B. Phosphate metabolism in the setting of chronic kidney disease: significance and recommendations for treatment. *Seminars in dialysis* 2007;**20**:286–94.

52. Kates DM, Sherrard DJ, Andress DL. Evidence that serum phosphate is independently associated with serum PTH in patients with chronic renal failure. *Am J Kidney Dis* 1997;**30**:809–13.

53. Malluche HH, Ritz E, Lange HP *et al*. Bone histology in incipient and advanced renal failure. *Kidney Int* 1976;**9**:355–62.

54. Kurz P, Monier-Faugere MC, Bognar B *et al*. Evidence for abnormal calcium homeostasis in patients with adynamic bone disease. *Kidney Int* 1994;**46**:855–61.

55. Kusano K, Saito H, Segawa H, Fukushima N, Miyamoto K. Mutant FGF23 prevents the progression of chronic kidney disease but aggravates renal osteodystrophy in uremic rats. *J Nutr Sci Vitaminol (Tokyo)* 2009;**55**:99–105.

56. Wesseling-Perry K, Pereira RC, Wang H *et al*. Relationship between Plasma Fibroblast Growth Factor-23 Concentration and Bone Mineralization in Children with Renal Failure on Peritoneal Dialysis. *The Journal of clinical endocrinology and metabolism* 2009;**94**:511–17.

57. Ott SM. Bone histomorphometry in renal osteodystrophy. *Semin Nephrol* 2009;**29**:122–32.

58. Feng JQ, Ye L, Schiavi S. Do osteocytes contribute to phosphate homeostasis?. *Curr Opin Nephrol Hypertens* 2009;**18**:285–91.

59. Bonewald, L.F. *Osteocytes*. In: Primer on Metabolic Bone Diseases and Disorders of Mineral Metabolism. (CJ Rosen, editor-in-chief) Published by the American Society for Bone and Mineral Research (Washington, DC) Seventh edition. 2008:Chapter 4; p.22–27.

Chapter 4

Calcium-sensing receptors (CaSR) in kidney, bone, and vessels

Ogo I. Egbuna and Edward M. Brown

Introduction

The calcium-sensing receptor (CaSR) plays key roles in the maintenance of a narrow range (1.1–1.3mM) of the ionized calcium concentration (Ca^{2+}_o) in extracellular fluids (ECF), including blood, primarily by modulating the function of the chief cells of the parathyroid gland. Here, it regulates the synthesis and secretion of parathyroid hormone (PTH) as well as parathyroid cellular proliferation,[1] inhibiting all three when Ca^{2+}_o is high and stimulating them when Ca^{2+}_o is low. Both very high and very low levels of Ca^{2+}_o can lead to serious clinical sequellae and, in some instances, can be life-threatening. Even minute alterations in Ca^{2+}_o from its normal level (e.g. of a few per cent) promote immediate physiological responses, especially reciprocal changes in PTH secretion, which operate to normalize the level of Ca^{2+}_o. Thus, the CaSR serves as a 'calciostat', informing the parathyroid glands and other regulatory tissues of the precise level of Ca^{2+}_o in the immediate extracellular environment and activating appropriate homeostatic responses.

There is only limited understanding of direct functions of the CaSR expressed in tissues other than the parathyroid. Several studies have supported a role of the CaSR in promoting the secretion of calcitonin by the C-cells of the thyroid gland,[2] and the CaSR plays several putative roles in regulating various aspects of renal function, as described in more detail below. There is also growing, albeit limited and/or controversial, evidence implicating the receptor in controlling the function of bone cells,[3] the gastrointestinal tract,[4] and the cardiovascular system.[5] Notably, recent studies in mice with conditional knockout of the receptor in chondrocytes or osteoblasts have implicated the CaSR as an important regulator of cartilage and bone. In any case, the implication(s) of the CaSR in controlling cellular processes unrelated to Ca^{2+}_o homeostasis, and the application of calcimimetics and various molecular tools in the investigation of these functions suggests that the biological roles of the CaSR may not be exclusively calcium-centric.

The CaSR (also known as CaSR1 and GPRC2A) was cloned using the expression-cloning technique in *Xenopus laevis* oocytes.[6] Analysis of its nucleotide and amino acid sequences place the CaSR within family C of the superfamily of seven transmembrane, G protein-coupled receptors (GPCRs). Other members of this family include the G protein-coupled, so-called metabotropic receptors for glutamate (mGluRs) and for gamma-aminobutyric acid (GABA), as well as GPCRs that sense pheromones and odorants (in fish). Recently, another member of family C, GPRC6A, has been found to share several pharmacological properties with the CaSR.[7] Like the CaSR, GPRC6A is sensitive towards certain L-amino acids, although unlike the CaSR, which senses predominantly aromatic amino acids, GPRC6A is most responsive to basic amino acids. Subsequent studies showed that this receptor is also activated by high concentrations of extracellular calcium (e.g. 10–20mM) and calcimimetics, which are allosteric activators of the CaSR that will be discussed later. These data have implicated GPRC6A as a second calcium-sensing receptor (CaSR2), potentially playing key roles in bone. Two recent studies of GPRC6A knockout mice, however, reached opposite conclusions, one finding a bone phenotype[8] and the other not.[9] In addition, establishing a direct connection between GPRC6A and bone has been complicated by a complex phenotype affecting multiple other organs in one of the knockout models.[8]

The physiological relevance of the CaSR in humans was proven by the identification of inherited disorders caused by mutations in the receptor leading to either loss- or gain-of-function.[10] Heterozygous (e.g. the mutation is present in only one allele) gain-of-function mutations (CaSR activating) cause a form of autosomal dominant hypoparathyroidism (ADH). Heterozygous loss-of-function (CaSR inactivating) mutations are the cause of a disorder called familial hypocalciuric hypercalcemia (FHH), also termed familial benign hypocalciuric hypercalcemia (FBHH), which typically manifests as asymptomatic hypercalcemia with relative or absolute hypocalciuria. When present in the homozygous or compound heterozygous state, in contrast, inactivating CaSR mutations produce neonatal severe primary hyperparathyroidism (NSHPT), a severe, sometimes lethal disease if left untreated. Mouse models with disruption of one or both CaSR genes produce biochemical and phenotypic features closely resembling those observed in FHH and NSHPT, respectively. Thus, our increasing understanding of inherited disorders of calcium-sensing, as well as the availability of mouse models with knockout of the receptor have illuminated not only the pathophysiology, but also the physiology of the CaSR in various tissues, as will be discussed in more detail below.

In addition to providing background information on the expression, function, and regulation of the CaSR in general, this chapter will pay particular attention to the known functions of the CaSR in kidney, bone, and blood vessels, and relate this knowledge to current clinical observations and potential clinical implications for patients, especially those with uremia in whom dysregulation of expression of the CaSR in a number of tissues has been clearly documented. In particular, the use of calcimimetics (CaSR activators) in patients with end-stage renal disease may potentially impact the cardiovascular system resulting from their direct actions on the heart and blood vessels in addition to indirect actions mediated, for example, by changes in circulating PTH levels.

Expression, structure, and signaling of the extracellular CaSR

The *CaSR* gene (Fig. 4.1) in humans is located on chromosome 3q21.1 and spans 7 exons. The *CaSR* gene has two promoters, p1 and p2, residing within non-coding

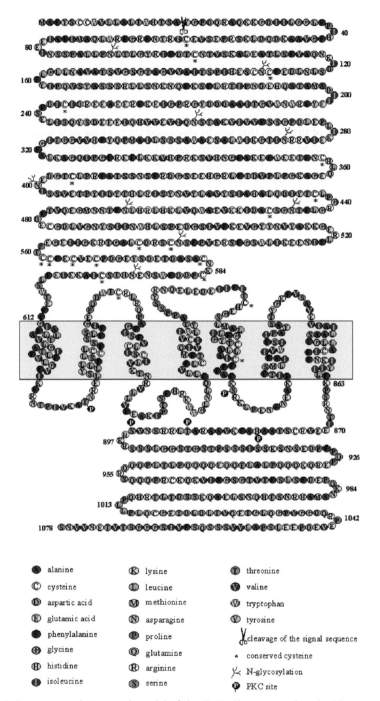

Fig. 4.1 Sequence and structural model of the CaSR. Figure reproduced with permissions from Dr G. N. Hendy. CaSR database. Available at: http://www.casrdb. mcgill.ca/?Topic=CasrGraph

exons 1A and 1B, respectively, which undergo alternative splicing to exon 2, which contains the translational start site of the receptor. Exons 1A and 1B each have a vitamin D response element (VDRE) that positively regulates *CaSR* gene expression in response to binding of the vitamin D-vitamin D receptor (VDR) complex. Expression of the CaSR is greatest in the parathyroid glands, and the calcitonin-secreting C-cells of the thyroid gland and kidney. The CaSR is also found in several other organs not known to be involved in calcium homeostasis, such as the hematopoietic and cardio-vascular systems. Available data have demonstrated that the CaSR participates in Ca^{2+}_o homeostasis not only in the organs that secrete calcium-regulating hormones (e.g. the parathyroid glands and C-cells), but also in target tissues for these hormones, such as the kidney, intestines, and bone. By acting on both hormone-secreting and hormone-responsive tissues, through its own cell surface receptor, Ca^{2+}_o acts, in effect, as another Ca^{2+}_o-regulating 'hormone' (in this case Ca^{2+}_o–lowering) or 'first messenger'.

The human CaSR functions as a homodimer, linked together by two intermolecular disulphide bonds that link the large (612 amino acid residues) extracellular C-terminal domains (ECD) of the two CaSR monomers. In addition to the ECD, the CaSR has a transmembrane domain (TMD) of 250 amino acids containing the 7-membrane spanning helices characteristic of the GPCRs and an intracellular C-terminal domain (ICD) of 216 amino acids. The ECD of each CaSR monomer is predicted to exist as a bi-lobed, so-called Venus fly trap motif (VFTM), with a crevice between the lobes likely participating in ligand binding.

The ECD of the CaSR likely contains more than one binding site for Ca^{2+}_o, because the Hill coefficient (a measure of co-operativity in binding of a ligand to its receptor) for the activation of the receptor by Ca^{2+}_o is 3–4, consistent with the presence of positive co-operativity among at least this number of binding sites within the dimeric CaSR, presumably 2 or more per monomer. The TMD is also apparently involved in Ca^{2+}_o-sensing, since a mutant CaSR lacking the ECD also responds to Ca^{2+}_o and other polyvalent cations.

Extracellular calcium is the prototypical ligand that activates the CaSR, although several other polyvalent cations and polycationic amine ligands, as well as hydropho-bic compounds have been identified that activate, inactivate, or allosterically modu-late the receptor. CaSR agonists are described as type I or type II. Type I agonists are direct agonists, listed here in order of potency $Gd^{3+} \geq La^{3+} >> Ca^{2+} = Ba^{2+} > Sr^{2+} > Mg^{2+}$, while type II agonists serve as allosteric modulators, requiring the presence of calcium in order to stimulate the CaSR. The best characterized type I organic polycationic CaSR agonists are neomycin, spermine, and amyloid β-peptides. The use of newer, more specific approaches, such as pharmacological activators (calcimimetics) or inhibitors (calcylitics) of the receptor, dominant negative constructs or RNA silenc-ing, offer better opportunities for specifying the functional activity of the receptor experimentally.

Agonists of the CaSR activate phospholipases A_2, (PLA_2), D and C, as well as various mitogen-activated protein kinases (MAPK). MAPK activation is involved in high Ca^{2+}_o-induced cell proliferation in rat-1 fibroblasts and other mammalian cell types, including human parathyroid cells, thus supporting the view that the CaSR can modulate both cellular proliferation and hormonal secretion through MAPK activation. The receptor also inhibits adenylate cyclase, either via activation of the inhibitory G protein, $G\alpha_{i/o}$, or by inhibiting adenylate cyclase through a $G\alpha_q$- and PLC-mediated increase in the cytosolic Ca^{2+} concentration Ca^{2+}_i with resultant inhibition of a Ca^{2+}-inhibitable isoform of adenylate cyclase.

The ICD of the CaSR binds directly or indirectly to the scaffolding proteins, filamin-A and caveolin-1; both of these proteins also bind signaling partners activated by the CaSR, such as components of the MAPK pathways. The interaction of the CaSR with filamin-A has been shown to protect the CaSR from intracellular degradation; and calcimimetics have been shown to increase surface expression of the CaSR *in vivo*. These observations may explain why some studies have found that the CaSR exhibits limited internalization following binding to its ligands, presumably an important way of maintaining sustained responsiveness to changes in Ca^{2+}_o in homeostatic tissues, such as the parathyroid and kidney.

CaSR in the kidney

The kidney plays several critical roles in calcium homeostasis. The CaSR is not to any significant extent expressed in the glomerulus but is widely expressed along essentially the whole nephron. The cellular localization and putative function(s) of the CaSR in the kidney varies depending upon the region of the nephron in which the receptor resides (Table 4.1). Expression of CaSR transcripts along the nephron has been studied using *in situ* hybridization, as well as reverse transcriptase-polymerase chain reaction (RT-PCR) of micro-dissected nephron segments.[11] Later, the cellular localization and regional distribution of receptor protein along the nephron was examined using immunofluorescence.[12] One outcome of these studies was the recognition that the polarity of CaSR protein varies along the nephron. In the proximal tubule, the receptor is present on the apical surface of the proximal tubular epithelial cells where it putatively participates in the modulation of calcium reabsorption. On the contrary, in the cells of the cortical thick ascending limb (CTAL), the receptor is localized in the basolateral membrane where it augments the hypercalciuric effect of hypercalcemia. Similarly, predominantly basolateral staining for the CaSR was observed in the medullary thick ascending limb (MTAL), macula densa, and the distal convoluted tubule (DCT) where it participates in the dilution of the hypertonic medullary interstitium in hypercalcemia. In the cortical collecting duct, immunostaining for the CaSR is located on some intercalated cells, while in the inner medullary collecting duct (IMCD) the receptor has primarily an apical distribution. In the lMCD, the CaSR participates in osmotic regulation by regulating the expression of the protein but not the mRNA of the aquaporin-2 channel for water transport.[13] The CaSR is also expressed in juxtaglomerular (JG) cells of the kidney and *in vitro* has been shown to regulate release of renin through inhibition of adenylate cyclase-dependent pathways in isolated mouse JG cells.[14] This direct effect, as well as indirect effects of the CaSR to increase VDR expression through presumably p38 MAPK-dependent pathways in the parathyroid and kidney may synergistically with vitamin D modulate the renin-angiotensin axis, where activation of the VDR with vitamin D agonists has been shown to decrease JG apparatus hypertrophy and renin secretion[15] with potential impacts on vascular smooth muscle and cardiomyocyte function.

Table 4.1 Key definitive and postulated∗ roles of the calcium-sensing receptor in the kidney, bone and cardiovascular system

Kidney

(1) Proximal tubule—blunt PTH-induced phosphaturia

(2) MTAL—inhibit NaCl reabsorption

(3) CTAL—inhibit reabsorption of Ca^{2+} and Mg^{2+}

(4) IMCD—inhibit vasopressin-elicited water reabsorption

Bone∗ (osteoblasts, chondrocytes, osteoclasts, hematopoietic stem cell)

(1) Stimulate chemotaxis and proliferation of preosteoblasts

(2) Increase expression/synthesis of osteoblastic differentiation markers and bone matrix

(3) Promote chondrogenesis in the growth plate and enhance longitudinal bone growth

(4) Modulate formation, activity and apoptosis of osteoclasts

Cardiovascular tissue∗ (endothelium, vascular smooth muscle, and cardiomyocyte)

(1) Modulate production of vasoactive substances by vascular endothelium

(2) Endothelium-independent modulation of vascular smooth muscle tone

(3) Inhibit endothelial cell proliferation

(4) Inhibit medial vascular calcification by direct and/or indirect mechanisms

(5) Modulate cardiomyocyte growth and apoptosis

∗Postulated effects of CaSR activation in kidney, bone, and cardiovascular tissue based on animal and/or human *in vitro* and *ex vivo* data. The term 'modulation' refers to circumstances where definitive statements on the role of the CaSR cannot be made. PTH, parathyroid hormone; MTAL, medullary thick ascending limb; CTAL, cortical thick ascending limb; IMCD, inner medullary collecting duct. See text for details as well as selected references addressing these points that are included in the reference list.

There has been relatively little work characterizing the factors that regulate the CaSR's expression in the kidney. A recent report demonstrated that in rat kidney, C-cell and parathyroid *in vivo*, as well as in a human proximal tubule cell line *in vitro*, transcription of the *CaSR* gene was increased about two-fold following 8 and 12h after treatment with $1,25(OH)_2D_3$, acting via the two promoters in exons 1A and 1B, respectively, which lie upstream of the translational start site of the *CaSR* gene in exon 2.[16] A low phosphate diet had no effect on CaSR expression along the nephron in one study, while Riccardi et al. demonstrated *in vivo* in rats that a low phosphate diet, as well as treatment with PTH, down-regulated CaSR protein in the proximal tubule.[17] Thus, CaSR expression in the proximal tubule of the rat kidney is modulated by $1,25(OH)_2D_3$ and PTH and, perhaps, by dietary phosphate.[18] One other study on the regulation of the CaSR's expression along the nephron demonstrated that the level of CaSR protein in the cTAL, was increased and the level of Na+ transporters decreased in rats rendered hypercalcemic by exogenous PTH administration.[19]

To summarize, the CaSR's roles along the nephron include:

- modulating the effect of PTH on renal calcium and phosphate reabsorption in the proximal tubule;

- inhibiting renal tubular reabsorption of calcium and probably Mg^{2+} and Na^+ in the cTAL;

- inhibiting salt transport in the MTAL as a contributor to the dilution of the hypertonic interstitium in hypercalcemia;

- reducing urinary concentrating ability in the IMCD by antagonizing the action of vasopressin and inhibiting renin secretion from the juxtaglomerular apparatus.

CaSR and bone

Bone is the major sink and store for calcium, and it fulfils essential roles in the maintenance of Ca^{2+}_o within its homeostatic range. The molecular mechanisms that enable bone cells to sense and respond to Ca^{2+}_o are not fully understood, but like the parathyroid cells, bone cells also express the CaSR, and accumulating data indicates that the CaSR is expressed in and regulates the functions of both osteoclasts and osteoblasts (Table 4.1).[3] This is potentially of significance in the osteoblast-like cells that develop from vascular smooth muscle cells in uremic patients as the CaSR may also mediate responses in these osteoblast-like cells in response to Ca^{2+}_o and other agonists of the CaSR.

The first evidence for the existence of a G protein-coupled, cation-sensing mechanism in osteoblasts was presented shortly after the cloning of the CaSR. Since then, some, but not all studies have found that the CaSR is expressed in various osteoblastic cell lines and primary osteoblasts, as well as in sections of intact bone.[3] Studies *in vitro* have indicated that the receptor may stimulate the chemotaxis and proliferation of preosteoblasts, increase expression of osteoblastic differentiation markers and bone matrix (e.g. osteocalcin, alkaline phosphatase and type 1 collagen), and increase the mineralization of bone nodules *in vitro*. The most definitive data thus far for the importance of the CaSR in osteoblast function has come from studies of mice with conditional knockout of exon 7 (encoding the entire transmembrane domain and C-tail) in osteoblasts.[20] These mice were runted with a severe mineralization defect, documenting that the CaSR in the osteoblast is essential for the mineralization and growth of bone in normal mice. One study demonstrated that osteoblasts from CaSR knock-out mice still had a promitogenic response to Ca^{2+}_o, supporting the presence of a calcium-sensing mechanism other than the full length CaSR. The latter could potentially be accounted for by GPRC6A, although the latter is responsive to calcimimetics, and the actions of extracellular calcium on the CaSR knockout osteoblasts were not.[21] Furthermore, these latter studies were carried out with mice in which the CaSR was knocked out by disruption of exon 5. These mice produce a shortened, alternatively spliced CaSR lacking exon 5 in some tissues. This exon-5-less CaSR apparently 'rescues' osteoblast function, given the severe bone phenotype of mice with osteoblast-specific CaSR KO compared with the relatively normal bones of mice with homozygous KO of exon 5 of the CaSR combined with KO of the *PTH* gene or the parathyroid glands (to obviate the lethal hyperparathyroidism in mice with KO only of exon 5 of the CaSR).

The CaSR is also present in articular and hypertrophic chondrocytes. Utilising a type II CaSR agonist in organ culture (fetal rat metatarsal bones) to study the possible role of the CaR in bone growth, Wu et al.[22] demonstrated that the receptor modulates chondrogenesis in the growth plate and enhances longitudinal bone growth. In addition, recent studies have shown the presence of embryonic lethality in mice in which exon 7 of the CaR was conditionally knocked out in chondrocytes, suggested a critical role for the receptor in cartilage development.

Regarding the signaling mechanism(s) utilized by the CaSR in osteoblasts, available data are equivocal regarding the involvement of the PLC pathway, a prominent signal transduction pathway in parathyroid and kidney. Whereas one report showed activation of PLC, another failed to shown such an effect. In MC3T3-E1 cells, elevated Ca^{2+}_o and other type I calcimimetics activated the p42/44 MAPK and p38 MAP kinase pathways. In rat primary osteoblasts, CaSR-stimulated proliferation is mediated via a JNK pathway.

The CaSR is expressed by some, but not all osteoclasts, and at higher levels in some species (e.g. rabbit) than in others (i.e. human, bovine, and rat), as well as by monocytes, which are of the same lineage as osteoclast precursors. The CaSR appears to be permissive for the formation of osteoclasts in some systems (Mentaverri), while in others, at higher concentrations of Ca^{2+}_o, it inhibits both the formation and activity of osteoclasts.[23] Very high levels of extracellular calcium (e.g. 10–20mM) have been shown to promote osteoclast apoptosis, a known downstream feature of the osteoclastic phase of the bone remodelling cycle that plays a key role in the regulation of bone resorption. It should be pointed out, however, that while these levels of Ca^{2+}_o may seem unphysiologically high, they may be similar to those encountered by osteoclast at resorptive surfaces of the bone. The signaling pathways associated with CaSR-induced osteoclast apoptosis likely include PLC and NF-κB. However, the calcimimetic, AMG 073, produced none of the actions of elevated extracellular calcium on osteoblast proliferation, or osteoclast formation and resorption in one study. Another possible mechanism that has been suggested to mediate calcium-sensing in osteoclasts is a plasma membrane, ryanodine-like receptor that couples to increases in the intracellular calcium concentration. Therefore, although the CaSR and other calcium-sensing mechanisms may participate in the regulation of bone cell and cartilage function, further studies are clearly required to clarify the divergent results observed in the studies to date.

The bone marrow compartment has gained increasing recognition not only as an environment for osteoblast–osteoclast interaction with implications for bone-mineral homeostasis, but also as an essential environment that is a prerequisite for normal medullary hematopoiesis following investigations in the nascent, but rapidly maturing field of osteoimmunology. A characteristic of the endosteal surface of the bone, where active bone modeling and remodeling take place, and which is thought to serve as a niche for hematopoietic stem cells, is an increased Ca^{2+}_o concentration, which reaches 40mM near resorbing osteoclasts, a level that is about 33-fold more than serum calcium levels. The CaSR could be a sensor of this unusual micro-environment and, indeed, CaSR expression has been shown on hematopoietic cells, including cells of the monocyte/macrophage lineage. CaSR activation of these cells induces their transmigration *in vitro* and *in vivo*, and a recent report by Adams et al. revealed that neonatal mice lacking the *CaSR* gene had hematopoietic stem cells in the circulation and spleen, whereas a lower than normal number of these cells were found in bone marrow.[24] In addition, bone marrow of CaSR deficient (CaSR–/–) mice exhibited hypocellularity and there was expanded extramedullary hematopoiesis. HSCs obtained from CaSR–/– mice exhibited chemotaxis in response to stromal-derived growth factor-1 (SDF-1) that was comparable to that observed with HSCs from CaSR +/+ mice. However, CaSR–/– HSCs cells were unable to engraft efficiently within the endosteal HSC niche. This defect could be due to the reduced capacity of the CaSR–/– HSCs to adhere to collagen I, which is the most abundant bone matrix protein produced by osteoblasts. Therefore, the CaSR could importantly participate in maintaining HSCs within their niche in the bone marrow and thereby modulate hematopoiesis. There is apparently a close relationship between bone physiology involving the endosteum and hematopoiesis under normal conditions. In view of the altered modeling invariably found in renal osteodystrophy and the effect of the CaSR on HSC engraftment, the CaSR may potentially have an impact in medullary hematopoiesis in this setting and may, therefore, participate in the multifactorial anemia and relative resistance to erythropoietin stimulating agents seen in uremic patients.

The CaSR and blood vessels

Cardiovascular disease is a major cause of morbidity and mortality in patients with kidney impairment through pathological processes that involve the endothelium, vascular smooth muscle, and cardiomyocytes. These pathological processes often manifest as increased vascular smooth muscle tone, atherosclerotic change, intimal and medial calcification, cardiomyocyte hypertrophy, and increased apoptosis of cardiomyocytes to ischemia reperfusion injury, as is commonly seen in ischemic cardiomyopathy. Excessive PTH levels in patients with primary or secondary hyperparathyroidism have been associated with permissive effects on elevating blood pressure, and promoting cardiac fibrosis, micro-vessel disease, and dyslipidemia. However, direct effects of the CaSR, independent of its regulatory effect on PTH secretion are recently being recognized as participating in the pathogenesis of cardiovascular pathology with potential implications for therapeutic manipulation of the CaSR in cardiovascular disease.

Several investigators have shown that the CaSR is expressed in rodent and human vascular endothelium, vascular smooth muscle and cardiomyocytes using a variety of techniques (Table 4.1). One of the earliest reports of expression of the CaSR in VSMCs was made by Wonneberger and colleagues, where CaSR mRNA was identified using RT-PCR in the gerbil spiral modiolar artery, producing the expected 448bp product (confirmed to be derived from the CaSR by sequencing) that was identical to that obtained from gerbil kidney.[25] RT-PCR and immunohistochemistry (IHC) were utilized by Smajilovic and colleagues to confirm the expression of CaSR transcript and protein in rat aortic VSMCs.[26] Since then other investigators have identified the CaSR in rat mesenteric and porcine coronary arteries,[27,28] human endothelial and VSMCs,[29,30] and rat cardiomyocytes[31] using combinations of RT-PCR, IHC, western blotting or CaSR-specific functional assays. Interestingly, the difficulty encountered by some investigators in identifying the CaSR in vascular tissues appears to be dependent on the species, biological milieu or physiological state of the tissue, with smaller/

undetectable amounts found in animals subjected to burns, or in calcified tissues, or those derived from osteogenic/uremic environments.[29,32] These observations suggest potential roles for the CaSR in these situations. The CaSR has also been shown to be expressed by macrophages, a key player in the active cellular process of atherosclerosis and vascular calcification.[33] Of note, the function of monocytes and the level of CaSR expression in these cells have been shown to be increased not only by inflammatory cytokines (e.g. IL-6, IL-1β), which are known to be relevant in atherosclerosis and vascular calcification, but also by ambient extracellular calcium concentrations, which are increased in inflamed and calcified vascular tissue.[34] As a follow-up to these observations, an impressive body of *in vitro* evidence has been generated, making plausible a causal relationship between CaSR function, and modulation of vascular tone, calcification, and atherosclerotic change. Exciting *in vivo* evidence is also accumulating through the use of systemic CaSR specific agonists and antagonists on the role of the CaSR in vascular function, but is confounded by concomitant changes in PTH, which are known to have direct effects on vascular function as well.

While there is no clinical evidence in humans for an effect of calcimimetics on blood pressure, there is a growing body of evidence supporting a potential role of the CaSR in regulating vascular smooth muscle tone in other mammals by modulating endothelial function through nitric oxide-dependent pathways.[35] Recent evidence suggests that the CaSR agonist, spermine, induces production of nitric oxide in aortic endothelial cells, which was abrogated by CaSR knockdown.[36] Endothelium-independent mechanisms of VSMC relaxation mediated by peripheral sensory nerves expressing the CaSR have also been shown to occur *in vitro* through phospholipids-dependent pathways.[37] In human aortic endothelial cells, an alternatively spliced variant of the CaSR has been noted to respond to polycationic amines and not to Ca^{2+}. The effects of the CaSR on vascular smooth muscle tone appear to depend on the experimental conditions (*in vitro* or *in vivo* experimentation), as acute administration of a calcimimetic was associated *in vivo* with an increase of mean arterial pressures (MAP), and probably related to splanchnic and limb vasoconstriction in uremic and non-uremic rats that was abrogated by ganglionic blockade.[38] However, *in vitro*, pre-contracted rat subcutaneous small arteries responded by dilatation (and, by extension, possibly a decrease in peripheral vascular resistance) to CaSR activation using a number of known CaSR agonists.[28] In parathyroid-intact animals, calcilytic administration, in addition to increasing PTH levels, increased MAP, a response that was abrogated by thyroparathyroidectomy.[33] Further studies by the same group using calcimimetics demonstrated a hypotensive effect of CaSR activation.

Rybczynska and colleagues, in addition to highlighting the confounding effects of PTH in these studies of CaSR activation on vascular tone, suggest hypotheses on the possible role of parathyroid hypertensive factor. This is an incompletely defined peptide produced by the parathyroid gland in spontaneously hypertensive rats and in 30–40% of hypertensive patients; its secretion appears to be regulated by vitamin D and possibly by the CaSR.[39] A recent study by Nakagawa et al. in rats using the active (R-) form of the calcimimetic NPS-568 and its inactive enantiomer, NPS S-568, demonstrated that at rates of infusion capable of inhibiting PTH secretion, no acute effects on blood pressure or heart rate were seen for either NPS R- or NPS S-568. However, at a 3-fold higher rate of infusion, both enantiomers lowered MAP and heart rate suggesting that NPS R-568, through CaSR-independent mechanisms, exerts a vasodilatory and negative chronotropic effect at concentrations higher than those needed to lower PTH secretion. These observations may explain the relative lack of efficacy on cardiovascular outcomes in human populations treated with Cinacalcet where it is primarily used at doses just sufficient to inhibit PTH secretion. Their observations also raise questions about the relative sensitivity of CaSR-expressing tissues to effects of calcimimetics that may be explained by the higher receptor expression density in the parathyroid compared with vascular tissues or tissue-specific signaling pathways.

An inhibitory effect of the CaSR on aortic endothelial cell proliferation in uremic rats has also been observed[38] complementing potential effects of the CaSR in regulating the well known macrophage-mediated intimal proliferation.[40] Ivanovski et al. used calcimimetics in uremic apoE knockout mice to show that CaSR activation reduced not only aortic plaque and non-plaque calcification compared with calcitriol or vehicle, but decreased atherosclerotic plaque area—an effect that was abolished in CaSR-SiRNA transfected cells. These observations suggest potential CaSR-based therapeutic interventions in atherosclerosis based on known effects of the CaSR in modulating monocyte function and the role of these cells in atherosclerosis.[41]

Medial vascular calcification, and its effects on vascular compliance and coronary perfusion pressures have also come to the forefront of investigation of the pathogenesis of cardiovascular disease in patients with kidney disease. The expression of the CaSR in VSMCs, known effects of the CaSR and VDR on each other's expression, known effects of agonists of the VDR on expression of promoters and inhibitors of vascular calcification *in vitro* and in *in vivo* animal models provide the rationale for the proposed role of the CaSR in vascular calcification.[42] Matrix Gla protein is a well recognized player in VSMC calcification responses in uremic conditions and has also been shown in *in vitro* models to be regulated by a mechanism functionally related to the CaSR.[43] Recent *in vitro* studies, using calcimimetics, mineralizing medium and calcified or non-calcified human blood vessels, support the role of the CaSR in medial calcification and highlight the potential therapeutic application of calcimimetics in retarding vascular calcification.[44] Lopez and colleagues showed that the co-administration of a calcimimetic (AMG 641) with calcitriol or paricalcitol reduced soft tissue calcification,[45] but studies by Henley et al. found that co-administration of calcitriol with Cinacalcet did not reduce aortic calcification.[46] The differences between these two studies appear to lie in the doses of vitamin D given, suggesting that the ability of CaSR modulation to impact phenotypical changes associated with VDR activation are dose-dependent.

A potential role for the CaSR in cardiomyocyte function has become known only recently and *in vitro* investigations have shown that the receptor is involved in apoptosis and hypertrophy of the cardiomyocyte through angiotensin II and calcineurin dependent pathways under ischemia/reperfusion conditions that are a hallmark of ischemic cardiomyopathy. The receptor, on the other hand, in other *in vitro* studies under defined conditions of ischemic pre-conditioning has been shown to protect against ischemia/reperfusion injury. These observations *in vitro*[47] are contradictory and the operational conditions that may lend themselves to therapeutic manipulation *in vivo* are yet to be identified.

Over the past few years, these basic and clinical studies have spurred efforts at translating these laboratory observations to clinical benefit for patients by therapeutic interventional trials and observational studies in the CKD and general population. The largest of these clinical efforts was reported by Cunningham and colleagues,[41] where they undertook a *post hoc* analysis of safety data from large double-blind, placebo-controlled randomized clinical trials of the calcimimetic Cinacalcet HCl in dialysis patients. This analysis showed that there was not only a decrease in risk for parathyroidectomy and fracture, but a significant decrease in the risk of cardiovascular hospitalizations in the treatment versus placebo groups. This has lead to the initiation of the Evaluation of Cinacalcet HCl therapy to Lower Cardiovascular Events (EVOLVE) trial, an ongoing large prospective trial in ~4000 patients with end-stage renal disease, specifically designed to address cardiovascular outcomes in the dialysis population. In a similar vein the 'ADVANCE' trial is an ongoing open-label randomized parallel arm trial, evaluating the effects of Cinacalcet HCl and low dose vitamin D on the progression of coronary artery calcification in about 400 patients with end-stage renal disease.

Finally, other clinical efforts recognizing a potential role of the CaSR in cardiovascular disease have focused on observational studies of the effects of single nucleotide polymorphisms (SNP's) on cardiovascular outcomes that could potentially guide individualized therapeutic interventions. Some of these observational association studies have suggested that:

- differences exist in 24-h ambulatory systolic and diastolic blood pressure readings for specific SNP's of the CaSR;[43]

- the A986S polymorphism of the CaSR may be an independent genetic predictor of angiographic coronary artery disease, previous myocardial infarction and cardiovascular mortality;[44]

- there is no difference in urinary sodium excretion as an explanation for the increased prevalence of hypertension in black vs. white cohorts in the general population for three of the most common allelic variant of the CaSR.[48]

At the present time, there is no confirmatory evidence that SNPs of the CaSR are directly disease-causing,[10] but there is the possibility that they may be associated with increased risk for disease and any conclusions that SNP's are independent predictors of the often complex polygenic phenotypes of cardiovascular disease will require more extensive investigation.

Summary

The CaSR is expressed not only in the parathyroid gland, kidney, and bone, where it is primarily involved in calcium homeostasis, but also in a number of tissues including the cardiovascular system not known to participate in calcium homeostasis. In these 'traditional' and 'non-traditional' tissues, the CaSR regulates a number of newly identified cellular processes ranging from modulation of water channels in the kidney, to vascular smooth muscle relaxation and calcification, endothelial proliferation, and apoptosis in several cell types including cardiomyocytes. The relative sensitivities of these tissues to CaSR agonism or antagonism may, in part, be related to tissue receptor density, expression in physiologically protected sites, and cell-specific signaling pathways that explain, at least in part, why any dose of a CaSR agonist or antagonist may have effects of varying magnitude in the growing number of potential target tissues. These findings have refined the definition of 'on' and 'off' target effects of agonists and antagonists of the CaSR, and provide the basis for exciting hypotheses that are already in the various stages of clinical translation from the bench to the bedside.

References

1. Tfelt-Hansen J, Brown EM. The calcium-sensing receptor in normal physiology and pathophysiology: a review. *Crit Rev Clin Lab Sci* 2005;**42**:35–70.

2. Fudge NJ, Kovacs CS. Physiological studies in heterozygous calcium sensing receptor (CaSR) gene-ablated mice confirm that the CaSR regulates calcitonin release *in vivo*. *Br Med Council Physiol* 2004;**4**:5.

3. Sharan K, Siddiqui JA, Swarnkar G, Chattopadhyay N. Role of calcium-sensing receptor in bone biology. *Ind J Med Res* 2008;**127**(3):274–86.

4. Kirchhoff P, Geibel JP. Role of calcium and other trace elements in the gastrointestinal physiology. *World J Gastroenterol* 2006;**12**:3229–36.

5. Al-Aly Z. The new role of calcimimetics as vasculotropic agents. *Kidney Int* 2009;**75**:9–12.

6. Brown EM, Gamba G, Riccardi D, et al. Cloning and characterisation of an extracellular Ca(2+)-sensing receptor from bovine parathyroid. *Nature* 1993;**366**(6455):575–80.

7. Wellendorph P, Hansen KB, Balsgaard A, Greenwood JR, Egebjerg J, Brauner-Osborne H. Deorphanisation of GPRC6A: a promiscuous L-alpha-amino acid receptor with preference for basic amino acids. *Mol Pharmacol* 2005;**67**:589–97.

8. Pi M, Chen L, Huang MZ, et al. GPRC6A null mice exhibit osteopenia, feminisation and metabolic syndrome. *PLoS ONE* 2008;**3**(12):e3858.

9. Wellendorph P, Johansen LD, Jensen AA, et al. No evidence for a bone phenotype in GPRC6A knockout mice under normal physiological conditions. *J Mol Endocrinol* 2009;**42**(3):215–23.

10. Egbuna OI, Brown EM. Hypercalcemic and hypocalcemic conditions due to calcium-sensing receptor mutations. *Best Pract Res Clin Rheumatol* 2008;**22**: 129–48.

11. Riccardi D, Lee WS, Lee K, Segre GV, Brown EM, Hebert SC. Localisation of the extracellular Ca(2+)-sensing receptor and PTH/PTHrP receptor in rat kidney. *Am J Physiol* 1996;**271**(4 Pt 2):F951-6.

12. Riccardi D, Hall AE, Chattopadhyay N, Xu JZ, Brown EM, Hebert SC. Localisation of the extracellular Ca2+/polyvalent cation-sensing protein in rat kidney. *Am J Physiol* 1998;**274**(3 Pt 2):F611–22.

13. Sands JM, Flores FX, Kato A, et al. Vasopressin-elicited water and urea permeabilities are altered in IMCD in hypercalcemic rats. *Am J Physiol* 1998;**274**(5 Pt 2):F978–85.

14. Ortiz-Capisano MC, Ortiz PA, Garvin JL, Harding P, Beierwaltes WH. Expression and function of the calcium-sensing receptor in juxtaglomerular cells. *Hypertension* 2007;**50**:737–43.

15. Li YC, Kong J, Wei M, Chen ZF, Liu SQ, Cao LP. 1,25-Dihydroxyvitamin D(3) is a negative endocrine regulator of the renin-angiotensin system. *J Clin Invest* 2002;**110**: 229–38.

16. Canaff L, Hendy GN. Human calcium-sensing receptor gene. Vitamin D response elements in promoters P1 and P2 confer transcriptional responsiveness to 1,25-dihydroxyvitamin D. *J Biol Chem* (2002);**277**:30337–50.

17. Sands JM, Naruse M, Baum M, et al. Apical extracellular calcium/polyvalent cation-sensing receptor regulates vasopressin-elicited water permeability in rat kidney inner medullary collecting duct. *J Clin Invest* 1997;**99**:1399–405.

18. Riccardi D, Traebert M, Ward DT, et al. Dietary phosphate and parathyroid hormone alter the expression of the calcium-sensing receptor (CaR) and the Na+-dependent Pi transporter (NaPi-2) in the rat proximal tubule. *Pflügers Arch* 2000;**441**:379–87.

19. Wang W, Li C, Kwon TH, et al. Reduced expression of renal Na+ transporters in rats with PTH-induced hypercalcemia. *Am J Physiol Renal Physiol* 2004;**286**:F534–45.

20. Chang W, Tu C, Chen TH, Bikle D, Shoback D. The extracellular calcium-sensing receptor (CaSR) is a critical modulator of skeletal development. *Sci Signal* 2008;**1**(35):ra1.

21. Kanatani M, Sugimoto T, Kanzawa M, Yano S, Chihara K. High extracellular calcium inhibits osteoclast-like cell formation by directly acting on the calcium-sensing receptor existing in osteoclast precursor cells. *Biochem Biophys Res Commun* 1999;**261**:144–8.

22. Wu S, Palese T, Mishra OP, Delivoria-Papadopoulos M, De Luca F. Effects of Ca2+ sensing receptor activation in the growth plate. *FASEB J* 2004;**18**:143–5.

23. Mentaverri R, Yano S, Chattopadhyay N, et al. The calcium sensing receptor is directly involved in both osteoclast differentiation and apoptosis. *FASEB J* 2006;**20**:2562–4.

24. Adams GB, Chabner KT, Alley IR, et al. Stem cell engraftment at the endosteal niche is specified by the calcium-sensing receptor. *Nature* 2006;**439**(7076):599–603.

25. Wonneberger K, Scofield MA, Wangemann P. Evidence for a calcium-sensing receptor in the vascular smooth muscle cells of the spiral modiolar artery. *J Membr Biol* 2000;**175**(3):203–12.

26. Smajilovic S, Hansen JL, Christoffersen TE, et al. Extracellular calcium sensing in rat aortic vascular smooth muscle cells. *Biochem Biophys Res Commun* 2006;**348**:1215–23.

27. Weston AH, Absi M, Ward DT, et al. Evidence in favor of a calcium-sensing receptor in arterial endothelial cells: studies with calindol and Calhex 231. *Circ Res* 2005;**97**(4):391–8.

28. Ohanian J, Gatfield KM, Ward DT, Ohanian V. Evidence for a functional calcium-sensing receptor that modulates myogenic tone in rat subcutaneous small arteries. *Am J Physiol Heart Circ Physiol* 2005;**288**(4):H1756–62.

29. Alam MU, Kirton JP, Wilkinson FL, et al. Calcification is associated with loss of functional calcium-sensing receptor in vascular smooth muscle cells. *Cardiovasc Res* 2009;**81**:260–8.

30. Berra Romani R, Raqeeb A, Laforenza U, et al. Cardiac microvascular endothelial cells express a functional Ca+ -sensing receptor. *J Vasc Res* 2009;**46**:73–82.

31. Zhang WC, Zhang WH, Wu B, Zhao YJ, Li QF, Xu CQ. [The role of calcium-sensing receptor on ischemia/reperfusion-induced rat cardiomyocyte apoptosis]. *Zhonghua Xin Xue Guan Bing Za Zhi* 2007;**35**(8):740–4.

32. Klein GL, Enkhbaatar P, Traber DL, et al. Cardiovascular distribution of the calcium sensing receptor before and after burns. *Burns* 2008;**34**:370–5.

33. Malecki R, Adamiec R. [The role of calcium ions in the pathomechanism of the artery calcification accompanying atherosclerosis]. *Postepy Hig Med Dosw* 2005;**59**:42–7 (online).

34. Olszak IT, Poznansky MC, Evans RH, et al. Extracellular calcium elicits a chemokinetic response from monocytes *in* vitro and in vivo. *J Clin Invest* 2000;**105**:1299–305.

35. Rybczynska A, Lehmann A, Jurska-Jasko A, et al. Hypertensive effect of calcilytic NPS 2143 administration in rats. *J Endocrinol* 2006;**191**:189–95.

36. Ziegelstein RC, Xiong Y, He C, Hu Q. Expression of a functional extracellular calcium-sensing receptor in human aortic endothelial cells. *Biochem Biophys Res Commun* 2006;**342**:153–63.

37. Rybczynska A, Boblewski K, Lehmann A, et al. Calcimimetic NPS R-568 induces hypotensive effect in spontaneously hypertensive rats. *Am J Hypertens* 2005;**18**:364–71.

38. Koleganova N, Piecha G, Ritz E, Schmitt CP, Gross ML. A calcimimetic (R-568), but not calcitriol, prevents vascular remodelling in uremia. *Kidney Int* 2009;**75**:60–71.

39. Farzaneh-Far A, Proudfoot D, Weissberg PL, Shanahan CM. Matrix Gla protein is regulated by a mechanism functionally related to the calcium-sensing receptor. *Biochem Biophys Res Commun* 2000;**277**:736–40.

40. Takahashi K, Takeya M, Sakashita N. Multifunctional roles of macrophages in the development and progression of atherosclerosis in humans and experimental animals. *Med Electron Microsc* 2002;**35**(4)**:**179–203.

41. Cunningham J, Danese M, Olson K, Klassen P, Chertow GM. Effects of the calcimimetic cinacalcet HCl on cardiovascular disease, fracture, and health-related quality of life in secondary hyperparathyroidism. *Kidney Int* 2005;**68**:1793–800.

42. Chertow GM, Pupim LB, Block GA, et al. Evaluation of Cinacalcet Therapy to Lower Cardiovascular Events (EVOLVE): rationale and design overview. *Clin J Am Soc Nephrol* 2007;**2**:898–905.

43. Tobin MD, Tomaszewski M, Braund PS, et al. Common variants in genes underlying monogenic hypertension and hypotension and blood pressure in the general population. *Hypertension* 2008;**51**:1658–64.

44. Marz W, Seelhorst U, Wellnitz B, et al. Alanine to serine polymorphism at position 986 of the calcium-sensing receptor associated with coronary heart disease, myocardial infarction, all-cause, and cardiovascular mortality. *J Clin Endocrinol Metab* 2007;**92:** 2363–9.

45. Lopez I, Mendoza FJ, Aguilera-Tejero E, et al. The effect of calcitriol, paricalcitol, and a calcimimetic on extraosseous calcifications in uremic rats. *Kidney Int* 2008;**73**:300–7.

46. Henley C, Colloton M, Cattley RC, et al. 1,25-Dihydroxyvitamin D3 but not cinacalcet HCl (Sensipar/Mimpara) treatment mediates aortic calcification in a rat model of secondary hyperparathyroidism. *Nephrol Dial Transplant* 2005;**20**:1370–7.

47. Zhang W, Xu C. Calcium sensing receptor and heart diseases. *Pathophysiology* 2009.

48. Pratt JH, Ambrosius WT, Wagner MA, Maharry K. Molecular variations in the calcium-sensing receptor in relation to sodium balance and presence of hypertension in blacks and whites. *Am J Hypertens* 2000;**13**(6 Pt 1):654–8.

Chapter 5

Regulation of parathyroid hormone biosynthesis and gene expression

Tally Naveh-Many and Justin Silver

Introduction

Parathyroid hormone (PTH) is at the centre of the intricate hormonal and cellular responses to changes in mineral metabolism. The parathyroid senses small changes in serum calcium to alter PTH secretion, which then binds to its receptor in its target tissues, the bone, and kidney to correct serum calcium. The parathyroid responds to changes in calcium, phosphate (Pi), $1,25(OH)_2$ vitamin D (1,25D), and fibroblast growth factor 23 (FGF23). Parathyroid cells have few secretory granules as compared with other endocrine cells and, therefore, PTH production is regulated largely at the levels of *PTH* gene expression and parathyroid cell proliferation. In this chapter we discuss the mechanisms of how 1,25D, calcium, Pi, and FGF23 regulate *PTH* gene expression.

Regulation of PTH expression by $1,25(OH)_2$ vitamin D

1,25D has independent effects on calcium and phosphate levels and also participates in a well-defined feedback loop between 1,25D and PTH. PTH increases the renal synthesis of 1,25D, which then increases blood calcium largely by increasing the efficiency of intestinal calcium absorption. 1,25D also potently decreases transcription of the *PTH* gene. This action was first demonstrated *in vitro* in bovine parathyroid cells in primary culture, where 1,25D led to a marked decrease in PTH mRNA levels and a consequent decrease in PTH secretion.[1] The physiological relevance of these findings was established by *in vivo* studies in rats.[2] The expression of 1,25D receptor (vitamin D receptor, VDR) mRNA in the parathyroid was demonstrated by *in situ* hybridization.[3] Rats injected with amounts of 1,25D that did not increase serum calcium had marked decreases in PTH mRNA levels, reaching <4% of control at 48 h. This effect was shown to be transcriptional both in *in vivo* studies in rats[2] and in *in vitro* studies with primary cultures of bovine parathyroid cells.[4]

A further level at which 1,25D might regulate the PTH gene would be at the level of the VDR. 1,25D in physiologically relevant doses led to an increase in VDR mRNA levels in the parathyroid glands in contrast to the decrease in PTH mRNA levels.[3] 1,25D may also amplify its effect on the parathyroid by increasing the activity of the calcium receptor (CaR). There are vitamin D response elements (VDREs) in the human CaR promoter. Functional VDREs in the CaR gene probably provide the mechanism whereby 1,25D up-regulates parathyroid CaR expression.[5] Extracellular calcium increases parathyroid VDR mRNA *in vitro* suggesting that activation of the CaR up regulates the parathyroid VDR mRNA.[7]

Weanling rats fed a diet deficient in calcium were markedly hypocalcemic at 3 weeks and had very high serum 1,25D levels. Despite the chronically high serum 1,25D levels, PTH mRNA levels did not fall and were increased markedly.[6] The lack of suppression of PTH synthesis in the setting of hypocalcemia and increased serum 1,25D is relevant physiologically because it allows an increase in both PTH and 1,25D at a time of chronic hypocalcemic stress.

The action of 1,25D to decrease serum PTH is used therapeutically in the management of patients with CKD. They are treated with 1,25D or its prodrug $1\alpha(OH)$-vitamin D_3 in order to treat or prevent the secondary hyperparathyroidism of CKD. The poor response in some patients who do not respond may well result from poor control of serum Pi, decreased VDR concentration in the patients' parathyroids,[8] an inhibitory effect of a uremic toxin(s) on VDR-VDRE binding,[9] or tertiary hyperparathyroidism with monoclonal parathyroid tumors.[10]

PTH promoter sequences

Regions upstream of the transcribed structural gene often determine tissue specificity and contain many of the regulatory sequences for the gene. For PTH, analysis of this region has been hampered by the lack of a parathyroid cell line. 5kb of DNA upstream of the start site of the human *PTH* gene was able to direct parathyroid gland-specific expression in transgenic mice.[11] The human PTH promoter region has a number of consensus sequences.[12] These include a sequence resembling the canonical cAMP-responsive element 5'-TGACGTCA-3' at position -81 with a single residue deviation. Specificity protein (Sp) and the nuclear factor-Y (NF-Y) complex are ubiquitously expressed transcription factors which co-operatively enhance transcription of target genes. There is a highly conserved Sp1 DNA element present in mammalian PTH promoters.[13] Co-expression of Sp proteins and NF-Y complex lead to synergistic transactivation of the hPTH promoter, with alignment of the Sp1 DNA element essential for full activation.[13]

Several groups have identified DNA sequences that might mediate the negative regulation of *PTH* gene transcription by 1,25D. When 684 bp of the 5'-flanking region of the human *PTH* gene was linked to a reporter gene and transfected into a rat pituitary cell line (GH4C1), gene expression was lowered by 1,25D.[14] Specific DNA sequences in the human *PTH* gene bind the VDR. There are two negative (n) VDREs in the rat PTH gene.[15] One is situated at −793 to −779 and bound a VDR/RXR heterodimer with high affinity, and the other at −760 to −746 bound the heterodimer with a lower affinity. Transfection studies with VDRE-CAT constructs showed that they had an additive effect. The chicken *PTH* gene VREs have been demonstrated and their functionality studied.[16] Selective mutations in the VDRE converted the negative activity imparted by the PTH VDRE to a positive transcriptional response. Further work is needed to demonstrate the function of the VDREs in parathyroid cells.

The transrepression by 1,25D has also been shown to be dependent upon another promoter element. An E-box (CANNTG)-like motif as another class of negative VDRE in the human 1α(OH)ase promoter has been identified.[17,18] A basic helix-loop-helix factor, designated VDR interacting repressor (VDIR), transactivates through direct binding to this E-box-type element (1αnVDRE). The functions of VDIR and E-box motifs in the human (h) PTH and *hPTHrP* gene promoters were characterized.[19] E-box-type elements acting as nVDREs in both the hPTH promoter (hPTHnVDRE; −87 to −60 bp) and in the hPTHrP promoter (hPTHrPnVDRE; −850 to −600 bp; −463 to −104 bp) in a mouse renal tubule cell line were described. These studies were specific to a mouse proximal tubule cell line and await the development of a parathyroid cell line to confirm them in a homologous cell system.

Post-transcriptional regulation of *PTH* gene expression by calcium, phosphate, and CKD

In contrast to the transcriptional effect of 1,25D on *PTH* gene expression,[2] the regulation of *PTH* gene expression by hypocalcemia, hypophosphatemia, and CKD is post-transcriptional. This regulation of PTH mRNA stability is mediated by protein-PTH mRNA interactions that determine the susceptibility of PTH mRNA to the degradation machinery. The balanced interaction of stabilizing and destabilizing proteins with the PTH mRNA determines PTH stability, PTH mRNA levels, serum PTH levels, and the resultant response of the parathyroid to hypocalcemia, hypophosphatemia, and CKD.

Structure of the PTH mRNA

PTH mRNAs are typical eukaryotic mRNAs that contain a 7-methylguanosine cap at the 5' terminus and a polyadenylic acid (poly A) stretch at the 3' terminus. The PTH mRNA consists of three exons coding for the 5'-UTR (exon I), the prepro region (exon II) and the structural PTH hormone, together with the 3'-UTR (exon III). The PTH mRNAs are twice as long as necessary to code for the primary translational product, due to 5' and 3' untranslated regions (UTRs) at both ends of the mRNA (Fig. 5.1). All PTH mRNA 3'-UTRs have a particularly large portion of A and U nucleotides, ranging from 68 to 74% of the nucleotides.[20,21] Interestingly, a 26 nucleotide *cis*-acting functional protein binding element at the distal region of the 3'-UTR is highly conserved in the PTH mRNA 3'-UTRs of rat, mouse, man, dog, and cat. The identity amongst species varies between 73 and 89%. In particular, there is a stretch of 14 nucleotides within the element that is present in all these species[22] (Fig. 5.1). This 26-nucleotide (26nt) element in the rat PTH mRNA 3'-UTR is a *cis*-acting sequence that determines PTH mRNA stability and its regulation by calcium, Pi and CKD (see below).[22] In addition, a 22 nucleotide proximal protein binding element in the 3' UTR was identified in bovine and porcine, as well as man, non-human primates, horse, dog, and cat, but not in rat and mouse PTH mRNAs.[21,23] The functionality of the proximal element remains to be determined. The conservation of sequences within the non-coding 3'-UTRs suggests that the binding element represents a functional unit that has been evolutionarily conserved.

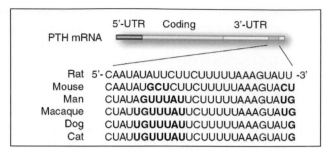

Fig. 5.1 Schematic representation of the PTH mRNA and the pressserved *cis* acting element in the PTH mRNA 3'-untranslated region (UTR). PTH mRNA including the 5'-UTR (red), coding region (orange) and the 3'-UTR (white) are shown with the 26 nucleotide *cis* acting element (green). The nucleotide sequence of the element in different species is shown. Nucleotides that differ from the rat sequence are in bold. Reproduced with permission of *Kidney International*.[65]

Regulation of PTH mRNA stability by calcium, phosphate, and CKD

Dietary induced hypocalcemia markedly increases PTH secretion, mRNA levels and after prolonged stimulation, parathyroid cell proliferation.[24,25] In the rat, hypocalcemia leads to a >10-fold increase in PTH mRNA levels and this increase in PTH mRNA levels is post-transcriptional affecting mRNA stability.[24,26] Serum Pi in turn, has a direct effect on PTH secretion, PTH mRNA levels and parathyroid cell proliferation.[25,26] Careful *in vivo* studies showed that the regulation of *PTH* gene expression by hypophosphatemia is independent of changes in serum calcium and 1,25D.[26] *In vitro* studies, when tissue architecture was maintained, confirmed the direct effect of Pi on the parathyroid. This was shown in whole glands or tissue slices of parathyroids from different sources, but not in isolated cells.[27–31] *In vivo* studies showed that dietary induced hypophosphatemia leads to a dramatic decrease in rat PTH mRNA levels and that this effect is post-transcriptional as is the effect of hypocalcemia to increase PTH mRNA levels.[24,26] There is a ~60-fold difference in PTH mRNA levels between hypocalcemic and hypophosphatemic rats, and these dietary models were used as tools to define the mechanism of the post-transcriptional regulation of PTH gene expression.[24,32]

CKD patients often develop secondary hyperparathyroidism (2HPT).[33] In these patients, calcimimetics and oral Pi binders are effective drugs used to control the 2HPT. In a rat model of renal failure, induced by an adenine high Pi diet, PTH mRNA levels were increased already after 3 days of the diet and more so at 7 and 21 days. The addition of the calcimimetic R-568 or an oral Pi binder, lanthanum carbonate (La), decreased PTH mRNA and serum PTH levels in the CKD rats at both 7 and 21 days.[34,35] The effects of the adenine diet and the calcimimetic or La, as the effects of calcium or Pi depletion, were all shown to be post-transcriptional and to correlate with differences in parathyroid protein- PTH mRNA 3'-UTR binding that determine PTH mRNA decay and thereby PTH mRNA levels.[32,34,36]

Protein-mRNA binding and mRNA stability

Post-transcriptional regulation of gene expression is often associated with protein–RNA interactions that determine mRNA stability. Critical *cis*-acting elements, mostly in UTRs of many mRNAs are targets for *trans*-acting proteins regulating mRNA stability and translation.[37] AU-rich elements (ARE) are a well defined family of *cis*-acting elements critical for the expression of many unstable mRNAs that code for cytokines, transcription factors, proto-oncogenes, and other mRNAs.[38] Three classes of AREs have been characterized, two of which contain several scattered or overlapping copies of the pentanucleotide AUUUA. The class III AREs lack the AUUUA motif, but require a U-rich sequence and possibly other unknown determinants.[39] A number of ARE binding proteins have been identified that can interact with AU- and U-rich regions. Tristetraprolin (TTP), butyrate response factor-1 (BRF1)-type splicing regulatory protein (KSRP) are examples for decay promoting factors.[37,40] Others, such as the ELAV protein family members (mainly HuR), are stabilizing factors and AU rich binding factor 1 (AUF-1) promotes either decay or stabilization, depending on the mRNA and cell type.[41]

The PTH mRNA 3'-UTR *cis*-acting protein binding element

A specific sequence in the rat PTH mRNA 3'-UTR was identified as a *cis* acting element that determines PTH mRNA stability and its regulation by calcium and Pi.[22] There is no parathyroid cell line; therefore, a cell-free mRNA *in vitro* degradation assay (IVDA) was utilized to demonstrate the factors involved in PTH mRNA decay. In this method, *in vitro* transcribed transcripts for PTH mRNA are incubated with cytosolic parathyroid proteins from rats on different diets and, at timed intervals, samples are removed and run on agarose gels to measure the amount of intact PTH transcript remaining with time. Parathyroid protein extracts from hypocalcemic rats stabilized and extracts from hypophosphatemic rats destabilized the PTH transcript compared with parathyroid extracts from control rat, correlating with mRNA levels *in vivo*. Calcium and Pi did not regulate the stability of a truncated transcript that did not include the 60 terminal nucleotide protein-binding region of the PTH mRNA 3'-UTR.[24] Similarly, PTH mRNA stability by IVDAs was increased by parathyroid cytosolic extracts from CKD rats and decreased by extracts from CKD rats after R568 or La.[34,36] Therefore, the IVDA reproduces the *in vivo* stabilizing effect of low calcium and CKD, and the destabilizing effects of low Pi, R568 and La on PTH mRNA levels, and this is dependent upon sequences in the terminal portion of the PTH mRNA 3'-UTR.

Protein-PTH mRNA binding experiments showed that there is specific binding of rat and human parathyroid extracts to an *in vitro* transcribed probe for the rat and human PTH mRNA 3'-UTR. This binding was regulated by calcium or Pi depletion and correlated with PTH mRNA levels and stability.[24] A 26nt element was the minimal protein binding element in the PTH mRNA.[22] Sequence analysis revealed preservation of the 26 nucleotide protein-binding element in rat, mouse, human, cat, and canine PTH mRNA 3'-UTRs (Fig. 5.1).[23] To demonstrate the functionality of the protein binding sequence in the context of another RNA, a 63 bp PTH cDNA sequence consisting of the 26 nucleotides and flanking regions was fused to the growth hormone (GH) cDNA. IVDAs were performed to determine the effect of parathyroid cytosolic proteins from rats fed the different diets on the stability of RNA transcripts for GH and the chimeric GH-PTH 63 nucleotide.[22,42] The GH transcript was more stable than PTH RNA and was not affected by parathyroid protein extracts from the different diets. The chimeric GH PTH 63 nucleotide transcript, like the full-length PTH transcript, was stabilized by parathyroid extracts from rats fed a calcium-depleted diet and destabilized by proteins from rats fed a Pi-depleted diet. Therefore, the 63nt protein binding region of the PTH mRNA 3'-UTR is both necessary and sufficient to regulate RNA stability and to confer responsiveness to changes in parathyroid proteins by calcium and Pi.[22] This PTH mRNA 3'-UTR cis element is AU rich and is a type III ARE.[37] Structural analysis of the element by RNase H, primer extension, and computer modeling showed that PTH mRNA 3'-UTR and, in particular, the region of the 63 nucleotide cis acting ARE is dominated by significant open regions with little folded base pairing. Mutation analysis of the 26nt core element demonstrated the importance of defined nucleotides for protein-RNA binding. This was the first study of an ARE that relates function to structure.[43] Therefore, the PTH mRNA 3'-UTR cis acting element is an open region that utilizes the distinct sequence pattern to determine mRNA stability by its interaction with trans acting factors.[43]

The PTH mRNA trans acting stabilizing proteins

Two PTH mRNA 3'-UTR binding and stabilizing proteins have been identified by PTH RNA affinity chromatography. These trans acting proteins are AUF1 and Up-stream of N-ras (Unr).[44,45] The two proteins bind the PTH mRNA 3'-UTR and are part of the PTH mRNA-parathyroid protein binding complex. Addition of recombinant AUF1 to parathyroid extracts from Pi depleted rats prevented the rapid degradation of the PTH RNA in IVDAs.[44] AUF1 is modified post-translationally in the parathyroids of rats fed a calcium or a Pi-depleted diet or CKD rats.[34,46] These modifications could lead to differences in AUF1-PTH mRNA binding affinity and PTH mRNA stability. Over-expression of AUF1 or Unr in human embryonic kidney (HEK) 293 cells co-transfected with expression plasmids for the PTH gene or a chimeric GH gene containing the rat 63 nucleotide PTH mRNA 3'-UTR cis-acting element, stabilized the PTH mRNA and chimeric reporter mRNA, but not a PTH mRNA lacking the cis element nor a reporter mRNA containing a truncated PTH element.[23,45] Knockdown of AUF1 or Unr by siRNA led to the opposite effect, decreasing PTH mRNA levels.[45,46] AUF1 also stabilized a reporter mRNA containing the bovine PTH mRNA protein-binding element that is different from the one characterized in rat.[23] These results identified AUF1 and Unr as PTH mRNA stabilizing proteins (Fig. 5.2). The question then was what is the mechanism of PTH mRNA decay and how do these stabilizing proteins affect it.

mRNA decay mechanisms

For many mRNAs decay begins with shortening of the poly(A) tail. Upon deadenylation, ARE-containing mRNAs are degraded in either a 3' to 5' or a 5' to 3' direction by

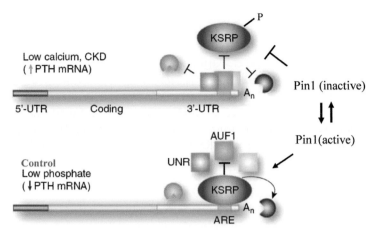

Fig. 5.2 Model for the regulation of PTH mRNA stability by changes in calcium and Pi levels, and CKD, the role of PTH mRNA interacting proteins. In experimental CKD and in rats fed a low calcium diet there is increased *PTH* gene expression, and this is associated with decreased interaction of the destabilizing protein KSRP with the ARE (green) in the PTH mRNA 3'-UTR (white) and increased interaction of the ARE with the protective proteins, AUF1 and Unr. In control or in rats fed a low Pi diet, there is increased association of PTH mRNA with KSRP, and decreased association with AUF1 and Unr. KSRP may then recruit the exosome to PTH mRNA leading to decreased PTH mRNA stability and levels. There is upstream regulation of these protein-PTH mRNA interactions by the peptidyl prolyl *os/trans* isomerase Pin1, which interacts with KSRP and regulates KSRP-PTH mRNA interaction in parathyroid cells. In hypocalcemia or CKD, Pin1 is inactive resulting in KSRP phosphorylation and, hence, its inactivation. This would allow AUF1 and Unr to bind the PTH mRNA 3'-UTR ARE with a greater affinity leading to increased PTH mRNA stability. Modification of a model shown in *Kidney International*.[65] ARE: AU rich element; UTR: Untranslated regions; AUF1: AU rich binding factor 1; Unr: Up-stream of N-*ras*; KSRP: KH-type splicing regulatory protein.

two distinct exoribonucleolytic pathways mediated by the multiprotein 3'–5' exoribonuclease complex, exosome, and XrnI, respectively.[47,48] It has been recently demonstrated that these two pathways are functionally linked.[49] ARE-binding proteins, like KSRP or TTP, interact with the exosome and recruit it to target ARE containing mRNAs, thereby promoting their rapid degradation.[50,51] Mammalian mRNAs are also subject to endoribonuclease-mediated decay by endonucleases that initiate decay by cleaving within the body of the mRNA.[52] In *Xenopus* hepatocytes, mRNAs encoding the majority of serum proteins are destabilized by estrogen through the activation of a polysome associated endonuclease, polysomal ribonuclease 1 (PMR1), which forms a selective complex with its substrate mRNA to initiate decay by cleaving within the mRNA.[53]

KSRP is a PTH mRNA *trans* acting destabilizing protein

The decay promoting protein KSRP binds PTH mRNA both *in vivo* in the parathyroid and *in vitro*. In HEK293 cells, KSRP over-expression and knock down experiments showed that KSRP decreases co-transfected PTH mRNA steady-state levels through the PTH mRNA ARE. Over-expression of the PTH mRNA stabilizing protein AUF1 blocked KSRP-PTH mRNA binding and partially prevented the KSRP mediated decrease in PTH mRNA levels.[32] KSRP and AUF1 protein-PTH mRNA interactions in the parathyroid were studied using a RNA immunoprecipitation (RIP) assay which provides a measure of protein-mRNA interactions at a specific time point *in vivo*. In this assay the parathyroid glands were cross-linked, AUF1 or KSRP immunoprecipitated using anti-AUF1 or anti KSRP antibodies, and the amount of PTH mRNA associated with each of the proteins determined by PTH mRNA qRT-PCR analysis. KSRP-PTH mRNA interaction was decreased in glands from calcium depleted or CKD rats where PTH mRNA is more stable, compared with parathyroid glands from controls. KSRP-PTH mRNA interactions were increased in parathyroids from Pi-depleted rats, where PTH mRNA is less stable. In contrast, AUF1-PTH mRNA interactions were increased by hypocalcemia and CKD, and decreased in the Pi-depleted rat parathyroids.[32] The regulation of PTH mRNA half-life is thus mediated by the balanced interactions of AUF1 functioning as a stabilizing protein and the destabilizing protein, KSRP, with the PTH mRNA (Fig. 5.2). These results indicate that KSRP and AUF1, directly or indirectly, respond to changes in serum calcium and Pi concentrations, and renal failure by altering their association with PTH mRNA. AUF1, as part of a stabilizing complex protects PTH mRNA from degradation.[44] KSRP recruits a degradation complex to PTH mRNA resulting in PTH mRNA decay.[32]

KSRP-PTH mRNA interaction was also increased by both R568 and La, which decrease PTH mRNA levels in CKD rats. IVDAs showed that PTH mRNA is destabilized by parathyroid extracts from CKD rats treated with R568 or La compared with parathyroid extracts from untreated CKD rats. This destabilizing effect by R568 and La was dependent upon KSRP and the PTH mRNA 3'-UTR. Therefore, the calcimimetic R568 and correction of serum phosphorus by La determine PTH mRNA stability through KSRP-mediated PTH mRNA decay, thereby decreasing PTH expression.[36] The changes in binding of the *trans* acting factors to the PTH mRNA therefore determine *PTH* gene expression in CKD and after management of the 2HPT by both calcimimetics or oral phosphorus binders (Fig. 5.2).

The mechanism of PTH mRNA degradation is not clear. KSRP recruits the exosome, which exonucleolytically cleaves mRNAs from the 3' end. It was shown that the exosome is necessary for the KSRP-mediated PTH mRNA decay *in vitro*. The exosome interacts with KSRP in parathyroid extracts and is necessary for PTH mRNA decay by parathyroid proteins.[32] Interestingly, PTH mRNA is a substrate for the endoribonuclease PMR1, which cleaved PTH mRNA *in vitro* and in transfected cells in an ARE-dependent manner. Moreover, PMR1 co-immunoprecipitated with PTH mRNA, the exosome, and KSRP in these cells. siRNA mediated knock-down of either exosome components or KSRP prevented PMR1-mediated decay of PTH mRNA in intact cells. These findings suggest that the degradation complex recruited by KSRP to PTH mRNA comprises of both endo- and exo-ribonucleases. They represent an unanticipated mechanism by which the decay of a mRNA is facilitated by KSRP, and is dependent on both the exonuclease complex exosome and an endoribonuclease.[66]

The peptidyl-prolyl isomerase Pin1 determines parathyroid hormone mRNA levels and stability in secondary hyperparathyroidism

The peptidyl prolyl *cis/trans* isomerase Pin1 specifically binds phosphorylated Ser/Thr-Pro protein motifs and catalyses the *cis/trans* isomerization of the peptide bonds thereby changing the biological activity, phosphorylation, and turnover of its target proteins.[54,55] Pin1-catalysed conformational regulation has a profound impact on many key proteins involved in various cell functions.[56,57] Pin1 was recently shown to regulate the turnover of ARE containing mRNAs, mainly cytokine mRNAs, through the interaction and isomerization of ARE binding proteins. Pin1 interacts with AUF1, and thereby stabilizes both GM-CSF and TGFβ mRNAs.[58,59] We have recently identified the peptidyl-prolyl isomerase Pin1 as a PTH mRNA destabilizing protein in rat parathyroids and transfected cells.[60] Pin1 activity is decreased in parathyroid protein extracts from hypocalcemic or CKD rats. Pharmacologic inhibition of Pin1 increases PTH mRNA levels post-transcriptionally *in vivo* in the parathyroid and in transfected cells. Pin1 regulates PTH mRNA stability and levels through the PTH mRNA 3'-untranslated region (UTR) *cis* acting element. Interestingly, Pin1 interacts with the PTH mRNA destabilizing protein, KSRP, and leads to KSRP dephosphorylation and activation. In the parathyroid, Pin1 inhibition decreases the KSRP-PTH mRNA interaction which contributes to the increased *PTH* gene expression. Furthermore, $Pin1^{-/-}$ mice have increased serum PTH and PTH mRNA levels. Therefore, Pin1 determines basal PTH expression *in vivo* and *in vitro* and decreased Pin1 activity correlates with increased PTH mRNA levels in CKD and hypocalcemic rats. These results demonstrate that Pin1 is a key mediator of PTH mRNA stability and indicate a role for Pin1 in the pathogenesis of the secondary hyperparathyroidism of CKD.[60]

Fibroblast growth factor-23 and *PTH* gene expression

Phosphate homeostasis is maintained by a counterbalance between efflux from the kidney and influx from intestine and bone. FGF23 is a bone-derived phosphaturic hormone that acts on the kidney to increase phosphate excretion and suppress biosynthesis of 1,25D. FGF23 signals through fibroblast growth factor receptors (FGFR) bound by the transmembrane protein Klotho.[61] Since most tissues express FGFRs, expression of Klotho virtually determines FGF23 target organs. Klotho protein is expressed not only in the kidney, but also in the parathyroid, pituitary, and sino-atrial node.[62] Since most tissues express FGFR, expression of Klotho virtually determines FGF23 target organs. We identified the parathyroid as a new target organ for FGF23. We showed that the rat parathyroid gland expresses Klotho and that the administration of recombinant FGF23 leads to an increase in parathyroid Klotho levels. In addition, FGF23 activates the MAP kinase pathway in the parathyroid through ERK1/2 phosphorylation and increases Egr-1 mRNA levels. Importantly, FGF23 suppresses the *PTH* gene expression and secretion *in vivo* and in *in vitro* models. The FGF23-induced decrease in PTH secretion was prevented by a MAPK inhibitor. FGF23 also led to a decrease in PTH secretion in bovine parathyroid primary cultures.[64] These data indicate that FGF23 acts directly on the parathyroid through the MAPK pathway to

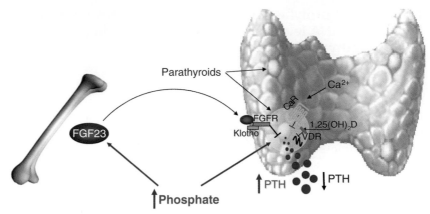

Fig. 5.3 FGF23 acts on the parathyroid to decrease parathyroid hormone (PTH) synthesis and secretion—a novel bone-parathyroid endocrine axis. FGF23 is secreted by bone after the stimulus of a high Pi by acting on the Klotho-FGFR1c. In addition to FGF23's action on the kidney to cause Pi excretion and decrease the synthesis of 1,25D, it acts on the parathyroid to decrease PTH synthesis and secretion. This new endocrine axis contributes to our understanding of how the metabolism of bone, Pi, and calcium are so tightly regulated. PTH is a major regulator of calcium, FGF23 of Pi and together with 1,25D they contribute to normal mineral and bone metabolism. FGF23, fibroblast growth factor 23; FGFR, fibroblast growth factor receptor; CaR, calcium receptor; VDR, vitamin D receptor. Reproduced with permission of *Kidney International*.[65]

decrease serum PTH. This novel bone-parathyroid endocrine axis adds a new dimension to the understanding of mineral homeostasis (Fig. 5.3).[63]

Conclusions

1,25D decreases *PTH* gene transcription and, hence, PTH secretion and this effect is the scientific basis for the treatment of CKD patients with 1,25D analogs. Dietary-induced hypocalcemia, hypophosphatemia, and CKD determine *PTH* gene expression post-transcriptionally. The regulation of PTH mRNA stability is mediated by the balance between stabilizing and decay promoting factors that interact with the PTH mRNA 3'-UTR. In hypocalcemia increased binding of the protective factors, AUF1 and Unr, prevents PTH mRNA degradation resulting in higher levels of PTH mRNA. In hypophosphatemia there is decreased binding of the protective factors and increased interaction of the decay promoting protein KSRP that recruit a degradation ribonuclease complex leading to PTH mRNA decay and decreased PTH mRNA levels. Pin1 is a regulator of *PTH* gene expression that determines basal PTH levels, and the response of the parathyroid to chronic hypocalcemia and CKD by post-translational modification of KSRP and changes in PTH mRNA protein interactions (Fig. 5.2). FGF23 decreases PTH expression through the MAPK pathway. The stimulus to PTH expression is a low serum calcium and high serum Pi as in CKD. 1,25D and FGF23 act together to suppress PTH levels (Fig. 5.3). A model depicting the interactions amongst calcium, Pi, and the calciotrophic hormones is shown in Fig. 5.4.

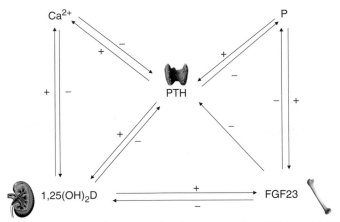

Fig. 5.4 Interrelationships of Ca^{2+}, Pi and their hormones, PTH, FGF23 and $1,25(OH)_2$ vitamin D. There is a network of endocrinological feedback loops that govern mineral homeostasis. Not shown is the effect of calcium to increase serum FGF23 levels, a low Pi to increase serum $1,25(OH)_2D$, and a high Pi to decrease serum $1,25(OH)_2D$. Reproduced with permission of *Kidney International*.[65]

References

1. Silver J, Russell J, Sherwood LM. Regulation by vitamin D metabolites of messenger ribonucleic acid for preproparathyroid hormone in isolated bovine parathyroid cells. *Proc Natl Acad Sci USA* 1985;**82**:4270–3.

2. Silver J, Naveh-Many T, Mayer H, Schmelzer HJ, Popovtzer MM. Regulation by vitamin D metabolites of parathyroid hormone gene transcription *in vivo* in the rat. *J Clin Invest* 1986;**78**:1296–301.

3. Naveh-Many T, Marx R, Keshet E, Pike JW, Silver J. Regulation of 1,25-dihydroxyvitamin D3 receptor gene expression by 1,25-dihydroxyvitamin D3 in the parathyroid *in vivo*. *J Clin Invest* 1990;**86**:1968–75.

4. Russell J, Lettieri D, Sherwood LM. Suppression by 1,25(OH)2D3 of transcription of the pre-proparathyroid hormone gene. *Endocrinol* 1986;**119**:2864–6.

5. Canaff L, Hendy GN. Human calcium-sensing receptor gene. Vitamin D response elements in promoters P1 and P2 confer transcriptional responsiveness to 1,25-dihydroxyvitamin D. *J Biol Chem* 2002;**277**:30337–50.

6. Naveh-Many T, Silver J. Regulation of parathyroid hormone gene expression by hypocalcemia, hypercalcemia, and vitamin D in the rat. *J Clin Invest* 1990;**86**:1313–19.

7. Garfia B, Canadillas S, Canalejo A, et al. Regulation of parathyroid vitamin D receptor expression by extracellular calcium. *J Am Soc Nephrol* 2002;**13**:2945–52.

8. Fukuda N, Tanaka H, Tominaga Y, et al. Decreased 1,25-dihydroxyvitamin D3 receptor density is associated with a more severe form of parathyroid hyperplasia in chronic uremic patients. *J Clin Invest* 1993;**92**:1436–43.

9. Patel S, Rosenthal JT. Hypercalcemia in carcinoma of prostate. *Its cure by orchiectomy*. *Urology* 1985;**25**:627–9.

10. Arnold A, Brown MF, Urena P, et al. Monoclonality of parathyroid tumors in chronic renal failure and in primary parathyroid hyperplasia. *J Clin Invest* 1995;**95:** 2047–53.

11. Imanishi Y, Hosokawa Y, Yoshimoto K, et al. Dual abnormalities in cell proliferation and hormone regulation caused by cyclin D1 in a murine model of hyperparathyroidism. *J Clin Invest* 2001;**107:**1093–102.

12. Kel A, Scheer M, Mayer H. In silico analysis of regulatory sequences in the human parathyroid hormone gene. In: T. Naveh-Many (ed.) *Molecular Biology of the Parathyroid.* New York: Landes Bioscience and Kluwer Academic/Plenum Publishers, 2005:68–83.

13. Alimov AP, Park-Sarge OK, Sarge KD, Malluche HH, Koszewski NJ. Transactivation of the parathyroid hormone promoter by specificity proteins and the nuclear factor Y complex. *Endocrinol* 2005;**146:**3409–16.

14. Okazaki T, Igarashi T, Kronenberg HM. 5'-flanking region of the parathyroid hormone gene mediates negative regulation by 1,25-(OH)2 vitamin D3. *J Biol Chem* 1988;**263:** 2203–8.

15. Russell J, Ashok S, Koszewski NJ. Vitamin D receptor interactions with the rat parathyroid hormone gene: synergistic effects between two negative vitamin D response elements. *J Bone Miner Res* 1999;**14:**1828–37.

16. Liu SM, Koszewski N, Lupez M *et al.* Characterisation of a response element in the 5'-flanking region of the avian (chicken) parathyroid hormone gene that mediates negative regulation of gene transcription by 1,25-dihydroxyvitamin D3 and binds the vitamin D3 receptor. *Mol Endocrinol* 1996;**10:**206–15.

17. Murayama A, Kim MS, Yanagisawa J, Takeyama K, Kato S. Transrepression by a liganded nuclear receptor via a bHLH activator through co-regulator switching. *EMBO J* 2004;**23:**1598–608.

18. Fujiki R, Kim MS, Sasaki Y, et al. Ligand-induced transrepression by VDR through association of WSTF with acetylated histones. *EMBO J* 2005;**24:**3881–94.

19. Kim MS, Fujiki R, Murayama A, et al. 1Alpha,25(OH)2D3-induced transrepression by vitamin D receptor through E-box-type elements in the human parathyroid hormone gene promoter. *Mol Endocrinol* 2007;**21:**334–42.

20. Kemper B. Molecular biology of parathyroid hormone. *CRC Crit Rev Biochem* 1986;**19:**353–79.

21. Bell O, Silver J, Naveh-Many T. Parathyroid hormone, from gene to protein. In: T. SNaveh-Many (ed.), *Molecular Biology of the Parathyroid.* New York: Landes Bioscience and Kluwer Academic/Plenum Publishers, 2005:8–28.

22. Kilav R, Silver J, Naveh-Many T. A conserved cis-acting element in the parathyroid hormone 3'-untranslated region is sufficient for regulation of RNA stability by calcium and phosphate. *J Biol Chem* 2001;**276:**8727–33.

23. Bell O, Silver J, Naveh-Many T. Identification and characterisation of *cis*-acting elements in the human and bovine parathyroid hormone mRNA 3'-untranslated region. *J Bone Min Res* 2005;**20:**858–66.

24. Moallem E, Silver J, Kilav R, Naveh-Many T. RNA protein binding and post-transcriptional regulation of PTH gene expression by calcium and phosphate. *J Biol Chem* 1998;**273:**5253–9.

25. Naveh-Many T, Rahamimov R, Livni N, Silver J. Parathyroid cell proliferation in normal and chronic renal failure rats: the effects of calcium, phosphate and vitamin D. *J Clin Invest* 1995;**96:**1786–93.

26. Kilav R, Silver J, Naveh-Many T. Parathyroid hormone gene expression in hypophosphatemic rats. *J Clin Invest* 1995;**96**:327–33.

27. Almaden Y, Canalejo A, Hernandez A, et al. Direct effect of phosphorus on parathyroid hormone secretion from whole rat parathyroid glands *in vitro*. *J Bone Miner Res* 1996;**11**:970–6.

28. Almaden Y, Hernandez A, Torregrosa V, et al. High phosphate level directly stimulates parathyroid hormone secretion and synthesis by human parathyroid tissue *in vitro*. *J Am Soc Nephrol* 1998;**9**:1845–52.

29. Nielsen PK, Feldt-Rasmusen U, Olgaard K. A direct effect of phosphate on PTH release from bovine parathyroid tissue slices but not from dispersed parathyroid cells. *Nephrol Dial Transplant* 1996;**11**:1762–8.

30. Slatopolsky E, Finch J, Denda M, et al. Phosphate restriction prevents parathyroid cell growth in uremic rats. High phosphate directly stimulates PTH secretion *in vitro*. *J Clin Invest* 1996;**97**:2534–40.

31. Rodriguez M, Almaden Y, Hernandez A, Torres A. Effect of phosphate on the parathyroid gland: direct and indirect? *Curr Opin Nephrol Hypertens* 1996;**5**:321–8.

32. Nechama M, Ben Dov IZ, Briata P, Gherzi R, Naveh-Many T. The mRNA decay promoting factor K-homology splicing regulator protein post-transcriptionally determines parathyroid hormone mRNA levels. *FASEB J* 2008;**22**:3458–68.

33. Silver J, Kilav R, Naveh-Many T. Mechanisms of secondary hyperparathyroidism. *Am J Physiol Renal Physiol* 2002;**283**:F367–76.

34. Levi R, Ben Dov IZ, Lavi-Moshayoff V, et al. Increased parathyroid hormone gene expression in secondary hyperparathyroidism of experimental uremia is reversed by calcimimetics: correlation with posttranslational modification of the trans acting factor AUF1. *J Am Soc Nephrol* 2006;**17**:107–12.

35. Ben Dov IZ, Pappo O, Sklair-Levy M, et al. Lanthanum carbonate decreases PTH gene expression with no hepatotoxicity in uremic rats. *Nephrol Dial Transplant* 2007;**22**:362–8.

36. Nechama M, Ben Dov IZ, Silver J, Naveh-Many T. Regulation of PTH mRNA stability by the calcimimetic R568 and the phosphorus binder lanthanum carbonate in CKD. *Am J Physiol Renal Physiol* 2009;**296**:F795–800.

37. Barreau C, Paillard L, Osborne HB. AU-rich elements and associated factors: are there unifying principles? *Nucl Acids Res* 2006;**33**:7138–50.

38. Brewer G. Messenger RNA decay during aging and development. *Ageing Res Rev* 2002; **1**: 607–25.

39. Chen CY, Shyu AB. AU-rich elements: characterisation and importance in mRNA degradation. *Trends Biochem Sci* 1995;**20**:465–70.

40. Gherzi R, Lee KY, Briata P, et al. A KH domain RNA binding protein, KSRP, promotes ARE-directed mRNA turnover by recruiting the degradation machinery. *Mol Cell* 2004;**14**:571–83.

41. Wilusz CJ, Wilusz J. Bringing the role of mRNA decay in the control of gene expression into focus. *Trends Genet* 2004;**20**:491–7.

42. Naveh-Many T, Bell O, Silver J, Kilav R. Cis and trans acting factors in the regulation of parathyroid hormone (PTH) mRNA stability by calcium and phosphate. *FEBS Lett* 2002;**529**:60–4.

43. Kilav R, Bell O, Le SY, Silver J, Naveh-Many T. The parathyroid hormone mRNA 3'-untranslated region AU-rich element is an unstructured functional element. *J Biol Chem* 2004;**279**:2109–16.

44. Sela-Brown A, Silver J, Brewer G, Naveh-Many T. Identification of AUF1 as a parathyroid hormone mRNA 3'-untranslated region binding protein that determines parathyroid hormone mRNA stability. *J Biol Chem* 2000;**275**:7424–9.

45. Dinur M, Kilav R, Sela-Brown A, Jacquemin-Sablon H, Naveh-Many T. *In vitro* evidence that upstream of N-ras participates in the regulation of parathyroid hormone messenger ribonucleic acid stability. *Mol Endocrinol* 2006;**20**:1652–60.

46. Bell O, Gaberman E, Kilav R, et al. The protein phosphatase calcineurin determines basal parathyroid hormone gene expression. *Mol Endocrinol* 2005;**19**:516–26.

47. Chen CY, Gherzi R, Ong SE, et al. AU binding proteins recruit the exosome to degrade ARE-containing mRNAs. *Cell* 2001;**107**:451–64.

48. Orban TI, Izaurralde E. Decay of mRNAs targeted by RISC requires XRN1, the Ski complex, and the exosome. *RNA*. 2005;**11**:459–69.

49. Murray EL, Schoenberg DR. A+U-rich instability elements differentially activate 5'-3' and 3'-5' mRNA decay. *Mol Cell Biol* 2007;**27**:2791–9.

50. Linker K, Pautz A, Fechir M, et al. Involvement of KSRP in the post-transcriptional regulation of human iNOS expression-complex interplay of KSRP with TTP and HuR. *Nucleic Acids Res* 2005;**33**:4813–27.

51. Chou CF, Mulky A, Maitra S, et al. Tethering KSRP, a decay-promoting AU-rich element-binding protein, to mRNAs elicits mRNA decay. *Mol Cell Biol* 2006;**26**:3695–706.

52. Chernokalskaya E, Dubell AN, Cunningham KS, et al. A polysomal ribonuclease involved in the destabilisation of albumin mRNA is a novel member of the peroxidase gene family. *RNA* 1998;**4**:1537–48.

53. Peng Y, Schoenberg DR. c-Src activates endonuclease-mediated mRNA decay. *Mol Cell* 2007;**25**:779–87.

54. Wulf GM, Liou YC, Ryo A, Lee SW, Lu KP. Role of Pin1 in the regulation of p53 stability and p21 transactivation, and cell cycle checkpoints in response to DNA damage. *J Biol Chem* 2002;**277**:47976–9.

55. Zhou XZ, Kops O, Werner A *et al.* Pin1-dependent prolyl isomerisation regulates dephosphorylation of Cdc25C and tau proteins. *Mol Cell* 2000; **6**: 873-883.

56. Winkler KE, Swenson KI, Kornbluth S, Means AR. Requirement of the prolyl isomerase Pin1 for the replication checkpoint. *Science* 2000;**287**:1644–7.

57. Lu PJ, Wulf G, Zhou XZ, Davies P, Lu KP. The prolyl isomerase Pin1 restores the function of Alzheimer-associated phosphorylated tau protein. *Nature* 1999;**399**:784–8.

58. Shen ZJ, Esnault S, Malter JS. The peptidyl-prolyl isomerase Pin1 regulates the stability of granulocyte-macrophage colony-stimulating factor mRNA in activated eosinophils. *Nat Immunol* 2005;**6**:1280–7.

59. Shen ZJ, Esnault S, Rosenthal LA, et al. Pin1 regulates TGF-beta1 production by activated human and murine eosinophils and contributes to allergic lung fibrosis. *J Clin Invest* 2008;**118**:479–90.

60. Nechama, M., Uchida, T., Mor Yosef-Levi, I., Silver, J., Naveh-Many, T. The peptidyl-prolyl isomerase Pin1 determines parathyroid hormone mRNA levels and stability in secondary hyperparathyroidism. *J Clin Invest* 2009;**119**:3102–14.

61. Kurosu H, Ogawa Y, Miyoshi M, et al. Regulation of fibroblast growth factor-23 signaling by klotho.*J Biol Chem* 2006;**281**:6120–3.

62. Takeshita K, Fujimori T, Kurotaki Y, et al. Sinoatrial node dysfunction and early unexpected death of mice with a defect of klotho gene expression. *Circulation* 2004;**109**:1776–82.

63. Ben Dov IZ, Galitzer H, Lavi-Moshayoff V, et al. The parathyroid is a target organ for FGF23 in rats. *J Clin Invest* 2007;**117**:4003–8.

64. Krajisnik T, Bjorklund P, Marsell R, et al. Fibroblast growth factor-23 regulates parathyroid hormone and 1alpha-hydroxylase expression in cultured bovine parathyroid cells. *J Endocrinol* 2007;**195**:125–31.

65. Silver J, Naveh-Many T. Phosphate and the parathyroid. *Kidney Int* 2009;**75**: 898–905.

66. Nechama M, Peng Y, Bell O, Briata P, Gherzi R, Schoenberg D, Naveh-Many T. KSRP-PMRI-exosome association determincs parathyroid hormone mNRA levels and stability in transfected cclls. *BMC Cell Biol* 2009;**10**:70.

Chapter 6

Abnormal parathyroid gland function in CKD

Ewa Lewin and Mariano Rodriguez

Introduction

Secondary hyperparathyroidism (2HPT) develops early in renal insufficiency and may affect the function of several organs beside the skeleton. The stimuli for the development of 2HPT of relevance to renal failure are hypocalcemia, hyperphosphatemia and low levels of 1,25(OH)$_2$D. Hypocalcemia increases parathyroid hormone (PTH) gene expression per parathyroid cell, increases secretion of PTH 1–84 from the parathyroid cells, and increases the number of parathyroid cells.[1,2] The effect of low calcium on *PTH* gene expression is post-transcriptional. The suppression of PTH secretion induced by high extracellular calcium is mediated via the calcium-sensing receptor (CaR) that is located on the surface of the parathyroid cells.[3] Expression of the CaR mRNA and protein is diminished in human parathyroid glands of advanced uremia and in rat parathyroids of 5/6 nephrectomized rats kept on high phosphorus diet; this reduced expression of CaR may impair the sensitivity of parathyroid cells to extracellular calcium in uremia.[4] Hyperphosphatemia, besides reducing the plasma Ca^{2+} concentration exerts a direct, calcium independent effect, on the stimulation of PTH secretion and PTH mRNA through post-transcriptional mechanisms. This has been demonstrated in *in vitro* models in rat, bovine, and human parathyroid glands.[5–8] The cellular target for phosphate is still unknown. 1,25(OH)$_2$D$_3$ (calcitriol) is an important regulator of the *PTH* gene.[9] Pharmacological doses of calcitriol decrease *PTH* gene expression at the transcriptional level by binding of the 1,25(OH)$_2$D receptor (VDR) to a vitamin D-responsive element on the *PTH* gene promoter.[10] The levels of calcitriol in mild and moderate uremia are maintained within the normal range at the expense of elevated PTH levels. In uremia, low levels of VDR have been demonstrated in the parathyroid cells,[11] together with an impaired affinity of vitamin D to its receptor, resulting in a reduced activity of calcitriol.[12] Furthermore, uremia *per se* enhances the stability of PTH mRNA by a post-transcriptional mechanism that decreases the degradation of RNA.[13]

Regulation of *PTH* gene transcription in CKD

The human *PTH* gene is located on the short arm of chromosome 11. The expression of the gene occurs primarily in the parathyroid cells, but has been shown in rodent hypothalamus and thymus as well. It has been shown that transgenic mice (deficient in the *Gcm2*-gene, a master regulatory gene of parathyroid gland development) that are lacking the parathyroid glands, had circulating PTH secreted from the thymus.[14] The DNA sequences determining the tissue specificity of the *PTH* gene has not been established. The expression of the *PTH* gene can probably be disrupted in severe nodular hyperplasia of the parathyroid glands in CKD, as PTH protein is not expressed in some nodular areas (please, see Fig. 6.5).[15] A calcium responsive element of several thousand base pair upstream from the start site of the *PTH* gene transcription has been identified, but the importance of this potential regulatory region has not been fully established.

1,25(OH)$_2$D regulates *PTH* gene transcription. The VDR responsive element (VDRE), mediating the negative regulation of calcitriol on PTH synthesis, is located in the 5'-flanking region of the *PTH* gene. A specific inhibitory effect of uremic plasma ultrafiltrate on this binding of VDR to VDRE has been demonstrated and the low serum calcium in uremia may further modulate the effect of calcitriol at the transcriptional level. Thus, it has been shown that nuclear calreticulin in the parathyroids prevents the binding of the VDR-retinoid X-receptor to the *PTH* gene during hypocalcemia, and thereby inhibits the down-regulatory function of the sterol. The direct effect of 1,25(OH)$_2$D, rapidly lowering *PTH* gene transcription rate, was first shown by Silver et al., using primary parathyroid cells in culture.[16] The isolated pathophysiological effect of low levels of 1,25(OH)$_2$D of relevance for CKD on *PTH* gene transcription has not been studied extensively in animal models, as the results will be difficult to interpret since changes in 1,25(OH)$_2$D will be associated to changes in calcium and phosphate that, in turn, affect parathyroid function.

Regulation of PTH release in CKD

Calcium-sensing by the parathyroid cells in CKD

In vitro studies

Plasma Ca^{2+} is the major determinant of the secretion of PTH from the parathyroid glands. The cloning and characterization of CaR in the plasma membrane of parathyroid cells brought important information on the mechanisms by which Ca^{2+} and other ions control the parathyroid function.[3] The detailed mechanism behind the complexity of the calcium regulated PTH secretion is, however, not yet well understood.[3,17] The parathyroid glands express abundant CaR mRNA and protein.[3,4,17] The CaR belongs to the superfamily of G-protein-coupled receptors.[3] CaR agonists activate phospholipase C (PLC), phospholipase A$_2$ (PLA$_2$) and phospholipase D (PLD) in the parathyroid cell.[17] Activation of PLA$_2$ and PLD involve protein kinase C dependent pathways that are activated by the CaR, presumably via PLC (Fig. 6.1).[17] High extracellular Ca^{2+} elicits a transient rise in intracellular Ca^{2+}, probably as a result of PLC activation and the inositol-tri-phosphate (IP$_3$)-mediated release of Ca^{2+} from the intracellular stores.[17] The high extracellular Ca^{2+} likewise induces a sustained increase in intracellular Ca^{2+} through incompletely defined Ca^{2+} influx pathways. PTH secretion is inhibited by the elevated intracellular Ca^{2+}.[17] Several lines of evidence

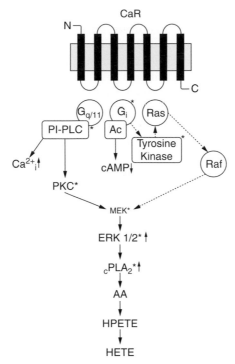

Fig. 6.1 Proposed model for mechanisms underlying CaR-induced activation of ERK1/2 and cPLA$_2$ in parathyroid cells. Activation of the 7-membrane-spanning CaR by Ca$_o^{2+}$ results in a G$_{q/11}$-mediated activation of PI-PLC, leading to intracellular calcium (Ca$_i^{2+}$) mobilization, PKC activation, and resultant PKC-mediated stimulation of the mitogen-activating protein kinase (MAPK) cascade. The CaR also activates MAPK and subsequent downstream activation of a tyrosine kinase-dependent process. Activated MAPK then phosphorylates and activates cPLA$_2$, which releases free arachidonic acid (AA) that can be metabolized to biologically active mediators, such as hydroxyperoxyeicosatetranoic acid (HPETE) or hydroxyeicosatetranoic acid (HETE). Modified from Kifor O, et al., *Am J Physiol* 2001;**280**:F291–302.[61]

support the role of the CaR as the key mediator of the inhibitory action of elevated extracellular Ca^{2+} on secretion of PTH. In *in vitro* studies it has been well documented that cultured parathyroid cells loose their Ca^{2+} sensitivity very fast,[18] and that a high calcium containing medium can only suppress PTH secretion by approximately 50–75 % of the maximal low Ca^{2+} stimulated secretion.[7] Brown et al.[18] reported, that the CaR mRNA declined by 70% during the first 4 h in a culture of bovine parathyroid cells and remained very low for the following 24 h of culture. Thus, loss of calcium responsiveness in cultured parathyroid cells and, as such, the non-suppressibility might be due to a dramatic drop in the expression of the CaR, supporting the notion that the sensitivity of the parathyroid cell to extracellular Ca^{2+} depends upon the dose of CaR on the cell surface.

Parathyroid glands from patients with severe secondary or tertiary HPT have elevated set-points for Ca^{2+} (the level of calcium required to induce 50% of maximal PTH secretion).[19] This was shown *in vitro* already in 1982 by Brown et al. and indicates an impaired sensitivity to extracellular calcium in uremia. Furthermore, the disturbed set-point correlated with an impairment in the increase of intracellular calcium in response to a high calcium concentration in the medium.[19]

A substantial reduction in the expression of the CaR protein and mRNA has been demonstrated in hyperplastic parathyroid glands from uremic patients by Gogusev et al. (Fig. 6.2).[4] This reduction was more marked in nodular areas than in diffusely hyperplastic tissue. Canadillas et al. examined the CaR gene expression and PTH secretion *in vitro* in 50 hyperplastic glands from 23 patients on hemodialysis[20] and found that the larger the gland, the lower the CaR mRNA expression. Parathyroid tissue with the lowest CaR expression secreted more PTH than those with relatively high CaR expression. Furthermore, glands with low CaR expression demonstrated a blunted inhibitory effect of high extracellular calcium on PTH secretion. As such, low CaR expression is related to several abnormalities in the function of the uremic parathyroid glands. However, in experimental 2HPT, the CaR is only decreased in the

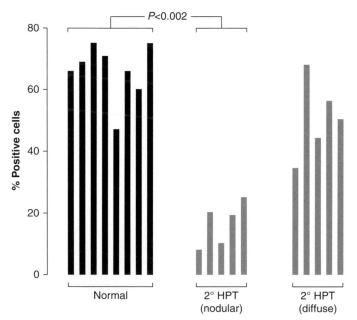

Fig. 6.2 A decrease in the expression of CaR protein, as demonstrated by immunohistochemistry, in secondary uremic hyperplastic parathyroid gland tissue (the two panels on the right) compared with normal parathyroid tissue (left panel). The decrease is more marked in nodular areas (characteristic of advanced hyperplasia) than in diffusely hyperplastic tissue. From Gogusev J, et al., *Kidney Int* 1997;**51**:328–36.[4]

hyperplastic parathyroid glands of hyperphosphatemic uremic rats, but not in glands obtained from uremic rats kept on standard diet. This indicates that the phenomenon of down-regulation of parathyroid CaR expression might be related to the increased parathyroid cell proliferation observed in severe 2HPT.[11,21]

In vivo studies

The Ca^{2+}/PTH relationship is described by a sigmoidal Ca^{2+}/PTH curve,[22] as shown in Fig. 6.3. The linear part of this curve is very steep. This means that just a small decline in Ca^{2+} below normal levels will result in a dramatic increase of PTH secretion. The maximal secretory rate (the maximal PTH) is accordingly achieved after just a mild degree of hypocalcemia. Induction of even mild hypercalcemia will, in contrast, result in a modest decline of PTH secretion, as indicated at the lower part of the curve (minimal PTH). It is, however, questioned whether PTH secretion can be totally suppressed, even at very high Ca^{2+} concentrations.[22–24]

The Ca^{2+}/PTH relationship is disturbed in CKD.[23–25] In a study on the development of CKD, a progressive increase of the maximal PTH values was observed as creatinine

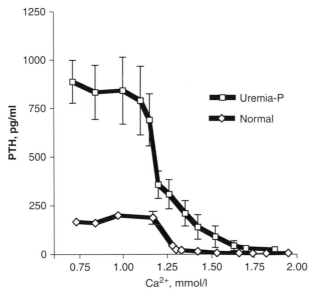

Fig. 6.3 Ca^{2+}/PTH relationship during acute inductions of hypocalcemia and hypercalcemia in uremic rats kept on high P diet (Uremia-P) and in normal control rats (Normal). The maximal PTH secretory response to hypocalcemia of the uremic rats was significantly higher ($p < 0.001$) than that of the normal rats. The minimal PTH in response to hypercalcemia was significantly higher ($p < 0.05$) in the uremic, hyperphosphatemic rats than in the normal rats. The Ca^{2+}/PTH curve of uremic, hyperphosphatemic rats is shifted to the right. Data from Lewin et al., *Kidney Int* 1997;**52**:1232–41.[24]

clearance decreased.[26] Minimal PTH was raised in CKD patients with severe 2HPT[25] with phosphorus retention being associated with impaired suppressibility of PTH secretion in CKD.[24]

Considerable controversy exists on the results and interpretations of *in vivo* assessments of parathyroid gland function in patients with uremia. Focus below will be on the complexity of the Ca^{2+}/PTH relationship, such as intraglandular/intracellular degradation, recruitment of parathyroid cells in an active state, autocrine/paracrine factors, hysteresis, rate-dependent control of the PTH response, and on the transient nature of the initial increase in the PTH response to a reduction of Ca^{2+}.

The *intracellular degradation of PTH within the parathyroid cell* appears to be regulated.[27] When secretion is stimulated by low ambient calcium most of the hormone is in the form of the PTH 1–84 molecule. By contrast, when the secretion is suppressed by high ambient calcium most of the secreted hormone consists of fragments.[27] Santamaria et al.[28] demonstrated that, although hypercalcemia reduces the secretion of both PTH 1–84 and C-PTH, the reduction of PTH 1–84 secretion is more marked than that of C-PTH. This may have important clinical implications because C-PTH may act on C-terminal PTH receptors and antagonize the calcemic effect of PTH 1–84.

Another intraglandular regulatory mechanism of possible importance for the secretion of PTH is the *recruitment of parathyroid cells,* as shown by Ritchie et al.,[29] who demonstrated that parathyroid cells may cycle between active and inactive secretory states. As such, the secretory response of PTH to changes in Ca^{2+} may be altered by the fraction of parathyroid cells in an active secretory state.[30] The possible influence of the number of cells in an active secretory state on the acute response of PTH to fluctuations in Ca^{2+} in uremia has, however, not yet been established.

Hysteresis describes the phenomenon that the parathyroid cells are sensing the direction of changes of Ca^{2+}.[31] The levels of PTH are higher during induction of hypocalcemia, than at the same level of Ca^{2+}, when the Ca^{2+} levels are returned toward normal. This results in two different curves.[31] The question, therefore, is which of the two curves—obtained during induction of hypocalcemia or during recovery from hypocalcemia—should be chosen as the one, which best is representing the parathyroid function? This was studied by Felsenfeld et al.[32] in 19 hemodialysis patients. Two different curves were obtained for each patient, clearly demonstrating the phenomenon of hysteresis and further showing that the set-points for calcium derived from the individual Ca^{2+}/PTH curves were higher in all patients during induction of hypocalcemia, than during recovery from hypocalcemia. Interestingly, when the patients were divided according to their basal Ca^{2+} concentrations, then the Ca^{2+}/PTH relationship showed much greater variation during induction of hypocalcemia than during recovery from hypocalcemia. Therefore, if the differences in the secretory responses of PTH do not result from different rates of Ca^{2+} reduction between the groups, then the conclusion must be that investigations on the Ca^{2+}/PTH relationship should start at basal Ca^{2+} level.

Rate-dependent control of the PTH response indicates that a rapid decrement of Ca^{2+} results in a higher PTH response than the response obtained during a slow decrement of Ca^{2+}, even when reaching at the same level of Ca^{2+}.[33]

Thus, a more rapid change in the rate of Ca^{2+} is associated with a higher shift upward and to the right of the relationship between PTH and Ca^{2+}.[34] It is therefore a question whether it is possible to determine the sensitivity of the parathyroid glands to Ca^{2+} by making Ca^{2+}/PTH curves and whether from such curves the set-point for calcium can be estimated. The answer to this question is very important for the nephrologists in order to obtain a better understanding of the mechanisms that are involved in uremic 2HPT and to obtain a better evaluation of the resulting treatment. The results of several clinical and experimental investigations are conflicting.[25] An abnormal Ca^{2+} set-point in uremic parathyroid glands was found in an *in vitro* investigation, although a wide range of set-points appeared.[19] Studies *in vivo* are difficult to evaluate due to the different responses to induction of hypocalcemia and hypercalcemia that exist among uremic patients. Only a few studies provide data on the differences in time required to obtain a certain level of hypo- and hypercalcemia. Kwan et al.[35] showed that the duration required to increase or decrease p-Ca^{2+} was dramatically different between patients on hemodialysis and concluded that according to the rate-dependency of the PTH response to Ca^{2+}, the Ca^{2+}/PTH curves of these patients were obtained during significantly different circumstances and therefore the authors subsequently abstained from any estimation of the Ca^{2+} set-points. McCarron et al.[36] examined the parathyroid function in normal subjects, and in kidney transplanted patients with persistent HPT and hypercalcemia, and noted significantly different decreases in Ca^{2+} during a 2 h of a fixed dose of EDTA infused in the two groups (0.45 versus 0.96 mEq/l). Thus, disturbances of the Ca^{2+} homeostasis might have resulted in different rates of change in p-Ca^{2+} in response to EDTA or calcium infusions. Most other studies describe the Ca^{2+}/PTH relationship by a 2-dimensional model, which is omitting the time factor.[23] Therefore, when considering the present knowledge on the Ca^{2+}/PTH relationship, most of these interpretations must be taken with some precaution. Nonetheless, at present the Ca^{2+}/PTH curve with its limitations is the only method to estimate the Ca^{2+} sensitivity (set-point) of the parathyroid glands in uremic patients.

The 'maximal' secretory response.

The PTH secretory response to hypocalcemia in uremia is enhanced and the maximal response of PTH secretion to hypocalcemia is dependent upon the rate of reducing the Ca^{2+} levels.[34] It is, therefore, a question whether the *in vivo* studies on the maximal secretory of PTH to hypocalcemia always have been performed at the 'maximal' rate and, as such, will result in a 'maximal' response. The transient nature of PTH secretion during induction of hypocalcemia adds difficulties to the interpretation of the maximum. During a severe and rapid decrease of Ca^{2+} an initial rapid increase of the PTH levels is seen, which soon declines to a lower level, despite a continuous fall in Ca^{2+}. The PTH levels remain, however, considerably higher than before stimulation.[37]

What level should be considered as the maximum? To answer this question we need to understand the cause of the transient elevation of PTH. This is not known as yet. Some investigators interpret the elevation as due to emptying the stores of preformed PTH and the subsequent levels of PTH secretion should express the ongoing biosynthesis of the hormone. This is in contrast to the accumulating knowledge on the complexity of the regulation of PTH secretion.[37] Thus, our results, which showed a dramatic, immediate and sustained enhancement of the low Ca^{2+}-induced PTH secretion by parathyroid hormone related peptide (PTHrP), are in contrast to the assumption of an initial emptying of all stored and preformed PTH during acute induction of hypocalcemia (Fig. 6.4).[37]

Furthermore, it has been assumed that the 'maximal' PTH level in response to hypocalcemia reflects the 'maximal secretory capacity' of the parathyroid glands and as such should be an indicator of the mass of the parathyroids.[38] Our results from both *in vivo* and *in vitro* experiments demonstrated that PTHrP significantly, and within minutes, enhanced the low Ca^{2+} stimulated 'maximal' PTH secretion by more than additional 300%, in normal, as well as in uremic rats (Fig. 6.4).[37,39] Another example, which illustrates that the so called 'maximal PTH' is not a correct expression for the maximal PTH secretory response, is demonstrated by the doubling of the response by induction of acute metabolic acidosis.[40] As such, these results clearly demonstrate that the level of PTH, which previously has been considered as an expression of the 'maximal secretory capacity' of the parathyroid cells, in fact is not the maximum, but that even the enhanced 'maximal' PTH secretion in uremia can be increased further by several fold. Thus, the maximal PTH response to hypocalcemia in a given patient is not a fixed value, that solely reflects the parathyroid glandular mass; instead the maximal PTH in response to hypocalcemia may vary in a same individual, depending upon a number of factors such as rate of calcium decrease, pH, regulation by paracrine factors and other unknown factors still to be identified.

The 'minimal' secretion of PTH.

It is generally accepted, that PTH secretion can not be totally suppressed even at very high concentrations of Ca^{2+}.[23,41] Not all evidence is, however, in accordance with this point of view and it is a question, whether the non-suppressible secretion of PTH 1–84 exists at all in normal subjects. The observation, that PTH secretion can not be completely suppressed by Ca^{2+} was obtained in *in vivo* studies at a time, when the available assays were co-measuring PTH fragments and later confirmed in *in vitro* studies on cultured parathyroid cells.[19] The non-suppressible secretion of PTH shown in several *in vivo* studies might represent PTH fragments resulting from intraglandular degradation of PTH during the condition of hypercalcemia. More recent studies on uremic patients with parathyroid hyperplasia have, however, shown that hypercalcemia can not totally suppress PTH 1–84 levels.[28,42]

There might be non-parathyroid sources of some of the circulating PTH, such as thymus or hypothalamus where the *PTH* gene is expressed.[43] However, total parathyroidectomy in patients and animals results in almost undetectable levels of PTH. Similarly, in patients with malignancy induced hypercalcemia PTH levels are totally suppressed in most cases. *In vitro* studies are not reliable methods to evaluate maximal PTH inhibition (minimal PTH), since it has been well documented that cultured parathyroid cells loose their Ca^{2+} sensitivity very fast.[18] Thus, loss of calcium responsiveness and non-suppressibility in cultured parathyroid cells might be due to a dramatic drop in the expression of the CaR.

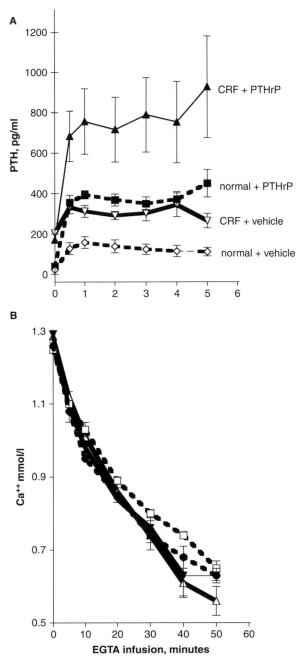

Fig. 6.4 Effect of PTHrP on the secretory response of PTH to an acute induction of hypocalcemia by an EGTA infusion in normal and uremic rats. The rate of reduction of p-Ca^{2+} induced was similar in all groups of rats. A bolus of PTHrP 1–40 or vehicle was injected at time 0. The maximal PTH was significantly increased in uremic rats. PTHrP further significantly enhanced ($p < 0.001$) the low-Ca^{2+} stimulated PTH secretion. Modified from Lewin et al., *Kidney Int* 2003;**64**:63–70.[39]

The interpretation of the minimal level of PTH, which is obtained during suppression of PTH secretion by calcium contributes another controversial aspect to the understanding of the Ca^{2+}/PTH relationship. An enhancement of 'minimal' PTH levels has by several investigators been taken as an expression of increased parathyroid mass.[23,36,44,45] Results from our laboratory,[24] however, in rats with significantly increased parathyroid mass [i.e. with 20 parathyroid glands implanted (a normal rat only has two glands)], clearly showed that PTH secretion can be suppressed to the same low level as that observed in normal rats.[24,44] It is therefore likely that for a given mass of parathyroid tissue maximal suppression of PTH may not be totally dependent on the number of cells, but on their ability to respond to maximal CaR activation. For example, it has been shown that the different parathyroid glands with nodular hyperplasia from the same uremic patient are not equipped with the same amount of CaR. Thus, the maximal inhibition of PTH should not be exactly the same for all of different parts of the parathyroid glands. Presently, we do not have a method to determine to what extent the minimal PTH secretion is related to other factors, beside the number of parathyroid cells.

We conclude, that the Ca^{2+}/PTH concept, beside being influenced by rate and/or direction of changing the Ca^{2+} concentration also might be the result of an interaction between Ca^{2+}, and several autocrine or paracrine factors, and of changes in the metabolism of PTH. It is still an unresolved question, how the regulation of these factors interplay in uremia and how they may affect the curves that are representing the detailed Ca^{2+}/PTH relationship.

The concept of a 'set point' for Ca^{2+} in parathyroids, kidneys, and bone.

The conceptual framework on how plasma calcium is held constant was outlined by Kurokawa.[46] He described a concept, which combined the 'set point' for the calcium flux between extracellular fluid (ECF) and bone, and the 'set point' for renal tubular calcium reabsorption in relation to the 'set point' for the calcium regulated PTH secretion from the parathyroids.[46] The interplay between PTH and $1,25(OH)_2D$ will set the ECF calcium effectively by adjusting the 'set points' in the different organs to the same level of calcium. As such the 'set points' of the calcium regulating tissues correspond to the resulting plasma Ca^{2+} level. This elegant concept is strongly supported by results from studies on the regulation of renal tubular reabsorption of calcium.[46] The site along the nephron where the 'set point' for calcium reabsorption is present and regulated appears to be in the distal nephron segments, where the PTH/PTHrP receptor and the VDR are located, together with the vitamin D inducible calcium-binding protein, calbindin-D_{28K} and CaR.[47]

How and where the calciotropic hormones are setting the 'set point' for calcium between bone and the ECF interphase are less clarified. The existence of such a calcium 'set point' in bone, which is regulated by PTH and $1,25(OH)_2D$, is supported by results from our group,[48] which showed that acute deviations in plasma Ca^{2+} levels were rapidly corrected back to a level determined by the PTH and/or $1,25(OH)_2D$ status. Kurokawa assumes that PTH and $1,25(OH)_2D$, in concert, adjust the 'set point' for calcium by regulating the rate of the coupled bone resorption and formation.[46]

A calcium-sensing mechanism at the quiescent bone surface will represent an attractive model for the rapid minute-to-minute regulation of plasma Ca^{2+}. Despite evidence for an important role of the CaR in recognizing and responding to changes in plasma Ca^{2+} at the level of the parathyroids and kidneys, the evidence for a calcium sensor at the level of bone is largely indirect.[49] The emerging understanding of the parathyroid-kidney-bone axis in the regulation of mineral homeostasis in uremia might further supports the concept of coordinated regulation of calcium set-points.

Phosphate and abnormal PTH synthesis and secretion in CKD

Studies in patients and animals have shown that 2HPT in chronic renal failure is stimulated by dietary phosphate loading and ameliorated by dietary phosphate restriction.[50,51] The effect of phosphate on parathyroid function is both indirect and direct—indirect, through the inhibition of vitamin D synthesis and the induction of hypocalcemia due to a decreased skeletal calcemic response to PTH and the precipitation of calcium; and direct via the direct effect of phosphate on parathyroid function that has been shown in *in vivo* and *in vitro* studies, demonstrating a direct effect on PTH synthesis, secretion and parathyroid cell proliferation.[5–7] The direct effect of phosphate *in vitro* was observed mainly in tissue preparations with intact architecture and not in dispersed parathyroid cells[7] suggesting the importance of a paracrine interaction in between parathyroid cells. Further demonstration of a direct effect of phosphate on PTH secretion was obtained *in vitro* in hyperplastic parathyroid tissue from hemodialysis patients with severe hyperparathyroidism[8] and in *in vivo* studies on hemodialysis patients[52] and dogs.[53]

The direct stimulatory effect of phosphate on PTH secretion is relatively rapid. It was observed after 2 h in the *in vitro* setting (personal observation). Intravenous infusion of sodium phosphate increased PTH within 10 min, whereas infusion of sodium chloride had no effect.[54] A new mechanism of regulation of PTH secretion by phosphate was addressed by the group of Slatopolsky. They showed that oral or intraduodenal phosphate administration increased PTH release rapidly. In uremic rats, adapted to a high phosphate diet, caused a switch to a low phosphate diet an 80% decrease in PTH within the 2-h with no change in plasma calcium, but a 1mg/dL fall in plasma phosphate. In contrast, gavage with a high phosphate diet (HPD) increased PTH by 80% within 15 min, with no change in either plasma phosphate or calcium. These results indicated the existence of an intestinal factor (hormone) that was regulated by the amount of phosphate ingested and that affected the secretion of PTH.[54] Phosphate does not only stimulate PTH secretion, but also its synthesis, thus *in vivo* studies in rats showed that HPD produced an elevation in serum PTH, as well as an increase in PTHmRNA,[55,56] and in hyperplastic parathyroid tissue from hemodialysis patients with severe hyperparathyroidism a high phosphate concentration *in vitro* stimulated both PTH secretion and PTHmRNA, Almaden et al.[8] The mechanisms of PTH mRNA regulation by phosphate was characterized by the group of Silver and Naveh-Many who demonstrated that phosphate regulates the *PTH* gene post-transcriptionally by modulation of the binding of parathyroid cytosolic proteins, trans factors, to a defined cis sequence in the PTH mRNA 3'-untranslated region (UTR), and thereby determining the stability of the PTHmRNA.[57]

Phosphate and parathyroid cell signaling

The effects of phosphate on parathyroid function may be mediated through a specific molecule capable of sensing variations in phosphate levels. The existence of such a sensing mechanism for phosphate still has, however, to be demonstrated. One candidate molecule would be a Na^+-Pi co-transporter, such as rat PiT-1, that has been isolated from rat parathyroids.[58] The amount of PiT-1 mRNA in the parathyroids was much greater in rats fed a LPD than in those fed a HPD, indicating that PiT-1 may contribute to the effects of phosphate on parathyroid function. Thus, it has been proposed that this transporter may function as a putative 'phosphate sensor' for the parathyroid cell.

The signal transduction mechanisms involved in the stimulation of PTH release by low extracellular calcium are increasingly understood; however, little is known about the intracellular signaling system involved in the regulation of PTH secretion by extracellular phosphate. Activation of the G-protein-coupled CaR results in hydrolysis of membrane phospholipids by phospholipase C, phospholipase D, and phospholipase A_2 (PLA_2) generating the appropriate intracellular signals.[59] The activation of PLA_2 leads to the formation of arachidonic acid (AA), a potent inhibitor of PTH release, which acts via the 12- and 15-lipoxygenase pathway.[60] A study by Kifor et al.[61] in bovine parathyroid cells, suggested that activation of CaR mediated the activation of PLA_2 through the MAP kinase cascade (Fig. 6.1). Recently, we have also observed the involvement of the ERK1/2-MAPK in the regulation by calcium of both the PTH secretion and VDR gene expression via PLA_2-AA; the production of AA leads to ERK1/2-MAPK activation (unpublished data). Results from our group showed that high phosphate regulates PTH secretion through the PLA_2-AA signaling system. The results of an *in vitro* study in parathyroid tissue[5] showed that despite the presence of high phosphate in the medium, the addition of exogenous AA to the medium restored the capacity of a high calcium to inhibit PTH secretion. Therefore, addition of AA reversed the stimulatory effect of phosphate on PTH secretion. In a different study,[62] it was demonstrated that the increase in PTH secretion induced by high extracellular phosphate was associated with a decrease in AA production by parathyroid cell. While in the presence of normal phosphate, exogenous PLA_2 decreased PTH secretion a high phosphate concentration prevented the inhibition of PTH secretion by exogenous PLA_2. This inhibitory effect of phosphate on AA production was not observed in another AA-producing tissue, such as rat adrenal glomerulosa tissue. Finally, we showed that in rat parathyroid tissue an increase in intracellular calcium activated PLA_2 resulted in increased AA production.[63] Then, the effect of an elevation of the intracellular calcium on AA production in the presence of high extracellular phosphate levels was evaluated. The results demonstrated that both an ionophore and thapsigargin were capable of inducing a marked increase in AA production, which was associated with a decrease in PTH secretion. These results support the hypothesis that the reduction in AA production induced by high extracellular phosphate is due to an inadequate increase in cytosolic calcium in response to stimulation of CaR by calcium.

Vitamin D and abnormal PTH synthesis and secretion in CKD

Reduced renal $1,25(OH)_2D$ synthesis in CKD is an important factor in the pathogenesis of 2HPT. $1,25(OH)_2D$ acts via VDR in both the parathyroid gland and the intestine. In the intestine, low $1,25(OH)_2D$ levels result in impaired calcium absorption contributing to hypocalcemia and hereby to disturbed parathyroid function.

It is well documented that $1,25(OH)_2D$ in pharmacological doses is an important inhibitor of the *PTH* gene.[16] It reduces the transcription of *PTH* gene.[10,64] It is uncertain whether this is an expression of a physiological role of $1,25(OH)_2D$ in the regulation of parathyroid function and it is also a question, whether the physiological effect of $1,25(OH)_2D$ is directly on the *PTH* gene or mediated mainly via it's calcemic effect. Thus, in VDR deficient mice normal circulating levels of PTH and normal histology of the parathyroids could be maintained, as long as the mice were kept normocalcemic by providing them a special rescue diet,[65] while the control group of untreated VDR deficient mice developed HPT and hyperplasia of the parathyroid glands.[65] It has been found in several investigations[2,24] that circulating $1,25(OH)_2D$ levels are normal in hyperparathyroid uremic models of 5/6 nephrectomized rats. The activity of the sterol might, however, be decreased due to reduced VDR expression in the parathyroid glands.

Reduced VDR expression in the parathyroids

In uremic rat models a reduced VDR mRNA has been shown in the parathyroids[11] and a low expression of VDR protein and mRNA has further been demonstrated in hyperplastic parathyroid glands from uremic patients.[66]

The low levels of plasma Ca^{2+} in CKD might be of importance for the reduced *VDR* gene expression.[67] Brown et al. found that vitamin D-depleted rats, which received a high calcium containing diet, had VDR mRNA levels similar to those of rats on a normal vitamin D containing diet and they suggested that the up-regulation of VDR mRNA in the parathyroid glands by pharmacological doses of $1,25(OH)_2D$ was mainly due to increased plasma calcium levels.[67] This concept has later been supported by results of other *in vitro* studies.[68]

After experimental kidney transplantation of previously uremic, severe hyperparathyroid, rats, it was found that the circulating levels of PTH rapidly became normal, despite low and unchanged expression of the VDR mRNA.[11] This could be due to the rapid normalization of plasma Ca^{2+}, that took place after the transplantation.[24,68] Thus, recent results underline the complexity of the co-ordinated regulation of the function of the parathyroid glands by calcium and $1,25(OH)_2D$.

Vitamin D and parathyroid CaR

Regulation of the *CaR* gene by vitamin D has been suggested by Brown et al.,[69] who found that the expression was affected by the vitamin D nutritional status and, as such, was decreased in rats kept on a vitamin D deficient diet. It was shown in the same study that parathyroid CaR mRNA was up-regulated by pharmacological doses of $1,25(OH)_2D$. Canaff et al.[70] showed that a bolus of $1,25(OH)_2D$ up-regulated CaR mRNA in the rat parathyroids already after 12 h. Furthermore, a functional vitamin D response element has been identified in the *CaR* gene.[70] This provides an understanding of the mechanism, of importance for CKD, by which 1,25(OH)$_2$D is involved in the regulation of the expression of CaR. However, in a model of uremic rats, that were given a standard diet, the *VDR* gene expression in the parathyroids was decreased, while the *CaR* gene expression was normal.[11] Therefore, a link between the activity of 1,25(OH)$_2$D and the expression of the CaR may be of limited physiological significance and may require pharmacological levels of the sterol.

Abnormal PTH synthesis and secretion due to other factors

The parathyroids are not controlled by a superior 'hypothalamic-pituitary axis', as seen in other endocrine glands. Changes in the intracellular and peripheral PTH metabolism might have a significant impact and the parathyroid glands are likely to use autocrine/paracrine regulatory mechanisms, such as chromogranin A (CgA), chromogranin A related peptides and endothelin-1, which all have been suggested as factors that might influence the PTH secretion.[71,72]

Chromogranin A

CgA is an acidic glycoprotein of about 450 amino acids, which together with PTH is a major secretory product of the parathyroid glands. CgA is co-stored and co-secreted with PTH. Fascito et al. showed that CgA strongly inhibited low calcium-stimulated PTH secretion in cultured porcine parathyroid cells, while addition of antisera to CgA potentiated the stimulatory effect of low calcium on PTH secretion.[71]

In the parathyroid cells CgA secretion and gene expression are up-regulated by 1,25(OH)$_2$D,[73] which at the same time down-regulate PTH mRNA. Exposure to high or low calcium has no effect on CgA mRNA.[73] Similarly, in an *in vivo* study on rats the reciprocal regulation of CgA and PTH mRNA's by 1,25(OH)$_2$D was demonstrated and it was further shown that parathyroid CgA mRNA levels were 50% lower in uremic rats, than in sham operated rats, suggesting a pathophysiological relevance of these early *in vitro* observations for 2HPT in CKD.[74]

Chromogranin A-related peptides

CgA might be a prohormone for smaller biologically active peptides that may function as autocrine or paracrine regulators of PTH secretion.[71] Such peptides are pancreastatin and parastatin that *in vitro* inhibit low calcium-stimulated secretion of both PTH and CgA.[71] The physiological importance of these CgA related peptides on PTH secretion and especially in CKD remains to be clarified.

Endothelin-1

Endothelin-1 (ET-1) is a potent vasoconstrictive peptide, that participates in the regulation of growth and function of various endocrine tissues. ET-1 mRNA is synthesized in rat parathyroid epithelial cells and in bovine parathyroid chief cells. Human parathyroid tissue, both adenoma and hyperplasia, expresses prepro-ET-1, and ET_A and ET_B receptor subtypes and ET-1 inhibits PTH secretion in bovine parathyroid cells, coupled dose-dependently to intracellular calcium signaling.[72] The possible physiological effect of ET-1 on PTH synthesis and secretion has, however, not yet been evaluated.

FGF23

The parathyroid cell is a target for a new phosphatonin, FGF23. The co-receptor for the FGF receptor, klotho, is highly expressed in the parathyroid gland, which indicates that FGF23 should have an effect on parathyroid function. Circulating levels of FGF23 are severely increased in uremia. PTH was shown to stimulate FGF23 secretion in a model of primary hyperparathyroidism. Surprisingly, the effect of FGF23 on PTH secretion and biosynthesis was inhibitory. As such there might be a feed-back regulation. The reader is kindly referred to chapter 24 on FGF23 in uremia.

PTH/PTHrP receptor targeting molecules

The PTH/PTH-related peptide (PTHrP) receptor has been demonstrated in human parathyroid tissue by Matsushita et al.[15] and by us in rat parathyroids.[39] This supports the possibility that N-terminal PTH and PTHrP, as ligands for the same receptor, might be involved in the regulation of parathyroid cell function (Fig. 6.5).

A direct inhibitory effect of PTH 1-34 on PTH secretion from bovine parathyroid primary cultured cells was first reported by Fugimi et al.,[75] who suggested, that amino-terminal PTH in the circulation might act *in vivo* as physiological inhibitor of the PTH secretion and thereby exert a negative feedback mechanism on the regulation of PTH secretion. A major difficulty in the interpretation of those results was due to the cross-reactivity of PTH fragments in the PTH assays. We tested the hypothesis in a simple *in vivo* model by reducing parathyroid mass by 50% by acute unilateral PTX and found no sign of a negative feedback regulation of circulating PTH on PTH secretion.[24]

PTH might, however, have a paracrine/autocrine role in higher concentrations at the glandular level and N-terminal PTHrP, used as a surrogate for PTH, was shown to enhance the secretory response of PTH to hypocalcemia by several fold.[37] The direct effect of PTHrP on the parathyroids was further confirmed in *in vitro* experiments on whole rat parathyroid glands.[37] The observation, that the activation of the PTH/PTHrP receptor increases PTH secretion by several fold, but only during hypocalcemia opens up for the possibility of amplification of PTH release by PTH itself, when an increased level is needed.[39] Thus, a model on the existence of a positive auto feedback regulatory mechanism of N-terminal PTH on its own secretion was proposed.[39]

C-terminal PTH fragments

Inomata et al. showed that C-terminal PTH fragments might have an autoregulatory role in the parathyroids[76] and they proposed a novel PTH receptor, not yet cloned, with specificity for the C-terminal region of PTH 1–84. Finally, synthetic hPTH 7–84 has been shown to induce hypocalcemia and to inhibit the PTH 1–84 secretory response to hypocalcemia in rats with intact parathyroid glands.[77]

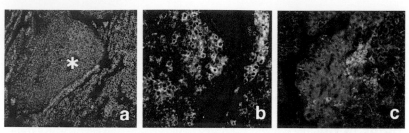

Fig. 6.5 Different parathyroid noduli expressing different proteins. Distribution of PTH and PTHrP in parathyroid hyperplasia secondary to chronic renal failure. Hyperplastic parathyroid tissues were double immunostained for PTH (green fluorescence) and for PTHrP (red fluorescence). The distribution of PTH and PTHrP was heterogeneous in nodular hyperplasia, although each nodule was homogeneously composed of one type of parathyroid cells, entirely PTH-positive cells (a), positive for both PTH and PTHrP (b), or positive only for PTHrP (c). From Matsushita H et al., *Kidney Int* 1999;**55**:130–8.[15]

PTHrP and other cytokines

PTHrP is an important cytokine that is expressed in essentially every tissue and organ at some point in the fetal development or in adult life. PTHrP mRNA is expressed in normal human, bovine, and rat parathyroid tissue,[15] and abnormal expression of PTHrP mRNA and protein has been demonstrated in human parathyroid adenomas, hyperplasia, and carcinomas.[15] PTH and PTHrP are co-localized in the same secretory granules and secreted simultaneously. In severe human parathyroid hyperplasia due to uremia[15] a majority of the glands were positive for PTHrP staining in the diffuse, as well as in the nodular type of hyperplasia and double immunofluorescent-staining for PTH and PTHrP revealed distinct differences in parathyroid nodular hyperplasia, where each nodule homogeneously comprised of one type of parathyroid cells, that were either exclusively PTH positive, exclusively PTHrP positive, or positive for PTH as well as for PTHrP (Fig. 6.5).[15] Our results, which clearly showed a strong stimulatory effect of PTHrP on the secretion of PTH in normal and uremic rats, further support the possibility of an autocrine/paracrine function of PTHrP in the parathyroids.[37]

Pro-inflammatory cytokines, such as interleukin-8 and interleukin-6 have also been shown to affect PTH secretion and PTH mRNA levels. An inhibitory effect of interleukin-1β on PTH secretion was shown in an *in vitro* model of bovine parathyroid tissue slices. The expression of PTHmRNA was unchanged, while an up-regulation of CaR expression was found.[78]

Post-transcriptional modulation of PTH synthesis in CKD

Uremia *per se* enhances the stability of PTH mRNA by a posttranscriptional mechanism that decreases the degradation of RNA, independent of changes in circulating levels of calcium and phosphate,[13] but mediated via cytosolic endonucleases,[79] factors that are selectively decreased in uremia. Hypocalcemic stress in uremia might further influence *PTH* gene expression. The post-transcriptional effect of low calcium on *PTH* gene expression involves protein-RNA interactions at the 3′untranslated region (UTR) of PTHmRNA.[80] The UTR of mRNAs interacts with proteins which determine localization and stability of mRNA. Naveh-Many et al. has shown that the stability of PTH transcript was increased by low extracellular calcium.[80]

Changes in the intracellular and peripheral metabolism of PTH in CKD

The parathyroid glands control the amount of hormone available for secretion by regulating the fraction of PTH that is either exocytosed or degraded. Habener et al.[27] showed that the intracellular degradation of newly synthesized PTH was regulated by the extracellular Ca^{2+} concentration. When bovine glands were incubated in a low calcium medium, almost all of the newly synthesized PTH was secreted as intact PTH. When exposed to a high calcium medium most of the newly synthesized PTH was degraded within the glands. In accordance with this observation, it was demonstrated *in vivo* that PTH secreted into the parathyroid venous blood of calves mainly consisted of hormonal fragments, when hypercalcemia was induced.[27]

Intact PTH is rapidly cleared from the circulation, the disappearance half-time is about 2 min. Clearance from the blood occurs mainly in the liver by 70%, and to a less extend in the kidneys. The Kuppfer cells in the liver are responsible for the rapid, high capacity, and non-saturable uptake of intact PTH and the following extensive proteolysis.[81] The Kuppfer cells also appear to be the source of circulating C-terminal PTH fragments. In contrast, N-terminal fragments are degraded *in situ* and do not re-enter the circulation. Renal clearance of intact PTH occurs by glomerular filtration. The hormone is further reabsorbed and extensively degraded by renal tubules. Quantitatively the kidneys are of paramount importance in removing C-terminal PTH fragments.[82]

There is no evidence for physiologically regulation of the peripheral metabolism of PTH *in vivo* in response to alterations in serum calcium, vitamin D, or parathyroid status.[83] In contrast, in the isolated perfused rat liver model, the clearance of intact PTH was 60% faster at high than at low Ca^{2+}.[84] Daugaard et al. also studied the metabolism of intact PTH in isolated livers obtained from chronic uremic rats, and found no difference in the clearance rate of intact PTH between uremic and normal control livers, releasing equal amounts of C-terminal PTH fragments and no detectable N-terminal fragments.[85]

Despite only 10–20% of secreted intact PTH is converted to circulating C-terminal fragments, these fragments represent 80% of total circulating PTH in normal individuals and up to 95% in renal failure patients. This discrepancy might be explained by a clearance of C-terminal fragments occurring via glomerular filtration in the kidneys that is slower than the hepatic clearance of intact PTH and might further be due to the amount of C-terminal fragments that are secreted by the parathyroid glands. Some circulating C-terminal fragments are large fragments with partially preserved amino-terminal structure. The longest fragment starts at position 4. A peptide starting at position 7 appears as the major component of these non-1–84 PTH fragments.[86] Synthetic hPTH 7–84 has been demonstrated to exert biologic effects, that are opposite to those of PTH 1–84. Parathyroids glands from advanced uremic nodular hyperplasia may overproduce and secrete a novel, biologically active form of PTH with an intact 1-6 region, but a presumably modified 12–18 region.[87]

Hyperplasia of parathyroid glands in CKD

Parathyroid tissue is a discontinuous replicator tissue, which is characterized by a low cell turnover, a low rate of mitosis, and no separate stem cells.[1] As estimated by Parfitt the mean life span of normal parathyroid cell is 20 years in humans and 2 years in rats.[1,88] Mitosis can be stimulated by functional demand. In human subjects parathyroid growth progresses in response to chronic renal failure through several stages from diffuse hyperplasia to different patterns of nodular hyperplasia.[1] Diffuse hyperplasia is probably initiated by hypocalcemia and phosphorus retention and becomes more severe as the result of calcitriol deficiency.[89] The next stage is that hyperplasia becomes nodular (Fig. 6.6). The nodules are encapsulated and consist of cells that are closely packed, free of fat and with an increased prevalence of mitosis and depletion of VDR and CaR.[4,90] Similarity exists in the gene expression between the cells in each nodule, while differences are found between nodules.[15,90] Monoclonal growth of the parathyroid cells has been demonstrated in a majority of the uremic patients with refractory hyperparathyroidism.[91] The genes responsible for monoclonality have not been identified. Apparently, somatic mutations confer a growth advantage to clones of parathyroid cells, which are causing monoclonal growth and nodular parathyroid hyperplasia, although these two phenomena are not strictly linked. The next stage is uninodular hyperplasia and emergence of a large adenoma-like nodulus, as an expression of a mutation in one of the cells that are undergoing the most rapid proliferation. In some cases there is a loss of a tumor suppressor gene on chromosome 11, a molecular defect with the potential for disrupting the control of the cell cycle.[92] Malignant transformation leading to parathyroid carcinoma is not common. It seems that at the initial stages development of parathyroid hyperplasia is a regulatory phenomenon, but that it during the progression escapes from normal growth control. The main factors responsible for parathyroid hyperplasia appear to be the same as those responsible for the enhanced PTH biosynthesis and secretion.[1]

The precise role of the disturbances in calcium, phosphorus and calcitriol levels for the development of abnormal parathyroid growth in uremia, as well as the precise role of these factors in the regulation of normal parathyroid growth have not been well established.[93] A decrease in the expressions of CaR and VDR as described in the parathyroid glands of uremic rats[11,18] and chronic dialysis patients,[4] should theoretically enhance parathyroid cell proliferation. This was proven indirectly by the observation that administration of a calcium-sensing receptor agonists or calcitriol led to the inhibition of parathyroid cell proliferation in uremic rats.[94,95] It remains, however, unclear, what molecular mechanisms that are involved in the CaR regulated parathyroid cell proliferation in uremia. It is furthermore not quite clear, whether down-regulated

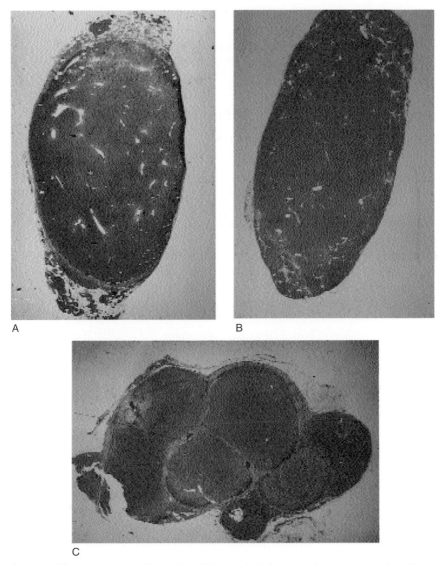

Fig. 6.6 Different patterns of parathyroid hyperplasia in secondary hyperparathyroidism. Macroscopical cross-sectional aspects of diffuse hyperplasia (a), uninodular hyperplasia (b), and multinodular hyperplasia (c) in parathyroid glands removed from dialysis patients with severe secondary hyperparathyroidism.

expression of CaR is inducing proliferation or whether increased proliferation is inducing down regulation of CaR. Recent studies might indicate that proliferation of the parathyroid gland may precede the down regulation of the CaR.[96] *In vitro* studies were unable to demonstrate any effect of low calcium on proliferation of human parathyroid cells in long-term culture system.[97]

The role of phosphorus accumulation on parathyroid cell growth is well documented in several studies in uremic rats where it also has been shown that early dietary phosphate restriction prevented parathyroid cell proliferation and development of 2HPT.[6,50,98] Furthermore, hyperphosphatemia-induced parathyroid cell proliferation, even when changes in plasma calcium and calcitriol were avoided, pointed towards a direct effect of phosphorus on cell proliferation,[1] which was confirmed *in vitro*.[97] The precise molecular mechanism involved in the parathyroid hyperplasia is sparsely clarified.

The expression of cyclin-dependent kinase inhibitors, p21 and p27, were examined in hyperplastic parathyroid glands from uremic patients.[99] The expression was reduced in a manner dependent upon VDR expression and it was significantly less in nodular hyperplasia than in diffuse hyperplasia. In uremic rats dietary phosphate restriction prevented parathyroid hyperplasia by inducing the cell cycle inhibitor p21.

An enhanced expression of transforming growth factor-α (TGF-α), known to promote cell growth, has been found in parathyroid hyperplasia in uremia.[100,101] The enhanced expression of both TGF-α and its receptor, the epidermal growth factor receptor (EGFR), was demonstrated early after onset of uremia in rats, and clearly aggravated by high phosphorus or low calcium diets.[100] The enhanced expression of TGF-α in the uremic parathyroid glands lead to its own up-regulation, generating a feed-forward loop for activation of EGFR. Parathyroid growth arrest induced by phosphate restriction, high dietary Ca, or prophylactic calcitriol administration induced a decrease in parathyroid TGF-α. Suppression of activation of the EGFR by erlotinib, a potent and specific EGFR-tyrosine kinase inhibitor, arrested not only parathyroid growth, but also TGF-α upregulation and the reduction of VDR expression.[102] Recently, activator protein 2α (AP2), an inducer of TGF-α gene transcription, was shown to mediate parathyroid TGF-α self-induction in uremic rats. In human hyperplastic parathyroid glands AP2 expression correlated directly with TGF-α expression and cell proliferation as estimated by PCNA expression.[102]

A role of ET-1 in parathyroid hyperplasia has been suggested. In hypocalcemic rats, cell proliferation and ET-1 immunoreactivity increased in parallel in the parathyroid cells, an effect that could be blocked by an ET-1 receptor antagonist. In uremic rats on a standard diet, developing 2HPT, did treatment with an ET-1 receptor antagonist, bosentan, resulted in a reduced increase in parathyroid gland weight and in reduction of ET-1 expression. In contrast, bosentan did not reduce parathyroid cell proliferation or parathyroid gland weight in uremic rats on a high phosphorus diet.[103]

PTHrP exhibits biological similarities to transforming growth factor-ß (TGF-ß) and may have effects on cell growth or differentiation. The proliferative activity of the parathyroid cells, as evaluated by the expression of PCNA, correlated negatively with the expression of PTHrP in human parathyroid hyperplasia. Therefore, an inhibitory effect of PTHrP on parathyroid cell proliferation has been postulated.[15]

Parathyroid function and VDR polymorphisms

Allelic polymorphisms in intron 8 (B/b and A/a alleles), exon 9 (T/t alleles), and in the translation start codon (F/f alleles) of the *VDR* gene have been associated with peak bone mass and bone loss, and a possible association between VDR polymorphisms and parathyroid function has been searched for in patients with primary and secondary HPT. In hemodialysis patients the BB genotype and the B allele were significantly more frequent in those with low PTH than high PTH, suggesting that VDR gene polymorphism might influence parathyroid function in chronic renal failure. HD patients with BB genotype responded to calcitriol administration with a significant decrease in PTH, whereas the bb did not.[104] A relationship between Apa I polymorphism (A/a alleles) and the severity of HPT has also been examined in Japanese hemodialysis patients.[105] In chronic renal failure patients serum PTH was significantly higher in the FF genotype than Ff and ff groups. Several studies have evaluated the loss of bone mass after renal transplantation and found that VDR polymorphism was related to bone density.[106] Nevertheless, although VDR polymorphism in some clinical conditions may be associated with variations of the half life of the VDR gene transcript or of VDR function,[107] no report has so far showed that the density of parathyroid cell VDR in uremic patients with 2HPT varies with the different VDR genotypes. Although VDR genotypes may have some influence on the degree of secondary parathyroid hyperplasia, the mechanism by which this may occur remains unknown.

Control of increased parathyroid mass

In the management of 2HPT it is of great importance to prevent the development of non-suppressible and non-reversible changes in the parathyroid glands. In CKD patients it is necessary to accept a certain degree of 2HPT, as enhanced PTH levels early in uremia have important homeostatic functions by stimulating the 1α-hydroxylase activity and by increasing the renal phosphorus excretion. In more advanced uremia, the development of adynamic bone disease should be avoided and, therefore, also in this condition it is necessary to accept some degree of 2HPT. Thus, 2HPT should be controlled at a level that permits normal bone turnover.

The important observation from several experimental studies on 2HPT is that the increased proliferation of parathyroid cells, induced by uremia, can be arrested again. Administration of CaR agonists (calcimimetics), calcitriol, or low phosphorus diet led to the suppression of parathyroid cell proliferation in uremic rats.[94,95,100,108] This opens a possibility for controlling the degree or severity of the increase in parathyroid mass in uremia. Furthermore, it has been shown that PTH secretion from increased parathyroid mass could be controlled, according to the 'functional demand' (Fig. 6.7). In two models of parathyroid hyperplasia, 20 normal isogenic parathyroid glands or eight isogenic parathyroid glands from uremic rats were implanted into one normal recipient rat after removal of its own two parathyroid glands.[24] Within 2 weeks plasma calcium became normal and remained so. PTH levels became normal from the third day after implantation of the parathyroid glands and remained normal.[24] Subsequently, parathyroid function was examined and normal suppressibility of PTH secretion by calcium was demonstrated in the rats with 20 parathyroid glands implanted (10 times increased parathyroid mass).[24]

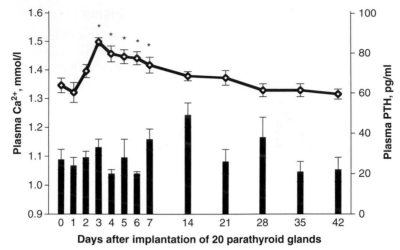

Fig. 6.7 PTH secretion depends primarily upon the functional demand. Despite a 10 times increase in parathyroid mass normal PTH and Ca^{2+} levels are obtained. Plasma Ca^{2+} and plasma PTH levels in rats with 20 isogenic parathyroid glands implanted are shown. PTX of their own parathyroid glands was performed on day 0, before the implantation of 20 glands. The line depicts plasma Ca^{2+} levels, while the bars depict PTH levels. Modified from Lewin et al., *Kidney Int* 1997;**52**:1232–41.[24]

In another model,[24] severe 2HPT, due to long-term uremia and associated with hypocalcemia and hyperphosphatemia, was reversible very fast after reversal of uremia by an experimental, isogenic kidney transplantation. The circulating levels of PTH became normal very early, within one week after normalization of GFR, plasma calcium, and plasma phosphorus levels (Fig. 6.8). The precise mechanism behind this rapid reversal of 2HPT after normalization of GFR is not completely clear. A reduction of CaR and VDR mRNA was demonstrated in parathyroid glands obtained from uremic rats with severe 2HPT. The dramatic decrease of PTH secretion, which took place after reversal of uremia, occurred, however, with unchanged and significantly diminished expression of *CaR* and *VDR* genes in the parathyroid glands.[11,44] In uremic rats on a high phosphorus diet the circulating levels of PTH increased 20 times and CaR mRNA levels decreased by 60%. One week after kidney transplantation PTH levels became normal, despite low remaining expression of CaR mRNA, similar to levels in the uremic rats. Surprisingly, normalization of circulating PTH levels after transplantation was not associated with normalization of the parathyroid *CaR* gene expression. This might indicate the existence of a secretory mechanism in the parathyroid cells, that is not coupled to CaR, and which responds to reversal of uremia or to the simultaneous normalization of plasma Ca^{2+} and phosphorus levels. In uremic hyperphosphatemic rats high plasma calcium did not suppress PTH secretion to the same extent as seen in normal and uremic normophosphatemic rats. Three weeks after an experimental kidney transplantation normal suppressibility by calcium of

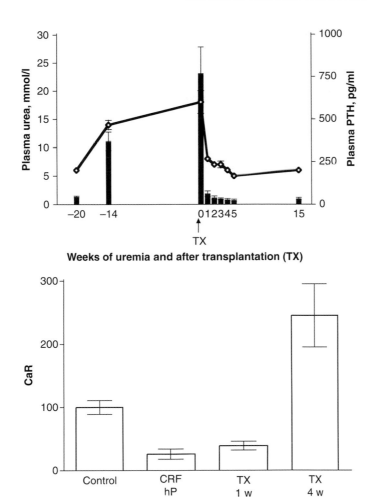

Fig. 6.8 Rapid normalization of PTH levels after reversal of uremia despite persistent increased mass of the parathyroid glands and significantly suppressed CaR mRNA. Kidney function and basal PTH levels are shown before introduction of uremia by 5/6 nephrectomy (–20 weeks), during uremia (–20 weeks to 0 weeks), and after reversal of uremia by an isogenic kidney transplantation (TX). The line depicts kidney function expressed as plasma urea, and the bars depict PTH levels in this model of severe secondary hyperparathyroidism in uremic rats on a high P diet. The dramatic decrease of PTH secretion, which took place 1 week after reversal of uremia, occurred with unchanged and significantly diminished expression of CaR gene in the parathyroid glands. Up-regulation of *CaR* gene was first detected at 4 weeks after kidney transplantation. Modified from Lewin et al., *Kidney Int* 1997;**52**:1232–41.[24]

PTH secretion was, however, restored and 4 weeks after the experimental kidney transplantation was the parathyroid *CaR* gene expression up-regulated.[44]

Support for the existence of a strong secretory regulation, which is independent of the level of expression of the parathyroid CaR, can be deduced from results by Takahashi et al.[109] They showed in uremic rats on a high phosphorus diet that PTH levels decreased, despite remaining high content of PTH in the parathyroid cell secretory granules, when the same uremic rats had the phosphorus content of their diet switched to low phosphorus. The expression of parathyroid CaR was low in the same model of uremic rats and remained low immediately after reducing the phosphorus content in the diet[110]. The time course of an upregulation of the CaR gene expression was rather slow, between one week[110] and 4 weeks [44]. These results clearly demonstrate that even considerable parathyroid hyperplasia can be controlled, when the 'functional demand' for increased PTH levels is abolished by normalization of GFR, plasma calcium, and phosphorus levels.

Parathyroid tissue apoptosis and necrosis

An important question is, whether regression of parathyroid hyperplasia can be induced. Can the increased glandular mass—during uremia—again be reduced? Such a reduction would call for massive apoptosis to take place in the parathyroids. This question has not yet been solved. Examination for apoptosis in the parathyroids is not an easy task.[1] The parathyroids have an extremely low cell turnover and, therefore, probably a poorly developed program for cell deletion. The number of apoptotic cells in normal human parathyroids is very low, 1/10000 parathyroid cells.[111] In rat models several research groups have been unable to find evidence of a programmed parathyroid cell death in normal and hyperplastic parathyroid tissue.[88,112] Experimental studies document that parathyroid hyperplasia can easily be prevented, but is poorly reversible,[94] or that reversal by apoptosis at least must be an extremely slow process.[88] There are no known stimuli for apoptosis in the parathyroid cell,[1] although vitamin D still is not completely excluded.[113,114] Evidence for induction of massive apoptosis by calcitriol is indirect and uncertain. Thus, Fukagawa et al.[113] found in patients on long-term dialysis that oral calcitriol pulse therapy induced a 40% reduction of the parathyroid volume, as measured by ultrasound. Already in 1977 Henry et al.[114] studied parathyroid glands of 3-month-old vitamin D deficient chicken that received vitamin D replacement and found evidence for a significant reduction in the number of parathyroid cells, based upon a reduction in glandular weight and similar reductions in protein and DNA content.[114] The changes were detectable already within 4 days and could have resulted from apoptosis only. Not all studies have, however, found similar positive results.[94,115] When the process of apoptosis was assessed directly by the TUNEL method or by the detection of DNA fragmentation,[116] no apoptosis of the parathyroids was induced in uremic rats, even by extreme high doses of calcitriol. *In vitro*, however, calcitriol has been shown to inhibit both parathyroid cells apoptosis and proliferation[117] and, more recently, Colloton et al.[95] showed that administration of cinacalcet to uremic rats significantly reduced parathyroid weight, although no apoptotic cells were found at the end of the study.

Summary

The abnormal function of the parathyroid glands in CKD is resulting in increased PTH biosynthesis and secretion and parathyroid cell hyperplasia. At the molecular level development of 2HPT is related to changes in CaR and VDR signaling and disturbances in the regulation of PTH mRNA. Other factors of importance for the regulation of parathyroid function and cell proliferation include some of autocrine or paracrine nature. The expression of all these factors is influenced by CKD. As such, hyperparathyroidism associated with chronic uremia results from a combination of functional and structural changes in the parathyroid glands.

References

1. Drueke TB. Cell biology of parathyroid gland hyperplasia in chronic renal failure. *J Am Soc Nephrol* 2000;**11**:1141–52.

2. Silver J, Kilav R, Naveh-Many T. Mechanisms of secondary hyperparathyroidism. *Am J Physiol Renal Physiol* 2002;**283**:F367–76.

3. Brown EM, Gamba G, Riccardi D, et al. Cloning and characterisation of an extracellular Ca(2+)-sensing receptor from bovine parathyroid. *Nature* 1993;**366**:575–80.

4. Gogusev J, Duchambon P, Hory B, et al. Depressed expression of calcium receptor in parathyroid gland tissue of patients with hyperparathyroidism. *Kidney Int* 1997;**51**:328–36.

5. Almaden Y, Canalejo A, Hernandez A, et al. Direct effect of phosphorus on PTH secretion from whole rat parathyroid glands *in vitro*. *J Bone Miner Res* 1996;**11**:970–6.

6. Slatopolsky E, Finch J, Denda M, et al. Phosphorus restriction prevents parathyroid gland growth. High phosphorus directly stimulates PTH secretion *in vitro*. *J Clin Invest* 1996;**97**:2534–40.

7. Nielsen PK, Feldt-Rasmussen U, Olgaard K. A direct effect *in vitro* of phosphate on PTH release from bovine parathyroid tissue slices but not from dispersed parathyroid cells. *Nephrol Dial Transplant* 1996;**11**:1762–8.

8. Almaden Y, Hernandez A, Torregrosa V, et al. High phosphate level directly stimulates parathyroid hormone secretion and synthesis by human parathyroid tissue *in vitro*. *J Am Soc Nephrol* 1998;**9**:1845–52.

9. Naveh-Many T, Marx R, Keshet E, Pike JW, Silver J. Regulation of 1,25-dihydroxyvitamin D3 receptor gene expression by 1,25-dihydroxyvitamin D3 in the parathyroid *in vivo*. *J Clin Invest* 1990;**86**:1968–75.

10. Demay MB, Kiernan MS, DeLuca HF, Kronenberg HM. Sequences in the human parathyroid hormone gene that bind the 1,25-dihydroxyvitamin D3 receptor and mediate transcriptional repression in response to 1,25-dihydroxyvitamin D3. *Proc Natl Acad Sci USA* 1992;**89**:8097–101.

11. Lewin E, Garfia B, Recio FL, Rodriguez M, Olgaard K. Persistent down regulation of calcium-sensing receptor mRNA in rat parathyroids when severe secondary hyperparathyroidism is reversed by an isogenic kidney transplantation. *J Am Soc Nephrol 1* 2002;**3**:2110–16.

12. Korkor AB. Reduced binding of [3H]1,25-dihydroxyvitamin D3 in the parathyroid glands of patients with renal failure. *N Engl J Med* 1987;**316**:1573–7.

13. Yalcindag C, Silver J, Naveh-Many T. Mechanism of increased parathyroid hormone mRNA in experimental uremia: roles of protein RNA binding and RNA degradation. *J Am Soc Nephrol* 1999;**10**:2562–8.

14. Gunther T, Chen ZF, Kim J, et al. Genetic ablation of parathyroid glands reveals another source of parathyroid hormone. *Nature* 2000;**406:**199–203.

15. Matsushita H, Hara M, Endo Y, et al. Proliferation of parathyroid cells negatively correlates with expression of parathyroid hormone-related protein in secondary parathyroid hyperplasia. *Kidney Int* 1999;**55:**130–8.

16. Silver J, Russell J, Sherwood LM. Regulation by vitamin D metabolites of messenger ribonucleic acid for preproparathyroid hormone in isolated bovine parathyroid cells. *Proc Natl Acad Sci USA* 1985;**82:**4270–3.

17. Kifor O, Kifor I, Brown EM: Signal transduction in the parathyroid. *Curr Opin Nephrol Hypertens* 2002;**11:**397–402.

18. Brown AJ, Zhong M, Ritter C, Brown EM, Slatopolsky E. Loss of calcium responsiveness in cultured bovine parathyroid cells is associated with decreased calcium receptor expression. *Biochem Biophys Res Commun* 1995;**212:**861–7.

19. Brown EM, Wilson RE, Eastman RC, Pallotta J, Marynick SP. Abnormal regulation of parathyroid hormone release by calcium in secondary hyperparathyroidism due to chronic renal failure. *J Clin Endocrinol Metab* 1982;**54:**172–9.

20. Canadillas S, Canalejo A, Santamaria R, et al. Calcium-sensing receptor expression and parathyroid hormone secretion in hyperplastic parathyroid glands from humans. *J Am Soc Nephrol* 2005;**16:**2190–7.

21. Brown AJ, Ritter CS, Finch JL, Slatopolsky EA. Decreased calcium-sensing receptor expression in hyperplastic parathyroid glands of uremic rats: role of dietary phosphate. *Kidney Int* 1999;**55:**1284–92.

22. Brown EM. Four-parameter model of the sigmoidal relationship between parathyroid hormone release and extracellular calcium concentration in normal and abnormal parathyroid tissue. *J Clin Endocrinol Metab* 1983;**56:**572–81.

23. Lewin E, Nielsen PK, Olgaard K. The calcium/parathyroid hormone concept of the parathyroid glands. *Curr Opin Nephrol Hypertens* 1995;**4:**324–33.

24. Lewin E, Wang W, Olgaard K. Reversibility of experimental secondary hyperparathyroidism. *Kidney Int* 1997;**52:**1232–41.

25. Felsenfeld AJ, Rodriguez M, Aguilera-Tejero E. Dynamics of parathyroid hormone secretion in health and secondary hyperparathyroidism. *Clin J Am Soc Nephrol* 2007;**2:**1283–305.

26. Cardinal H, Brossard JH, Roy L, Lepage R, Rousseau L, D'Amour P. The set point of parathyroid hormone stimulation by calcium is normal in progressive renal failure. *J Clin Endocrinol Metab* 1998;**83:**3839–44.

27. Habener JF, Rosenblatt M, Potts JT, Jr. Parathyroid hormone: biochemical aspects of biosynthesis, secretion, action, and metabolism. *Physiol Rev* 1984;**64:**985–1053.

28. Santamaria R, Almaden Y, Felsenfeld A, et al. Dynamics of PTH secretion in hemodialysis patients as determined by the intact and whole PTH assays. *Kidney Int* 2003;**64:**1867–73.

29. Ritchie CK, Cohn DV, Maercklein PB, Fitzpatrick LA. Individual parathyroid cells exhibit cyclic secretion of parathyroid hormone and chromogranin-A (as measured by a novel sequential hemolytic plaque assay). *Endocrinology* 1992;**131:**2638–42.

30. Sun F, Ritchie CK, Hassager C, Maercklein P, Fitzpatrick LA. Heterogeneous response to calcium by individual parathyroid cells. *J Clin Invest* 1993;**91:**595–601.

31. Conlin PR, Fajtova VT, Mortensen RM, Leboff MS, Brown EM. Hysteresis in the relationship between serum ionized calcium and intact parathyroid hormone during

recovery from induced hyper- and hypocalcemia in normal humans. *J Clin Endocrinol Metab* 1989;**69:**593–9.

32. Felsenfeld AJ, Ross D, Rodriguez M. Hysteresis of the parathyroid hormone response to hypocalcemia in hemodialysis patients with low turnover aluminum bone disease. *J Am Soc Nephrol* 1991;**2:**1136–43.

33. Estepa JC, Aguilera-Tejero E, Almaden Y, Rodriguez M, Felsenfeld AJ. Effect of rate of calcium reduction and a hypocalcemic clamp on parathyroid hormone secretion: a study in dogs. *Kidney Int* 1999;**55:**1724–33.

34. Grant FD, Conlin PR, Brown EM. Rate and concentration dependence of parathyroid hormone dynamics during stepwise changes in serum ionized calcium in normal humans. *J Clin Endocrinol Metab* 1990;**71:**370–8.

35. Kwan JT, Beer JC, Noonan K, Cunningham J. Parathyroid sensing of the direction of change of calcium in uremia. *Kidney Int* 1993;**43:**1104–9.

36. McCarron DA, Muther RS, Lenfesty B, Bennett WM. Parathyroid function in persistent hyperparathyroidism: relationship to gland size. *Kidney Int* 1982;**22:**662–70.

37. Lewin E, Almaden Y, Rodriguez M, Olgaard K. PTHrP enhances the secretory response of PTH to a hypocalcemic stimulus in rat parathyroid glands. *Kidney Int* 2000;**58:**71–81.

38. Ramirez JA, Goodman WG, Gornbein J, et al. Direct *in vivo* comparison of calcium-regulated parathyroid hormone secretion in normal volunteers and patients with secondary hyperparathyroidism. *J Clin Endocrinol Metab* 1993;**76:**1489–94.

39. Lewin E, Garfia B, Almaden Y, Rodriguez M, Olgaard K. Autoregulation in the parathyroid glands by PTH/PTHrP receptor ligands in normal and uremic rats. *Kidney Int* 2003;**64:**63–70.

40. Lopez I, Aguilera-Tejero E, Felsenfeld AJ, Estepa JC, Rodriguez M. Direct effect of acute metabolic and respiratory acidosis on parathyroid hormone secretion in the dog. *J Bone Miner Res* 2002;**17:**1691–700.

41. Brown EM. Mechanisms underlying the regulation of parathyroid hormone secretion *in vivo* and *in vitro*. *Curr Opin Nephrol Hypertens* 1993;**2:**541–51.

42. Valle C, Rodriguez M, Santamaria R, et al. Cinacalcet reduces the set point of the PTH-calcium curve. *J Am Soc Nephrol* 2008;**19:**2430–6.

43. Fraser RA, Kronenberg HM, Pang PK, Harvey S. Parathyroid hormone messenger ribonucleic acid in the rat hypothalamus. *Endocrinology* 1990;**127:**2517–22.

44. Lewin E, Olgaard K. Influence of parathyroid mass on the regulation of PTH secretion. *Kidney Int* 2006;Suppl. S16–21.

45. Indridason OS, Heath H, III, Khosla S, Yohay DA, Quarles LD. Non-suppressible parathyroid hormone secretion is related to gland size in uremic secondary hyperparathyroidism. *Kidney Int* 1996;**50:**1663–71.

46. Kurokawa K. How is plasma calcium held constant? Milieu interieur of calcium. *Kidney Int* 1996;**49:**1760–4.

47. Hemmingsen C, Staun M, Lewin E, Nielsen PK, Olgaard K. Effect of parathyroid hormone on renal calbindin-D28k. *J Bone Miner Res* 1996;**11:**1086–93.

48. Wang W, Lewin E, Olgaard K. 1,25(OH)2D3 only affects long-term levels of plasma Ca2+ but not the rapid minute-to-minute plasma Ca2+ homeostasis in the rat. *Steroids* 1999;**64:**726–34.

49. Huan J, Martuseviciene G, Olgaard K, Lewin E. Calcium-sensing receptor and recovery from hypocalcemia in thyroparathyroidectomised rats. *Eur J Clin Invest* 2007;**37:**214–21.

50. Slatopolsky E, Caglar S, Gradowska L, Canterbury J, Reiss E, Bricker NS. On the prevention of secondary hyperparathyroidism in experimental chronic renal disease using 'proportional reduction' of dietary phosphorus intake. *Kidney Int* 1972;**2**:147–51.

51. Lopez-Hilker S, Dusso AS, Rapp NS, Martin KJ, Slatopolsky E. Phosphorus restriction reverses hyperparathyroidism in uremia independent of changes in calcium and calcitriol. *Am J Physiol* 1990;**259**:F432–7.

52. de Francisco AL, Cobo MA, Setien MA, et al. Effect of serum phosphate on parathyroid hormone secretion during hemodialysis. *Kidney Int* 1998;**54**:2140–5.

53. Estepa JC, Aguilera-Tejero E, Lopez I, Almaden Y, Rodriguez M, Felsenfeld AJ. Effect of phosphate on parathyroid hormone secretion *in vivo*. *J Bone Miner Res* 1999;**14**:1848–54.

54. Martin DR, Ritter CS, Slatopolsky E, Brown AJ. Acute regulation of parathyroid hormone by dietary phosphate. *Am J Physiol Endocrinol Metab* 2005;**289**:E729–34.

55. Hernandez A, Concepcion MT, Rodriguez M, Salido E, Torres A. High phosphorus diet increases preproPTH mRNA independent of calcium and calcitriol in normal rats. *Kidney Int* 1996;**50**:1872–8.

56. Kilav R, Silver J, Naveh-Many T. Parathyroid hormone gene expression in hypophosphatemic rats. *J Clin Invest* 1995;**96**:327–33.

57. Kilav R, Silver J, Naveh-Many T. A conserved cis-acting element in the parathyroid hormone 3'-untranslated region is sufficient for regulation of RNA stability by calcium and phosphate. *J Biol Chem* 2001;**276**:8727–33.

58. Tatsumi S, Segawa H, Morita K, et al. Molecular cloning and hormonal regulation of PiT-1, a sodium-dependent phosphate cotransporter from rat parathyroid glands. *Endocrinology* 1998;**139**:1692–9.

59. Kifor O, Diaz R, Butters R, Brown EM. The Ca2+-sensing receptor (CaR) activates phospholipases C, A2, and D in bovine parathyroid and CaR-transfected, human embryonic kidney (HEK293) cells. *J Bone Miner Res* 1997;**12**:715–25.

60. Bourdeau A, Moutahir M, Souberbielle JC, et al. Effects of lipoxygenase products of arachidonate metabolism on parathyroid hormone secretion. *Endocrinology* 1994;**135**:1109–12.

61. Kifor O, MacLeod RJ, Diaz R, et al. Regulation of MAP kinase by calcium-sensing receptor in bovine parathyroid and CaR-transfected HEK293 cells. *Am J Physiol Renal Physiol* 2001;**280**:F291–302.

62. Almaden Y, Canalejo A, Ballesteros E, Anon G, Rodriguez M. Effect of high extracellular phosphate concentration on arachidonic acid production by parathyroid tissue *in vitro*. *J Am Soc Nephrol* 2000;**11**:1712–18.

63. Almaden Y, Canalejo A, Ballesteros E, et al. Regulation of arachidonic acid production by intracellular calcium in parathyroid cells: effect of extracellular phosphate. *J Am Soc Nephrol* 2002;**13**:693–8.

64. Silver J, Yalcindag C, Sela-Brown A, Kilav R, Naveh-Many T. Regulation of the parathyroid hormone gene by vitamin D, calcium and phosphate. *Kidney Int* 1999;Suppl 73:S2–7.

65. Li YC, Amling M, Pirro AE, et al. Normalisation of mineral ion homeostasis by dietary means prevents hyperparathyroidism, rickets, and osteomalacia, but not alopecia in vitamin D receptor-ablated mice. *Endocrinology* 1998;**139**:4391–6.

66. Carling T, Rastad J, Szabo E, Westin G, Akerstrom G. Reduced parathyroid vitamin D receptor messenger ribonucleic acid levels in primary and secondary hyperparathyroidism. *J Clin Endocrinol Metab* 2000;**85**:2000–3.

67. Brown AJ, Zhong M, Finch J, Ritter C, Slatopolsky E. The roles of calcium and 1,25-dihydroxyvitamin D3 in the regulation of vitamin D receptor expression by rat parathyroid glands. *Endocrinology* 1995;**136**:1419–25.

68. Garfia B, Canadillas S, Canalejo A, et al. Regulation of parathyroid vitamin D receptor expression by extracellular calcium. *J Am Soc Nephrol* 2002;**13**:2945–52.

69. Brown AJ, Zhong M, Finch J, et al. Rat calcium-sensing receptor is regulated by vitamin D but not by calcium. *Am J Physiol* 1996;**270**:F454–60.

70. Canaff L, Hendy GN. Human calcium-sensing receptor gene. Vitamin D response elements in promoters P1 and P2 confer transcriptional responsiveness to 1,25-dihydroxyvitamin D. *J Biol Chem* 2002;**277**:30337–50.

71. Fasciotto BH, Denny JC, Grecley Jr GH, Cohn DV. Processing of chromogranin A in the parathyroid: generation of parastatin-related peptides. *Peptides* 2000;**21**:1389–401.

72. Kanesaka Y, Tokunaga H, Iwashita K, Fujimura S, Naomi S, Tomita K. Endothelin receptor antagonist prevents parathyroid cell proliferation of low calcium diet-induced hyperparathyroidism in rats. *Endocrinology* 2001;**142**:407–13.

73. Russell J, Lettieri D, Adler J, Sherwood LM. 1,25-Dihydroxyvitamin D3 has opposite effects on the expression of parathyroid secretory protein and parathyroid hormone genes. *Mol Endocrinol* 1990;**4**:505–9.

74. Soliman E, Canaff L, Fox J, Hendy GN. *In vivo* regulation of chromogranin A messenger ribonucleic acid in the parathyroid by 1,25-dihydroxyvitamin D: studies in normal rats and in chronic renal insufficiency. *Endocrinology* 1997;**138**:2596–600.

75. Fujimi T, Baba H, Fukase M, Fujita T. Direct inhibitory effect of amino-terminal parathyroid hormone fragment [PTH(1-34)] on PTH secretion from bovine parathyroid primary cultured cells *in vitro*. *Biochem Biophys Res Commun* 1991;**178**:953–8.

76. Inomata N, Akiyama M, Kubota N, Juppner H. Characterisation of a novel parathyroid hormone (PTH) receptor with specificity for the carboxyl-terminal region of PTH-(1–84). *Endocrinology* 1995;**136**:4732–40.

77. Huan J, Olgaard K, Nielsen LB, Lewin E. Parathyroid hormone 7-84 induces hypocalcemia and inhibits the parathyroid hormone 1–84 secretory response to hypocalcemia in rats with intact parathyroid glands. *J Am Soc Nephrol* 2006;**17**:1923–30.

78. Nielsen PK, Rasmussen AK, Butters R, ct al. Inhibition of PTH secretion by interleukin-1 beta in bovine parathyroid glands in vitro is associated with an up-regulation of the calcium-sensing receptor mRNA. *Biochem Biophys Res Commun* 1997;**238**:880–5.

79. Kilav R, Silver J, Naveh-Many T. A conserved cis-acting element in the parathyroid hormone 3'-untranslated region is sufficient for regulation of RNA stability by calcium and phosphate. *J Biol Chem* 2001;**276**:8727–33.

80. Naveh-Many T, Silver J. Regulation of parathyroid hormone gene expression by hypocalcemia, hypercalcemia, and vitamin D in the rat. *J Clin Invest* 1990;**86**:1313–19.

81. Bringhurst FR, Segre GV, Lampman GW, Potts JT, Jr. Metabolism of parathyroid hormone by Kupffer cells: analysis by reverse-phase high-performance liquid chromatography. *Biochemistry* 1982;**21**:4252–8.

82. Segre GV, D'Amour P, Hultman A, Potts JT, Jr. Effects of hepatectomy, nephrectomy, and nephrectomy/uremia on the metabolism of parathyroid hormone in the rat. *J Clin Invest* 1981;**67**:439–48.

83. Bringhurst FR, Stern AM, Yotts M, Mizrahi N, Segre GV, Potts JT, Jr. Peripheral metabolism of [35S]parathyroid hormone *in vivo*: influence of alterations in calcium availability and parathyroid status. *J Endocrinol* 1989;**122**:237–45.

84. Daugaard H, Egfjord M, Olgaard K. Influence of calcium on the metabolism of intact parathyroid hormone by isolated perfused rat kidney and liver. *Endocrinology* 1990;**126:**1813–20.

85. Daugaard H, Egfjord M, Lewin E, Olgaard K. Metabolism of intact PTH by isolated perfused kidney and liver from uremic rats. *Exp Nephrol* 1994;**2:**240–8.

86. D'Amour P, Brossard JH, Rousseau L, et al. Structure of non-(1–84) PTH fragments secreted by parathyroid glands in primary and secondary hyperparathyroidism. *Kidney Int* 2005;**68:**998–1007.

87. Arakawa T, D'Amour P, Rousseau L, et al. Overproduction and secretion of a novel amino-terminal form of parathyroid hormone from a severe type of parathyroid hyperplasia in uremia. *Clin J Am Soc Nephrol* 2006;**1:**525–31.

88. Wang Q, Palnitkar S, Parfitt AM. Parathyroid cell proliferation in the rat: effect of age and of phosphate administration and recovery. *Endocrinology* 1996;**137:**4558–62.

89. Rodriguez M, Canalejo A, Garfia B, Aguilera E, Almaden Y. Pathogenesis of refractory secondary hyperparathyroidism. *Kidney Int* 2002;**61**(Suppl 80):155–60.

90. Valimaki S, Farnebo F, Forsberg L, Larsson C, Farnebo LO. Heterogeneous expression of receptor mRNAs in parathyroid glands of secondary hyperparathyroidism. *Kidney Int* 2001;**60:**1666–75.

91. Arnold A, Brown MF, Urena P, Gaz RD, Sarfati E, Drueke TB. Monoclonality of parathyroid tumors in chronic renal failure and in primary parathyroid hyperplasia. *J Clin Invest* 1995;**95:**2047–53.

92. Falchetti A, Bale AE, Amorosi A, et al. Progression of uremic hyperparathyroidism involves allelic loss on chromosome 11. *J Clin Endocrinol Metab* 1993;**76:**139–44.

93. Naveh-Many T, Rahamimov R, Livni N, Silver J. Parathyroid cell proliferation in normal and chronic renal failure rats. The effects of calcium, phosphate, and vitamin D. *J Clin Invest* 1995;**96:**1786–93.

94. Szabo A, Merke J, Beier E, Mall G, Ritz E. 1,25(OH)2 vitamin D3 inhibits parathyroid cell proliferation in experimental uremia. *Kidney Int* 1989;**35:**1049–56.

95. Colloton M, Shatzen E, Miller G, et al. Cinacalcet HCl attenuates parathyroid hyperplasia in a rat model of secondary hyperparathyroidism. *Kidney Int* 2005;**67:**467–76.

96. Ritter CS, Finch JL, Slatopolsky EA, Brown AJ. Parathyroid hyperplasia in uremic rats precedes down-regulation of the calcium receptor. *Kidney Int* 2001;**60:**1737–44.

97. Nakajima K, Umino KI, Azuma Y, et al. Stimulating parathyroid cell proliferation and PTH release with phosphate in organ cultures obtained from patients with primary and secondary hyperparathyroidism for a prolonged period. *J Bone Miner Metab* 2009;**27:**224–33.

98. Dusso AS, Pavlopoulos T, Naumovich L, et al. p21(WAF1) and transforming growth factor-alpha mediate dietary phosphate regulation of parathyroid cell growth. *Kidney Int* 2001;**59:**855–65.

99. Tokumoto M, Tsuruya K, Fukuda K, Kanai H, Kuroki S, Hirakata H. Reduced p21, p27 and vitamin D receptor in the nodular hyperplasia in patients with advanced secondary hyperparathyroidism. *Kidney Int* 2002;**62:**1196–207.

100. Cozzolino M, Lu Y, Sato T, et al. A critical role for enhanced-TGFαand EGFR expression in the initiation of parathyroid hyperplasia in experimental kidney disease. *Am J Physiol Renal Physiol*, 2005.

101. Gogusev J, Duchambon P, Stoermann-Chopard C, Giovannini M, Sarfati E, Drueke TB. *De novo* expression of transforming growth factor-alpha in parathyroid gland tissue of

patients with primary or secondary uremic hyperparathyroidism. *Nephrol Dial Transplant* 1996;**11**:2155–162.

102. Arcidiacono MV, Cozzolino M, Spiegel N, et al. Activator protein 2alpha mediates parathyroid TGF-alpha self-induction in secondary hyperparathyroidism. *J Am Soc Nephrol* 2008;**19**:1919–28.

103. Jara A, von Hoveling A, Jara X, et al. Effect of endothelin receptor antagonist on parathyroid gland growth, PTH values and cell proliferation in azotemic rats. *Nephrol Dial Transplant* 2006;**21**:917–23.

104. Marco MP, Martinez I, Betriu A, Craver L, Fibla MJ, Fernandez E. Influence of Bsml vitamin D receptor gene polymorphism on the response to a single bolus of calcitrol in hemodialysis patients. *Clin Nephrol* 2001;**56**:111–16.

105. Yokoyama K, Shigematsu T, Kagami S, et al. Vitamin D receptor gene polymorphism detected by digestion with Apa I influences the parathyroid response to extracellular calcium in Japanese chronic dialysis patients. *Nephron* 2001;**89**:315–20.

106. Torres A, Garcia S, Gomez A, et al. Treatment with intermittent calcitriol and calcium reduces bone loss after renal transplantation. *Kidney Int* 2004;**65**:705–12.

107. Hawa NS, Cockerill FJ, Vadher S, et al. Identification of a novel mutation in hereditary vitamin D resistant rickets causing exon skipping. *Clin Endocrinol (Oxf)* 1996;**45**:85–92.

108. Wada M, Nagano N, Furuya Y, Chin J, Nemeth EF, Fox J. Calcimimetic NPS R-568 prevents parathyroid hyperplasia in rats with severe secondary hyperparathyroidism. *Kidney Int* 2000;**57**:50–8.

109. Takahashi F, Denda M, Finch JL, Brown AJ, Slatopolsky E. Hyperplasia of the parathyroid gland without secondary hyperparathyroidism. *Kidney Int* 2002;**61**:1332–8.

110. Ritter CS, Martin DR, Lu Y, Slatopolsky E, Brown AJ. Reversal of secondary hyperparathyroidism by phosphate restriction restores parathyroid calcium-sensing receptor expression and function. *J Bone Miner Res* 2002;**17**:2206–13.

111. Zhang P, Duchambon P, Gogusev J, et al. Apoptosis in parathyroid hyperplasia of patients with primary or secondary uremic hyperparathyroidism. *Kidney Int* 2000;**57**:437–45.

112. Wada M, Furuya Y, Sakiyama Ji, et al. The calcimimetic compound NPS R-568 suppresses parathyroid cell proliferation in rats with renal insufficiency. Control of parathyroid cell growth via a calcium receptor. *J Clin Invest* 1997;**100**:2977–83.

113. Fukagawa M, Okazaki R, Takano K, et al. Regression of parathyroid hyperplasia by calcitriol-pulse therapy in patients on long-term dialysis. *N Engl J Med* 1990;**323**:421–2.

114. Henry HL, Taylor AN, Norman AW. Response of chick parathyroid glands to the vitamin D metabolites, 1,25-dihydroxycholcalciferol and 24,25-dihydroxycholalciferol. *J Nutr* 1977;**107**:1918–26.

115. Quarles LD, Yohay DA, Carroll BA, et al. Prospective trial of pulse oral versus intravenous calcitriol treatment of hyperparathyroidism in ESRD. *Kidney Int* 1994;**45**:1710–21.

116. Jara A, Gonzalez S, Felsenfeld AJ, et al. Failure of high doses of calcitriol and hypercalcemia to induce apoptosis in hyperplastic parathyroid glands of azotemic rats. *Nephrol Dial Transplant* 2001;**16**:506–12.

117. Almaden Y, Felsenfeld AJ, Rodriguez M, et al. Proliferation in hyperplastic human and normal rat parathyroid glands: role of phosphate, calcitriol, and gender. *Kidney Int* 2003;**64**:2311–17.

Chapter 7

PTHrP physiology and pathophysiology, and the PTH/PTHrP receptor

David Goltzman

Introduction

In the 1920s Zondek et al.[1] first noted the association between elevated blood calcium and neoplastic disease and it was postulated that release of calcium from bone by the direct osteolytic action of malignant cells was responsible for hypercalcemia associated with malignancy. In 1941 Albright,[2] on the basis of observations in a patient with hypercalcemia associated with a renal cell carcinoma, suggested that the clinical manifestations in his patient, which also included hypophosphatemia, resembled that of primary HPT, and theorized that a circulating parathyroid hormone (PTH)-like factor produced by the tumor was responsible. After the biochemical isolation and sequencing of PTH and the development of antisera and immunoassays for its measurement, investigators concluded that it was a PTH-like factor, rather than native PTH that was produced by tumors associated with hypercalcemia.[3] In the late 1980s, the active moiety produced by tumors and responsible for this syndrome was identified as PTH-related peptide (PTHrP).[4–6] This peptide was noted to have close homology in its amino (N)-terminal domain to the N-terminal domain of PTH, the region of PTH known to contain most or all of its bioactivity. This analysis therefore predicted the biological basis of the similarity in action of PTHrP and PTH.

Characteristics of the *PTHrP* gene

The genes encoding PTH and PTHrP have been localized to the short arms of human chromosomes 11 and 12, respectively, placing them among syntenic groups of functionally related genes and suggesting a common ancestral origin.[7] The similarities in their structural organization and in the functional properties of their N terminal regions provide further support for the hypothesis that *PTH* and *PTHrP* are members of a single gene family. The human *PTHrP* gene is a complex unit that spans more than 15kb of DNA. Its mRNA is transcribed from at least three promoters and undergoes differential splicing, giving rise to several mRNA species. The cDNA encodes a prototypical secretory protein with predicted mature isoforms of 139, 141, and 173 amino acids. Species conservation of PTHrP is evident with high homology across a variety of mammalian species.[8]

Regulation of PTHrP production

PTHrP is widely distributed in embryonic and adult tissues and has essential functions in development and growth. In view of its broad distribution pattern in many cell types, overproduction of PTHrP by malignant cells most likely results from deregulated expression of endogenous PTHrP during the process of malignant transformation, that is, 'eutopic' rather than 'ectopic' production. Several factors have implicated in its regulation, chiefly in cell models *in vitro* and mainly in transformed cells.

Growth factors, cytokines, and other small molecules

A variety of growth factors have been found to be potent stimulators of *PTHrP* gene transcription including EGF,[9,10] and insulin-like growth factor I (IGF-I).[11] Both have been reported to increase basal levels of mRNA, and release of PTHrP into conditioned medium of various transformed and non-transformed cell lines. Signaling by growth factors acting through receptor tyrosine kinases (RTKs) appears to be an important mechanism for regulating *PTHrP* gene expression and studies have also demonstrated an important role for Ras in enhancing PTHrP production in transformed cells.[12] Other growth factors and cytokines have also been found to play a critical role in PTHrP over-production, notably transforming growth factor β (TGF β). PTHrP mRNA is typically unstable with a short half-life, but cytokines such as TGF β increase PTHrP mRNA stability.[13] Among the most potent inducers of PTHrP in vascular smooth muscle are vasoconstrictors including angiotensin II,[14] serotonin, endothelin, noradrenaline, bradykinin, and thrombin.

Steroid hormones

Several steroid hormones have been reported to influence the production of PTHrP. Thus, oestradiol has been reported to inhibit *PTHrP* gene promoter activity in breast cancer cell models *in vitro* and to diminish PTHrP production *in vivo*.[15] Similarly, androgens (dihydrotestosterone) have also been shown to inhibit PTHrP production in models of prostate cancer both *in vitro* and *in vivo* at least in part via a transcriptional mechanism.[16] Glucocorticoids[11,17] and the secosteroid 1,25 dihydroxyvitamin D $(1,25(OH)_2D)$[10] can inhibit *PTHrP* gene transcription and a $1,25(OH)_2$ D-responsive repressor sequence has been identified between bases -1121 to -1075 upstream of the single promoter in the rat *PTHrP* gene.[18] Analogues of vitamin D (EB1089) were also found to inhibit PTHrP production and prevent the development of malignancy-associated hypercalcemia in an animal model *in vivo*.[19]

Viral proteins

Viral proteins, notably Tax, have been implicated in transcriptional stimulation of PTHrP production in malignant states, such as acute T-cell leukemia (ATL),[20] in which human T-cell leukemia virus type I (HTLV-I) infection has a documented pathogenetic role. TAX is a 40-kDa nuclear phosphoprotein that transactivates its own promoter, as well as those of a number of host genes, and interacts with a variety of transcription complexes that bind to DNA consensus elements in the *PTHrP* promoter including the cAMP response element, Ets-1, serum response element, and the AP-1 binding site.[21]

Calcium

Various well-established breast and cancer cell lines have been found to express the calcium sensing receptor (CaSR) mRNA and protein.[22] Both pharmacological and molecular evidence indicates that elevated calcium up-regulates PTHrP synthesis and release via CaSR activation in these cell lines. Consequently, elevated calcium induced by circulating PTHrP may have a stimulatory effect on further PTHrP release by the tumor. Furthermore, bone-derived calcium released during skeletal resorption, which results in an increase in extracellular calcium in the local microenvironment, may be 'sensed' by cancer cells metastatic to bone and could enhance further PTHrP release from tumor cells metastatic to bone.

Overall, therefore, these studies indicate that PTHrP production may be modulated by alterations in the interaction between stimulatory and inhibitory signaling pathways in malignant cells and probably in normal cells as well.

Processing and degradation of PTHrP

Like PTH, PTHrP is synthesized as a prohormone with an N-terminal extension. The biological potency of pro-PTHrP is considerably less than that of PTHrP-(1–34).[23] A furin recognition sequence is found between the propeptide and the mature protein, and studies[23] have shown that pro-PTHrP was indeed a substrate for the prohormone convertase furin. PTHrP appears to undergo endoproteolytic cleavage in the secretory pathway, resulting in the release of multiple fragments. In studies in a rat model of hypercalcemia associated with malignancy,[24] biosynthetic labeling of nascent PTHrP revealed rapid processing into three distinct amino-terminal species of 1–36, 1–86, and 1–141 amino acids, which were constitutively released into the extracellular environment. These observations were in agreement with similar studies that had been performed in malignant human cells.[25]

Physiological actions of PTHrP

PTHrP was initially discovered through its 'endocrine' effects, that is, it is released from tumors into the circulation and acts at distant sites, such as the skeleton and kidneys, however, unlike PTH, PTHrP does not circulate in appreciable amounts in normal subjects. Consequently this route of action is generally considered to be the exception rather than the rule. The majority of the actions of PTHrP are believed to occur in a paracrine/autocrine fashion, particularly in fetal development and physiology. In keeping with the widespread cellular distribution of PTHrP, it has been implicated in multiple functions in a variety of tissue and organs. These include, but may not be restricted to, roles in the normal development of:

- the cartilaginous growth plate;[26]
- in bone anabolism;[27,28]
- in tooth eruption;[29]

- in skin and hair follicle development;[30]
- in mammary gland development including the development of mammary ducts and nipple formation;[31]
- in calcium transport across the placenta;[32]
- in smooth muscle relaxation;[33]
- in vasodilatation;[34]
- in heart development and function;[35]
- in kidney maturation, glomerular development, and renal function;[36]
- in lung development;[37]
- in delaying beta cell apoptotic death and increasing beta cell mass and insulin secretion.[38]

PTHrP actions in development of the cartilaginous growth plate

Perhaps the most prominent physiological function of PTHrP was disclosed by targeted ablation in mice of the gene encoding PTHrP.[26,39] PTHrP null mice die in the immediate postnatal period, with widespread abnormalities of endochondral bone development. The abnormalities in the cartilaginous growth plate are characterized by diminished chondrocyte proliferation, accelerated chondrocyte differentiation, and premature apoptotic death of chondrocytes. Consequently, the proliferative zone of the growth plate is narrowed and the architecture of the hypertrophic zone is markedly distorted.[26] This form of chondrodysplasia results in the untimely and rapid maturation of the skeleton. Indian hedgehog (Ihh), a member of the hedgehog family of secreted signaling molecules, is also required for normal skeletal development, and a model has been proposed in which Ihh, produced by prehypertrophic chondrocytes promotes PTHrP expression in perichondrium (PC) and in chondrocytes in the periarticular cartilage.[40] PTHrP, by acting in proliferating/prehypertrophic chondrocytes, would then delay maturation and ensure a supply of proliferating chondrocytes, which is essential for skeletal growth. Cells apparently not acted on by PTHrP could withdraw from the cell cycle and begin terminal differentiation. PTHrP appears to promote chondrocyte proliferation and delay differentiation by several mechanisms. For example, it appears to regulate the transcription factor Sox9 by enhancing its phosphorylation, which increases its transcriptional efficiency of cartilage-specific genes such as collagen II, and decreases terminal differentiation.[41] Additionally, PTHrP decreases production of the transcription factor Runx2.[42]

PTHrP action in bone

Although PTHrP homozygous null mice die shortly after birth, heterozygotes survive and appear to grow normally. They do, however, manifest haploinsufficiency, a phenotypic consequence of which is osteoporosis.[27] Conditional 'knockout' studies have shown that the source of the PTHrP required for modulation of normal bone formation is PTHrP locally synthesized in cells of the osteoblast phenotype.[28] Consequently, locally produced PTHrP appears to have a role in bone formation as does circulating PTH, suggesting that the action of both peptides in this respect is via the activation of PTH1R via their homologous N-terminal domains. The contribution of this action of PTHrP to the spectrum of renal osteodystrophy remains unknown.

PTHrP actions in vascular smooth muscle cells (VSMCs) and vascular calcification

PTHrP is produced in abundance in smooth muscle including vascular smooth muscle cells where the protein functions to regulate contractility and proliferation. PTHrP has been shown to replicate the vasorelaxant activity of PTH in many vascular beds, including heart,[43] kidney,[44] placenta,[45,46] and mammary gland,[47] and therefore appears to exert its vasodilatory actions through its N-terminal domain.

In addition to its effects on vascular tone, PTHrP also modulates VSMC proliferation. The trans-endothelial influx of low density lipoprotein (LDL) particles and the action of subsequently oxidized LDL particles can produce inflammation in vascular (mostly arterial) walls and heart valves with a resulting chemo-attraction for monocytes and T cells, and the conversion of LDL-laden macrophages to foam cells in the sub-endothelial intima. Cytokines and growth factors [notably bone morphogenetic protein (BMP)-2] released by foam cells and endothelial cells can enhance the expression of PTHrP by VSMCs. PTHrP, through its N-terminal domain can also stimulate the expression of the chemokine MCP-1, which would further augment the migration of circulating monocytes through the vascular endothelium and consequently increase foam cells in the vascular intima and thereby increase pro-inflammatory and osteo-inductive factors (Fig. 7.1).[48,49] Increasing evidence also indicates that endogenous PTHrP stimulates VSMC proliferation[50] and migration of proliferating VSMCs from the media to the intima to thicken the intima and form an atheromatous plaque (Fig. 7.1). Some VSMCs can apparently also differentiate from muscle cells to osteoblast-mimicking calcifying vascular cells (CVCs) and create bone by endochondral ossification.

Medial artery calcification (MAC), as well as atherosclerotic types of calcification is a common occurrence in chronic kidney disease (CKD), and both arise independently in the same or anatomically similar arterial segments. The concentric nature of MAC is distinct from the eccentric, calcified atherosclerotic plaque. In CKD and diabetes mellitus, MAC appears to occur via matrix vesicle-nucleated mineralization, with apatitic calcium phosphate deposition in the tunica media of blood vessels, in the absence of atheroma and neo-intima. It has been suggested[51] that in MAC inflammation and oxidative stress, macrophage, and T cell infiltration appears to occurs first in the adventitia, and up-regulates expression of TNF-α, BMP2, Msx2, and osteopontin (OPN) gene expression. BMP2 and Msx2 expression occur in adventitial pericytic myofibroblasts. OPN expression is up-regulated in medial VSMCs, where expression enhances adventitial myofibroblast (osteoprogenitor) migration, proliferation, medial thickening, matrix deposition and matrix metalloproteinase (MMP)-dependent matrix turnover. The mineralization process resembles intramembranous bone formation. Hyperphosphatemia, a common feature of CKD, promotes osteogenic 'transdifferentiation' of VSMCs via Runx2. The relative extent to which CVC recruitment

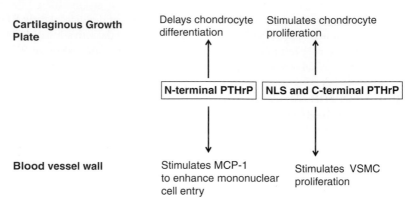

Fig. 7.1 Model of the actions of PTHrP domains in the normal growth plate and in atheromatous blood vessels. In the cartilaginous growth plate, the N-terminal domain of PTHrP acts predominantly to regulate the pace of chondrocyte differentiation, whereas the NLS and C-terminal domains are required for chondrocyte proliferation. In atheromatous blood vessels, the N-terminal domain appears to increase the chemokine MCP-1 to enhance mononuclear cell entry into the vessel wall. The NLS and C-terminal domains seem to be required for VSMC proliferation.

versus VSMC 'trans-differentiation' mechanisms contribute to the osteogenic calcification in MAC has yet to be determined, and the precise role of PTHrP in the increase and differentiation of ossifying cells in MAC remains to be determined.

Mechanisms of action of PTHrP

Interaction of amino-terminal PTHrP with cell surface G-protein coupled receptors

Sequence homology between PTH and PTHrP is restricted to only eight of the first 13 residues; however, this domain is known to be required for activation of signal transduction cascades. Additional conformational similarities in the 14–34 region, a domain that appears critical for peptide binding to the receptor, permit amino-terminal fragments of the proteins to act as equivalent agonists for their common receptor, the type 1 PTH/PTHrP receptor (PTH1R). The PTH1R is a seven-transmembrane G-protein linked receptor that has the 'signature' G protein-coupled receptor (GPCR) topology, a seven-membrane-spanning, 'serpentine' domain, as well as a large extracellular ligand-binding domain and an intracellular COOH-terminal domain.[52] The receptor couples to Gs and Gq leading to activation of the protein kinase A (PKA) and protein kinase C (PKC) pathways[52] and, like other GPCRs, undergoes cyclical receptor activation, desensitization, and internalization.[53] After ligand binding and endocytosis, the PTH1R is either recycled to the cell membrane or targeted for degradation. Arrestins contribute to the desensitization of both Gs and Gq mediated PTH1R signaling. PTH1R activation and internalization can be selectively dissociated.[54] PTH1R signaling can be modified by scaffolding proteins such as the Na⁺/H⁺ exchanger regulatory factor (NHERF) 1 and 2 through PDZ1 and PDZ2 domains.[55] PTH1R signaling via the cAMP pathway, leading to PKA activation and phosphorylation of the cyclic AMP response element binding protein (CREB), has been extensively documented. CREB binds to the cyclic AMP response element (CRE) in the promoter region of many genes and transcriptionally modulates their expression. PTH1R, as with PTHrP, is expressed in a wide variety of embryonic and adult tissues, including cartilage and bone, and therefore mediates the autocrine/paracrine actions of locally produced and secreted PTHrP.

Jansen chondrodysplasia is an autosomal dominant disorder characterized by short-limbed dwarfism associated with hypercalcemia and hyperphosphatemia which is independent of circulating PTH levels.[56] Three heterozygous nucleotide substitutions in the PTH1R were initially identified in this disorder; these included a histidine at position 223 to arginine (exon M2) (H223R), a threonine at position 410 to proline (T410P) (exon M5), and an isoleucine at position 458 to arginine (I458R) (exon M7).[57] The three mutated residues are strictly conserved in all mammalian forms of PTH1R, suggesting an important functional role for these three residues. Furthermore, transient over expression of PTH1R with either the H223R, T410P, or I458R mutation in a heterologous system, showed significantly higher basal accumulation of cyclic AMP than cells expressing the wild-type PTH1R.[57] Consequently, this disorder is caused by gain-of-function mutations in the PTH1R. The targeted over expression of such constitutively active receptors to the growth plate of transgenic mice[58] result in delayed endochondral bone formation; therefore, either over expression of PTHrP[59] or the presence of a constitutively active PTHR1 in the growth plate (either naturally or by transgenic technology), ultimately results in a similar pattern of abnormalities in endochondral bone formation.

Blomstrand lethal chondrodysplasia (BLC) is an autosomal recessive disease that typically results in fetal death during the last trimester of pregnancy and is characterized by short stature, extremely short limbs, generalized osteosclerosis and advanced skeletal maturation,[60] a phenotype similar to that observed in the PTHR1-null mice. BLC is associated with compound heterozygous or homozygous mutations that lead to mutant PTH1R with severely impaired functional properties.[61,62]

These findings emphasize the importance of PTH1R signaling in human fetal skeletal development and support the thesis that this receptor mediates most of the cartilaginous effects of PTHrP. Additionally, in keeping with the role of PTH1R/PTHrP signaling described in mammary gland and tooth development of genetically manipulated mice[29,31] defects in the development of these tissues have been recently demonstrated in two human fetuses with BLC.[63] In these fetuses, nipples were absent, and no subcutaneous ductal tissue could be identified by histochemical analysis. Tooth buds were present, but developing teeth were severely impacted within the surrounding alveolar bone, leading to distortions in their architecture and orientation. However, there are subtle differences in the receptor-deficient and in the PTHrP-null mice. These include, for example, a delay in vascular invasion in the growth plate of PTH1R mice not shared by the PTHrP null mice. These differences may stem in part from the absence of PTH actions via the PTH1R in the PTH1R null mice that are not present in the PTHrP null mice, but may also suggest that PTHrP may exert additional biological functions via other domains in the molecule.[64]

Actions of carboxy-terminal PTHrP

In the past, several investigators have reported a variety of functions for fragments of PTHrP that are C-terminal to the domain that is homologous with PTH.[65] These include the pentapeptide PTHrP-(107–111), which was named osteostatin for its potential to inhibit osteoclastic bone resorption in culture. Other studies using C-terminal fragments of PTHrP have shown that such fragments inhibit production of the early osteoblast marker osteopontin in isolated osteoblasts and are almost as effective as PTHrP-(1–34) in stimulating functional osteoclast formation from progenitor cells. These studies support *in vivo* observations demonstrating decreased osteoblastic and increased osteoclastic activity in association with elevated circulating levels of C-terminal fragments of PTHrP in patients with hypercalcemia associated with malignancy. Several reports have reported the presence of cell surface binding proteins for C-terminal fragments of PTHrP on skeletal cells. To date, however, the molecular nature of these binding proteins remains unclear.

Intracellular mechanism of PTHrP action

Although most of the cellular actions of PTHrP have been attributed to the interaction of its N- terminus with the cell surface PTH1R, there is now good evidence that PTHrP also has a direct, intracellular mode of action. There are at least three potential mechanisms that have been described for the translocation of PTHrP, a prototypical secretory protein, into the cytoplasmic compartment of target cells. One involves retrograde transport of nascent PTHrP from the endoplasmic reticulum (ER)[66,67] into the cytoplasm. Thus, under some circumstances, PTHrP within the ER may be translocated back to the cytoplasm by specific ER sequestering proteins or chaperones, and from there have access to the nucleus or be degraded by the ubiquitin-mediated proteasomal pathway. A second involves internalization of secreted PTHrP via a cell-surface binding protein for PTHrP, which might be PTH1R or an unrelated protein.[68] The possibility that an endocytosed form of PTHrP could reach the nucleus by binding to an intracellular form of the PTH1R also exists because a novel splice variant of the PTH1R, which preferentially localizes to the cytoplasm has been described[69] and PTH1R also contains a nuclear localization signal (NLS).[70] The third mechanism involves the alternative initiation of PTHrP translation to exclude the 'pre' or leader sequence, which is necessary for entry of the molecule into the endoplasmic reticulum and secretory pathway.[71] Thus, PTHrP mRNA contains four CUG codons within the secretory signal that all have the potential to serve as alternative post-translational start sites.

The intracrine action of PTHrP appears to be mediated at least in part, through residues 87–107 in the mid-region of the protein.[72] This region shares sequence homology with a lysine-rich bipartite nuclear localization sequence (NLS) in nucleolin and with an arginine-rich NLS in the retroviral regulatory protein TAT. The PTHrP NLS is both necessary and sufficient to direct the passage of PTHrP to the nuclear compartment of transfected cells and can localize endogenously expressed PTHrP to nucleoli in chondrocytes and osteoblasts *in vitro* and *in vivo*.[72] Nuclear localization of PTHrP occurs in a cell cycle dependent manner with higher expression in the G2 and

M phases of the cycle.[73] The cell cycle-dependent localization of PTHrP appears to be regulated by the activity of the cyclin-dependent kinases (cdk) cdc2 and cdk2, which phosphorylate PTHrP at threonine 85 within a consensus cdc2/cdk2 site.[74] Phosphorylation increases as cells progress from G1 to G2 and M of the cell cycle, and leads to decreased nuclear entry, perhaps by enhancing binding to a cytoplasmic retention factor. PTHrP appears to bind with high affinity to importin β1 and the GDP-bound protein, Ran. PTHrP nuclear import seems dependent on microtubular integrity, implying a role for the cytoskeleton in transport to the nucleus.[75] After translocation across the nuclear envelope, PTHrP may apparently act in the nucleolus to bind RNA, thereby regulating mRNA processing or mRNA transport.[76]

Functionally, intranuclear PTHrP has been shown in studies *in vitro* to increase cell proliferation and to delay apoptosis. Thus, endogenous PTHrP with its intact NLS stimulates proliferation, for example in VSMC *in vitro*, via intranuclear targets that inactivate retinoblastoma protein (Rb), the inhibitory G_1/S checkpoint regulator, by stimulating its hyperphosphorylation.[77] Nuclear localization of PTHrP was initially shown to delay apoptosis in chondrocytes *in vitro*[72] and, subsequently, was also found to be protective for apoptosis in prostate and breast cancer cells.

These *in vitro* studies showing the functional significance of the nuclear localization of PTHrP have now been confirmed *in vivo*.[78] After inserting a premature stop codon at position 85 of PTHrP, a 'knock-in' (KI) mouse was engineered which expressed PTHrP(1-84) but not the NLS or C-terminal portion of PTHrP.[78] Consequently the N terminal domain of PTHrP was expressed and retained the capacity of interacting with the PTH1R, but the truncated peptide could no longer localize to the nucleus. This mouse KI model manifested growth retardation and evidence of premature senility, and died with multiple organ involvement at 2–3 weeks of age. The skeletal growth retardation included abnormalities in the growth plate, which predominantly were manifested by a reduction in the proliferative zone. Although the hypertrophic zone was narrowed due to the reduction in proliferating chondrocytes, the architecture was normal. Consequently, the N-terminal domain of PTHrP appears to be involved in delaying accelerated chondrocyte differentiation, whereas the NLS and C-terminus appears to be involved in enhancing chondrocyte proliferation (Fig. 7.1).

In addition to developing growth retardation, KI mice also developed kyphosis, and evidence of premature osteoporosis associated with a reduction in bone formation. Consequently, the NLS and C-terminus of PTHrP maybe act in concert with the N-terminal domain in modulating normal bone acquisition.

A number of potential downstream molecular targets of the NLS and C-terminus of PTHrP were identified in these *in vivo* studies. One was the polycomb protein Bmi-1 which appeared to require nuclear localization of PTHrP to facilitate its entry into the nucleus (Fig. 7.2). In the absence of Bmi-1 nuclear uptake, there can be a number of consequences. These include the failure of phosphorylation of Rb, with resulting cell cycle arrest and premature senility. These alterations as well as alterations in cell patterning and cell commitment due to alterations in additional downstream intracellular targets of the NLS and C-terminus of PTHrP may explain the multiple abnormalities observed in these mice.

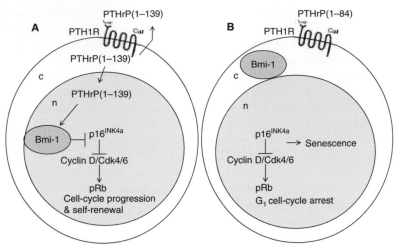

Fig. 7.2 Model of the mechanism of action of PTHrP. Under normal conditions (A), intact PTHrP (e.g. PTHrP(1-139)) may be secreted from a cell and act on the cell surface GPCR (PTH1R) in a paracrine and/or autocrine mode. Alternatively, intact PTHrP, in the cytoplasm (c), containing the NLS, may be translocated to the nucleus (n), where it may have several downstream targets. One is the polycomb protein Bmi-1, whose nuclear entry is facilitated by PTHrP. Bmi-1 itself has several downstream targets one of which is the cyclin-dependent kinase inhibitor, INK^{4a}, which normally inhibits cyclin-dependent phosphorylation (via Cyclin D/cdk4/6) of Rb. Nuclear Bmi-1 can inhibit INK^{4a} and allow phosphorylation of Rb to pRb and facilitate cell cycle progression and stem cell renewal. In the PTHrP KI mouse[78] PTHrP(1-84) is secreted and acts on PTH1R, but in the absence of the NLS and C-terminus of PTHrP, Bmi-1 nuclear entry is prevented. Consequently, pRb is inhibited leading to cell cycle arrest in G_1 and senescence.

PTH/PTHrP receptor expression in renal osteodystrophy

A number of studies have reported that PTH1R is generally down-regulated in CKD. This includes PTH1R expression in kidney and bone,[79–81] but also in non-traditional cells for PTH action, such as heart and liver where the natural ligand may be PTHrP.[82]

PTH1R in cells of the osteoblast lineage transmit the signal for PTH-induced bone formation, but also can transduce the signal for increased expression of RANK ligand and decreased expression of osteoprotegerin, thus establishing the conditions for osteoclastogenesis and increased osteoclastic bone resorption. It has been postulated that the reduction in PTH1R expression in osteoblastic cells, which has been reported may contribute to skeletal resistance to PTH in CKD and potentially to the pathogenesis of adynamic bone disease.

The PTH1R appears to be expressed in parathyroid glands. PTHrP mRNA and protein have also been reported in human parathyroid adenomas, hyperplasia, and carcinomas,[83,84] but may also play a role in normal physiology.[85] It has been reported that the N-terminal domain of PTHrP could significantly increase hypocalcemia-induced PTH secretion in normal rats and could also enhance PTH secretion in uremic rats. These observations are consistent with the thesis that PTHrP in a normal gland or in a hyperplastic gland as in CKD, might play a role via the PTH1R in modulating PTH secretion. Alternatively, it is consistent with the thesis that PTH per se during hypocalcemia might have a positive auto-feedback regulatory role on its own secretion.[85]

Summary

Although PTHrP was initially discovered as the cause of hypercalcemia-associated with malignancy, this calcium modulating effect of PTHrP appears to be a minor component of its significance in physiology and pathophysiology. PTHrP is a widely expressed modulator of cell growth, differentiation, apoptosis, and differentiated function, with critical roles in skeletal growth and development, and potentially key roles in the function of many other organ systems including blood vessels, breast, and skin both *in utero* and in the post-natal state. The cell surface GPCR, PTH1R is critical for the function of PTHrP as a paracrine/autocrine regulator, and allows cross-over with the function of PTH, particularly when PTH is present in high circulating concentrations. Increasing evidence both *in vitro* and now *in vivo* are accumulating that demonstrates its important intracrine roles, and further studies are required to define the interaction of intracrine functions of PTHrP with its role in activating the PTH1R. Although evidence indicates that the PTH1R may be substantially reduced in multiple tissues in CKD the broad implications for dysfunction of PTHrP, as well as for PTH, and the effects of CKD on the intracrine actions of PTHrP in multiple tissues need further definition.

References

1. Zondek H, Petrow H, Siebert W. Die Bedeutung der Calcium-Bestimmung im Blute fur die Diagnose der Nierrenin-siffizientz. *Z Clin Med* 1923;**99**:129–32.
2. Albright F. Case records of the Massachusetts General Hospital (Case 27461). *N Engl J Med* 1941;**225**:789–91.
3. Powell D, Singer FR, Murray TM, Minkin C, Potts JT. Non-parathyroid humoral hypercalcemia in patients with neoplastic diseases. *N Engl J Med* 1973;**289**:176–80.
4. Suva LJ, Winslow GA, Wettenhall REH, et al. A parathyroid hormone-related protein implicated in malignant hypercalcemia: Cloning and expression. *Science* 1987;**237**:893–6.
5. Burtis WJ, Wu T, Bunch C, et al. Identification of a novel 17,000-dalton parathyroid hormone-like adenylate cyclase-stimulating protein from a tumor associated with humoral hypercalcemia of malignancy. *J Biol Chem* 1987;**262**:7151–6.
6. Strewler GJ, Stern PH, Jacobs WJ, et al. Parathyroid hormone-like protein from human renal carcinoma cells: Structural and functional homology with parathyroid hormone. *J Clin Invest* 1987;**80**:1803–7.
7. Goltzman D, Hendy, GN, Banville D. Parathyroid hormone-like peptide: molecular characterisation and biological properties. *Trends Endocrinol Metab* 1989;**1**:39–44.
8. Burtis WJ. Parathyroid hormone-related protein: structure, function, and measurement. *Clin Chem* 1992;**38**:2171–83.

9. Henderson JE, Sebag M, Rhim J, Goltzman D, Kremer R. Dysregulation of parathyroid hormone-like peptide expression and secretion in a keratinocyte model of tumor-progression. *Cancer Res* 1991;**51**:6521–8.

10. Kremer R, Karaplis AC, Henderson JE, et al. Regulation of parathyroid hormone-like peptide in cultured normal human keratinocytes. *J Clin Invest* 1991;**87**:884–93.

11. Sebag M, Henderson JE, Goltzman D, Kremer R. Regulation of parathyroid hormone-related peptide production in normal human mammary epithelial cells *in vitro*. *Am J Physiol* 1994;**267**:C723–30.

12. Aklilu F, Park M, Goltzman D, Rabbani SA. Induction of parathyroid hormone related peptide by the Ras oncogene: role of Ras farnesylation inhibitors as potential therapeutic agents for hypercalcemia of malignancy. *Cancer Res* 1997;**57**:4517–22.

13. Sellers RS, Luchin AI, Richard V, Brena RM, Lima D, Rosol TJ. Alternative splicing of parathyroid hormone related protein mRNA: Expression and stability. *J Mol Endocrinol* 2004;**33**:227–41.

14. Pirola CJ, Wang HM, Kamyar A, et al. Angiotensin II regulates parathyroid hormone-related protein expression in cultured rat aortic smooth muscle cells through transcriptional and post-transcriptional mechanisms. *J Biol Chem* 1993;**268**: 1987–94.

15. Rabbani SA, Khalili P, Arakelian A, Pizzi H, Chen G, Goltzman D. Regulation of parathyroid hormone related peptide by estrogen: effect on tumor growth and metastasis *in vitro* and *in vivo*. *Endocrinology* 2005;**146**: 2885–94.

16. Pizzi H, Gladu J, Carpio L, Miao D, Goltzman D, Rabbani SA. Androgen regulation of parathyroid hormone-related peptide production in human prostate cells. *Endocrinology* 2003;**144**:858–67.

17. Glatz JA, Heath JK, Southby J, et al. Dexamethasone regulation of parathyroid hormone-related protein (PTHrP) expression in a squamous cancer cell line. *Mol Cell Endocrinol* 1994;**101**:295–306.

18. Kremer R, Sebag M, Champigny C, et al. Identification and characterisation of 1,25-dihydroxyvitamin D3-responsive repressor sequences in the rat parathyroid hormone-related peptide gene. *J Biol Chem* 1996;**271**:16310–16.

19. Haq M, Kremer R, Goltzman D, Rabbani SA. A vitamin D analogue (EB1089) inhibits parathyroid hormone-related peptide production and prevents the development of malignancy-associated hypercalcemia *in vivo*. *J Clin Invest* 1993;**91**: 2416–22.

20. Motokura T, Fukumoto S, Matsumoto T, et al. Parathyroid hormone-related protein in adult T-cell leukemia-lymphoma. *Ann Intern Med* 1989;**111**:484–8.

21. Ejima E, Rosenblatt JD, Massari M, et al. Cell-type-specific trans-activation of the parathyroid hormone-related protein gene promoter by the human T-cell leukemia virus type I (HTLV-I) tax and HTLV-II tax protein. *Blood* 1993;**81**:1017–24.

22. Cattopadhyay N. Effects of calcium-sensing receptor on the secretion of parathyroid hormone-related peptide and its impact on humoral hypercalcemia of malignancy. *Am J Physiol Endocrinol Metab* 2006;**290**:E761–70.

23. Liu B, Goltzman D, Rabbani SA. Processing of pro-PTHrP by the prohormone convertase, furin: effect on biological activity. *Am J Physiol* 1995;**268**:E832–8.

24. Rabbani SA, Haq M, Goltzman D. Biosynthesis and processing of endogenous parathyroid hormone-related peptide (PTHrP) by the rat Leydig cell tumor H-500. *Biochemistry* 1993;**32**:4931–7.

25. Soifer NE, Dee KE, Insogna KL, et al. Parathyroid hormone-related protein. Evidence for secretion of a novel mid-region fragment by three different cell types. *J Biol Chem* 1992;**267**:18236–43.

26. Amizuka N, Warshawsky H, Henderson JE, Goltzman D, Karaplis AC. Parathyroid hormone-related peptide-depleted mice show abnormal epiphyseal cartilage development and altered endochondral bone formation. *J Cell Biol* 1994;**126**:1611–23.

27. Amizuka N, Karaplis AC, Henderson JE, et al. Haploinsufficiency of parathyroid hormone-related peptide (PTHrP) results in abnormal postnatal bone development. *Dev Biol* 1996;**175**:166-76.

28. Miao D, He B, Jiang Y, et al. Osteoblast-derived PTHrP is a potent endogenous bone anabolic agent that modifies the therapeutic efficacy of administered PTH 1–34. *J Clin Invest* 2005;**115**:2402–11.

29. Philbrick WM, Dreyer BE, Nakchbandi IA, Karaplis A. PTHrP is required for tooth eruption. *Proc Natl Acad Sci USA* 1998;**95**:11846–51.

30. Foley J, Longely BJ, Wysolmerski JJ, Dreyer BE, Broadus AE, Philbrick WM. PTHrP regulates epidermal differentiation in adult mice. *J Invest Dermatol* 1998;**111**:1122–8.

31. Foley J, Dann P, Hong J, et al. Parathyroid hormone-related protein maintains mammary epithelial fate and triggers nipple skin differentiation during embryonic breast development. *Development* 2001;**128**: 513–25.

32. Kovacs CS, Lanske B, Hunzelman JL, Guo J, Karaplis AC, Kronenberg HM. Parathyroid hormone-related peptide (PTHrP) regulates fetal-placental calcium transport through a receptor distinct from the PTH/PTHrP receptor. *Proc Natl Acad Sci USA* 1996;**93**:15233–8.

33. Botella A, Rekik M, Delvaux M, et al. Parathyroid hormone (PTH) and PTH-related peptide induce relaxation of smooth muscle cells from guinea pig ileum: interaction with vasoactive intestinal peptide receptors. *Endocrinology* 1994;**135**:2160–7.

34. Maeda S, Sutliff RL, Qian J, et al. Targeted over expression of parathyroid hormone-related protein (PTHrP) to vascular smooth muscle in transgenic mice lowers blood pressure and alters vascular contractility. *Endocrinology* 1999;**140**:1815–25.

35. Schlueter K, Katzer C, Frischkopf K, Wenzel S, Taimor G, Piper HM. Expression, release, and biological activity of parathyroid hormone-related peptide from coronary endothelial cells. *Circ Res* 2000;**86**:946–51.

36. Massfelder T, Stewart AF, Endlich K, Soifer N, Judes C, Helwig JJ. Parathyroid hormone-related protein detection and interaction with NO and cyclic AMP in the renovascular system. *Kidney Int* 1996;**50**:1591–603.

37. Hastings RH, Berg JT, Summers-Torres D, Burton DW, Deftos LJ. Parathyroid hormone-related protein reduces alveolar epithelial cell proliferation during lung injury in rats. *Am J Physiol Lung Cell Mol Physiol* 2000;**279**:L194–200.

38. Porter SE, Sorenson RL, Dann P, Garcia-Ocana A, Stewart AF, Vasavada, RC. Progressive pancreatic islet hyperplasia in the islet-targeted, parathyroid hormone-related protein-overexpressing mouse. *Endocrinology* 1998;**139**:3743–51.

39. Karaplis AC, Luz A, Glowacki J, et al. Lethal skeletal dysplasia from targeted disruption of the parathyroid hormone-related peptide gene. *Genes Dev* 1994;**8**:277–89.

40. Lanske B, Karaplis AC, Lee K, et al. PTH/PTHrP receptor in early development and Indian hedgehog-regulated bone growth. *Science* 1996;**273**:663–6.

41. Huang W, Chung UI, Kronenberg HM, de Crombrugghe B. The chondrogenic transcription factor Sox9 is a target of signaling by the parathyroid hormone-related peptide in the growth plate of endochondral bones. *Proc Natl Acad Sci USA* 2001;**98**:160–5.

42. Guo J, Chung UI, Yang D, Karsenty G, Bringhurst FR, Kronenberg HM. PTH/PTHrP receptor delays chondrocyte hypertrophy via both Runx2-dependent and –independent pathways. *Dev Biol* 2006;**292:**116–28.

43. Nickols GA, Nana AD, Nickols MA, DiPette DJ, Asimakis GK. Hypotension and cardiac stimulation due to the parathyroid hormone-related protein, humoral hypercalcemia of malignancy factor. *Endocrinology* 1989;**125:**834–41.

44. Musso MJ, Plante M, Judes C, Barthelmebs M, Helwig JJ. Renal vasodilatation and microvessel adenylate cyclase stimulation by synthetic parathyroid hormone-like protein fragments. *Eur J Pharmacol* 1989;**174:**139–51.

45. Macgill K, Moseley JM, Martin TJ, Brennecke SP, Rice GE, Wlodek ME. Vascular effects of PTHrP (1-34) and PTH (1-34) in the human fetal-placental circulation. *Placenta* 1997;**18:**587–92.

46. Mandsager NT, Brewer AS, Myatt L. Vasodilator effects of parathyroid hormone, parathyroid hormone-related protein, and calcitonin gene-related peptide in the human fetal-placental circulation. *J Soc Gynecol Invest* 1994;**1:**19–24.

47. Prosser CG, Farr VC, Davis SR. Increased mammary blood flow in the lactating goat induced by parathyroid hormone-related protein. *Exp Physiol* 1994;**79:**565–70.

48. Martín-Ventura JL, Ortego M, Esbrit P, Hernández-Presa MA, Ortega L, Egido J. Possible role of parathyroid hormone-related protein as a proinflammatory cytokine in atherosclerosis. *Stroke* 2003;**34:**1783–9.

49. Whitfield JF. Osteogenic PTHs and vascular ossification-Is there a danger for osteoporotics? *J Cell Biochem* 2005;**95:**437–44.

50. Massfelder T, Dann P, Wu TL, Vasavada R, Helwig JJ, Stewart AF. Opposing mitogenic and anti-mitogenic actions of parathyroid hormone related protein in vascular smooth muscle cells: a critical role for nuclear targeting. *Proc Natl Acad Sci USA* 1997;**94:**13630–5.

51. Vattikuti R, Towler DA. Osteogenic regulation of vascular calcification: an early perspective. *Am J Physiol Endocrinol Metab* 2004;**286:**E686–96.

52. Mannstadt M, Jüppner H, Gardella TJ. Receptors for PTH and PTHrP: their biological importance and functional properties. *Am J Physiol* 1999;**277:**F665–75.

53. Weinman, EJ, Hall RA, Friedman PA, Liu-Chen LY, Shenolikar S. The association of NHERF adaptor proteins with G protein-coupled receptors and receptor tyrosine kinases. *Ann Rev Physiol* 2006;**68:**491–505.

54. Sneddon WB, Syme CA, Bisello A, et al. Activation independent parathyroid hormone receptor internalisation is regulated by NHERF1 (EBP50). *J Biol Chem* 2003;**278:**43787–96.

55. Mahon MJ, Donowitz M, Yun CC, Segre GV. Na$^+$/H$^+$ exchanger regulatory factor 2 directs parathyroid hormone 1 receptor signaling. *Nature* 2002;**417:**858–61.

56. Schipani E, Langman CB, Parfitt AM, et al. Constitutively activated receptors for parathyroid hormone and parathyroid hormone-related peptide in Jansen's metaphyseal chondrodysplasia. *N Engl J Med* 1996;**335:**708–14.

57. Calvi LM, Schipani E. The PTH/PTHrP receptor in Jansen's metaphyseal chondrodysplasia. *J Endocrinol Invest* 2000;**23:**545–54.

58. Schipani E, Lanske B, Hunzelman J, et al. Targeted expression of constitutively active receptors for parathyroid hormone and parathyroid hormone-related peptide delays endochondral bone formation and rescues mice that lack parathyroid hormone-related peptide. *Proc Natl Acad Sci USA* 1997;**94:**13689–94.

59. Weir EC, Philbrick WM, Amling M, Neff LA, Baron R, Broadus AE. Targeted over expression of parathyroid hormone-related peptide in chondrocytes causes

chondrodysplasia and delayed endochondral bone formation. *Proc Natl Acad Sci USA* 1996;**93:**10240–5.

60. Blomstrand S, Claeesson I, Saeve-Soederbergh J. A case of lethal congenital dwarfism with accelerated skeletal maturation. *Pediatr Radiol* 1985;**15:**141–3.

61. Jobert AS, Zhang P, Couvineau A, et al. Absence of functional receptors for parathyroid hormone and parathyroid hormone-related peptide in Blomstrand chondrodysplasia. *J Clin Invest* 1998;**102:**34–40.

62. Karaplis AC, He B, Nguyen MT, et al. Inactivating mutation in the human parathyroid hormone receptor type 1 gene in Blomstrand chondrodysplasia. *Endocrinology* 1998;**139:**5255–8.

63. Oostra RJ, Van der Harten JJ, Rijnders WP, Scott RJ, Young MP, Trump D. Blomstrand osteochondrodysplasia: three novel cases and histological evidence for heterogeneity. *Virchows Arch* 2000;**436:**28–35.

64. Goltzman D. Studies on the mechanisms of the skeletal anabolic action of endogenous and exogenous parathyroid hormone. *Arch Biochem Biophys* 2008;**473:**218–24.

65. Clemens TL, Cormier S, Eichinger A, et al. Parathyroid hormone-related protein and its receptors: nuclear functions and roles in the renal and cardiovascular systems, the placental trophoblasts and the pancreatic islets. *Br J Pharmacol* 2001;**134:**1113–36.

66. Meerovitch K, Wing S, Goltzman D. Preproparathyroid hormone related protein, a secreted peptide, is a substrate for the ubiquitin proteolytic system. *J Biol Chem* 1997;**272:**6706–13.

67. Meerovitch K, Wing S, Goltzman D. Proparathyroid hormone related protein is associated with the chaperone protein BiP and undergoes proteasome mediated degradation. *J Biol Chem* 1998;**134:**1113–36.

68. Aarts M, Guo R, Bringhurst R, Henderson JE. The nucleolar targeting signal (NTS) of parathyroid hormone related protein (PTHrP) mediate endocytosis and nuclear translocation. *J Bone Miner Res* 1999;**14:** 1493–503.

69. Joun H, Lanske B, Karperien M, Qian F, Defise L, Abou-Samra A. Tissue-specific transcription start sites and alternative splicing of the parathyroid hormone (PTH)/PTH-related peptide (PTHrP) receptor gene: a new PTH/PTHrP receptor splice variant that lacks the signal peptide. *Endocrinology* 1997;**138:**1742–9.

70. Watson PH, Fraher LJ, Hendy GN, et al. Nuclear localisation of the type 1 PTH/PTHrP receptor in rat tissues. *J Bone Miner Res* 2000;**15:**1033–44.

71. Nguyen MT, Karaplis AC. The nucleus: a target site for parathyroid hormone-related peptide (PTHrP) action. *J Cell Biochem* 1998;**70:**193–9.

72. Henderson, JE, Amizuka N, Warshawsky, H, et al. Nucleolar targeting of PTHrP enhances survival of chondrocytes under conditions that promote cell death by apoptosis. *Mol Cell Biol* 1995;**15:**4064–75.

73. Okano K, Pirola CJ, Wang HM, Forrester JS, Fagin JA, Clemens TL. Involvement of cell cycle and mitogen-activated pathways in induction of parathyroid hormone-related protein gene expression in rat aortic smooth muscle cells. *Endocrinology* 1995;**136:**1782–9.

74. Lam MH, Thomas RJ, Martin TJ, Gillespie MT, Jans DA. Nuclear and nucleolar localisation of parathyroid hormone-related protein. *Immunol Cell Biol* 2000;**78:**395–402.

75. Lam MH, Thomas RJ, Loveland KL, et al. Nuclear transport of parathyroid hormone (PTH)-related protein is dependent on microtubules. *Mol Endocrinol* 2002;**16:**390–401.

76. Aarts MM, Levy D, He B, et al. Parathyroid hormone related (PTHrP) interacts with RNA. *J Biol Chem* 1999;**274:**4832–8.

77. Fiaschi-Taesch N, Takane KK, Masters S, Lopez-Talavera JC, Stewart AF. Parathyroid-hormone-related protein as a regulator of pRb and the cell cycle in arterial smooth muscle. *Circulation* 2004;**110:**177–85.

78. Miao D, Su H, He B, et al. Severe growth retardation and early lethality in mice lacking the nuclear localisation sequence and C-terminus of PTH-related protein. *Proc Natl Acad Sci USA* 2008;**105:**20309–14.

79. Urena P, Kubrusly M, Mannstadt M, et al. The renal PTH/PTHrP receptor is down-regulated in rats with chronic renal failure. *Kidney Int* 1994;**45:**605–11.

80. Tian J, Smogorzewski M, Kedes L, Massry SG. PTH-PTHrP receptor mRNA is downregulated in chronic renal failure. *Am J Nephrol* 1994;**14:**41–6.

81. Picton ML, Moore PR, Mawer EB, et al. Down-regulation of human osteoblast PTH/PTHrP receptor mRNA in end-stage renal failure. *Kidney Int* 2000;**58:**1440–9.

82. Massry SG, Smogorzewski M. PTH-PTHrP receptor in chronic renal failure. *Nephrol Dial Transplant* 1998;**13**(Suppl. 1): 50–7.

83. Danks JA, Ebeling PR, Hayman JA, et al. Immunohistochemical localisation of parathyroid hormone-related protein in parathyroid adenoma and hyperplasia. *J Pathol* 1990; **161:** 27–33.

84. Matsushita H, Usui M, Hara M, et al. Co-secretion of parathyroid hormone and parathyroid-hormone-related protein via a regulated pathway in human parathyroid adenoma cells. *Am J Pathol* 1997;**150:**861–71.

85. Lewin E, Garfia B, Almaden Y, Rodriguez M, Olgaard K. Autoregulation in the parathyroid glands by PTH/PTHrP receptor ligands in normal and uremic rats. *Kidney Int* 2003;**64:**63–70.

Chapter 8

Vitamin D metabolism and action in CKD

Ishir Bhan, Kevin J. Martin, and Ravi Thadhani

Introduction

The kidney is central to the normal metabolism of vitamin D, converting the most prevalent circulating form, 25-hydroxyvitamin D, to the 'active' 1,25-dihydroxyvitamin D. This highly-regulated activity, which is carried out by the renal 1-α hydroxylase enzyme, is disrupted as chronic kidney disease (CKD) progresses and, along with associated changes in mineral metabolism, leads to disordered calcium and phosphate homeostasis, secondary hyperparathyroidism, and bone disease. An increasing amount of data points to additional effects on multiple organ systems previously thought to function independently of vitamin D. As a result, changes in vitamin D metabolism may have broad and consequential effects on health in CKD.

25-Hydroxyvitamin D deficiency in CKD

Although decreased production of 1,25-dihydroxyvitamin D is classically viewed as the predominant CKD-associated deficit in vitamin D metabolism, deficiency of 25-hydroxyvitamin D is both common and potentially consequential. Approximately 70–85% of individuals with moderate to severe CKD were found to have 25-hydroxyvitamin D insufficiency (defined as 25-hydroxyvitamin D≤30ng/mL);[1,2] among those with end-stage renal disease (ESRD) on hemodialysis vitamin D insufficiency may be found in 70% to as high as 97% of patients.[2,3] Diabetics appear to be at particularly high risk of vitamin D deficiency, as are individuals with hypoalbuminemia.[4]

The reasons for the high rates of 25-hydroxyvitamin D insufficiency are likely to be multifactorial. Vitamin D can be acquired from the diet, and the malnutrition that often accompanies advanced CKD may contribute to its deficiency. However, a significant amount of vitamin D is generated from the skin as ultraviolet (UV) light exposure facilitates the conversion of 7-dehydrocholesterol to previtamin D (Fig. 8.1). This process appears to be impaired in advanced CKD.[5] Urinary loss of vitamin D binding protein (DBP), the major carrier protein for 25-hydroxyvitamin D, may also contribute to the risk of deficiency, particularly in the setting of high-grade proteinuria.

Deficiency of 25-hydroxyvitamin D may have an important effect on biological outcomes. With respect to the traditional actions of vitamin D, treatment with

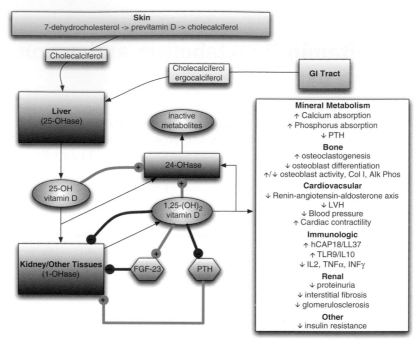

Fig. 8.1 The metabolism and actions of vitamin D.

ergocalciferol or cholecalciferol (which can boost 25-hydroxyvitamin D levels) is effective at suppressing parathyroid hormone (PTH) in early CKD, potentially reducing the risk of bone disease. In addition to effects on mineral metabolism, however, 25-hydroxyvitamin D may have more broad-reaching effects. In a study of the general population, the risk of developing a cardiovascular event was significantly higher in individuals' 25-hydroxyvitamin D deficiency.[6] This risk correlated with severity of deficiency and was independent of other risk factors. While this population presumably had intact vitamin D metabolism, deficiency of 25-hydroxyvitamin D has also been associated with an increased risk of both all-cause and cardiovascular mortality in dialysis.[3] The importance of 25-hydroxyvitamin D levels in advanced CKD is the topic of ongoing research.

Calcitriol production in CKD

While 25-hydroxyvitamin D is the form of vitamin D traditionally used to measure adequacy of vitamin D stores in the general population, 1,25-dihydroxyvitamin D (calcitriol) is the active, hormonal form. In addition to the high prevalence of 25-hydroxyvitamin D deficiency, 1,25-dihydroxyvitamin D levels in CKD are adversely affected by a number of processes. Renal 1-α hydroxylase is the primary route through which 25-hydroxyvitamin D is converted to 1,25-dihydroxyvitamin D, and its activity declines in concert with the reduction in renal mass that accompanies CKD. Recent discoveries, however, suggest that the physiology is more complex than a simple reduction in the amount of enzyme available.

As glomerular filtration rate (GFR) declines, so too does the kidney's ability to clear phosphate. Hyperphosphatemia has been associated with suppression of 1-α hydroxylase, while hypophosphatemia is typically linked to increased activity. This phenomenon may reflect the actions of the phosphaturic hormone fibroblast growth factor-23 (FGF23). CKD is associated with elevated production of FGF23 even prior to the development of overt hyperphosphatemia. As hypophosphatemia induced by FGF23 results in increased, rather than decreased activity of 1-α hydroxylase, it is likely FGF23, rather than the serum phosphate level itself, is a key regulator of the 1,25-dihydroxyvitamin D production. This hormonal regulation of vitamin D metabolism is likely central to the metabolic abnormalities of CKD, as 1,25-dihydroxyvitamin D production declines out of proportion to the absolute amount of 1-α hydroxylase.[7]

The physiology of DBP may also be an important contributor to the metabolism of vitamin D in CKD. DBP is a major carrier of vitamin D in the circulation, and some studies suggest that DBP-bound vitamin D is relatively inaccessible to cells and, hence, less active, than the free form of vitamin D. However, 25-hydroxyvitamin D bound to DBP is readily filtered through the glomerulus. In the proximal tubule, this complex then binds to megalin, allowing for endocytosis. This pathway appears to deliver 25-hydroxyvitamin D to 1-α hydroxylase for conversion. CKD-associated reduction in GFR decreases the filtration of DBP-bound 25-hydroxyvitamin D and, thus, restricts the availability of 25-hydroxyvitamin D to renal 1-hydroxylase.[8]

Metabolic acidosis commonly accompanies the development of CKD and may further influence this balance. Induction of metabolic acidosis has been shown to increase production of 1,25-dihydroxyvitamin D in humans without CKD, possibly by promoting renal phosphate wasting.[9] The link between metabolic acidosis and vitamin D metabolism in advanced CKD is less clear.

Although renal 1-α hydroxylase activity garners the greatest attention, this enzyme is also found outside the kidney. Studies have identified expression in skin, lymph nodes, gastrointestinal (GI) tract, pancreas, adrenal glands, brain, and other sites.[10] Local conversion of 25-hydroxyvitamin D to 1,25-dihydroxyvitamin D may be important in the non-traditional activities of vitamin D (those outside the realm of calcium and phosphorous metabolism) and may be increasingly important as renal conversion declines. This extrarenal activity also highlights the potential importance of 25-hydroxyvitamin D levels in CKD, as local production of 1,25-dihydroxyvitamin D at specific sites may not be adequately addressed by systemic treatment with activated vitamin D analogs. While these alternative sources of 1-α hydroxylase may help to buffer declining renal conversion, this may be offset by loss of 25-dihydroxyvitamin D to an alternative metabolic pathway.

1-α hydroxylase competes for 25-hydroxyvitamin D with CYP24A1, also known as 24-hydroxylase, which is widely expressed both in the kidney and other tissues. This enzyme converts 25-hydroxyvitamin D to the relatively inactive 24,25-dihydroxyvitamin D, effectively serving as a degradation pathway for the vitamin. 24-hydroxylation of 1,25-dihydroxyvitamin D can also occur. Both 25-hydroxyvitamin D and

1,25-dihydroxyvitamin D appear to stimulate 24-hydroxylase, while PTH leads to supression.[4,11,12] While the exact role of 24-hydroxylase activity in CKD is still uncertain, preferational metabolism of 25-hydroxyvitamin D via this pathway may an important contributor to calcitriol deficiency in CKD.[4]

The vitamin D receptor

Vitamin D's actions are effected via binding to the vitamin D receptor (VDR), a steroid hormone receptor with an N-terminal activation domain, a DNA-binding region, a hinge region, and a lateral binding domain. Once bound to 1,25-dihydroxyvitamin D, VDR forms a heterodimer with the retinoic X receptor (RXR) and binds to vitamin D response elements (VDRE) in DNA, where it can influence gene expression.[13] In an animal model, uremia was associated with decreased concentration of the VDR in the parathyroid.[14] Patients with renal failure were found to have impaired 1,25-dihydroxyvitamin D binding in parathyroid glands, likely driven by reduced concentrations of the vitamin D receptor (VDR).[15] In addition, animal models suggest that uremia leads to impaired binding of the VDR to VDRE.[16]

Effects of declining 1,25-dihydroxyvitamin D on mineral metabolism

One of the most widely recognized functions of vitamin D relates to its effect on intestinal transport of calcium. 1,25-dihydroxyvitamin D increases expression of the transient receptor potential vanilloid 6 (TRPV6). This allows for passage of calcium from the intestinal lumen to the intracellular compartment. Calcium then binds calbindin and is directed to the plasma membrane calcium ATPase (PMCA), which allows for transfer of calcium into the circulation; both these proteins are also regulated by 1,25-dihydroxyvitamin D, which allows for transfer of calcium into the circulation.[17,18] As levels of the active form of vitamin D fall, calcium transport in the intestine is reduced, which may lead to subclinical or overt hypocalcemia. This promotes increased production of PTH, which helps to maintain serum calcium through increased release from bone. This secondary hyperparathyroidism is exacerbated by the decreased suppression of PTH by both low circulating 1,25-dihydroxyvitamin D and a decline in vitamin D receptor (VDR) expression in the parathyroid gland that accompanies CKD.

Chronic elevation in circulating PTH is thought to contribute to the most common form of renal osteodystrophy, osteitis fibrosa cystica. This disorder is characterized by increased rates of bone turnover despite preserved mineralization. Lamellar bone is lost and replaced by increased amounts of woven bone, which is weaker and predisposes to fracture out of proportion to bone density.[19] Vitamin D deficiency itself is likely to a direct role in the development of bone disease. Vitamin D has a number of effects on osteoblasts, including induction of matrix Gla protein and osteopontin, as well as either stimulatory and inhibitory effects on type I collagen and alkaline phosphatase, depending on the stage of osteoblast maturation.[20] Osteoblast differentiation appears to be suppressed by vitamin D, while effects on osteoblast activity may depend on state of maturation.[18] Vitamin D also appears to increase expression of RANK-ligand, thus promoting osteoclastogenesis. In total, vitamin D appears to be important for both bone formation and remodelling, and its deficiency in CKD likely contributes to the high prevalence of bone disease.

Phosphate retention is a common problem in CKD, and relative deficiency of 1,25-dihydroxyvitamin D would, at first blush, appear to be beneficial. Intestinal phosphate absorption occurs largely via sodium-phosphate co-transporters, and the type IIb Na-P transporter is regulated in part by 1,25-dihydroxyvitamin D.[21] Similarly, 1,25-dihydroxyvitamin D increases sodium-phosphate reabsorption in the proximal tubule.[22] Therefore, vitamin D deficiency should reduce absorption of phosphate from dietary sources, as well as reabsorption in the kidney. In CKD, however, the associated decline in calcium absorption and consequent secondary hyperparathyroidism cause release of both calcium and phosphate from bone, exacerbating the hyperphosphatemia. This initiates a vicious cycle as hyperphosphatemia itself stimulates PTH production. Vitamin D appears to promote expression of FGF23 in osteoblasts, and thus its deficiency would appear to impair excretion of phosphate.[23] However, hyperphosphatemia stimulates FGF23, which rises with progressive CKD; thus the potentially beneficially effects of vitamin D deficiency on phosphate metabolism appear to be overcome by limited excretory capacity in CKD. Elevated FGF23, in contrast, suppresses renal 1-α hydroxylase, and thus further perpetuates 1,25-dihydroxyvitamin D deficiency. Of note, uremia itself does not appear to affect the physiology of renal or intestinal phosphate transport independently of vitamin D.[24]

Given the central role of 1,25-dihydroxyvitamin D in secondary hyperparathyroidism and consequent bone disease, therapeutic use of calcitriol has become an essential component of the therapeutic armamentarium in ESRD. Administration of calcitriol and similar vitamin D analogues are associated with significant decreases in PTH levels and improvement in bone disease.[25–29]

Non-traditional actions of vitamin D

While vitamin D's effects on mineral metabolism, particularly that of calcium and phosphorus, are the best studied, numerous other actions have come to light in recent years (Fig. 8.1). Vitamin D receptors are broadly distributed in a wide range of tissues and this, in concert with the result of observational studies on clinical outcomes, suggests that these 'non-traditional' roles may have important clinical significance.

Cardiac effects of calcitriol

In CKD, cardiovascular mortality occurs at a rate 10–20 times higher than that seen in the general population; cardiovascular disease is the leading cause of death in this population and often associated with the development of left ventricular hypertrophy (LVH).[30–32] Several biological effects linked to vitamin D action suggest that it could have beneficial effects on the cardiovascular system, including observations in children noting the association between cardiac dysfunction and rickets.[33,34] 1,25-dihydroxyvitamin D blocked hypertrophy in an *in vitro* rat model,[35] while a vitamin D deficient diet lead to altered cardiac contractility *in vivo*.[36] Dahl salt-sensitive rats, when fed a high-salt diet, develop LVH and heart failure. Coincidentally, they also develop profound renal wasting of DBP and become vitamin D deficient. When these animals are treated with paricalcitol, a synthetic analog of calcitriol, they demonstrate improved cardiac contractility and smaller cardiac dimensions than the control rats.[37] Gene expression profiling suggests that these effects are mediated by a direct effect of vitamin D on cardiac myocytes. Additional recent animal studies have provided further support for a direct effect of 1,25-dihydroxyvitamin D on cardiac contractility.[38,39] Small retrospective human studies have demonstrated increased E/A ratios and ejection fractions, and decreased lower posterior wall thickness by echocardiogram in those treated with paricalcitol.[37]

The cardiac actions of vitamin D have also been studied in knockout mice lacking the 1-α hydroxylase enzyme (and thus unable to synthesize 1,25-dihydroxyvitamin D).[40] These animals were found to have hypertension, cardiac hypertrophy, and reduced cardiac function. Dietary modifications to normalize calcium and phosphorus levels failed to ameliorate these changes. Exogenous administration of calcitriol, on the other hand, appeared to correct hypertension, and improve cardiac structure and function.

These effects of calcitriol in these animals were similar to those of an angiotensin converting enzyme (ACE) inhibitor and an angiotensin receptor blocker (ARB). Indeed, 1,25-dihydroxyvitamin D appears to suppress the renin-angiotensin-aldosterone axis; mice lacking the VDR demonstrate increased renin expression and this may be an important mechanism underlying its cardiac effects.[41,42] Given that LVH is present in over 70% of individuals initiating hemodialysis and is associated with an increased risk of cardiovascular mortality in this population, there has been increased interest in validating these effects in large prospective trials. The paricalcitol benefits in renal failure induced cardiac morbidity (PRIMO) study is a multi-national, double blinded randomized controlled trial in both advanced pre-dialysis CKD (PRIMO I) and end-stage renal disease (PRIMO II) examining the effect of paricalcitol versus placebo on LVH (clinicaltrials.gov NCT00497146 and NCT00616902). These and other studies will help to further define cardiovascular effects in the years to come.

Vitamin D and the immune system

Although cardiovascular disease is the greatest contributor to mortality in CKD, infectious disease represents a considerable burden in this population.[30] High rates of infection are due in part to access-related factors in dialysis, such as the frequent use of in-dwelling catheters. However, non-access related infections are also increased, suggesting additional risk factors are present.[43,44] One such risk factor may involve the human cationic antimicrobial peptide 18 (hCAP18, also referred to as LL-37), the only human member of a class of endogenous antimicrobial peptides called cathelcidins. These potent proteins are a central component of the innate immune system in most multicellular organisms and are active against both Gram positive and Gram-negative organisms.[45] In humans, expression hCAP18 appears to be regulated by 1,25-dihydroxyvitamin D, which may be in part be produced locally in macrophages via an extra-renal 1-α hydroxylase.[35] Recent retrospective data in the dialysis population suggests that low circulating levels of hCAP18 predicts death from infectious causes, suggesting another potential role of vitamin D in effecting clinical outcomes.[46]

Toll-like receptors (TLRs) are evolutionarily conserved cell-surface receptors that recognize molecular patterns present in pathogens and are thought to be important in stimulating the immune response to infection. Indeed, TLR-stimulation in macrophages is thought to lead to upregulation of macrophage 1-α hydroxylase and the vitamin D receptor, facilitating hCAP18 production in these cells as part of a pro-inflammatory cascade. However, vitamin D may also be important in control of inflammation. Recent data demonstrates treatment with 1,25-dihydroxyvitamin D can increase expression of TLR9 and IL-10, an anti-inflammatory cytokine, in human regulatory T-cells.[47] Indeed, vitamin D deficiency has been linked to an increased risk of asthma in the general population and may play a role in the development of inflammatory bowel disease and other autoimmune conditions.

A broad range of studies has shown an influence of vitamin D in various other inflammatory and hematopoietic pathways. These include induction of tolerogenic dendritic cells, promotion of myeloid differentiation, and inhibition of IL-2, TNF-α, and interferon-γ production.[48–51] One early human study suggested that vitamin D may improve the delayed hypersensitivity response in ESRD, though this effect fell short of statistical significance.[52] The immunologic role of vitamin D in CKD remains an area of active investigation.

Additional effects of vitamin D

Recent studies have suggested a broad scope for vitamin D action beyond that described above. Vitamin D deficiency has been linked to insulin resistance, obesity, hypertension, and diabetes.[53,54] Administration of calcitriol, in contrast, has been shown to improve insulin sensitivity and lipid abnormalities in advanced CKD.[55,56] Although vitamin D levels are clearly affected by CKD progression, the converse may also be true. Animal models suggest that vitamin D administration may improve proteinuria, glomerulosclerosis, glomerular hypertrophy, mesangial cell proliferation, podocyte hypertrophy, and interstitial fibrosis.[57–61]

Vitamin D and survival in CKD

In 2003, Teng et al. published the findings of an observational study involving over 60,000 hemodialysis patients that found lower rates of mortality in those treated with intravenous paricalcitol versus calcitriol.[62] These findings held up even after multivariate and stratified analysis adjusting for factors such as calcium, phosphorus, and PTH. A follow-up study by the same group found that those who received any form of active vitamin D had a 26% 2-year reduction in mortality compared with those who received none, and the cardiovascular mortality was nearly cut in half.[63]

These findings have been echoed by several other studies, including another cohort of 58,000 hemodialysis patients in the US, which showed a survival benefit for paricalcitol, and the Choices for Health Outcomes in Caring for ESRD (CHOICE) study that showed the same with injectable calcitriol.[64,65] Alfacalcidol (1α-hydroxyvitamin D, converted to 1,25-dihydroxyvitamin D by the liver) was associated with a similar survival benefit in Japan.[66] Many,[67–69] but not all[70,71] similar studies have supported these findings. Although the bulk of data are in patients on dialysis, recent studies have shown improved survival associated with activated vitamin D use in pre-dialysis CKD as well.[72–74]

These studies have generated considerably excitement, given that vitamin D is a widely-available and inexpensive therapy. However, the link between improved survival and vitamin D administration is drawn exclusively from observational studies. While these studies typically use statistical adjustment to account for potential confounding factors, there is always the possibility that residual confounding exists and that this, rather than any biological effect of the therapy, is responsible for the observed differences in survival. Indeed, a meta-analysis of 76 studies failed to find any survival effect of activated vitamin D.[75] The majority of these studies were not designed or powered adequately to assess mortality as a primary outcome, and this meta-analysis combined pre-dialysis and dialysis populations, as well as adult and pediatric populations, potentially masking true effects of vitamin D. However, these findings highlight the need for prospective, randomized controlled trials designed to assess how vitamin D affects survival.

Summary

Chronic kidney disease is associated with progressive derangement of several metabolic processes, including multiple stages of vitamin D metabolism. These changes lead to deficiency in both 25-hydroxyvitamin D and 1,25-dihydroxyvitamin D, which in turn can contribute to hypocalcemia, hyperphosphatemia, secondary hyperparathyroidism, and bone loss. Recent studies point to additional effects beyond the traditional axis of mineral metabolism. Active vitamin D appears to ameliorate LVH and may suppress activity of the renin-angiotensin-aldosterone axis. Vitamin D also appears to be important in the regulation of both antimicrobial peptides that contribute to innate immunity and to anti-inflammatory cytokines that moderate the immune response. Several retrospective observational studies in both dialysis and pre-dialysis CKD suggest a survival benefit associated with vitamin D use. Prospective randomized controlled trials, currently underway, are needed to better define the risks and benefits of exogenous vitamin D in CKD.

References

1. LaClair RE, Hellman RN, Karp SL, et al. Prevalence of calcidiol deficiency in CKD: a cross-sectional study across latitudes in the United States. *Am J Kidney Dis* 2005;**45**:1026–33.

2. González EA, Sachdeva A, Oliver DA, Martin KJ. Vitamin D insufficiency and deficiency in chronic kidney disease. A single center observational study. *Am J Nephrol* 2004;**24**: 503–10.

3. Wolf M, Shah A, Gutierrez O, et al. Vitamin D levels and early mortality among incident hemodialysis patients. *Kidney Int* 2007;**72**:1004–13.

4. Ishimura E, Nishizawa Y, Inaba M, et al. Serum levels of 1,25-dihydroxyvitamin D, 24,25-dihydroxyvitamin D, and 25-hydroxyvitamin D in nondialyzed patients with chronic renal failure. *Kidney Int* 1999;**55**:1019–27.

5. Jacob AI, Sallman A, Santiz Z, Hollis BW. Defective photoproduction of cholecalciferol in normal and uremic humans. *J Nutr* 1984;**114**:1313–19.

6. Wang TJ, Pencina MJ, Booth SL, et al. Vitamin D deficiency and risk of cardiovascular disease. *Circulation* 2008;**117**:503–11.

7. Gutierrez O, Isakova T, Rhee E, et al. Fibroblast growth factor-23 mitigates hyperphosphatemia but accentuates calcitriol deficiency in chronic kidney disease. *J Am Soc Nephrol* 2005;**16**:2205–15.

8. Nykjaer A, Dragun D, Walther D, et al. An endocytic pathway essential for renal uptake and activation of the steroid 25-(OH) vitamin D3. *Cell* 1999;**96**:507–15.

9. Krapf R, Schaffner T, Iten PX. Abuse of germanium associated with fatal lactic acidosis. *Nephron* 1992;**62**:351–6.

10. Zehnder D, Bland R, Williams MC, et al. Extrarenal expression of 25-hydroxyvitamin d(3)-1 alpha-hydroxylase. *J Clin Endocrinol Metab* 2001;**86**:888–94.

11. Tashiro K, Abe T, Oue N, Yasui W, Ryoji M. Characterisation of vitamin D-mediated induction of the CYP 24 transcription. *Mol Cell Endocrinol* 2004;**226**:27–32.

12. Zierold C, Mings JA, DeLuca HF. Regulation of 25-hydroxyvitamin D3-24-hydroxylase mRNA by 1,25-dihydroxyvitamin D3 and parathyroid hormone. *J Cell Biochem* 2003;**88**:234–7.

13. Ebert R, Schütze N, Adamski J, Jakob F. Vitamin D signaling is modulated on multiple levels in health and disease. *Mol Cell Endocrinol* 2006;**248**:149–59.

14. Merke J, Hügel U, Zlotkowski A et al. Diminished parathyroid 1,25(OH)2D3 receptors in experimental uremia. *Kidney Int* 1987;**32**:350–3.

15. Korkor AB. Reduced binding of [3H]1,25-dihydroxyvitamin D3 in the parathyroid glands of patients with renal failure. *N Engl J Med* 1987;**316**:1573–7.

16. Patel SR, Ke HQ, Vanholder R, Koenig RJ, Hsu CH. Inhibition of calcitriol receptor binding to vitamin D response elements by uremic toxins. *J Clin Invest* 1995;**96**:50–9.

17. Jurutka PW, Bartik L, Whitfield GK, et al. Vitamin D receptor: key roles in bone mineral pathophysiology, molecular mechanism of action, and novel nutritional ligands. *J Bone Miner Res* 2007;**22** Suppl 2:V2–10.

18. St-Arnaud R. The direct role of vitamin D on bone homeostasis. *Arch Biochem Biophys* 2008;**473**:225–30.

19. Hruska KA, Teitelbaum SL. Renal osteodystrophy. *N Engl J Med* 1995;**333**:166–74.

20. Owen TA, Aronow MS, Barone LM, Bettencourt B, Stein GS, Lian JB. Pleiotropic effects of vitamin D on osteoblast gene expression are related to the proliferative and differentiated state of the bone cell phenotype: dependency upon basal levels of gene expression, duration of exposure, and bone matrix competency in normal rat osteoblast cultures. *Endocrinology* 1991;**128**:1496–504.

21. Hattenhauer O, Traebert M, Murer H, Biber J. Regulation of small intestinal Na-P(i) type IIb cotransporter by dietary phosphate intake. *Am J Physiol* 1999;**277**:G756–62.

22. Sommer S, Berndt T, Craig T, Kumar R. The phosphatonins and the regulation of phosphate transport and vitamin D metabolism. *J Steroid Biochem Mol Biol* 2007;**103**:497–503.

23. Masuyama R, Stockmans I, Torrekens S et al. Vitamin D receptor in chondrocytes promotes osteoclastogenesis and regulates FGF23 production in osteoblasts. *J Clin Invest* 2006;**116**:3150–9.

24. Loghman-Adham M. Renal and intestinal Pi transport adaptation to low phosphorus diet in uremic rats. *J Am Soc Nephrol* 1993;**3**:1930–7.

25. Teitelbaum SL, Bone JM, Stein PM, et al. Calcifediol in chronic renal insufficiency. Skeletal response. *J Am Med Ass* 1976;**235**:164–7.

26. Andress D, Norris KC, Coburn JW, Slatopolsky EA, Sherrard DJ. Intravenous calcitriol in the treatment of refractory osteitis fibrosa of chronic renal failure. *N Engl J Med* 1989;**321**:274–9.

27. Hamdy NA, Kanis JA, Beneton MN, et al. Effect of alfacalcidol on natural course of renal bone disease in mild to moderate renal failure. *Br Med J* 1995;**310**:358–63.

28. Ritz E, Küster S, Schmidt-Gayk H et al. Low-dose calcitriol prevents the rise in 1,84-iPTH without affecting serum calcium and phosphate in patients with moderate renal failure (prospective placebo-controlled multicentre trial). *Nephrol Dial Transplant* 1995;**10**: 2228–34.

29. Coyne D, Acharya M, Qiu P, et al. Paricalcitol capsule for the treatment of secondary hyperparathyroidism in stages 3 and 4 CKD. *Am J Kidney Dis* 2006;**47**:263–76.

30. US Renal Data System: USRDS 2007 Annual Data Report. 2007

31. Silberberg JS, Barre PE, Prichard SS, Sniderman AD. Impact of left ventricular hypertrophy on survival in end-stage renal disease. *Kidney Int.* 1989;**36**:286–90.

32. Foley RN, Parfrey PS, Kent GM, Harnett JD, Murray DC, Barre PE. Serial change in echocardiographic parameters and cardiac failure in end-stage renal disease. *J Am Soc Nephrol.* 2000;**11**:912–16.

33. Gillor A, Groneck P, Kaiser J, Schmitz-Stolbrink A. [Congestive heart failure in rickets caused by vitamin D deficiency]. Monatsschrift Kinderheilkunde. *Org Deutsch Gesellsch Kinderheilk* 1989;**137**:108–10.

34. Uysal S, Kalayci AG, Baysal K. Cardiac functions in children with vitamin D deficiency rickets. *Pediatr Cardiol* 1999;**20**:283–6.

35. Liu PT, Stenger S, Li H, et al. Toll-like receptor triggering of a vitamin D-mediated human antimicrobial response. *Science* 2006;**311**:1770–3.

36. Weishaar RE, Simpson RU. Vitamin D3 and cardiovascular function in rats. *J Clin Invest* 1987;**79**:1706–12.

37. Bodyak N, Ayus JC, Achinger S, et al. Activated vitamin D attenuates left ventricular abnormalities induced by dietary sodium in Dahl salt-sensitive animals. *Proc Natl Acad Sci USA* 2007;**104**:16810–15.

38. Mancuso P, Rahman A, Hershey SD, Dandu L, Nibbelink KA, Simpson RU. 1,25-Dihydroxyvitamin-D3 treatment reduces cardiac hypertrophy and left ventricular diameter in spontaneously hypertensive heart failure-prone (cp/+) rats independent of changes in serum leptin. *J Cardiovasc Pharmacol* 2008;**51**:559–64.

39. Tishkoff DX, Nibbelink KA, Holmberg KH, Dandu L, Simpson RU. Functional vitamin D receptor (VDR) in the t-tubules of cardiac myocytes: VDR knockout cardiomyocyte contractility. *Endocrinology* 2008;**149**:558–64.

40. Zhou CL, Lu FX, Cao KX, Xu D, Goltzman D, Miao DS. Calcium-independent and 1,25(OH)(2)D(3)-dependent regulation of the renin-angiotensin system in 1alpha-hydroxylase knockout mice. *Kidney Int* 2008;**74**:170–9.

41. Li YC, Kong J, Wei M, Chen ZF, Liu SQ, Cao LP. 1,25-Dihydroxyvitamin D(3) is a negative endocrine regulator of the renin-angiotensin system. *J Clin Invest* 2002;**110**: 229–38.

42. Xiang W, Kong J, Chen S, et al. Cardiac hypertrophy in vitamin D receptor knockout mice: role of the systemic and cardiac renin-angiotensin systems. *Am J Physiol Endocrinol Metab* 2005;**288**:E125–32.

43. Sarnak MJ, Jaber BL. Pulmonary infectious mortality among patients with end-stage renal disease. *Chest.* 2001;**120**:1883–7.

44. Slinin Y, Foley RN, Collins AJ. Clinical epidemiology of pneumonia in hemodialysis patients: the USRDS waves 1, 3, and 4 study. *Kidney Int* 2006;**70**:1135–41.

45. Zasloff M. Inducing endogenous antimicrobial peptides to battle infections. *Proc Natl Acad Sci USA* 2006;**103**:8913–14.

46. Gombart AF, Bhan I, Borregaard N, et al. Low plasma level of cathelicidin antimicrobial peptide (hCAP18) predicts increased infectious disease mortality in patients undergoing hemodialysis. *Clin Infect Dis* 2009;**48**:418–24.

47. Urry Z, Xystrakis E, Richards D, et al. Ligation of TLR9 induced on human IL-10–secreting Tregs by 1α,25-dihydroxyvitamin D3 abrogates regulatory function. *J Clin Invest* 2009;**119**:387–98.

48. Adorini L, Penna G. Dendritic cell tolerogenicity: a key mechanism in immunomodulation by vitamin D receptor agonists. *Hum Immunol* 2009;**70**:345–52.

49. Manolagas SC, Yu XP, Girasole G, Bellido T. Vitamin D and the hematolymphopoietic tissue: a (1994) update. *Semin Nephrol* 1994;**14**:129–43.

50. Manolagas SC, Provvedini DM, Tsoukas CD. Interactions of 1,25-dihydroxyvitamin D3 and the immune system. *Mol Cell Endocrinol* 1985;**43**:113–22.

51. Müller K, Bendtzen K. 1,25-Dihydroxyvitamin D3 as a natural regulator of human immune functions. *J Invest Dermatol Symp Proc* 1996;**1**:68–71.

52. Moe SM, Zekonis M, Harezlak J et al. A placebo-controlled trial to evaluate immunomodulatory effects of paricalcitol. *Am J Kidney Dis* 2001;**38**:792–802.

53. Chonchol M, Scragg R. 25-Hydroxyvitamin D, insulin resistance, and kidney function in the Third National Health and Nutrition Examination Survey. *Kidney Int* 2007;**71**:134–9.

54. Martins D, Wolf M, Pan D, et al. Prevalence of cardiovascular risk factors and the serum levels of 25-hydroxyvitamin D in the United States: data from the Third National Health and Nutrition Examination Survey. *Arch Intern Med* 2007;**167**:1159–65.

55. Mak RH. 1,25-Dihydroxyvitamin D3 corrects insulin and lipid abnormalities in uremia. *Kidney Int* 1998;**53**:1353–7.

56. Kautzky-Willer A, Pacini G, Barnas U, et al. Intravenous calcitriol normalises insulin sensitivity in uremic patients. *Kidney Int* 1995;**47**:200–6.

57. Hirata M, Makibayashi K, Katsumata K, et al. 22-Oxacalcitriol prevents progressive glomerulosclerosis without adversely affecting calcium and phosphorus metabolism in subtotally nephrectomised rats. *Nephrol Dial Transplant* 2002;**17**:2132–7.

58. Kuhlmann A, Haas CS, Gross ML, et al. 1,25-Dihydroxyvitamin D3 decreases podocyte loss and podocyte hypertrophy in the subtotally nephrectomised rat. *Am J Physiol Renal Physiol* 2004;**286**:F526–33.

59. Panichi V, Migliori M, Taccola D, et al. Effects of 1,25(OH)2D3 in experimental mesangial proliferative nephritis in rats. *Kidney Int* 2001;**60**:87–95.

60. Tian J, Liu Y, Williams LA, de Zeeuw D. Potential role of active vitamin D in retarding the progression of chronic kidney disease. *Nephrol Dial Transplant* 2007;**22**:321–8.

61. Zhang Z, Zhang Y, Ning G, Deb DK, Kong J, Li YC. Combination therapy with AT1 blocker and vitamin D analog markedly ameliorates diabetic nephropathy: blockade of compensatory renin increase. *Proc Natl Acad Sci USA* 2008;**105**:15896–901.

62. Teng M, Wolf M, Lowrie E, Ofsthun N, Lazarus JM, Thadhani R. Survival of patients undergoing hemodialysis with paricalcitol or calcitriol therapy. *N Engl J Med* 2003;**349**:446–56.

63. Teng M, Wolf M, Ofsthun MN, et al. Activated injectable vitamin D and hemodialysis survival: a historical cohort study. *J Am Soc Nephrol* 2005;**16**:1115–25.

64. Melamed ML, Eustace JA, Plantinga L et al. Changes in serum calcium, phosphate, and PTH and the risk of death in incident dialysis patients: a longitudinal study. *Kidney Int* 2006;**70**:351–7.

65. Kalantar-Zadeh K, Kuwae N, Regidor DL, et al. Survival predictability of time-varying indicators of bone disease in maintenance hemodialysis patients. *Kidney Int* 2006;**70**: 771–80.

66. Shoji T, Shinohara K, Kimoto E, et al. Lower risk for cardiovascular mortality in oral 1alpha-hydroxy vitamin D3 users in a hemodialysis population. *Nephrol Dial Transplant* 2004;**19**:179–84.

67. Tentori F, Hunt WC, Stidley CA, et al. Mortality risk among hemodialysis patients receiving different vitamin D analogs. *Kidney Int* 2006;**70**:1858–65.

68. Naves-Díaz M, Alvarez-Hernández D, Passlick-Deetjen J, et al. Oral active vitamin D is associated with improved survival in hemodialysis patients. *Kidney Int* 2008;**74**:1070–8.

69. Shinaberger CS, Kopple JD, Kovesdy CP, et al. Ratio of paricalcitol dosage to serum parathyroid hormone level and survival in maintenance hemodialysis patients. *Clin J Am Soc Nephrol* 2008;**3**:1769–76.

70. St Peter WL, Li S, Liu J, Gilbertson DT, Arneson TJ, Collins AJ. Effects of monthly dose and regular dosing of intravenous active vitamin D use on mortality among patients undergoing hemodialysis. *Pharmacotherapy* 2009;**29**:154–64.

71. Tentori F, Albert JM, Young EW, et al. The survival advantage for hemodialysis patients taking vitamin D is questioned: findings from the Dialysis Outcomes and Practice Patterns Study. *Nephrol Dial Transplant* 2009;**24**:963–72.

72. Kovesdy CP, Ahmadzadeh S, Anderson JE, Kalantar-Zadeh K. Association of activated vitamin D treatment and mortality in chronic kidney disease. *Arch Intern Med* 2008;**168**:397–403.

73. Shoben A, Rudser K, De Boer I, Young B, Kestenbaum B. Association of oral calcitriol with improved survival in nondialyzed CKD. *J Am Soc Nephrol* 2008;7.

74. Levin A, Djurdjev O, Beaulieu M, Er L. Variability and risk factors for kidney disease progression and death following attainment of stage 4 CKD in a referred cohort. *Am J Kidney Dis* 2008;**52**:661–71.

75. Palmer SC, McGregor DO, Macaskill P, Craig JC, Elder GJ, Strippoli GF. Meta-analysis: vitamin D compounds in chronic kidney disease. *Ann Intern Med* 2007;**147**:840–53.

Chapter 9

Growth factors and cytokines in renal bone disease

Esther A. González and Kevin J. Martin

Introduction

Studies on the pathogenesis of abnormalities in bone, which are seen in association with kidney disease, have mainly focused upon abnormalities in the parathyroid hormone-vitamin D axis and have in recent years been expanded to consideration of calcifications at extraskeletal sites.[1,2] Thus, hyperparathyroidism can give rise to a high bone turnover state, which in its severe form is manifested as osteitis fibrosa cystica and, on the other hand, relatively low levels of parathyroid hormone (PTH) are associated with a low bone turnover state of adynamic bone. However, it is now clear that the wide variations in the manifestations of renal bone disease present in patients with end stage renal disease cannot be explained simply by abnormalities in PTH or vitamin D. Thus, measurements of parathyroid hormone correlate relatively weakly with the various parameters of bone histology and many investigators have shown that there is a wide scatter of data points of histomorphometric parameters for any given level of PTH.[3] The abnormalities in bone may also be modified by the administration of potent vitamin D metabolites given to control hyperparathyroidism, but this therapy may also potentially have direct consequences on the activity of bone cells, and by influencing the levels of calcium and phosphorus levels in serum, could conceivably affect calcification.

In the past two decades, there has been a remarkable increase in our understanding of the regulation of bone cell activity, and it is now clear that there is a multitude of local and circulating growth factors and cytokines which can influence the activity of the cells of bone.[4] Abnormalities in several of these factors have been demonstrated to occur during the course of chronic kidney disease and, therefore, have a potential to contribute to the protean manifestations of bone disease seen in this setting of kidney disease.[5,6]

The cells of bone

Bone remodeling is complex process by which old bone is removed and replaced by new bone, a process that requires interaction between different cell types, and is regulated by a variety of biochemical and mechanical factors. The remodeling process allows for the maintenance of the shape, quality, and strength, as well as size, of the skeleton. The process requires the coordinated actions of osteoclasts and osteoblasts.

Osteoblasts are responsible for the production of bone matrix. They originate from mesenchymal stem cells, which reside in the bone marrow and have the capacity to differentiate into either osteoblasts, adipocytes, chondrocytes, myoblasts, or fibroblasts (Fig. 9.1).[7] This process is under the influence of several growth factors including bone morphogenetic protein 2 (BMP-2), transforming growth factor–beta (TGF-β), insulin like growth factor-1 (IGF-1) and basic fibroblast growth factor (bFGF).[8] The activity of the mature osteoblast can be regulated by a variety of hormones, cytokines, and growth factors, some of which are secreted from the osteoblast itself, and act in an autocrine and paracrine manner. Thus, osteoblasts may produce insulin-like growth factors (IGF), platelet-derived growth factor (PDGF), transforming growth factor-beta (TGF-β), basic fibroblast growth factor (bFGF), and bone morphogenetic proteins (BMP). Regulation of osteoblast activity can be influenced by a variety of systemic hormones which include PTH, vitamin D, growth hormone, estrogen, androgen, thyroid hormone, and insulin.

Osteoclasts are derived from the hematopoietic cells of the monocyte macrophage lineage, and are the bone cells that are responsible for bone resorption. Like the osteoblast, osteoclast development and function is also regulated by a variety of locally acting cytokines at various stages of differentiation, as well as by systemic hormones (Fig. 9.2).[9] Osteoclast development is intimately involved with the osteoblast/stromal cells (see below).

Osteocytes are osteoblasts that have been trapped in the osteoid. These cells have numerous long cell processes and are organized during the formation of the bone matrix before it calcifies, and so have a network of connections that permeate the bone matrix. It is thought that the osteocytes are the cells of bone that respond to tissue

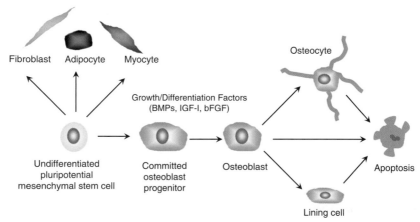

Fig. 9.1 Development and fate of the osteoblast. The pluripotential mesenchymal stem cell of the bone marrow gives rise to osteoblast precursors as well as to fibroblasts, adipocytes, and myocytes. The bone morphogenetic proteins, IGF-1, and bFGF favor differentiation into mature osteoblasts. Mature osteoblasts replace the bone resorbed by osteoclasts and go on to differentiate into lining cells, osteocytes, or undergo apoptosis.

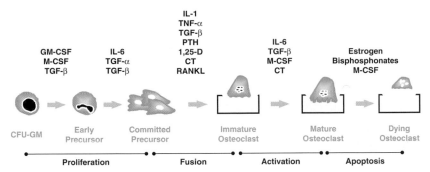

Fig. 9.2 Development and fate of the osteoclast. Osteoclast progenitors derive from the hematopoietic CFU-GM under the influence of M-CSF, and their further development requires interaction with cells of the osteoblastic lineage and the actions of a variety of cytokines and growth factors. The mature osteoclast resorbs bone and then undergoes apoptosis. (Modified from Roodman.[9])

strain and enhance bone remodeling activity by recruiting bone resorbing cells to areas where remodeling is required.

Bone remodeling

The bone remodeling process results from the coordinated action of osteoblasts and osteoclasts and is illustrated in Fig. 9.3. The normal remodeling cycling process requires the process of bone resorption and bone formation to take place in a co-ordinated fashion, which depends upon the orderly development and activation of osteoclasts and osteoblasts.[10] Activation of the remodeling cycle, for example, by PTH, results in retraction of the lining cells of bone and the secretion of collagenase, which degrades the collagen on the bone surface. This results in a chemotactic signal for osteoclasts which attach to the bone and begin to create a resorption cavity. These ultimately detach from the bone surface and are replaced by osteoblasts, which begin to fill the cavity with bone matrix that later becomes mineralized. Thus, bone remodeling is accomplished by resorption of old bone, followed by the formation of new bone. The osteoclasts that resorb a section of bone then detach from the bone surface and are replaced by osteoblasts, which initiate the process of bone formation and fill the resorption cavity by secreting bone matrix that later becomes mineralized. These complex series of events are under the regulation of a variety of systemic and local factors and is the integrated effect of these factors on cell differentiation, cell proliferation, and cellular activity that are responsible for the maintenance of a healthy skeleton.[11]

As noted above, it has been recognized for some time that the development of osteo-clasts requires a close interaction between the osteoclast precursor and osteoblastic stromal cells (Fig. 9.4). It now appears that the activation of the remodeling cycle begins with the activation of cells of the osteoblast lineage, which express RANKL

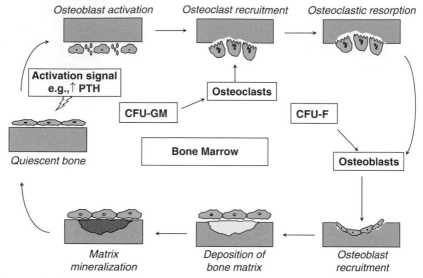

Fig. 9.3 The bone remodeling cycle. The cycle is initiated by an activation signal that results in a sequence of events leading to osteoclast recruitment and activation followed by bone resorption. The osteoclasts are subsequently replaced by osteoblasts and the latter fill the resorption lacuna with matrix, which later becomes mineralized. The new bone remains covered by a layer of quiescent cells until the cycle is reactivated. (Reproduced from Gonzalez et al.[29] with permission.)

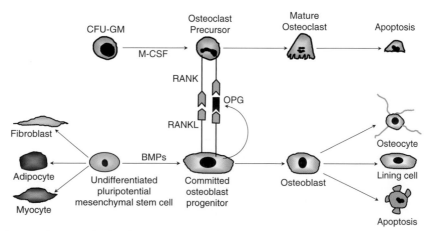

Fig. 9.4 The central role of the RANK/RANKL/OPG system in osteoclastogenesis. The development of the osteoclast requires interaction with osteoblastic precursors/stromal cell RANKL for development to mature osteoclasts. The osteoblast produces OPG, a decoy receptor for RANKL, which can inhibit the RANKL/RANK interaction.

(receptor activator of NF-κB ligand) on their surface.[12,13] RANKL then interacts with the receptor (RANK) on the osteoblast precursor. This RANK ligand and RANK interaction results in the activation, differentiation, and fusion of the osteoclast precursor to result in the generation of the mature osteoclast, which then initiates bone resorption. The interaction between RANK and RANKL can be influenced by a protein known as osteoprotegerin (OPG), which is secreted from the osteoblast, and acts as a decoy receptor for RANKL, and thus can inhibit the final differentiation and activation of osteoclasts.[14,15]

The importance of the effects of OPG have been demonstrated in experimental animals, where it can be shown that OPG inhibits osteoclast development and activity induced by RANKL, and can block the increase in serum calcium caused by administration of RANKL.[12] Thus, OPG should have a protective effect on bone by decreasing osteoclastogenesis and osteoclast-mediated bone resorption. In experimental animals, administration of OPG leads to increased bone mineral density and over expression of OPG has been shown to result in osteopetrosis, while conversely, disruption of the OPG gene results in osteoporosis.[16,17] The RANK/RANKL/OPG system appears to be of major importance in bone remodeling and is regulated by the actions of many cytokines and hormones, including PTH, calcitriol, prostaglandins, TNF-alpha, glucocorticoids, estrogens, bone morphogenetic protein-2, and TGF-β, as well as interleukin-1 and interleukin-11.

Effects of uremia on skeletal biology

There is increasing information to indicate that the various cytokine and growth factor systems involved in the regulation of the bone remodeling cycle may be disturbed in patients with chronic kidney disease, and accordingly, may potentially contribute to the variation in the histological abnormalities of bone in the setting of chronic kidney disease. Thus, the levels of interleukin-1 (IL-1), which has been demonstrated to be an important activator of the bone remodeling cycle and to influence the RANK/RANKL/OPG system, have been reported to be elevated in patients on dialysis.[18] However, the levels of IL-1 receptor antagonists have also been demonstrated to be increased in such patients and, accordingly, may also modify the effects of IL-1 on the remodeling cycle. Indeed, Ferrera and others have reported an inverse relationship between the levels of IL-1 receptor antagonists and osteoblast surface of bone.[19]

TNF-alpha is another important cytokine for the regulation of the activity of the bone remodeling cycle. This has also been found to circulate in high levels in patients with uremia.[18] This inflammatory cytokine may be increased because of a systemic inflammatory state that is not uncommon in patients with advanced kidney failure and may affect the skeleton, as well as calcification at extraskeletal sites.[20]

Interleukin-6 has been shown to regulate the RANK/RANKL/OPG system, and may also appear to influence osteoclastogenesis and osteoclast function by mechanisms, which are independent of the RANK/RANKL system.[21,22] Several abnormalities of the IL-6 system have been described in uremia, as well as in patients with chronic kidney disease. Montelban et al. found that IL-6 levels and bone remodeling markers were well correlated in patients with renal osteodystrophy.[23] Elevated levels of soluble IL-6 receptors, which can modulate the actions of IL-6, have been reported in patients on hemodialysis, and an inverse relationship between the soluble IL-6 receptor/IL-6 ratio and osteoclast surface in bone has also been demonstrated in uremic patients.[19] Studies by Langub et al. have demonstrated an increased expression of IL-6 receptor mRNA in osteoclasts in bone biopsies of patients with chronic kidney disease, and it appeared that the bone resorbing activity correlated with the levels of IL-6 receptor mRNA.[24] Although the exact contribution of abnormal IL-6 metabolism to the manifestations of renal bone disease is not entirely clear at the present time, it is likely to be important, based on the well established role of this cytokines in other states of abnormal bone resorption.

The components of RANK/RANKL/OPG system have not been well studied in the setting of decreased renal function, but alterations are expected, since this system is crucial in the regulation of bone cell metabolism and is clearly regulated by the calciotropic hormones PTH and calcitriol, as well as estrogen, androgen, and many of the cytokines that have been demonstrated to be abnormal in this clinical setting. Indeed, studies have demonstrated elevated levels of circulating OPG in uremic patients, and that the levels of OPG appear to be associated with histological parameters of bone resorption and bone formation.[25]

Other factors that are known to regulate osteoblast growth and differentiation have also been demonstrated in uremic patients. Levels of IGF-1 have been shown to be elevated and have been demonstrated to correlate with bone formation rate.[26]

TGF-β, as well as other members of the TGF-β family, such as BMP-7, which appears to be important in osteoblast differentiation, may also be abnormal in the setting of advanced kidney disease. A role for BMP-7 in the pathogenesis or modification of renal osteodystrophy is supported by studies in experimental animals, in which it has been demonstrated by BMP-7 administration, appears to modify the histological abnormalities of bone induced by renal failure.[27] Specifically, marrow fibrosis, an important feature of hyperparathyroid bone disease, appears to be attenuated in animals treated with BMP-7. Conversely, in a different model of chronic kidney disease, BMP-7 administration appeared to increase bone formation.[28] Further studies are required to define the role of BMP-7 in renal bone disease.

In summary, in addition to the effects of the well known calciotropic hormones, normal bone remodeling appears to depend on the integrated effects of a variety of growth factors and cytokine systems. There are many abnormalities in the setting of chronic kidney disease, not only in circulating hormones, but also in terms of systemic inflammatory responses associated with abnormalities in a variety of cytokines. Since these cytokines appear to impact upon the bone remodeling cycle, they are likely to modify the active cellular processes of bone, and thus alter the manifestations of renal osteodystrophy. Further work is required to specifically delineate their actions on bone, especially in the setting of renal bone disease and to investigate the potential of modifying these cytokine and growth factor pathways with specific therapeutic agents to improve not only the abnormalities of the skeleton, but which might also have the potential to influence calcifications at extraskeletal sites.

References

1. Martin KJ, Gonzalez EA, Slatopolsky E. Renal osteodystrophy. In: B. M. Brenner (ed.), The *Kidney*. Philadelphia: W.B. Saunders Company, 2004:2255–304.

2. Moe SM, Chen NX. Mechanisms of vascular calcification in chronic kidney disease. *J Am Soc Nephrol* 2008;**19**:213–6.

3. Drueke TB. Is parathyroid hormone measurement useful for the diagnosis of renal bone disease? *Kidney Int* 2008;**73**:674–6.

4. Manolagas SC, Jilka RL. Bone marrow, cytokines, and bone remodeling. Emerging insights into the pathophysiology of osteoporosis. *N Engl J Med* 1995;**332**:305–11.

5. Gonzalez EA. The role of cytokines in skeletal remodeling: possible consequences for renal osteodystrophy. *Nephrol Dial Transplant* 2000;**15**:945–50.

6. Monier-Faugere MC, Malluche HH. Role of cytokines in renal osteodystrophy. *Curr Opin Nephrol Hypertens* 1997;**6**:327–32.

7. Bianco P, Riminucci M, Gronthos S, et al. Bone marrow stromal stem cells: nature, biology, and potential applications. *Stem Cells* 2001;**19**:180–92.

8. Hughes FJ, Turner W, Belibasakis G, et al. Effects of growth factors and cytokines on osteoblast differentiation. *Periodontol* 2006;**41**:48–72.

9. Roodman GD. Advances in bone biology: the osteoclast. *Endocr Rev* 1996;**17**:308–32.

10. Hadjidakis DJ, Androulakis, II. Bone remodeling. *Ann NY Acad Sci* 2006;**1092**:385–96.

11. Hofbauer LC, Khosla S, Dunstan CR, Lacey DL, Boyle WJ, Riggs BL, et al. The roles of osteoprotegerin and osteoprotegerin ligand in the paracrine regulation of bone resorption. *J Bone Miner Res* 2000;**15**:2–12. Review.

12. Lacey DL, Timms E, Tan HL, et al. Osteoprotegerin ligand is a cytokine that regulates osteoclast differentiation and activation. *Cell* 1998;**93**:165–76.

13. Yasuda H, Shima N, Nakagawa N, et al. Osteoclast differentiation factor is a ligand for osteoprotegerin/osteoclastogenesis-inhibitory factor and is identical to TRANCE/RANKL. *Proc Nat Acad Sci USA* 1998;**95**:3597–602.

14. Kwon BS, Wang S, Udagawa N, et al. TR1, a new member of the tumor necrosis factor receptor superfamily, induces fibroblast proliferation and inhibits osteoclastogenesis and bone resorption. *FASEB J* 1998;**12**:845–54.

15. Tsuda E, Goto M, Mochizuki S, et al. Isolation of a novel cytokine from human fibroblasts that specifically inhibits osteoclastogenesis. *Biochem Biophys Res Comm* 1997;**234**:137–42.

16. Bucay N, Sarosi I, Dunstan CR, et al. osteoprotegerin-deficient mice develop early onset osteoporosis and arterial calcification. *Genes Dev* 1998;**12**:1260–8.

17. Simonet WS, Lacey DL, Dunstan CR, et al. Osteoprotegerin: a novel secreted protein involved in the regulation of bone density. *Cell, USA* 1997;**89**:309–19.

18. Herbelin A, Nguyen AT, Zingraff J, et al. Influence of uremia and hemodialysis on circulating interleukin-1 and tumor necrosis factor alpha. *Kidney Int* 1990;**37**:116–25.

19. Ferreira A, Simon P, Drueke TB, et al. Potential role of cytokines in renal osteodystrophy [letter]. *Nephrol Dial Transplant* 1996;**11**:399–400.

20. Al-Aly Z, Shao JS, Lai CF, et al. Aortic Msx2-Wnt calcification cascade is regulated by TNF-alpha-dependent signals in diabetic LDLr–/– mice. *Arterioscler Thromb Vasc Biol* 2007;**27**:2589–96.

21. Adebanjo OA, Moonga BS, Yamate T, et al. Mode of action of interleukin-6 on mature osteoclasts. Novel interactions with extracellular Ca2+ sensing in the regulation of osteoclastic bone resorption. *J Cell Biol* 1998;**142**:1347–56.

22. Dai JC, He P, Chen X, et al. TNFalpha and PTH utilize distinct mechanisms to induce IL-6 and RANKL expression with markedly different kinetics. *Bone* 2006;**38:**509–20.

23. Montalbán C, García-Unzueta MT, De Francisco AL, et al. Serum interleukin-6 in renal osteodystrophy: relationship with serum PTH and bone remodeling markers. *Hormone Metabol Res* 1999;**31:**14–17.

24. Langub MC, Jr., Koszewski NJ, Turner HV, et al. Bone resorption and mRNA expression of IL-6 and IL-6 receptor in patients with renal osteodystrophy. *Kidney Int* 1996;**50:** 515–20.

25. Coen G, Ballanti P, Balducci A, et al. Serum osteoprotegerin and renal osteodystrophy. *Nephrol Dial Transplant* 2002;**17:**233–8.

26. Andress DL, Pandian MR, Endres DB, et al. Plasma insulin-like growth factors and bone formation in uremic hyperparathyroidism. *Kidney Int* 1989;**36:**471–7.

27. Gonzalez EA, Lund RJ, Martin KJ, et al. Treatment of a murine model of high-turnover renal osteodystrophy by exogenous BMP-7. *Kidney Int* 2002;**61:**1322–31.

28. Davies MR, Lund RJ, Mathew S, et al. Low turnover osteodystrophy and vascular calcification are amenable to skeletal anabolism in an animal model of chronic kidney disease and the metabolic syndrome. *J Am Soc Nephrol* 2005;**16:**917–28.

29. González E, Martin K. Bone cell response in uremia. *Sem Dial* 1996;**9:**339–46.

Chapter 10

Bone histomorphometry in renal osteodystrophy

Arnold J. Felsenfeld* and Armando Torres

Historical perspective of renal osteodystrophy

The first descriptions of renal osteodystrophy preceded the dialysis era by many years. The earliest descriptions of bone disease associated with renal failure were in children. Subsequently, azotemic adults with abnormal bone histology were described. A detailed review of this topic has been performed previously[1] and only a brief review will be provided.

Renal rickets

The term 'renal rickets' was first used in the early 20th century to describe bone disease in children and adolescents with renal failure. In 1921, 10 cases of stunted development associated with bone deformities due to chronic nephritis were described. Subsequently, several different forms of renal rickets were described and attributed to acidosis or a combination of acidosis and hyperparathyroidism.

In the 1970s, studies from Heidelberg, Germany differentiated renal rickets from vitamin D deficiency. These studies showed that in contrast to children with vitamin D deficiency, the cartilagenous growth plate in uremic children was not widened, but rather was devoid of a well-ordered column of cartilage cells. In advanced stages, dense cellular fibrous tissue was present under the growth plate. Thus, in contrast to vitamin D deficiency in which the radiographic radiolucent area was due to the accumulation of non-mineralized irregularly structured cartilage, the radiolucent area in uremia resulted from the transformation of the zone of primary spongiosa into woven bone with a low mineral content. In severe renal rickets, epiphyseal slipping often developed and it was associated with hypocalcemia. However, epiphyseal slipping was rarely seen in children on dialysis probably because of improved calcium balance.

Calcium and phosphorus balance in renal failure

In 1943 Liu and Chu were the first to use balance studies to study calcium in renal failure. They showed that impaired intestinal calcium absorption was present and it failed to improve even after large doses of vitamin D. Dihydrotachysterol which does not require renal 1α-hydroxylation for activation, was shown to increase intestinal calcium.

Bone disease in the predialysis era

While symptomatic bone disease was observed in azotemic children in the predialysis era, clinical manifestations of bone disease were initially stated to be infrequent in the azotemic adult. However, in a study of renal osteodystrophy in the predialysis era published in 1966, Stanbury and Lumb correlated the plasma calcium and phosphorus values with the form of bone disease in 134 azotemic patients, who were mostly adults. Of the 134 patients, 40 were personal cases and 94 cases were compiled from the published literature. As shown in Fig. 10.1, the values (mean $\pm$ SD) of serum calcium (10.05 $\pm$ 1.25 versus 7.63 $\pm$ 1.47mg/dl, $p < 0.001$), phosphorus (8.79 $\pm$ 2.74 versus 6.03 $\pm$ 2.25mg/dl, $p < 0.001$) and the calcium-phosphorus product (86.5 $\pm$ 21.9 versus 45.7 $\pm$ 18.6, $p < 0.001$) were greater in patients with osteitis fibrosa ($n = 55$) than in patients with osteomalacia or rickets ($n = 79$). Thus, Stanbury and Lumb concluded that hypocalcemia contributed to the development of renal rickets and osteomalacia.

Support for this hypothesis was provided by Mora Palma et al.[2] and Nielsen et al.[3] In the former study of 327 predialysis patients, 54% of the bone biopsies showed osteitis fibrosa, 34% a combination of osteomalacia and osteitis fibrosa, and 12% neither abnormality. The combination of osteomalacia and osteitis fibrosa was strongly associated with interstitial kidney disease, hypocalcemia, normophosphatemia (in contrast to hyperphosphatemia seen in osteitis fibrosa), a lower calcium-phosphorus product, and acidosis. Similarly, Nielsen et al. reported that hypocalcemia in the predialysis patient was associated with osteoid accumulation and decreased bone formation. These clinical studies suggest that the availability of calcium and phosphorus are important for mineralization of bone in the azotemic patient.

Pathology of different forms of renal osteodystrophy

Renal osteodystrophy is a multifactorial disorder affecting bone and many different histological abnormalities of bone are observed in CKD patients. The four major types of bone disease that occur in CKD are: osteitis fibrosa (OF), mixed uremic osteodystrophy (MUO), low turnover osteomalacia (OM), and adynamic (AD) bone.[4] A description of normal bone remodeling is included to provide a better understanding of the different forms of renal osteodystrophy.

These 134 cases were published by Stanbury and Lumb in 1966, and reproduced in Felsenfeld and Torres.[1] In the top panel, the frequency of distribution of plasma calcium and phosphorus is shown for patients with renal rickets and osteomalacia, and for patients with osteitis fibrosa. In the bottom panel, the frequency of distribution of the calcium-phosphorus product is shown for patients with renal rickets and osteomalacia, and for patients with osteitis fibrosa. Cases of osteomalacia are shown as open squares, cases of rickets are shown as squares with diagonal, and cases of osteitis fibrosa are shown as stippled squares. The letters F and A refer, respectively, to cases with Fanconi syndrome and renal tubular acidosis. Reprinted with permission of the *Quarterly Journal of Medicine*.[64]

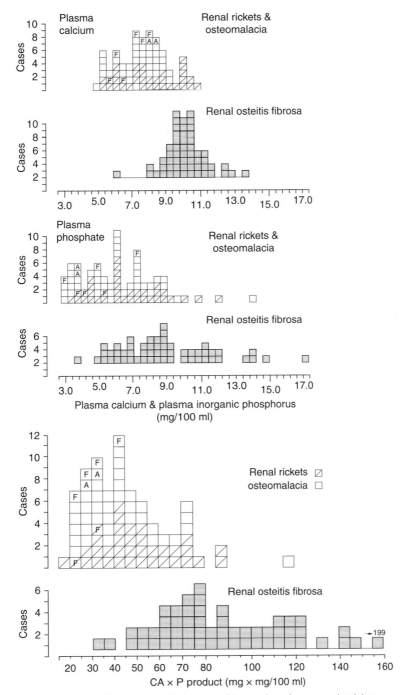

Fig. 10.1 Frequency of distribution of plasma calcium, phosphorus, and calcium-phosphate product in 134 cases of azotemic osteodystrophy in the predialysis era.

Normal bone

The adult skeleton undergoes continual remodeling, a dynamic process which allows for removal of older, potentially damaged bone and the formation of new bone. The remodeling cycle, which normally lasts from 4 to 8 months, encompasses several steps:

- an activation phase in which osteoclasts are recruited and the bone surface prepared;
- a resorption phase in which osteoclasts erode the bone surface;
- a reversal phase which begins when resorption ends and osteoblasts appear at the site;
- bone formation in which osteoid deposition by osteoblasts is followed by mineralization.

The amount of bone remodeled per unit depends both on osteoblastic and osteoclastic activity at each bone remodeling unit site, and on the number of active remodeling sites per unit of bone volume. In normal bone, osteoclasts are present on a small percentage of the bone surface (<2%), osteoid is lamellar and is present on a moderate amount of the bone surface (<25%), and osteoblasts cover 20–40% of the osteoid surface. Another cell, the osteocyte (Fig. 10.2A) has recently become the focus of great interest. The osteocyte besides being the site of FGF23 production,[5] is likely important in the signal to activate bone remodeling and is also involved in other metabolic activities.

Bone histomorphometric analysis is divided into four categories—(1) structural; (2) static formation; (3) dynamic formation; and (4) resorption. Table 10.1 shows the histomorphometric parameters and normal values following the American Society for Bone and Mineral Research (ASBMR) nomenclature.[6,7] The normative data shown in Table 10.2 come from relatively small and heterogenous series.[7–9] An international effort is needed to collect all currently available normative data and to prospectively obtain bone biopsy samples from healthy volunteers.

Tetracycline is used to assess bone formation because of its fluorescent properties and deposition at sites of bone mineralization. Before performing a bone biopsy, tetracycline is administered at two separate time intervals. The two time-spaced fluorescent labels in bone are used to measure the mineral apposition rate which is calculated from the distance between the midpoints of two tetracycline labels divided by the days between the two labels (Figure 10.3A). Four important dynamic measurements of bone[7,10]—(1) the bone formation rate, (2) the activation frequency, (3) the osteoid maturation time, and (4) the mineralization lag time—are derived from tetracycline labeling (Table 10.1). The first two parameters are used to evaluate bone turnover, primarily how much mineralized bone is being formed. The second two parameters are used to determine how well the osteoid is mineralising. The bone formation rate (BFR) is defined as the amount of bone being formed per unit of bone per unit of time (per day or year). It can be measured directly as the length of the tetracycline labels per bone surface (MS/BS) multiplied by the distance between labels (mineral appositional rate) and expressed in reference to the bone surface, bone volume, or tissue volume (Table 10.1).

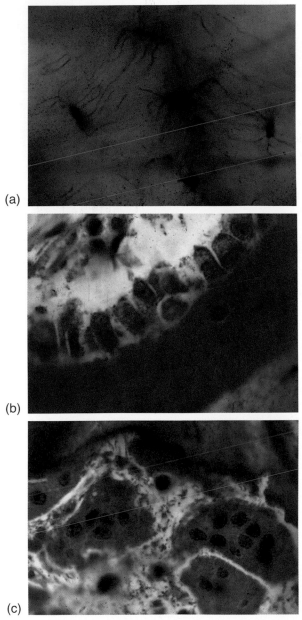

Fig. 10.2 Bone cells. (A) Shown is a high power view of osteocytes with their multiple canaliculi spreading throughout much of the bone. (B) A high power view of osteoblasts lining an osteoid seam (magenta color) in a hemodialysis patient with OF is shown. Also seen is an osteoblast migrating through the osteoid destined to become an osteocyte. An osteocyte can also be seen within the bone at the bottom right. (C) A high power view of several large multi-nucleated osteoclasts in a resorption cavity of a hemodialysis patient with OF is shown. The scalloped resorption surface of the bone is seen along the top quarter of the figure.

Table 10.1 Formulas used to calculate histomorphometric values from primary measurements[a,7] Reproduced from Glorieux FH, Travers R, Taylor A, et al. (2000) Normative data for iliac bone histomorphometry in growing children. *Bone* **26**:103–109, Copyright © 2000 with permission from Elsevier.

Abbreviation	Parameter	Unit	Formula
Structural			
Ct.Wi	Cortical width	Mm	Direct measurement
BV/TV	Bone volume/tissue volume	%	(bone area/tissue area) × 100
Md.V/TV	Mineralized volume/tissue volume	%	(BV/TV) − (OV/TV)
Tb.Th	Trabecular thickness	µm	(bone area/bone perimeter) × 2/1.2
Tb.N	Trabecular number	/mm	(BV/TV)/Tb.Th × 10
Tb.Sp	Trabecular separation	µm	(1000/Tb.N) − Tb.Th
BS/BV	Bone surface/bone volume	mm²/mm³	(bone perimeter/bone area) × 1.2
BS/TV	Bone surface/tissue volume	mm²/mm³	(bone perimeter/tissue area) × 1.2
Static formation			
O.Th	Osteoid thickness	µm	(osteoid area/osteoid perimeter) × 2/1.2
OS/BS	Osteoid surface/bone surface	%	(osteoid perimeter/bone perimeter) × 100
OS/TV	Osteoid surface/tissue volume	mm²/mm³	(osteoid perimeter/tissue area) × 1.2
OV/BV	Osteoid volume/bone volume	%	(osteoid area/bone area) × 100
OV/TV	Osteoid volume/tissue volume	%	(osteoid area/tissue area) × 100
Ob.S/BS	Osteoblast surface/bone surface	%	(osteoblast perimeter/bone perimeter) × 100
Ob.S/OS	Osteoblast surface/osteoid surface	%	(osteoblast perimeter/osteoid perimeter) × 100
Ob.S/TV	Osteoblast surface/tissue volume	mm²/mm³	(osteoblast perimeter/tissue area) × 1.2
W.Th	Wall thickness	µm	(distance between quiescent bone surface and change in lamellar direction)/1.2
Dynamic formation			
MS/BS	Mineralising surface/bone surface	%	(perimeter double label + 1/2 perimeter single label)/bone perimeter × 100
MS/OS	Mineralising surface/osteoid surface	%	(MS/BS)/(OS/BS)
MAR	Mineral apposition rate	µm/d	(distance between labels/marker interval)/1.2
Aj.AR	Adjusted apposition rate	µm/d	MAR × (MS/OS)/100
Mlt	Mineralization lag time	D	O.Th/Aj.AR
Omt	Osteoid maturation time	D	O.Th/MAR
BFR/BS	Bone formation rate/bone surface	µm³/µm²/y	MAR × (MS/BS) × 365
BFR/BV	Bone formation rate/bone volume	%/y	(BFR/BS) × (BS/BV)
BFR/TV	Bone formation rate/tissue volume	%/y	(BFR/BS) × (BS/TV)

Table 10.1 (continued) Formulas used to calculate histomorphometric values from primary measurements[a,7] Reproduced from Glorieux FH, Travers R, Taylor A, et al. (2000) Normative data for iliac bone histomorphometry in growing children. *Bone* **26**:103–109, Copyright © 2000 with permission from Elsevier.

Abbreviation	Parameter	Unit	Formula
Ac.F	Activation frequency	/y	(BFR/BS)/W.Th
FP	Formation period	D	W.Th/Aj.AR
Resorption			
ES/BS	Eroded surface/bone surface	%	(erosive perimeter/bone perimeter) × 100
ES/TV	Eroded surface/tissue volume	mm^2/mm^3	(erosive perimeter/tissue area) × 1.2
Oc.S/BS	Osteoclast surface/bone surface	%	(osteoclast perimeter/bone perimeter) × 100
Oc.S/TV	Osteoclast surface/tissue volume	mm^2/mm^3	(osteoclast perimeter/tissue area) × 1.2
N.Oc/B.Pm	Number of osteoclasts/bone perimeter	/mm	osteoclast number/bone perimeter
N.Oc/T.Ar	Number of osteoclasts/tissue area	$/mm^2$	osteoclast number/tissue area

[a]Reprinted with permission of Bone.

Table 10.2 Frequently applied histomorphometric parameters in normal individuals. Nomenclature of the ASBMR.[6] Data from Parfitt AM, Drezner MK, Glorieux FH, et al. Bone histomorphometry: standardization of nomenclature, symbols, and units: Report of the ASBMR Histomorphometry Nomenclature Committee. *J Bone Miner Res* 1987;**2**:595–610.

	Coen et al. (Italy)[8]	Dos Reis et al., (Brazil)[9]	Glorieux et al. (young adults 17–23 years; USA)[7]
BV/TV	19.01 ± 4.5	24.60 ± 7.10	27.80 ± 4.50
OV/BV	1.39 ± 1.08	2.30 ± 2.40	1.57 ± 0.67
O.Th	9.55 ± 3.32	11.2 ± 3.40	6.90 ± 1.2
OS/BS	9.58 ± 6.88	13.30 ± 11.10	16.50 ± 5.40
Ob.S/BS	0.20 ± 0.49	1.60 ± 3.30	5.30 ± 2.70
Ocl.S/BS	0.18 ± 0.19	0.03 ± 0.09	1.04 ± 0.41
N.Ocl/TA mm^2	0.05 ± 0.05	0.05 ± 0.05	0.92 ± 0.45
MAR (μm/day)	0.64 ± 0.13	NA	0.75 ± 0.09
FbV/BV	0	NA	0
Ac.fr (/yr)	NA	NA	0.54 ± 0.23
BFR/BS ($μm^3/μm^2$/day)	0.066 ± 0.037	NA	0.061 ± 0.025
MLT (days)	33.80 ± 10.18	NA	17.30 ± 6.5

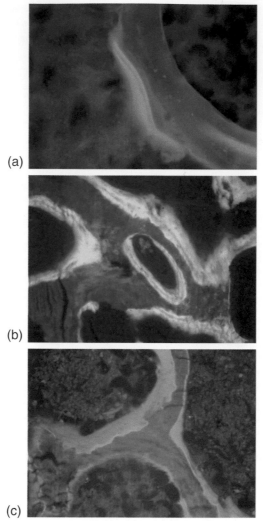

(a)

(b)

(c)

Fig. 10.3 Tetracycline labeling in the bone. (A) Two well demarcated tetracycline labels on the bone surface of a patient with a well-functioning, living related renal transplant of 14 years is shown. The tetracycline was given on days 14, 13, 4, and 3 before the bone biopsy. The tetracycline label deep inside in the bone is old. (B) Tetracycline labeling in a hemodialysis patient with severe OF is shown. The bone surface covered with tetracycline labels is extensive and reflects greatly increased osteoblast activity with ensuing mineralization. Also the two tetracycline labels are less well demarcated than those in (A) even though the time sequence of tetracycline administration was the same. This suggests the presence of disordered mineralization. (C) Tetracycline labeling in a hemodialysis patient with aluminum-induced OM is shown. Despite the sequential dosing of tetracycline administered as described in (A), only scanty deposition of tetracycline is seen at the interface of the large osteoid seams and mineralized bone.

The activation frequency (Acf) represents the rate at which each bone remodeling unit is initiated (expressed as number of times per year) and should not be confused with the frequency of originating new bone remodeling units. The Acf is the ratio between BFR and wall thickness (WTh), which in turns corresponds to the quantity of bone replaced or formed at any bone remodeling unit (Acf = BFR/WTh). Thus, Acf may increase though the BFR is unchanged merely by a decrease of WTh. However, in renal bone disease, the correlation between BFR and Acf is excellent (r = 0.95 in dialysis and r = 0.97 in predialysis patients).[11]

The osteoid maturation time is the mean time interval between the onset of matrix deposition and onset of mineralization at each bone forming site. It is calculated as the ratio of osteoid width divided by the distance between labels per day. The mineralization lag time (MLT) is defined as the mean time interval between the deposition of osteoid and its mineralization averaged over the entire life span of the osteoid surface. Thus, MLT is the osteoid maturation time adjusted for the percentage of osteoid surface that has a tetracycline label. If the entire osteoid surface is mineralising, then the osteoid maturation time and the mineralization lag time are the same. However, if much of the osteoid seam is not mineralising, then the mineralization lag time is many days longer than the osteoid maturation time.

Osteitis fibrosa

A markedly elevated PTH value is the driving force in OF which is characterized by a marked increase in bone turnover, increased osteoblast (Fig. 10.2B) and osteoclast (Fig. 10.2C) activity, and fibrosis of the bone marrow (Fig. 10.4A). The typical picture is a marked increase in osteoblasts, an increased deposition of osteoid resulting in an increase in the osteoid surface and to a lesser extent, an increase in osteoid seam width (Fig. 10.4B). Osteoclasts increase as does the resorption surface. Collagen also accumulates in the bone marrow leading to variable degrees of fibrosis. Initially, fibrosis is seen in a peritrabecular pattern. With more severe disease, bridging areas of fibrosis develop between trabeculae, and finally areas of consolidated fibrosis are seen (Fig. 10.4A). The bone formed is woven instead of the normal lamellar bone. Tetracycline labels are increased because of the increased osteoid surface resulting in an increased bone formation rate (Fig. 10.3B). In some studies, OF is graded based on severity.[4,12,13] In mild OF, marrow fibrosis is minimal (<0.5% of tissue area). Severe OF is present when marrow fibrosis exceeds 0.5% of tissue area (Fig. 10.4A).

Mixed uremic osteodystrophy

MUO has elements of both OF and OM. Elements of OF include a mild to moderate increase in osteoblasts and osteoclasts, and marrow fibrosis. Elements of OM include an increased osteoid volume and osteoid seam width. The bone formation rate may be mildly decreased, normal or mildly increased. However, osteoid accumulation develops because of a mismatch between the rate of osteoid deposition and mineralization in which the former exceeds the latter.[4,12,13]

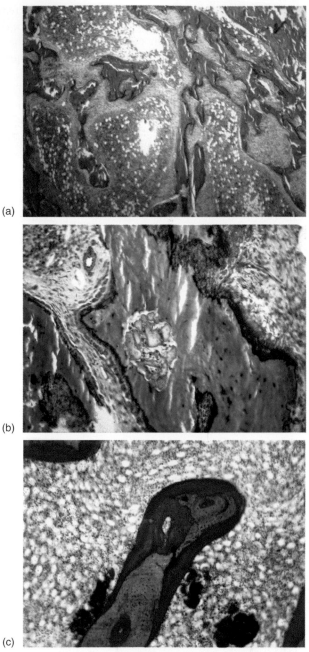

(a)

(b)

(c)

Fig. 10.4 Bone histology in renal osteodystrophy. (A) A low power view of a bone biopsy from a hemodialysis patient with severe OF is shown. Bands of marrow fibrosis extending from one trabeculum to another, as well as areas of consolidated fibrosis are seen. The red color is osteoid and the green is mineralized bone. While most of the

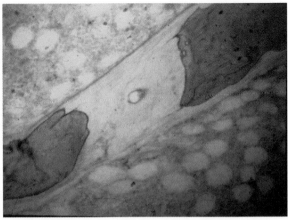

(d)

Fig. 10.4 (continued) biopsy is trabecular bone, cortical bone is present in the upper right corner. (B) A high power view of the same bone biopsy shown in (A) shows the presence of osteoclasts cutting through the bone, areas of peritrabecular fibrosis, and osteoblasts on the osteoid seams. In the top left corner, an area of normal bone marrow is present. (C) Shown is the bone biopsy of a hemodialysis patient with OM. The magenta stained area is osteoid which is devoid of osteoblasts. The osteoid seam is abnormally wide in most places and covers virtually all of the trabecular bone. Osteoclasts and marrow fibrosis are both absent. The large amorphous areas adjacent to the trabecular bone in the bottom half of the figure are staining artefacts. (D) Shown is the bone stained for aluminum. The thin red staining line at the interface of the osteoid (transparent area) and mineralized bone represents aluminum. A positive aluminum stain is also seen as a thin red line along the osteoid surface in the top half of the figure and within the mineralized bone to the right of the bridging osteoid seam at the site of an old resorption cavity which has since mineralized. The latter is known as a reversal line.

Low-turnover osteomalacia

The marked accumulation of osteoid together with the absence or near absence of osteoblasts, osteoclasts and mineralization are the hallmarks of OM (Fig. 10.4C). In OM, the mineralization defect is more pronounced than the inhibition of osteoid deposition because with time there is a marked accumulation of osteoid. Little or no tetracycline deposition is seen even when two-time spaced doses of tetracycline are given (Fig. 10.3C). OM is most often associated with excessive exposure to aluminum and its accumulation in bone (Fig. 10.4D).

Adynamic bone

AD is characterized by a defect of osteoid deposition that matches the mineralization defect. Thus, osteoid accumulation does not occur or is patchy. The latter is often associated with focal areas of osteomalacia. The osteoid seams lack osteoblasts and similarly osteoclasts are decreased and peritrabecular fibrosis is absent or minimal (<0.5%). Tetracycline labels are absent or barely visible.

Bone aluminum deposition

Aluminum deposition is seen at the osteoid-bone interface and along the surface of osteoid and mineralized bone. Aluminum deposits can be detected histologically by means of the aurintricarboxylic acid stain (aluminom; Fig. 10.4D). The evidence that OM is due to aluminum is quite strong with:

- its initial occurrence associated with aluminum contamination of the dialysis water supply;
- its virtual disappearance after removal of aluminum from the dialysate water;
- the demonstration in OM of aluminum deposition at critical sites in the bone;
- the induction of OM in animal models after aluminum administration.

Initially, it was also believed that aluminum was associated with the development of AD because of the accumulation of aluminum in AD. However, the low turnover state in this disorder may have resulted in aluminum accumulation. However, even in the absence of aluminum, there is a high incidence of AD. As will be discussed later, aluminum can also affect bone in high turnover states.

Traditional histomorphometric criteria

Sherrard et al. separated bone disease into five different categories based on histomorphometric criteria (Table 10.3).[4] To differentiate OM from AD, an osteoid volume of 15% was used; others have used a 12% value.[13] However, even an osteoid volume of 12% is much greater than that in normal subjects in whom the osteoid volume is less than 5%. Differences in the diagnostic criteria of MUO also exist in studies. To separate OF from MUO, Sherrard et al. (Table 10.3)[4] and others[12] used osteoid volume, which is higher in MUO, but this classification was independent of the bone formation rate.[4,12,13] In other studies, a mineralization defect determined by a low bone formation rate was used as an additional criteria. Finally, Malluche et al.[14] have used a more qualitative and broader criteria in which features include activation frequency, the co-existence of lamellar with woven osteoid and the presence of active mineralising surfaces in woven bone with reduced mineralization surfaces in lamellar bone.

TMV classification by KDIGO

At a recent KDIGO conference on renal osteodystrophy, the decision was made to recommend that bone biopsies in CKD patients be reported based on the turnover, mineralization, and volume (TMV) classification.[15] Bone turnover reflects the rate of bone remodeling in the coupled process of bone formation and resorption. Because bone resorption cannot be measured directly, measurement of bone formation is used to assess bone turnover. Bone formation is a dynamic measurement obtained by using tetracycline labeling (Table 10.1). Both the bone formation rate and the activation frequency are accepted markers of bone turnover. By using the lowest value observed in normal individuals, low bone turnover can be defined when the bone formation rate is <0.03 $\mu m^3/\mu m^2/day$ (<10.95 $\mu m^3/\mu m^2/year$)[4] or the activation frequency is <0.49 years.[16]

The second parameter of the TMV classification is mineralization, which evaluates osteoid. Parameters used to assess mineralization include the static measurement of osteoid volume, which reflects both the osteoid surface and osteoid thickness, and two dynamic, tetracycline-based measurements, osteoid maturation time, and mineralization lag time. Osteoid accumulation can be from a high rate of osteoid deposition, rather than abnormal mineralization. Both the osteoid maturation time and the mineralization lag time are used to show whether mineralization is normal or abnormal (see 'Normal bone'). A mineralization lag time in the range of 50-100 days is considered moderately prolonged. Values >100 days plus an osteoid thickness >20 μm[16] or an osteoid volume >15%,[4] are typical of osteomalacia.

The third parameter of the TMV classification is bone volume. The bone volume represents the balance between bone formation and resorption. When the former exceeds the latter, bone volume increases. Bone volume decreases when bone resorption exceeds formation. Normal or increased bone volume might suggest a decreased fracture risk, but the quality of bone, as reflected by bone turnover, adequacy of mineralization, and bone micro-architecture, is also an important determinant of fracture risk.

An example of how the TMV classification can be used to provide graphic information is shown in Fig. 10.5. In this three-dimensional representation, turnover can be low, normal, or high, mineralization can be normal or abnormal, and volume can be low, normal, or high. As is shown by this classification, the different types of renal osteodystrophy, OF, MUO, AD, OM and normal bone, separate into different positions in Fig. 10.5. It is now recommended that the TMV nomenclature be used for the assessment of renal osteodystrophy to promote a more widespread and consistent understanding of bone histomorphometry.

Measurement of PTH and indications for bone biopsy

PTH assay

The KDOQI guidelines published in 2003 recommended that the target goal for PTH be between 150 and 300pg/ml for dialysis patients.[17] This recommendation was based on studies that showed that normal bone remodeling in dialysis patients required PTH values that were 2–4 times the upper limit of normal for the Allegro immunoradiometric assay for intact PTH by Nichols.[12,18–20] This dual antibody assay for the measurement of intact (1–84) PTH was developed in the late 1980s. The assay was designed to measure intact PTH by its simultaneous recognition of a carboxy-terminal site and an amino-terminal site. The amino-terminal epitopes recognised by this assay were after the first six amino acids. Subsequently, it was shown that besides 1–84 PTH, the Nichols assay and other first generation intact PTH assays also measure large, truncated, amino-terminal PTH fragments of which 7–84 PTH is the prototype.[21] In dialysis patients, these large non 1–84 PTH fragments account for approximately 50% of the measured PTH. In the late 1990s, a second generation intact PTH assay was developed in which the amino-terminal antibody was directed against epitopes in the first six amino acids.[22] Thus, the second generation PTH assay eliminated the detection of the large, truncated amino-terminal PTH fragments, which were being measured

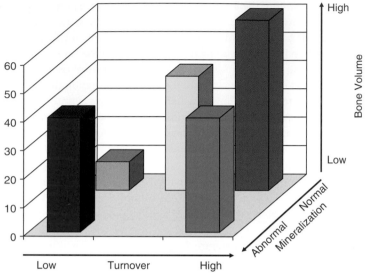

Fig. 10.5 TMV classification system for bone histomorphometry. The figure is a graphical example of how the TMV system provides more information than the present, commonly used classification scheme. Each axis represents one of the descriptors in the TMV classification: turnover (from low to high), mineralization (from normal to abnormal), and bone volume (from low to high). Individual patient parameters could be plotted on the graph, or means and ranges of grouped data could be shown. For example, many patients with renal osteodystrophy cluster in areas shown by the bars. The red bar (OM, osteomalacia) is currently described as low-turnover bone with abnormal mineralization, The bone volume may be low to medium, depending on the severity and duration of the process, and other factors that affect bone. The green bar (AD, adynamic bone disease) is currently described as low-turnover bone with normal mineralization, and the bone volume in this example is at the lower end of the spectrum, but other patients with normal mineralization and low turnover will have normal bone volume. The yellow bar (mild HPT, mild hyperparathyroid-related bone disease) and purple bar (OF, osteitis fibrosa or advanced hyperparathyroid-related bone disease) are currently used distinct categories, but in actuality represent a range of abnormalities along a continuum of medium to high turnover, and any bone volume depending on the duration of the disease process. Finally, the blue bar (MUO, mixed uremic osteodystrophy) is variably defined. In the present graph, it is depicted as high-turnover, normal bone volume, with abnormal mineralization. In summary, the TMV classification system more precisely describes the range of pathologic abnormalities that can occur in patients with CKD. *Definitions:* low-turnover: bone formation rate $<0.03\mu m^3/\mu m^2$-/day ($<10.95\mu m^3/\mu m^2$/year) or activation frequency <0.49 years. Abnormal mineralization: mineralization lag time >100 days (between 50–100 days is moderately abnormal) or in the absence of tetracycline uptake, osteoid volume >15% or osteoid thickness >20 μm. Reproduced from S Moe, T Drüeke, J Cunningham et al (2006). Definition, evaluation, and classification of renal osteodystrophy: A position statement from Kidney Disease: Improving Global Outcomes (KDIGO). *Kidney Int* **69:**1945–1953, with permission from Macmillan Publishers Ltd.

with the first generation intact PTH assay. However, more recent studies have shown that the second generation intact PTH assay also detects an N-form of PTH, different from 1–84 PTH.[23] In renal failure patients, the N-form of PTH accounts for approximately 15% of PTH. To date, the second generation intact PTH assay has not convincingly improved the prediction of bone disease or correlated better with biochemical markers.[24,25]

With the Allegro assay, the circulating intact PTH level was a useful marker of bone remodeling with reasonably good correlations with bone histomorphometric indices.[12,18,19] Both predialysis and dialysis patients with OM and AD had lower mean PTH levels than patients with OF or MUO.[12] However, in patients with mild OF, PTH values were often similar to those in patients with OM and AD. From studies performed in dialysis patients, several guidelines for the interpretation of PTH levels were developed. These included:

- PTH values >450pg/ml are almost 100% predictive of OF or MUO;

- PTH levels below 100–150pg/ml are associated with an increased incidence OM and AD;

- intermediate PTH levels (150–450pg/ml) do not predict the bone turnover state.

The above mentioned guidelines for PTH values interpretation are also applicable to stage 5 CKD patients.[12]

Factors affecting the relationship between PTH and bone histology

Previous studies of bone histomophometry in dialysis patients in which the Allegro PTH assay was used, have shown skeletal resistance to PTH because PTH values 2–4 times the upper limits of normal values were needed to maintain a normal osteoblast surface and bone formation rate. However, there is considerable evidence that many extrinsic factors modify this relationship, thus potentially confounding the interpretation of measured PTH values. These factors include uremia, calcitriol, age, diabetes, gender, and race. Finally, the phosphate burden is perhaps the most important modifier of skeletal resistance to PTH.

Uremia

With the Allegro PTH assay, good and similar correlations between circulating intact PTH levels and bone histomorphometric indices have been reported for both stage 5 and stage 5D CKD patients.[12] However, the slope of the regression line between PTH and different static and dynamic histomorphometric parameters was less steep in predialysis patients than in hemodialysis patients.[12] Thus, the optimum PTH levels to maintain a normal osteoblast surface and bone formation was higher in stage 5 CKD predialysis patients than in dialysis patients.

Calcitriol

In azotemic animals and humans, calcitriol administration at pharmacological doses has been shown to enhance the calcemic response to PTH. However, in azotemic patients, prolonged calcitriol administration has resulted in AD even when PTH values remained elevated and did not decrease.[13] The reason why prolonged calcitriol administration has resulted in AD bone in some dialysis patients even when PTH values did not decrease remains unexplained.

Age

In studies of PTH and calcium dynamics in normal young and old men and women, PTH values for a similar serum calcium level were greater in old individuals. This result suggests a degree of skeletal resistance to PTH in the elderly population. Supporting this interpretation is the finding that the calcemic response to a PTH infusion is less in old than in young men. Several studies in dialysis patients have also suggested that for a similar PTH value, age may independently affect bone histology in dialysis patients. Qi et al. showed that for a similar intermediate intact PTH values between 150 and 450pg/ml, bone turnover was lower after than before the age of 45 years.[19] In another study in dialysis patients, the slope of the regression line between PTH and both the osteoblast surface and bone formation rate was less in patients older than in those younger than 50 years.[26] Thus, these studies suggest that age directly affects bone histology in dialysis patients by reducing the bone response to PTH.

Race

In normal humans, the PTH response to induced hypocalcemia tends to be greater in black than in white men,[27] while the skeletal response to a PTH infusion, as measured by urinary telopeptides, is less in black than in white women.[28] Several studies have shown that for the same dietary calcium intake, black children absorb more and excrete less calcium resulting in a better calcium balance, and more dense bones than in white children. In CKD patients, PTH values are greater in black than in white patients at every stage of CKD including dialysis.[29] Also in dialysis patients, high PTH levels are less predictive of high bone turnover in black patients.[16] These results suggest that bone remodeling is more resistant to PTH in black than in white CKD patients.

Gender

In both old women and men, PTH values are greater than in their younger counterparts. Estrogen treatment in postmenopausal women lowers serum phosphorus without changes in PTH values.[30] It was recently shown in parathyroidectomised rats that estrogen treatment decreases the Na-Pi2a cotransporter on the luminal surface of the proximal tubule resulting in phosphaturia and a decrease in serum phosphorus.[31] Studies in dialysis patients have shown the need for parathyroidectomy is increased in females.[32] Female gender was also shown to contribute to the increased proliferative capacity of parathyroid cells in parathyroid glands harvested from dialysis patients at parathyroidectomy.[32] Whether the effect of female gender is only manifested via increased PTH values or also involves a separate bone effect, directly mediated by estrogen or by estrogen-induced changes in serum phosphorus, remains to be determined.

Diabetes

The azotemic diabetic patient is often characterized by a relative PTH deficiency and AD.[33] Thus, the matching of a relatively low PTH level with reduced bone remodeling would seem appropriate. Recently, it was shown in CKD patients starting hemodialysis that poor diabetic control was associated with lower PTH values than in diabetic patients with good control.[34] However, whether diabetes has a direct effect on bone independent of PTH is difficult to answer. In an *in vitro* study, it was shown that the addition of diabetic serum from patients with poorly controlled diabetes (Hgb A_1C 9%) to cultures of human osteoblasts, inhibited growth. After intensive treatment in these same patients reduced the Hgb A_1C value to 4.2%, the addition of diabetic serum no longer inhibited growth of human osteoblast cultures.[35] In a study in azotemic rats, it was shown that despite a similarly increased PTH level, the osteoblast surface and bone formation rate were less in the diabetic than in the non-diabetic rat.[36] Thus, besides the increased frequency of relative hypoparathyroidism in diabetic hemodialysis patients, poorly-controlled diabetes may also decrease the bone response to PTH.

Indications for a bone biopsy

Because the bone biopsy is an invasive test and requires a dedicated laboratory for its analysis, it is not recommended as part of the routine analysis of renal bone disease. Rather the PTH assay has been used as the standard test to decide on treatment for hyperparathyroidism. The KDOQI guidelines of maintaining a PTH value between 150 and 300pg/ml was based on the Allegro intact PTH assay described in the previous section. However, even with this tested assay, PTH values between 150 and 450pg/ml were a gray zone in which OF, MUO, OM, AD and normal bone could be found. With the discontinuation of the Allegro assay and the use of other first generation intact PTH assays and even second generation intact assays (see previous section), there is some uncertainty about the correlation between PTH and bone histomorphometry.

Clinical indications for a bone biopsy in CKD patients that are stated in the KDIGO position statement include:

- inconsistencies among biochemical parameters that preclude a definitive interpretation;
- unexplained skeletal fracture or bone pain;
- severe progressive vascular calcification;
- unexplained hypercalcemia;
- suspicion of overload or toxicity from aluminum and possibly other metals;
- previous significant exposure to aluminum when planning a parathyroidectomy;
- to be considered before beginning treatment with bisphosphonates.[15]

Furthermore, the bone biopsy remains a valuable research tool that could provide a better understanding in the link between renal bone disease and vascular calcification.

The spectrum of renal osteodystrophy

The extent to which changes in demographics and treatment modalities are responsible for changes in the incidence of different forms of renal osteodystrophy is difficult to know. Elderly and diabetic patients now comprise a large and growing percentage of the dialysis population. Awareness of aluminum toxicity resulted in the removal of aluminum from the dialysate water and the discontinuation of aluminum hydroxide as the phosphate binder of choice. As a result, first the use of calcium-based phosphate binders increased greatly and subsequently non-calcium-based phosphate binders, such as sevelamer and lanthanum have been introduced. Active vitamin D sterols are now frequently used to control hyperparathyroidism. The calcimimetic, cinacalcet, an important treatment for advanced hyperparathyroidism is now also used frequently. Finally, the standard calcium concentration of the dialysate has changed from 3.5–2.5 mEq/L during the past two decades. The effect that these changes have had on renal osteodystrophy is difficult to define.

Prevalence of different types of renal bone disease

In the KDIGO Clinical Practice Guidelines for Chronic Kidney Disease-Related Bone and Mineral Disorders,[37] a literature review of renal osteodystrophy (Table 10.3) between 1983 and 2003 evaluated the following four patient categories:

patients with CKD stages 3–5 (11 studies, $n = 711$);
peritoneal dialysis patients (7 studies, $n = 371$);
hemodialysis patients or combined dialysis modalities (31 studies, $n = 7909$);
children with CKD stage 5 or stage 5D (7 studies, $n = 325$).

The distribution of bone disease in each of the aforementioned four categories is shown in Table 10.4. In CKD stages 3–5, OF and MUO predominate. In patients on peritoneal dialysis, AD predominates, but OF and mild OF together compose a significant percentage. In hemodialysis patients, OF and MUO again predominate. Finally, in children with stage 5 or 5D CKD, OF predominates with minimal differences in the incidence of other forms of bone disease.

The results of this analysis show that disorders of high bone turnover (OF and mild OF) predominate over those of low bone turnover (AD and OM) in adults with CKD stages 3–5, hemodialysis patients, and children with CKD stage 5 or stage 5D. However, in peritoneal dialysis patients, disorders of low bone turnover, primarily AD, predominate. When MUO is included as a high turnover disorder, then the scale is

Table 10.3 Traditional histological classification of renal osteodystrophy[4] Reproduced from Sherrard DJ, Hercz G, Pei Y, et al. The spectrum of bone disease in end-stage renal failure—An evolving disorder. *Kidney Int* 1993;**43**:436–442. By permission from Macmillan Publishers Ltd.

Lesion	Area of fibrosis (% of tissue area)	Area of osteoid (% of total bone area)	Bone formation rate ($\mu m^2/\mu mm^2$ tissue area/day)
Mild	< 0.5%	< 15%	> 108
Osteitis fibrosa	> 0.5%	< 15%	X
Mixed	> 0.5%	> 15%	X
Osteomalacia	< 0.5%	> 15%	X
Aplastic	< 0.5%	< 15%	< 108
Normal range	0	1–7%	108–500

X is not a diagnostic criterion.

Table 10.4 Prevalence of different types of renal bone disease from KDIGO literature review of renal osteodystrophy between 1983 and 2003.[37]

	CKD stages 3 to 5 11 studies, n = 711	Peritoneal Dialysis (PD) 7 studies, n = 371	Hemodialysis (HD) or HD + PD 31 studies, n = 7909	Children with stage 5/5D CKD 7 studies, n = 325
OF	32%	18%	34%	41%
Mild OF	6%	20%	32%	10%
MUO	20%	5%	3%	10%
Normal	16%	2%	2%	17%
AD	18%	50%	19%	16%
OM	8%	5%	10%	6%

OF, osteitis fibrosa; MUO, mixed uremic osteodystrophy; AD, adynamic bone; OM, osteomalacia.

further tipped in favor of high bone turnover in patients with CKD stages 3–5, hemodialysis patients and children with CKD stage 5 or 5D, but remains essentially unchanged in peritoneal dialysis patients. In peritoneal dialysis patients, it is likely that the greater calcium transfer, lower PTH values, and better phosphate control contribute to the lower bone turnover in these patients.

The KDIGO evaluation of hemodialysis patients also separated patients who were referred for bone biopsy for a specific reason from those presumably biopsied for participation in a study. No differences in the pattern of bone histology were found. Patients were also separated before and after 1995. Aluminum intoxication decreased from 40 to 20% after 1995 and there was an approximately 15% increase in the incidence of OF and a similar decrease in MUO. OM did not decrease and there was a small increase in AD.

Two recent studies in which bone biopsies were obtained in hemodialysis patients illustrate the difficulty of correlating PTH values with bone histomophometry. In a study from Portugal ($n = 68$), the baseline intact PTH value (first generation intact assay) was in the mid-100s (pg/ml).[38] The percentage of patients with OF or mild OF was 37%, MUO 3%, AD 62%, and OM 1%. Three patients were not entered in the study because stainable aluminum exceeded 20%. Vitamin D use during the 12 months before study entry was 68%. Thus, in this study, low bone turnover predominated probably because at entry patients had relatively low PTH values and also many had been treated with vitamin D. However, excessive aluminum exposure was not a major factor.

In a second study from Brazil ($n = 97$) the mean PTH value was 392pg/ml and stainable aluminum was present on greater than 25% of the bone surface in 41% of the total patients, 46.5% in patients with low bone turnover and 36% in patients with high bone turnover.[39] Some patients were on calcitriol at the time of the bone biopsy, but a specific percentage was not stated. As would be expected, the mean calcitriol dosage was nine times greater in patients with high than low bone turnover. When PTH values were <150pg/ml ($n = 40$), 83% had low bone turnover, 14% had high bone turnover, and 3% had normal bone. When PTH values were between 150 and 300pg/ml, 64% had low bone turnover, 27% had high bone turnover, and 9% had normal bone. When PTH values were >300pg/ml, 63% had high bone turnover and 37% had low bone turnover.

As these studies show, there often are selection criteria for entry into a study such as aluminum burden, desirable PTH values and diabetic status. In the study from Brazil, the presence of aluminum appeared to increase the incidence of OM and AD and also changed OF to MUO. Thus, the effect of aluminum toxicity probably altered the comparison between PTH and bone. Finally, in both studies many patients had recently been or were being treated with active vitamin D sterols that are used to lower PTH values and may also directly affect bone turnover.

Osteitis fibrosa and mixed disease

Pathophysiology

A markedly elevated PTH value is the driving force for the development of OF leading to an increased bone formation rate, activation frequency, cellular activity, and marrow fibrosis. Patients with PTH values measured by the Allegro PTH assay by Nichols, who had values greater than 450pg/ml generally had OF while those with intermediate values (150–450pg/ml) could have either high or low bone turnover bone.[19] When PTH values are intermediate, bone alkaline phosphatase values may be helpful in separating high and low bone turnover.

The difference between OF and MUO includes a reduction in mineralization and osteoid accumulation. In some cases of MUO, the origin of the reduction in mineralization may be aluminum accumulation. However, in our series of predialysis and dialysis patients.[12] MUO was not associated with an increase in stainable aluminum. As with the MUO reported in the older studies of bone disease in the predialysis era, lower serum calcium values may favor the development of MUO in the dialysis patient. Similarly, a deficiency of 25OHD may also contribute to the development of MUO.[40,41]

Clinical manifestations

Studies of patients with stage 3 and 4 CKD have shown that the incidence of hip and other fractures are increased.[42,43] Similarly, the incidence of hip, spine, and other fractures are also increased in dialysis patients. In a retrospective study in 9000 hemodialysis patients a U-shaped bimodal relationship between fracture risk and PTH levels was observed.[44] Thus, both extremes of bone turnover may critically alter bone micro-architecture and stability. Finally, the presence of aluminum in bone likely will increase the risk of fracture.

Osteomalacia

Historical perspective

OM first appeared as a clinical entity in the 1970s with the advent of chronic hemodialysis.[1] In certain geographic areas, it occurred in epidemic proportions. Besides 'fracturing' bone disease, OM was often associated with:

- neurological findings such as dysarthria, myoclonic jerks, confusion, seizures and dementia, often termed 'dialysis dementia';
- microcytic anemia.[45]

The first complete descriptions of this devastating disorder were reported in Newcastle, England. It was recognised that OM was a new entity never seen before in predialysis patients. The incidence of OM began to increase about 6 months after the start of hemodialysis and by 2 years, approximately 75% of the patients had OM. Also, OM occurred in certain geographic areas that often were in close proximity to OM free areas. Support for a water-borne factor came from the geographic distribution of OM and the observation that OM did not develop in hemodialysis patients in whom deionized water was used.[46] Eventually epidemiological and experimental studies showed that aluminum was the cause of OM and dialysis encephalopathy.

Besides the epidemic form of OM, a sporadic form was subsequently recognised in which affected patients were from hemodialysis units with treated water.[47] On rare occasions, OM was even reported in predialysis patients. The cause for the sporadic form was attributed to the oral burden of aluminum from aluminum-based phosphate binders often in association with citrate containing solutions which enhance aluminum absorption.[48] Also relatively low PTH values in conjunction with low bone turnover contributed to the development of aluminum-induced OM.[49]

OM was also sometimes seen in geographic areas in which the aluminum concentration of the domestic water supply was not high, but periodic spikes in the aluminum concentration occurred because aluminum sulfate (alum) was added to the domestic water supply after heavy rains to precipitate flocculent material present. Unless the dialysate aluminum concentration is maintained below 5μg/L, there is transfer of aluminum from the dialysate to blood.[50] Intradialytic transfer of aluminum occurs at even relatively low dialysate aluminum concentrations because approximately 80% of serum aluminum is bound, mainly to transferring.[50] In the epidemic form of OM and dialysis encephalopathy, serum aluminum levels generally exceed 100μg/L with mean values in the 200–300μg/L range.

Aluminum-related bone disease

Aluminum accumulation has been shown to inhibit both bone mineralization and osteoblast function.[51] Even in OF, aluminum accumulation has been shown to reduce bone mineralization. In such cases, the presence of aluminum should affect the decision to proceed to parathyroidectomy because the marked reduction in PTH values following parathyroidectomy can result in the development of OM.[52]

Whether aluminum toxicity results in OM or AD depends on how aluminum affects the rate of osteoid deposition and the rate of bone formation (mineralization). Even though both are depressed by aluminum, when the rate of osteoid deposition exceeds that of bone formation, osteoid accumulates, and OM develops. When the rate of osteoid deposition and bone formation are in balance even though both are depressed, then AD develops because osteoid does not accumulate.

A brief review of the interaction between aluminum and PTH in animal models is instructive. In azotemic parathyroidectomised rats, aluminum administration proportionally reduced both the osteoblast surface and bone formation rate and produced bone that resembled AD.[51] This model suggests that, in the absence of PTH, aluminum proportionally reduces the rate of matrix deposition and bone formation. In a model of endogenous hyperparathyroidism induced by a high phosphate diet in azotemic rats, aluminum administration marginally decreased the osteoblast surface, but resulted in a profound decrease in the bone formation rate.[53] Thus, while hyperparathyroidism provided some protection against aluminum toxicity, the protective effect of PTH was greater for osteoblasts than for the bone formation rate.

Adynamic bone

Definition

AD is defined by the presence of low or absent bone formation as determined by tetracycline uptake in bone, in conjunction with a paucity of bone-forming osteoblasts and bone-resorbing osteoclasts. Using the TMV classification system (Turnover, Mineralization, and Volume), AD is characterized by low turnover associated with a preserved mineralization which avoids osteoid accumulation.[15] Bone volume, as well as trabecular connectivity are usually at the lower end of the spectrum, although many patients may exhibit normal values. The recent identification of *minimodeling*, which represents localized areas of bone formation within generalised adynamic bone, may explain the variability in trabecular bone volume among patients with AD.[54] Interestingly, *minimodeling* occurs over quiescent bone surfaces instead of over previously resorbed bone as is the case in bone remodelling.[55]

Etiology and pathogenesis

The causes of low bone formation in CKD patients are multifactorial (Table 10.5). Aluminum which has been shown to inhibit bone mineralization and to be toxic to the osteoblast was in the past the most common cause of AD. The importance of factors besides aluminium toxicity as a cause of AD is illustrated by the fact that AD with negative aluminium staining has occurred in at least one third of patients with stage 5 CKD.[12,56]

Table 10.5 Factors associated with a high prevalence of AD in ESRD

- ◆ Low PTH levels
- ◆ High calcium load
- ◆ Vitamin D over-treatment
- ◆ Increasing age
- ◆ Diabetes Mellitus
- ◆ CAPD compared with hemodialysis.
- ◆ Aluminum toxicity
- ◆ Other factors:
  - • Uremic toxins
  - • Decreased IGF-I and IGFBP-5 levels
  - • Malnutrition
  - • Premature hypogonadism
  - • Acidosis
  - • Glucocorticoid use

Three important clinical conditions have been associated with low bone formation: aging, diabetes, and an increased calcium load.[57] Thus, the recent increase in AD prevalence parallels the steady increase in elderly and diabetic patients with CKD beginning dialysis, many of whom having had received calcium-containing phosphate binders and active vitamin D sterols.

The mechanisms for the age-related reduction in bone formation are incompletely understood although reduced circulating sex steroids, oxidative stress and accumulation of advanced glycation end products (AGE) are potential candidates.[58] Low bone formation in diabetes may be related to the accumulation of AGEs and their induction of osteoblast apoptosis.[59]

A positive calcium balance due to the concomitant use of a high calcium concentration in the dialysate, calcium-containing phosphate binders, and active vitamin D sterols act to decrease circulating PTH levels and depress bone turnover.[57] A 'relative hypoparathyroidism' is regarded as an important risk factor for AD. It may due to low 1–84 PTH levels or to a relative excess PTH fragments (PTH 7–84) antagonising the effects of 1–84 PTH.[22] Furthermore, AD is frequently characterized by skeletal resistance to PTH via a down-regulation of the PTH/PTHrP receptor on osteoblasts.[60] Thus, PTH values 2–4-fold above the upper limit of normal are often needed to maintain normal bone formation in dialysis patients.[12,18,19]

Several studies have demonstrated a higher prevalence of AD in CAPD patients as compared with hemodialysis patients.[12,37] This result probably reflects a continuous positive calcium balance from a high dialysate calcium concentration in CAPD patients. In a prospective, controlled trial involving 51 CAPD patients with biopsy proven AD, normalization of bone turnover in 40% of the patients occurred after 16 months of using a low-calcium dialysate.[61] Other mediators of AD include uremic toxins, premature hypogonadism, and derangements in cytokines and growth factors, which may decrease osteoblast proliferation and function.[58]

Recent *in vitro* and *in vivo* evidence has shown that vitamin D receptor (VDR) activation is required for osteoblast development and normal bone formation, as well as for normal mineralization, probably by a calcium-independent pathway.[58] Interestingly, osteoblasts contain 1α-hydroxylase as well as megalin receptors, which are known to function as a 25OHD3 acceptor protein facilitating its incorporation into the cell. In addition, vitamin D analogs, similar to sex steroids, have been recognised as anti-apoptotic hormones for the osteoblast.[62] Thus, the correction of 25OHD3 deficiency/insufficiency in CKD patients is desirable. Whether the use of non-pharmacological and non-calcemic doses of VDR activators stimulate osteoblast activity and prevent low bone formation in ESRD should be addressed in properly designed clinical trials.

Clinical manifestations

AD is associated with a diminished ability to repair microdamage, which may result in an increase in fractures. In fact, a U-shaped bimodal relationship between fracture risk and PTH levels, has been described in hemodialysis patients.[44] AD is characterized by a reduced ability to incorporate calcium into the bone compartment. Thus, systemic exposure to calcium via the use of excessive calcium-containing phosphate binders and/or active vitamin D sterols, may increase the risk of ectopic, and particularly, vascular calcifications. In a cross-sectional study, London et al.[63] have shown that aortic stiffness and calcification were both positively associated with calcium load and negatively associated with bone activity. Interestingly, calcium load had a greater influence on aortic stiffness and calcification in the group of patients with AD. Consequently, a principle of AD management should be to minimize the calcium and vitamin D load.

Conclusions

Treatment for disorders of high bone turnover, OF and MUO, characterized by high PTH values include active vitamin D sterols, cinacalcet, parathyroidectomy, and in a limited number of centres direct injection of the parathyroid gland. OM is much less common than before because of strict standards for dialysate water preparation and the discontinuation of aluminum-based phosphate binders. However, in some areas of the world, aluminum exposure still remains a problem. AD is now a common disorder that is seen in the absence of aluminum. It is probably associated with an increased risk of fractures and even more important, a possible acceleration of vascular calcification. AD is associated with a relative deficiency of PTH and factors contributing to its development include old age, diabetes, and an increased calcium load. Treatment of AD is limited because it is difficult to increase PTH levels in patients with AD. It is generally accepted that PTH is the primary modifier of bone turnover. However, less well appreciated is that several factors may alter the bone response to PTH. Several studies of bone histology in dialysis patients have shown that the bone response to PTH as measured by the osteoblast surface and bone formation rate, decreases after age 45 or 50 years. Older patients also eat less protein resulting in a decreased phosphate load that, in turn, reduces the stimulus for PTH secretion. There is also increasing evidence that the bone response to PTH, as determined by bone turnover in histological studies, is decreased in black CKD patients. Attempts to use non-invasive means of assessing bone turnover, such as PTH values and bone alkaline phosphatase, have lacked sensitivity at intermediate PTH values between 150 and 450pg/ml. Finally, variability in PTH assays and problems associated with the collection of PTH samples have further complicated the ability to make therapeutic decisions based on PTH measurements.

* Dr Felsenfeld is an employee of the United States Government and his work is not subject to Copyright protection in the United States.

References

1. Felsenfeld AJ, Torres A. Osteitis fibrosa, osteomalacia, and mixed bone lesions. In T. B. Drüeke & I. Salusky (eds) *The Spectrum of Renal Osteodystrophy*, 1st edn. Oxford: Oxford University Press, 2001:185–226.
2. Mora-Palma FJ, Ellis HA, Cook DB, et al. Osteomalacia in patients with chronic renal failure before dialysis or transplantation. *Q J Med* 1983;**52**:332–48.
3. Nielsen HE, Melsen F, Christensen MS. Interrelationships between calcium-phosphorus metabolism, serum parathyroid hormone and bone histomorphometry in non-dialyzed and dialyzed patients with chronic renal failure. *Miner Electrolyte Metab* 1980;**4**:113–22.

4. Sherrard DJ, Hercz G, Pei Y, et al. The spectrum of bone disease in end-stage renal failure—an evolving disorder. *Kidney Int* 1993;**43:**436–42.

5. Strom TM, Jüppner H. PHEX, FGF23, DMP1 and beyond. *Curr Opin Nephrol Hypertens* 2008;**17:**357–62.

6. Parfitt AM, Drezner MK, Glorieux FH, et al. Bone histomorphometry: standardisation of nomenclature, symbols, and units: Report of the ASBMR Histomorphometry Nomenclature Committee. *J Bone Miner Res* 1987;**2:**595–610.

7. Glorieux FH, Travers R, Taylor A, et al. Normative data for iliac bone histomorphometry in growing children. *Bone* 2000;**26:**103–9.

8. Coen G, Mazzaferro S, Ballanti P, et al. Renal bone disease in 76 patients with varying degrees of predialysis chronic renal failure: a cross-sectional study. *Nephrol Dial Transplant* 1996;**11:**813–19.

9. Dos Reis LM, Batalha JR, Muñoz DR, et al. Brazilian normal static bone histomorphometry: effects of age, sex, and race. *J Bone Miner Metab* 2007;**25:**400–6.

10. Ott SM. Histomorphometric measurements of bone turnover, mineralization, and volume. *Clin J Am Soc Nephrol* 2008;**3** Suppl 3:S151–6.

11. Ballanti P, Coen G, Mazzaferro S, et al. Histomorphometric assessment of bone turnover in uremic patients: comparison between activation frequency and bone formation rate. *Histopathology* 2001;**38:**571–83.

12. Torres A, Lorenzo V, Hernandez D, et al. Bone disease in predialysis, hemodialysis, and CAPD patients: evidence of a better bone response to PTH. *Kidney Int* 1995;**47:**1434–42.

13. Goodman WG, Ramirez JA, Belin TR, et al. Development of adynamic bone in patients with secondary hyperparathyroidism after intermittent calcitriol therapy. *Kidney Int* 1994;**46:**1160–6.

14. Malluche HH, Faugere MC. The role of bone biopsy in the management of patients with renal osteodystrophy. *J Am Soc Nephrol* 1992;**4:**1631–2.

15. Moe S, Drüeke T, Cunningham J, et al. Kidney Disease. Improving Global Outcomes (KDIGO): Definition, evaluation, and classification of renal osteodystrophy: a position statement from Kidney Disease: Improving Global Outcomes (KDIGO). *Kidney Int* 2006;**69:**1945–53.

16. Sawaya BP, Butros R, Naqvi S, et al. Differences in bone turnover and intact PTH levels between African American and Caucasian patients with end-stage renal disease. *Kidney Int* 2003;**64:**737–42.

17. National Kidney Foundation: K/DOQI clinical practice guidelines for bone metabolism and disease in chronic kidney disease. *Am J Kidney Dis* 2003;**42:**S1–202.

18. Quarles LD, Lobaugh B, Murphy G. Intact parathyroid hormone overestimates the presence and severity of parathyroid-mediated osseous abnormalities in uremia. *J Clin Endocrinol Metab* 1992;**75:**145–50.

19. Qi Q, Monier-Faugere MC, Geng Z, Malluche HH. Predictive value of serum parathyroid hormone levels for bone turnover in patients on chronic maintenance dialysis. *Am J Kidney Dis* 1995;**26:**622–31.

20. Cohen-Solal ME, Sebert JL, Boudailliez B, et al. Comparison of intact, midregion, and carboxy terminal assays of parathyroid hormone for diagnosis of bone disease in hemodialyzed patients. *J Clin Endocrinol Metab* 1991;**73:**516–23.

21. Lepage, R, Roy, L, Brossard, JH, et al. A non-(1-84) circulating parathyroid hormone fragment interferes significantly with intact PTH commercial assay measurement in uremic samples. *Clin Chem* 1998;**44:**805–9.

22. Slatopolsky E, Finch J, Clay P, et al. A novel mechanism for skeletal resistance in uremia. *Kidney Int* 2000;**58:**753–61.

23. Arakawa T, D'Amour P, Rousseau L, et al. Overproduction and secretion of a novel amino-terminal form of parathyroid hormone from a severe type of parathyroid hyperplasia in uremia. *Clin J Am Soc Nephrol* 2006;**1:**525–31.

24. Lehmann G, Stein G, Hüller M, Schemer R, Ramakrishnan K, Goodman WG. Specific measurement of PTH (1–84) in various forms of renal osteodystrophy (ROD) as assessed by bone histomorphometry. *Kidney Int* 2005;**68:**1206–14.

25. Souberbielle JC, Boutten A, Carlier MC, et al. Inter-method variability in PTH measurement: implication for the care of CKD patients. *Kidney Int* 2006;**70:**345–50.

26. Jarava C, Armas JR, Palma A. Study of renal osteodystrophy by bone biopsy. Age as an independent factor. Diagnostic value of bone remodeling markers. *Nefrologia* 2000;**20:**362–72.

27. El-Hajj Fuleihan G, Gundberg CM, Gleason R, et al. Racial differences in parathyroid hormone dynamics. *J Clin Endocrinol Metab* 1994;**79:**1642–7.

28. Cosman F, Morgan DC, Nieves JW, et al. Resistance to bone resorbing effects of PTH in black women. *J Bone Miner Res* 1997;**12:**958–66.

29. Sawaya, BP, Monier-Faugere, M-C, Ratanapanichkich, P, et al. Racial differences in parathyroid hormone levels in patients with secondary hyperparathyroidism. *Clin Nephrol* 2002;**57:**51–5.

30. Packer E, Holloway L, Newhall K, Kanwar G, Butterfield G, Marcus R. Effects of estrogen on daylong circulating calcium, phosphorus, 1,25-dihydroxyvitamin D, and parathyroid hormone in postmenopausal women. *J Bone Miner Res* 1990;**5:**877–84.

31. Faroqui S, Levi M, Soleimani M, Amlal H. Estrogen downregulates the proximal tubule type IIa sodium phosphate cotransporter causing phosphate wasting and hypophosphatemia. *Kidney Int* 2008;**73:**1141–50.

32. Almaden Y, Felsenfeld AJ, Rodriguez M, et al. Proliferation in hyperplastic human and normal rat parathyroid glands: role of phosphate, calcitriol, and gender. *Kidney Int* 2003;**64:**2311–17.

33. Pei Y, Hercz G, Greenwood C. Renal osteodystrophy in diabetic patients. *Kidney Int* 1993;**44:**159–64.

34. Murakami R, Murakami S, Tsushima R, et al. Glycemic control and serum intact parathyroid hormone levels in diabetic patients on hemodialysis therapy. *Nephrol Dial Transplant* 2008;**23:**315–20.

35. Brenner RE, Riemenschneider B, Blum W, et al. Defective stimulation of proliferation and collagen biosynthesis of human bone cells by serum from diabetic patients. *Acta Endocrinol (Copenh)* 1992;**127:**509–14.

36. Jara A, Bover J, Felsenfeld AJ. The development of secondary hyperparathyroidism and bone disease in diabetic rats with renal failure. *Kidney Int* 1995;**47:**1746–51.

37. KDIGO. Clinical Practice Guidelines for Chronic Kidney Disease-Related Bone and Mineral Disorders. *Kidney Int* 2009;**76:**Supplement 113, S1–S130.

38. Ferreira A, Frazão JM, Monier-Faugere MC, et al. Sevelamer Study Group. Effects of sevelamer hydrochloride and calcium carbonate on renal osteodystrophy in hemodialysis patients. *J Am Soc Nephrol* 2008;**19:**405–12.

39. Barreto FC, Barreto DV, Moysés RM, et al. K/DOQI-recommended intact PTH levels do not prevent low-turnover bone disease in hemodialysis patients. *Kidney Int* 2008;**73:**771–7.

40. Ghazali A, Fardellone P, Pruna A, et al. Is low plasma 25-(OH)vitamin D a major risk factor for hyperparathyroidism and Looser's zones independent of calcitriol? *Kidney Int* 1999;**55:**2169–77.

41. Coen G, Mantella D, Manni M, et al. 25-hydroxyvitamin D levels and bone histomorphometry in hemodialysis renal osteodystrophy. *Kidney Int* 2005;**68:**1840–8.

42. Fried LF, Biggs ML, Shlipak MG, et al. Association of kidney function with incident hip fracture in older adults. *J Am Soc Nephrol* 2007;**18:**282–6.

43. Nickolas TL, Leonard MB, Shane E. Chronic kidney disease and bone fracture: a growing concern. *Kidney Int* 2008;**74:**721–31.

44. Danese MD, Kim J, Doan QV, et al. PTH and the risks for hip, vertebral, and pelvic fractures among patients on dialysis. *Am J Kidney Dis* 2006;**47:**149–56.

45. Parkinson IS, Ward MK, Kerr DN. Dialysis encephalopathy, bone disease and anemia: the aluminum intoxication syndrome during regular hemodialysis. *J Clin Pathol* 1981;**34:**1285–94.

46. Posen GA, Gray DG, Jaworski ZF, Couture R, Rashid A. Comparison of renal osteodystrophy in patients dialyzed with deionized and non-deionized water. *Trans Am Soc Artif Intern Organs* 1972;**18:**405–7.

47. Norris KC, Crooks PW, Nebeker HG, et al. Clinical and laboratory features of aluminum-related bone disease: differences between sporadic and 'epidemic' forms of the syndrome. *Am J Kidney Dis* 1985;**6:**342–7.

48. Coburn JW, Mischel MG, Goodman WG, Salusky IB. Calcium citrate markedly enhances aluminum absorption from aluminum hydroxide. *Am J Kidney Dis* 1991;**17:**708–11.

49. Andress DL, Kopp JB, Maloney NA, Coburn JW, Sherrard DJ. Early deposition of aluminum in bone in diabetic patients on hemodialysis. *N Engl J Med* 1987;**316:**292–6.

50. Cannata-Andía JB, Fernández-Martín JL. The clinical impact of aluminium overload in renal failure. *Nephrol Dial Transplant* 2002;**17** Suppl 2:9–12.

51. Cannata Andía JB. Hypokinetic azotemic osteodystrophy. *Kidney Int* 1998;**54:**1000–16.

52. Felsenfeld AJ, Harrelson JM, Gutman RA, Wells SA, Jr., Drezner MK. Osteomalacia after parathyroidectomy in patients with uremia. *Ann Intern Med* 1982;**960:**34–9.

53. Felsenfeld AJ, Machado L, Rodriguez M. The effect of high parathyroid hormone levels on the development of aluminum induced osteomalacia in the rat. *J Am Soc Nephrol* 1991;**1:**970–9.

54. Ubara Y, Tagami T, Nakanishi S, et al. Significance of minimodeling in dialysis patients with adynamic bone disease. *Kidney Int* 2005;**68:**833–9.

55. Yajima A, Inaba M, Tominaga Y, Ito A. Bone formation by minimodeling is more active than remodeling after parathyroidectomy. *Kidney Int* 2008;**74:**775–81.

56. Hernandez D, Concepcion MT, Lorenzo V, et al. Adynamic bone disease with negative aluminium staining in predialysis patients: prevalence and evolution after maintenance dialysis. *Nephrol Dial Transplant* 1994;**9:**517–23.

57. Brandenburg VM, Floege J. Adynamic bone disease-bone and beyond. *Nephrol Dial Transplant Plus* 2008;**3:**135–47.

58. Andress DL. Adynamic bone in patients with chronic kidney disease. *Kidney Int* 2008;**73:**1345–54.

59. Alikhani M, Alikhani Z, Boyd C, et al. Advanced glycation end products stimulate osteoblast apoptosis via the MAP kinase and cytosolic apoptotic pathways. *Bone* 2007;**40:**345–53.

60. Iwasaki-Ishizuka Y, Yamato H, Nii-Kono T, Kurokawa K, Fukagawa M. Downregulation of parathyroid hormone receptor gene expression and osteoblastic dysfunction associated with skeletal resistance to parathyroid hormone in a rat model of renal failure with low turnover bone. *Nephrol Dial Transplant* 2005;**20**:1904–11.

61. Haris A, Sherrard DJ, Hercz G. Reversal of adynamic bone disease by lowering of dialysate calcium. *Kidney Int* 2006;**70**:931–7.

62. Zhang X, Zanello LP. Vitamin D receptor-dependent 1 alpha,25(OH)2 vitamin D3-induced anti-apoptotic PI3K/AKT signaling in osteoblasts. *J Bone Miner Res* 2008;**23**:1238–48.

63. London GM, Marchais SJ, Guérin AP, Boutouyrie P, Métivier F, de Vernejoul MC. Association of bone activity, calcium load, aortic stiffness, and calcifications in ESRD. *J Am Soc Nephrol* 2008;**19**:1827–35.

64. Stanbury SW, Lumb GA. Parathyroid function in chronic renal failure. A statistical survey of the plasma biochemistry in azoremic renal osteodystrophy. *Q J Med* 1966;**35**:1–23.

Chapter 11

Biochemical markers of bone metabolism in CKD

Pablo Ureña, Klaus Olgaard, and Kevin J. Martin

Introduction

Bone is a specialized connective tissue composed of cells that produce an extracellular matrix that has the unique ability to mineralize, in conjunction with cartilage, forming the skeletal system. Two opposing processes, bone formation and bone resorption, characterize bone metabolism. Bone formation depends on osteoblasts that are bone-lining cells responsible for the production of bone matrix constituents: collagen and ground substances. Bone resorption depends on osteoclasts, giant multinucleated cells that are usually found in contact with a calcified bone surface and within the lacuna, resulting from its own resorption activity. The combination of these two processes is required for bone remodeling and is very well coupled in normal conditions. Even though they occur along the bone surface at random and bone formation mainly takes place where resorption of old bone has already occurred, it can sometimes be observed without previous resorption (called mini-modeling) as in cases after parathyroid-ectomy.[1] Of course, it is the equilibrium between bone resorption and bone formation that will determine the gain, loss, or balance of total bone mass.

An altered bone resorption/formation balance characterizes most of the metabolic bone diseases, including the abnormalities of bone that occur in chronic kidney disease (CKD). In CKD, bone turnover may be high, normal, or low, and may be associated with abnormal mineralization or with B2-microglobuline deposition in bone or with abnormal bone mass.[2]

Iliac bone biopsy after double tetracycline labeling, alone or in combination with clinical and radiographic signs, serum biochemical markers, and isotopic kinetic studies, has been used to try to distinguish between high (HTBD) and normal or low (N/LTBD) bone remodeling in CKD patients, and also to establish the absence or the presence of abnormal mineralization or any trace metal deposition. However, since bone biopsy is an invasive procedure, it is not widely used in clinical practice. Accordingly, there is a great need to develop reliable non-invasive methods for the assessment of bone metabolism in these patients.

Among these methods, the evaluation of several circulating molecules, which are either derived from bone structures itself or are closely related to bone metabolism, have been proposed as specific serum markers of bone remodeling for a variety of metabolic bone diseases (Table 11.1).

Calcium

Calcium is the most common divalent cation in the body, principally found in mineralized components of the skeleton (>99%, or ~25,000 mmol or 1kg). Calcium also plays a major role in many biological processes, including blood coagulation, neuromuscular conduction, skeletal and cardiac muscle tone and excitability, secretion of exocrine glands, and preservation of cell membrane integrity and permeability, particularly in terms of sodium and potassium exchange. What is measured in the circulation represents less than 1% of the total body calcium content and does not reflect the total calcium balance (Table 11.2).[3]

In blood, three distinct forms of calcium can be measured: ionized or free calcium (48%), protein (mostly albumin)-bound calcium (40%), and calcium bound to low molecular weight ligands, such as phosphate, lactate, citrate, and bicarbonate (12%). The amount of calcium bound to protein is dependent on plasma albumin concentration and on pH.[3,4]

Total serum calcium is the most common measurement of calcium status. While reference ranges vary between laboratories, normal values for total calcium in adults generally range from 8.4 to 10.2 mg/dL (2.10–2.60 mmol/L). The normal range for total plasma calcium is slightly higher in children, particularly in those under 6 years of age (Table 11.3).

As total calcium levels are affected by the degree of protein binding, in situations where plasma albumin levels are abnormal, total calcium may not accurately reflect the patient's calcium status. In an effort to account for this inaccuracy in total calcium values, several formulas have been devised. One of the more commonly used formulas to provide a 'corrected' calcium value is to add 0.8 mg/dL (0.02 mmol/L) to the measured total calcium for each 1.0 g/dL (1 g/L) decrease in albumin below 4.0 g/dL (40 g/L).[5] Thus, a patient with a normal total calcium concentration of 10.0 mg/dL (2.50 mmol/L) and a plasma albumin level of 2.0 g/dL (20 g/L) would have a corrected calcium concentration of 11.6 mg/dL (2.90 mmol/L), indicating a significantly high plasma calcium level. These corrections provide a better estimation of calcium status in some patients; however, they incorrectly predict calcium status in up to 30% of patients when correlated with actual ionized calcium levels.[4] Therefore, measurement of ionized calcium is preferable in the presence of altered plasma albumin concentration or plasma pH. The rationale for correcting a calcium measurement downwards in patients with albumin levels above 4.0 g/dL remains questionable.

Finally, another point that we need to take into consideration, when assessing serum calcium levels, is the accumulating evidences suggesting that high total serum calcium levels may be related or associated with a high relative risk (RR) of mortality in CKD dialysis patients. The values associated with this significantly increase in the RR of death is reported to be >11.4 mg/dL (>2.85 mmol/L).[6–10] Therefore, serum levels of calcium, should be measured in all patients with CKD and GFR<60 ml/min/1.73m[2] of total body surface (b.s.) at least every 3 months, then monthly in patients with CKD stage 5 or on dialysis.[11]

Table 11.1 Circulating bone biomarkers and their characteristics

Name	Method	Normal values of measurement
Bone formation		
Bone-specific alkaline phosphatase (BSAP)	IRMA	5.8–20.6 ng/ml
	Enzymatic activity	11.6–41.3 IU/L
	Electrophoresis	–
Intact osteocalcin (iOc)	IRMA	11–46 ng/mL
N-mid region osteocalcin (nmOC)	ELISA	23 ± 7 ng/mL
Procollagen type-I N-terminal extension peptide (PINP)	RIA	40–100 µg/mL
Procollagen type-I carboxy-terminal extension peptide (PICP)	ELISA	38–202 ng/mL
Bone resorption		
Tartrate resistant acid phosphatases 5b (TRAP 5b)	ELISA	2.5–45 IU/L
Deoxypyridinoline (DPD)	ELISA	–
Pyridinoline (PYD)	ELISA	1.59 ± 0.38 nmol/L
NTX	ELISA	6.2 ± 19.0 nmol/L
CTX (CrossLaps or C-Terminal Collagen cross linked peptide)	ELISA	1.74–3.01 nmol/L
Procollagen type-I cross-linked carboxy-terminal telopeptide (ICTP)	ELISA	1.8–5.0 ng/mL
Bone sialoprotein	RIA	5.0–21.6 ng/mL
Other markers related to bone metabolism		
Total calcium	Automated	92.20–2.26 mmol/L
Ionized calcium	Electrodes	1.15–1.35 mmol/L
Phosphate	Automated	0.85–1.45 mmol/L
Magnesium	Automated	0.65–1.05 mmol/L
Total alkaline phosphatases (TAP)	Automated	90–120 IU/L
Aluminum	Electrodes	< 0.30 µmol/l
Parathyroid hormone (PTH)	IRMA	15–65 pg/mL
Vitamin D $(25(OH)D_3)$	RIA	9–45 ng/mL
Calcitriol $(1,25(OH)_2D_3)$	RIA	25–45 pg/mL
Vitamin D binding protein (DBP)	RIA	333 ± 58 mg/L
Insulin growth factor I (IGF-I)	IRMA	<10 pg/mL
Insulin growth factor binding proteins	RIA	53–120 ng/mL
Fibroblast growth factor 23 (FGF23) (C-terminal)	ELISA	0–150 RU/mL
Fibroblast growth factor 23 (FGF23) (intact)	ELISA	29 ± 28 pg/mL
Osteoprotegerin (OPG)	ELISA	6–138 pg/mL
RANKL	ELISA	5.2–12.4 pg/mL
Cathepsin K	ELISA	3.1 ± 1.9 pmol/L
Fetuin A	ELISA	0.52 ± 0.15 g/L
Matrix Gla protein (MGP)	ELISA	6.2 ± 3.5 nmol/L
Parathyroid related peptide (PTHrP)	IRMA	<1.5 pmol/L

Abbreviations: RANKL, receptor activator of NK-κB ligand.

Table 11.2 Total serum calcium concentration does not always corresponds to the total calcium balance

| Calcium balance | Total serum calcium concentration | | |
	High	Normal	Low
Negative	Primary hyperparathyroidism Malignancy hypercalcemia Hyperthyroidism	Post-menopausal osteoporosis Aging related bone disorders Chronic kidney disease Osteomalacia Hyperthyroidism	Hypoparathyroidism Osteomalacia
Neutral	Primary hyperparathyroidism	Normal situation Chronic kidney disease Osteitis fibrosis	Hypoparathyroidism
Positive	Milk-alkali syndrome Chronic kidney disease	Normal growth 'Hungry-bone' syndrome	Hypoparathyroidism

Data from Parfitt A. *Metab Bone Dis Rel Res* 1979;**13**:279–93.

Houillier P, et al. *Nephrol Dial Transplant* 2006;**21**:29–32

Ionized calcium is the fraction of blood calcium that is critical to physiological processes. It is usually measured using ion-selective electrodes, which enable nearly all laboratories to measure ionized calcium accurately. However, its routine use is limited because it is technically more demanding and more costly. The normal reference range for ionized calcium concentration is approximately 4.6–5.4 mg/dL (1.10–1.30 mmol/L). Ionized calcium concentration inversely correlated with pH and this

Table 11.3 Reference values for serum calcium

| Age | Total calcium | |
	mg/dL	mmol/L
Children		
Under 28 days	7.1–10.8	1.75–2.70
1–12 months	8.2–10.8	2.05–2.70
1–20 years	8.6–10.6	2.14–2.65
Adults		
Normal GFR	8.8–10.4	2.20–2.26
CKD stages 1, 2, 3		
CKD stage 4		
CKD stage 5 and dialysis	8.5–10.5	2.13–2.55
Ionized calcium		
Adults (normal GFR) CKDs	4.6–5.4	1.15–1.35

dependence on pH is explained by the fact that hydrogen ions compete with calcium, as well as with magnesium, for binding sites on albumin and other proteins. Both ionized calcium and ionized magnesium concentrations tend to decrease as the pH increases, indicating the stronger binding of these ions with protein in alkaline milieu. In addition to these factors well known to influence serum ionized calcium concentration, serum phosphate concentration can also plays an important role as suggested by the observed inverse relationship between ionized calcium and phosphate levels at any pH values.

Phosphate

Phosphorus is one of the most common anions in the organism and a critical element in skeletal development, bone mineralization, storage and transfer of energy (ATP and GTP), pH regulation, intracellular signal transduction, cellular membrane composition, nucleic acids structures, vitamins, and in the oxygen dissociation from the hemoglobin. It represents approximately 1% of the total body weight (~20,000 mmol), distributed mainly in three compartments: 85% in mineralized bone, 14% in intracellular compartments of soft tissues (~2,000 mmol), and less than 1% in extracellular fluids (~15 mmol). Within the cell, phosphorus is one of the most abundant anions, assuring the intracellular electro-negativity, and found in two forms—inorganic (not bound to any carbon containing element) and organic (bound to carbohydrates, nucleotides, lipids, etc). In the blood, phosphorus circulates predominantly in its free form, with only 25% bound to proteins. Of ultra-filterable phosphate, approximately 60% is ionized and 40% is complexed with cations such as calcium, magnesium, and sodium. The fraction of the total ultra-filterable phosphate decreases when extracellular concentration of calcium increases, probably due to the formation of calcium-phosphate-proteinate complexes. It should be emphasized that clinical assays for 'phosphate' typically measure phosphate ion concentration and the results are reported as elemental phosphorus concentration. The measurement of circulating phosphate is based on the formation of phosphomolybdic acid determined by colorimetric methods in the presence of an excess of molybdic acid. Normal ranges for serum phosphate levels are laboratory-specific, with the typical range of 2.5–4.5 mg/dL (0.8–1.45 mmol/L). Since most of the extraskeletal phosphate resides within the cells; it is critical that specimens are processed correctly, with prompt separation of the red cells to minimize cell lysis that could result in falsely high levels. Serum phosphate levels can vary significantly depending on the time of the day and recent dietary phosphorus intake; however, the overall day-to-day concentration variation is 5–10%. It tends to be higher in summer and lower in winter. Interestingly, the results of the Third National Health and Nutrition Examination Survey (NHANES III) showed that serum phosphate concentration is weakly related to dietary phosphorus and not related to phosphorus-rich foods in the general population. Indeed, demographic, nutritional, cardiovascular and kidney function variables explained only 12% of variation in serum phosphate levels.[12] Serum phosphate levels are also higher in young children and in post-menopausal women, whereas they are lower in women during menstruation (Table 11.4). There is an inverse relationship between serum phosphate

Table 11.4 Reference values for serum phosphate

Age	Total phosphates	
	mg/dL	mmol/L
Children		
Under 28 days	4.9–9.6	1.60–3.10
1–12 months	4.9–10.8	1.60–2.70
>1 years	3.4–6.2	1.10–2.00
Adults		
Normal GFR	2.6–4.4	0.87–1.45
CKD stages 1, 2, 3		
CKD stage 4		
CKD stage 5 and dialysis	3.5–5.5	1.13–1.78
Ionized calcium		
Adults (normal GFR) CKDs	4.6–5.4	1.15–1.35

levels and pH; acidosis increases serum phosphate levels, whereas alkalosis decreases it. There are variations of serum phosphate levels during the day, with the nadir being observed in the morning, in fasting states. It is not unusual to see a transient postprandial decrease in plasma phosphorus levels. Thus, for maximum accuracy, phosphorus levels should ideally be evaluated with the patient fasting.

Increased serum levels of phosphate appear to be associated with a variety of deleterious endpoints in CKD patients including secondary hyperparathyroidism, arterial hypertension, extraskeletal calcifications, fracture rates, and all-cause and cardiovascular mortality.[6–10,13] The values associated with this increase in the RR of death is reported to be >5.5 mg/dL (>1.80 mmol/L). Low serum levels of phosphate are also associated with a high risk of mortality.[6–10] Serum levels of phosphate should be measured in all patients with CKD and GFR<60mL/min/1.73m^2 of b.s., at least every 3 months, then monthly in patients with CKD stage 5 or on dialysis.

Parathyroid hormone

Parathyroid hormone (PTH) is a polypeptide molecule of 84 amino acids with a molecular weight of 9500 Da. It is synthesized and secreted from the chief cells of the parathyroid glands. The mature peptide is stored in secretory granules that fuse with the cell membrane and release PTH in response to reduction in the extracellular ionized calcium concentration. Most of this PTH is secreted in its intact form 1–84; however, it can also be secreted as a variety of N-terminal truncated fragments or C-terminal fragments following intracellular degradation, as may occur in hypercalcemia.[14]

Normally, approximately 10–20% of the total circulating PTH molecules are in its intact and bioactive form (1–84; Fig. 11.2). Indeed, once the secreted 1–84 PTH reaches the circulation, liver and kidney metabolize it. This degradation gives rise to

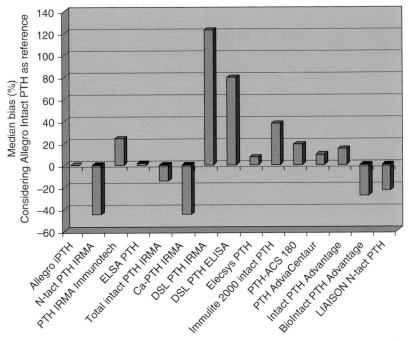

Fig. 11.1 Variability of serum parathyroid hormone (PTH) concentration with second- and third-generation PTH assays. From results of Table 3 of the article by Souberbielle et al. *Kidney Int* 2006;**70**:345–350.[21] DSL, Diagnostic Systems Laboratories; ELISA, enzyme-linked immunosorbent assay; IRMA, immunoradiometric assay.

several C-terminal fragments starting from residues at positions 34, 37, 41, and 43, and ending probably at position 84 or shorter, which often are released back into the circulation.[15] Because of the longer half-life of these fragments (5–10 times longer than the intact form), these C-terminal PTH fragments represent 80% of the total circulating PTH molecules in normal individuals (Fig. 11.1). Because the kidneys play an important role in the catabolism of intact PTH and of its fragments, when they fail, there is marked accumulation of circulating PTH fragments.

Since PTH is a major regulator of bone metabolism and since secondary hyperparathyroidism is a common feature of CKD, measurement of circulating PTH concentration has been widely used as a surrogate marker for the assessment of bone disease because of its correlation with the degree of bone turnover (Table 11.5).[16–18] However, recent experience has shown that there is wide variation in this correlation, which diminishes its predictive value when used alone. Many factors contribute to the variation including variation in blood sampling and storage procedures, and of the lack of reliable standardization of many PTH kits with regard to the degree of recognition of PTH fragments.[19] PTH values can be under- or over-estimated depending if they are measured in serum, citrate plasma, or EDTA plasma samples, if they are processed immediately or left at room temperature for more than 12h.[19–21]

Table 11.5 Predictive value of serum parathyroid hormone (PTH) levels in CKD-MBD

Author	Year	Number of patients	High bone turnover			Low bone turnover		
			Cut-off	PPV	Sensitivity	Cut-off	PPV	Sensitivity
Torres, A.	1995	119	≤450	100	43	<120	89	48
Couttenye, M.M.	1996	103				<150	65	81
Urena, P.	1996	42	>200	92	72	<150	51	70
Gerakis, A.	1996	114	>200	78	87	<65	45	69
Bervoets, A.R.	2003	84				<237	47	78
Barreto, F.C.	2008	97	>300	62	69	<150	83	50

Abbreviations: CKD-MBD, chronic kidney disease-mineral bone disorders; PPV: positive predictive value – the percentage of patients with high or low bone turnover rates if PTH is above or below the cut-off; Sensitivity, the % of patients that will be correctly detected

   The first generation of PTH assays were employed and developed through 1959 to 1987. They utilized a single antibody directed against PTH (epitopes on amino acids 39–84 or 53–84) in the radioimmunoassay (RIA) and measured many fragments of PTH, in addition to intact PTH.[22] The second generation PTH assays called 'intact' PTH assays have been developed from 1987.[23] They utilize two different antibodies, one directed against the C-terminal region of PTH (epitopes on amino acids 39–84, 44–84, 55–64, or 53–84), which is often immobilized onto plastic surfaces and binds intact PTH 1–84 and C-terminal PTH fragments. The second antibody is directed against the N-terminal region (epitopes on amino acids 13–34 'proximal epitope' as in the Allegro assay from Nichols Institute Diagnostics, San Clemente, CA, USA or 26–32 'distal epitope' as in the Elecsys assay from Roche Diagnostics, Meylan, France) and it is often radio-labeled, biotinylated, bound to an enzyme allowing to its easy detection and quantification or served as the coated antibody. These 'sandwich' assays were the first radio-immunometric assays (IRMA) and they were thought to only measure the full-length PTH 1–84, however they also measure large PTH fragments (such as PTH 7–84).[24] These N-terminal truncated PTH fragments may have some biological activity at a putative C-terminal PTH receptor and may have multiple not yet known biological functions in the skin, bone, hematopoietic system, and placenta.[15] The third generations of PTH assays have been developed since 2000, they utilize the same 'sandwich' and radio-immunometric techniques, with the first antibody directed against amino acids 39–84, but the second antibody has been restricted and directed against the first 6 N-terminal residues of PTH 1–84 (epitopes on amino acids 1–4 or 1–5).[25] They have been demonstrated to be most sensitive and more specific measuring bioactive intact PTH 1–84, but probably also another new form of PTH named amino-PTH recently identified in patients with parathyroid carcinoma, and in severe cases of primary and secondary hyperparathyroidism.

From the beginning, the utility of the third generation PTH assays has generated a highly charged debate. Many of the studies published found an excellent correlation of serum PTH values between the second and third generation PTH assays[25,26]) in CKD patients undergoing dialysis. However, mean circulating PTH levels are 30–60% lower[27] with the third generation PTH assays than those assessed with the second generation assays. Furthermore, most of uremic patients exhibit a normal ratio of intact to N-terminal truncated PTH fragments (intact PTH/N-terminal truncated PTH – intact PTH). However, in certain cases, this ratio can be abnormal, which has led several investigators to propose that a ratio lower than 1 could be the best predictor of a low turn-over bone disease (LBTD); however, other investigators have been unable to confirm these findings.

The inter-method variability in the measurement of circulating PTH concentration of 15 different PTH assays (13 second-generation and two third-generation PTH assays) was recently reported.[19,21] They demonstrate that, when using the second-generation Allegro Intact PTH assay from Nichols Institute as the reference assay, the median bias between the different PTH assays varied from –44.9% to +123.0% (Fig. 11.1). This implicates that the 'true' serum PTH concentration may be under- or over-estimating depending on the type of PTH assay chosen. A patient with a serum PTH value of 150 pg/mL or 300 pg/mL in one place may have values comprised between 83–323 pg/mL and 160–638 pg/mL, respectively, in another place. This clearly illustrates that the method used to measure circulating PTH concentration is a very important issue and that results from different laboratories are not interchangeable. While PTH is the primary biomarker used in the assessment of the degree of bone turnover, it might be a more appropriate strategy if it is combined with other specific markers of bone formation rate, such as bone-specific alkaline phosphatase, and bone resorption rate such as TRAP5b and collagen type-I breakdown cross-linked peptides (cross-laps), in order to gather more information about the bone response to a given serum PTH concentration.

Finally, similar to serum phosphate levels, both low and high serum levels of PTH appear to be associated with a variety of deleterious endpoints in CKD patients including extraskeletal calcifications, fracture rates, hospitalization rates, and all-cause and cardiovascular mortality.[7,8]

Circulating markers of bone formation

Total alkaline phosphatase and bone-specific alkaline phosphatase

Six alkaline phosphatase isoenzymes have been indentified: hepatic, intestinal, skeletal, renal, placental, and tumoural.[28] Such diversity is partly due to the existence of at least four human genes, three of them on chromosome 2q34–37 and the other one on chromosome 1p36.1–34. One single gene codes for the tissue non-specific group of alkaline phosphatase (AP) that consists of liver, bone, and kidney isoforms, and these isoenzymes differ only by post-transcriptional glycosylation. The physiological role of AP is yet to be fully understood. However, the *AP* gene seems to be essential in the process of bone mineralization since the transfection of its cDNA confers the capacity of mineralization to cells normally lacking this gene.[28]

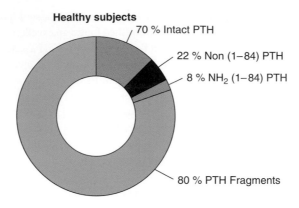

Healthy subjects
70 % Intact PTH
22 % Non (1–84) PTH
8 % NH$_2$ (1–84) PTH
80 % PTH Fragments

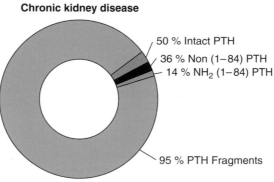

Chronic kidney disease
50 % Intact PTH
36 % Non (1–84) PTH
14 % NH$_2$ (1–84) PTH
95 % PTH Fragments

Fig. 11.2 The reduction in the glomerular filtration rate is associated with an decrease in the amount of circulating intact PTH and with an increase in PTH fragments. Adapted from Brossard, J.H., et al. *J Clin Endocrinol Metab* 1996;**81**:3923–3929.[24]

The bone-specific isoenzyme or BSAP has a molecular weight of 80kDa, is exclusively produced by osteoblast cells, and is neither dialysable nor filterable by the kidneys. Therefore, plasma BSAP concentration is not modified by variation in GFR, and its concentration depends on the rate of release from bone osteoblasts and on the rate of its hepatic degradation.[29] BSAP is a robust molecule since most of its activity is still found after 72h at 4°C, after several years stored at –20°C, and after several cycles of freezing and thawing. Different methods have been employed in order to measure plasma AP isoforms, among them, heat denaturation, chemical activators or inhibitors of specific AP isoforms, wheat germ lectin, or concanavalin-A precipitation, eventually associated with a separation by agarose-gel electrophoresis or by high performance affinity chromatography. However, these methods are expensive, laborious, time-consuming, and of too low sensitivity to be easily applied in clinical practice. Fortunately, specific monoclonal antibodies against BSAP have successfully been developed and reliably utilized in radio-immunological and immuno-enzymatic assays.[30] The values obtained using immunological assays such as Ostase®, IRMA from Hybritech which measures the mass of BSAP and Alkaphase®, ELISA from Metra Biosystems, Inc., which measures the activity are well correlated with the values obtained by separation methods, such as Isopal® from Beckman.[31] It seems, however, that the electrophoretical method is more sensitive than the other methods when measuring low concentrations of BSAP.[32]

As expected, using these new methods, recent observations showed that plasma BSAP is more sensitive than total AP, osteocalcin, and osteonectin in the evaluation of bone remodeling in CKD-MBD.[33] Furthermore, since the monoclonal antibody against BSAP exhibits a very low cross-reactivity with other alkaline phosphatases, it has become possible to differentiate the elevation of total AP due to liver disease from that due to bone diseases.[34] During life, there are two age-dependent physiological peaks of plasma BSAP, one during infancy and the other during puberty. Both peaks are disturbed in pediatric uremic patients in accordance with their altered longitudinal growth.[35] Nonetheless, in such children, plasma BSAP correlated with PTH and not with total AP, and showed a better correlation with height velocity than total AP. Plasma BSAP also correlates with bone trabecular density, the metabolically most active part of bone, pointing to its significance as a marker of bone formation.

Values of plasma BSAP > 20 ng/mL are constantly associated with either histological signs of secondary hyperparathyroidism or high bone turnover.[36] In addition, plasma BSAP correlates better with iPTH ($r = 0.82$) than total AP with iPTH ($r = 0.66$). Plasma BSAP also correlates better than PTH and total AP with most of bone histomorphometric parameters including osteoclast and osteoblast surfaces. Accordingly, when based on these bone parameters, the sensitivity and specificity of a plasma BSAP value > 20 ng/mL can reach 100% in the prediction of a high bone turnover disease.[16,36] This high specificity suggests, however, that plasma BSAP higher than 20 ng/mL formally excludes the existence of a low or normal bone turnover. In contrast, providing a plasma BSAP value below which there would be a great probability of low turnover bone disease appears to be more difficult. The two bone biopsy-based studies reported employed different and non-comparable methods of BSAP measurements,[16] and did not allow to obtain sensitive plasma BSAP value predictive of adynamic bone disease (ABD). However, from these observations, it can be proposed that the diagnosis of ABD in hemodialysis patients should be suspected when plasma PTH levels are less than 150 pg/mL and that BSAP levels are lower than 7 ng/mL (Ostase®) or 27 U/L (Isopal®).[16]

In some cases a discrepancy between plasma BSAP and PTH concentrations is found. Certain dialysed patients have high plasma concentrations of BSAP associated with plasma PTH levels either low or within the limits considered as normal.[33] Several hypotheses can be made to explain this phenomenon. First, the threshold of 20 ng/mL might be inadequate in the presence of a concomitant augmentation of total AP. Indeed, the antibodies against BSAP show a cross-reactivity of 16% with total AP. However, the radio-immunological measurement of BSAP can still be considered as reliable, if the increase of total AP does not exceed 2.6-fold the upper normal limit. Secondly, as the same gene encodes liver, kidney, and bone AP isoenzymes; there could be an extraskeletal synthesis of BSAP, either hepatic or renal.[28,37] Thirdly, the production of skeletal BSAP could be independent of PTH-stimulated osteoblastic activity. Several cytokines and growth factors have been shown to exert a PTH-like action on bone cells. Among them, IL-1, IL-6, and TNF are usually found increased in dialysis patients.[28] Fourthly, the serum concentration of certain electrolytes could influence the concentration of BSAP. It has been demonstrated that BSAP activity is proportional to the concentration of phosphate in the culture milieu (28). Likewise, an inverse relationship has been observed between plasma urea concentration and BSAP activity in the rat.

In approximately 20% of hemodialysis patients, low plasma BSAP concentrations are associated with PTH values higher than 200 pg/mL. First of all, it might suggest that the increased PTH is not always synonymous of high turnover bone disease in such patients. On the other hand, low plasma BSAP values reflect a decreased BSAP synthesis by osteoblastic cells. It could be explained, first, by a functional alteration of osteoblastic cells. Cultured osteoblasts from hemodialysis patients respond less well to several stimuli including PTH, than those from normal individuals.[38] Secondly, the poor response of osteoblasts to PTH and the low plasma BSAP may result from the PTH receptor down-regulation in these uremic cells.[39] Thirdly, the presence of a genetic alkaline hypophosphatemia may be responsible as well.[29,37] Finally, there is probably no direct correlation between plasma BSAP and PTH because we might have been overestimating the plasma concentration of the biologically active form of PTH with the assay methods used.[24,40]

After surgical parathyroidectomy (PTX), plasma BSAP concentration behaves like PTH, and decreases from often above 40 ng/mL before PTX to < 10 ng/mL 3 months after the PTX. After successful kidney transplantation, hypocalcemia, hyperphosphatemia, and calcitriol deficiency are commonly corrected and plasma PTH returns to normal values in 70–90% of patients after several months. Paradoxically, plasma BSAP levels show a tendency to increase probably because of the augmentation of bone turnover induced by most of the immunosuppressive drugs.[41] However, bone resorption rate appears to predominate over bone formation rate as evidenced by the important bone loss observed during the first year of kidney graft.

The response to medical treatments in uremic patients with secondary hyperparathyroidism, for instance, to intravenous bolus of calcitriol, has been based on the reduction of plasma PTH levels alone. However, it has been noted that calcitriol can have a direct effect on bone turnover independently of its effect on PTH synthesis.[42] Calcitriol decreases the expression of PTH receptor on osteoblastic cells and, thereby, the action of PTH on bone remodeling. Such effect could lead to the installation of a low bone turnover bone disease even in the presence of relatively high plasma PTH levels. We have observed that plasma BSAP levels can help in making a decision to decrease or to stop calcitriol. Recently, a *post hoc* analysis of pooled data from phase 3 randomized controlled trials using the calcimimetic cinacalcet HCl in dialysis patients with secondary hyperparathyroidism showed that serum total AP was reduced in a greater proportion of patients who were receiving cinacalcet compared with patients who received traditional care alone. The proportion of patients with total AP >120 U/L decreased during the course of the study in cinacalcet-treated patients but increased in control subjects.[43]

Altogether, the observations mentioned above suggest that in the absence of bone histology, plasma BSAP alone provides useful information about the rate of bone remodeling in hemodialysis patients. Its combination with PTH improves sensitivity, specificity, and the predictive value in the diagnosis of the type of bone turnover. Nevertheless, bone histomorphometry appears to be still indispensable to make the distinction between patients with normal bone and patients with adynamic bone disease, and in situations where there is discordance between plasma BSAP and PTH values. Again, it should be stressed that an independent augmentation of either plasma PTH or BSAP may not always correspond to an increased bone turnover. The idea that in hemodialysis patients one must try to maintain plasma PTH levels 2–5 times higher than the normal values has to be reconsidered and not necessarily generalized. As discussed before, paradoxically, histomorphometric signs of high bone remodeling can be seen in patients with normal or even low plasma PTH, and vice versa. Finally, it should also stressed that two recent studies reported that high levels of serum total AP, >120 U/L, are associated with higher risks of hospitalization and mortality in hemodialysis patients, independent of other liver enzymes, serum calcium, phosphorus, and PTH levels.[44,45] Similarly, in a prospective cohort study of 627 patients with CKD stages 1–5, increased serum BSAP levels predicted cardiovascular morbidity and mortality.[46]

Osteocalcin or bone Gla protein

Osteocalcin (OC) or bone Gla protein (protein containing γ carboxyglutamic acid, BGP) is the most abundant non-collagenic protein of the bone matrix.[47] Its gamma-carboxyglutamination occurs principally at the amino acids 17, 21, and 24, and depends on the presence of the cofactor, vitamin K. The gamma-carboxyglutamination of its glutamic acid at position 17 seems to be essential for the structural and spatial conformation of the molecule allowing the interaction with hydroxyapatite crystals.[48] When there is a deficiency in vitamin K (K1 or phylloquinone and K2; or menaquinones MK-4, MK-7, and MK-8), the carboxylate fraction of osteocalcin tends to decrease and can be associated with a reduced bone mass and a high risk of fractures.[49] Indeed, intestinal absorption of vitamin K is, in part, regulated by apolipoprotein E (ApoE). There is an association between the level of plasma vitamin K, bone density and the risk of fractures in hemodialysis patients and in post-menopausal women having the polymorphism E4 in the *Apo E* gene.[48,49] The physiological explanation of this is probably because the incorporation of vitamin K-charged lipoproteins into intestinal, hepatic, and bone cells depends exclusively on the fixation of ApoE on its specific receptor. In case of apoE4 phenotype the incorporation of vitamin K seems to be reduced.[49]

Human Oc possesses 49 amino acids, and is produced by only osteoblasts and odontoblasts under the control of 1,25-OH$_2$D$_3$. Incidentally, it was on the *Oc* gene where the sequence of DNA sensitive to the vitamin D-vitamin D receptor complex (VDR response element) was identified for the first time. It was also demonstrated that the regulation of the *Oc* gene by vitamin D was species specific. Vitamin D increased its expression in humans and in rats, whereas the opposite effect was observed in mice.[50] Osteocalcin and fragments of the peptide are released from bone matrix during bone resorption. Moreover, the intact molecule can be cleaved by cathepsins and plasmin. Plasmin cleaves it at position 43–44, giving rise to N-terminal (1–43) and C-terminal[44–49] fragments.[51] The C-terminal peptapeptide seems to be an important chemotactic bone factor since bone particles lacking it become resistant to resorption.[51] Likewise, extracellular calcium regulates the cleavage of Oc by plasmin probably through the induction of conformational changes.[51] The half-life of intact Oc in the circulation is of approximately 5 min. The physiological role of Oc is still not completely understood. Osteocalcin surely plays an important role in bone formation, perhaps favoring or preventing it. It was generally thought that osteocalcin stimulates bone formation, however, recent elegant studies have showed an impressive augmentation of bone formation and bone density in transgenic animals lacking the *Oc* gene. This led to the provoking hypothesis that osteocalcin might be an inhibitor of bone formation. The synthesis of osteocalcin by mature osteoblastic cells is probably one of the signals used by PTH to slow down osteoblastic activity and thereby bone formation.[52] Interestingly, Oc could also be the hormone through which the skeleton exert an endocrine regulation of sugar homeostasis and energy metabolism. Oc stimulates pancreatic beta-cell prolifération, insulin secretion, and improves peripheral insulin sensitivity by increasing the expression of adiponectin in fat cells.[53]

Numerous studies have used plasma Oc measurements in several metabolic bone disorders.[47] It has always been considered as a useful biomarker of the rate of bone formation. However, its use in the context of CKD-MBD is still limited by several problems. First, many Oc fragments of yet unknown function are retained in the plasma of uremic patients. Secondly, at least three forms of intact Oc can be measured in the plasma: total, carboxylated, and decarboxylated. Thirdly, the intact molecule is rapidly degraded at room temperature. Thus, the concentration measured depends on the type of antibodies used in the assay. Many of these antibodies recognized the intact molecule, but also some of the fragments. As already mentioned, Oc fragments are also liberated during bone matrix degradation. It is possible that in the future one or more of these fragments might turn out to be specific of bone resorption and measurable in the plasma.[54] Finally, there is great intra-assay variability in the levels of osteocalcin with most of the current assays.[47,54]

In CKD patients, circulating intact Oc represents 26% of total molecule. The remaining 74% comprises mainly four fragments: N-terminal, mid-region, mid-region C-terminal, and C-terminal. A study compared the dosage of osteocalcin using six different assays: ELSA-OST-NAT IRMA (Cis Bio Int), ELSA-OSTEO IRMA (Cis Bio Int), Osteocalcin IRMA (Nichols), OSTK-PR RIA (Cis Bio Int), OSCA Test Osteocalcin RIA (Henning) et Osteocalcin RIA (Nichols). The authors concluded that there was a good correlation of Oc values obtained with these kits when they examined normal individuals, pre-menopausal, and osteoporotic women. In contrast, there was no correlation when uremic patients and patients with Paget's disease were studied.[55]

Using the ELSA-OSTEO IRMA kit (Cis Bio Int), which utilizes two antibodies, one recognizing the end N-terminal fragment and the other recognizing a mid-region amino acid sequence, plasma Oc values were 4–6 Z-scores higher in hemodialysis patients than in normal individuals were found.[56] In spite of this accumulation, plasma Oc concentration demonstrated good sensitivity in the distinction between patients with high bone turnover due to hyperparathyroidism and those with normal or low bone turnover. As with other biochemical markers, the diagnostic sensitivity was low when the aim was to differentiate patients with adynamic bone disease from those with normal bone turnover. Although weaker than BSAP and PTH, the correlations of plasma Oc with bone histomorphometric parameters in hemodialysis patients were quite good.[56]

The results of these studies demonstrate the limitation of the use of plasma osteocalcin as a biochemical marker of bone remodeling in patients with impaired renal function[57] and in patients under hemodialysis treatment. Obviously, a clear understanding of the physiological role of osteocalcin and its fragments is still lacking. The development of new assays will certainly increase its sensitivity in the evaluation of CKD-MBD.

Matrix Gla protein

The matrix Gla protein (MGP) is a calcium-binding, 10 kDa molecular weight, vitamin K-dependent protein produced by osteoblastic cells.[58] It belongs to the family of mineral-binding Gla proteins that include osteocalcin (bone Gla protein), coagulation factors VII and IX, and anticoagulation factors protein S and C.[52,58] As other Gla proteins, MGP inhibits tissue mineralization by binding to mineral ions through γ-carboxylated glutamic acid residues γ-carboxylation. Thus, mice lacking the MGP gene develop strikingly arterial calcifications, which lead to blood-vessels rupture and death within the first 2 months of age. These animals also exhibit inappropriate calcification of cartilages, osteopenia, and fractures.[58] It has also been demonstrated that MGP together with fetuin-A bind to calcium and phosphate forming a complex, which is much more soluble that the complex calcium phosphate alone,[59] preventing crystal deposition in extraskeletal tissues.

Serum MGP levels can be measured by an enzyme-linked immunosorbent assay from Biomedica (Wien, Austria). The normal values, obtained from 25 healthy subjects, are of 6.2 ± 3.5 nmol/L. The first clinical studies assessing MGP with this assays found that serum MGP levels were inversely correlated with the severity of coronary calcifications in non-CKD patients. However, in CKD patients, no association has been observed between the presence of arterial calcification and the levels of serum MGP.[60] Disappointingly, serum MGP levels did not differ between CKD patients with low and high bone turnover.[61] Nevertheless, a significant correlation was evidenced between serum MGP levels and two histomorphometric parameters, namely BFR/BS and Tb.Th.[61]

In summary, circulating MGP concentration may certainly provide information about bone mineralization, as well as extraskeletal calcifications; however, the limited data so far reported plead for additional larger clinical studies.

Procollagen type I C-terminal extension peptide

Type I procollagen carboxy-terminal extension peptide (PICP) results from the extracellular cleavage of a molecule of type I procollagen at the time of its incorporation into the bone matrix. PICP has a molecular weight of approximately 100 kDa. Its plasma concentration is not altered by the decrease in glomerular filtration rate because its degradation takes place in the liver through the mannose-6-phosphate receptor.[62]

Specific antibodies against PICP have been developed and are actually employed to measure its plasma concentration.[56,62] Because PICP is produced by the osteoblastic cell lineage, its plasma concentration has been proposed as a biomarker of bone formation. CKD patients not yet treated by dialysis have significant increase in plasma PICP levels.[63] However, this increase does not correlate with other biomarkers of bone turnover or with bone histomorphometric parameters while patients treated with active vitamin D analogs had higher plasma PICP than patients without treatment.[64] In CKD patients already treated by dialysis, the results are contradictory. In some cases, plasma PICP levels provided useful information regarding the degree of bone formation, and showed a good correlation with plasma BSAP, Oc, and PTH,[62] while in other cases, no significant correlation between PICP levels and any of the bone histomorphometric parameters were observed.[56,62,63]

Procollagen type I N-terminal extension peptide

Like osteocalcin, type I procollagen type I amino-terminal extension peptide (PINP) is synthesized by osteoblastic cells and has been considered as a new marker of type I collagen synthesis as well as of bone turnover. Its can be measured by an ELISA method, utilizing an antibody against the alpha-chain of procollagen type I.[65] Increased plasma levels of PINP have been found in patients with hypovitaminosis D-induced hyperparathyroidism[65] and in dialysis patients with high bone turnover correlating significantly with serum PTH and BSAP.[66] Serum PINP also correlated negatively with the annual changes in BMD at the distal radius.[66] Thus, plasma PINP might be a useful marker of bone matrix synthesis, however, its utility in case of CKD-MBD requires further evaluation.

Circulating markers of bone resorption

Tartrate-resistant acid phosphatase

Acid phosphatases are lysosomial enzymes produced by osteoclasts, prostate, uterus, pancreas, spleen, blood red and white cells, and platelets. Analogous to total alkaline phosphatases, the different acid phosphatases can be separated and measured by enzymatic, electrophoretical, or chromatographic methods.[67] Thus, the bone-specific acid phosphatase (TRAP), or the purple acid phosphatase because of its iron content, has been proposed as a potential marker of bone resorption. TRAP has a molecular weight of 30 kDa but circulates in the plasma as a 250 kDa complex, non filterable by the kidney, which, among other elements, contains calcium.[67] Serum TRAP was previously determined by virtue of its' resistance to tartric acid. Many questions have however, been raised about its osteoclast specificity and even though TRAP appears to be essential in the process of bone resorption, its physiological role on the skeleton is yet poorly understood. TRAP dephosphorylates a variety of bone matrix protein such osteopontin and sialoprotein[68] and interacts with cathepsin K, which is a major collagenolytic cysteine proteinase expressed in osteoclasts, capable of proteolytically processing and activation of TRAP *in vitro*. The absence of cathepsin K in osteoclasts is associated with increased expression of TRAP mRNA, monomeric TRAP protein and total TRAP activity, cathepsin K is also involved in the intracellular trafficking of TRAP.[69] Transgenic mice with targeted disruption of *TRAP* gene develop an osteopetrotic phenotype with altered osteoclastic function.[70] The *TRAP* gene belongs to a family of genes coding for iron transport proteins, and it seems to be regulated, at the transcriptional level, by extracellular iron concentrations. It possesses an iron-sensitive DNA sequence (iron-response element) on its 5' unstranslated region.

The first studies on the utility of TRAP in the assessment of metabolic bone diseases demonstrated that the amount and the activity of TRAP correlated with rate of bone resorption. TRAP also correlated positively with serum PTH, total AP, BSAP, number of osteoclasts and percent of eroded bone surface in CKD patients. The stability of this enzyme is however limited and samples have to be separated rapidly from blood within the first 2h and frozen until being assayed.

Specific antibodies against the isoforms TRAP5b have successfully been developed and applied in an enzyme-linked immunoabsorbent assay (ELISA)[71,72] and elevated levels of TRAP5b have been demonstrated in primary hyperparathyroidism.[67] Normal subjects can have sensibly measurable amount of serum TRAP5b,[67] probably because of the recognition by the assay of other acid phosphatases or that TRAP5b is produced by certain blood cells. Serum TRAP5b is not affected by renal dysfunction, which has led to the assumption that it might be a useful marker of osteoclastic activity and bone resorption in CKD-MBD. Recent studies in dialysis patients have demonstrated that serum TRAP5b correlated significantly with BSAP, intact OC, PTH, and especially with serum NTX (N-terminal collagen cross-link peptides) another marker of bone resorption,[46,72] besides with the annual change in BMD. The sensitivity and specificity for detection of rapid bone loss were 58 and 77%, respectively, for serum TRAP5b levels.[72]

Finally, similar to other biomarkers such as BSAP, calcium, phosphate, and PTH, TRAP5b could also serve as a predictor of cardiovascular morbidity and mortality in CKD patients.[46] Thus, measurement of serum TRAP5b may in the future be a clinically relevant assay for estimation of CKD-MBD and its outcomes.

C-terminal cross-link telopeptides

CTX or CrossLaps

Telopeptides are small amino acid sequences generated from the degradation of non-helical ends of collagen molecules. Because of their low molecular weight they are normally cleared by the kidneys and accumulate in case of renal failure. Two types of immunoassays for measurements or C-telopeptides, the CTX and the ICTP, exist. Both assays recognize different domains of the C-terminal telopeptide region of the α1 chain of type-I collagen. The CTX assays are based on the CrossLaps antibodies, which recognize the EKAHD-β-GGR amino acid sequence where the aspartate residue is β-isomerized. The degree of isomerization of the aspartate residue correlates with bone age.[73] Serum should be separated from the whole blood immediately after coagulation and stored until analysis in a deep freezer.

Using the automated Elecsys analyser (Roche Diagnostics GmbH) for CrossLaps, it has been reported that both serum CTX and BSAP discriminate between bone turnover rates of adolescent young women of different ages and that serum β-CrossLaps concentrations were significantly increased in CKD dialysis patients and positively correlated with serum PTH and BSAP.[74] Inversely, serum β-CrossLaps concentrations negatively correlated with patients' age, and with bone mineral density at the midradius.[75] In kidney transplanted patients, and in parallel with serum Oc levels, a significant decrease in serum β-CrossLaps concentration was observed 6 months after transplantation, and also that a positive correlation exists between these two molecules at any time after transplantation.

In conclusion, serum CTX measurements may be a useful bone resorption marker in CKD-MBD and its use combined with bone formation markers may improve the management of this condition.

Type I collagen C-terminal cross-link telopeptide

Procollagen type I cross-linked carboxy-terminal telopeptide (ICTP) is a part of type I collagen released during bone resorption and containing cross-linking molecules. One molecule of ICTP is composed of two C-terminal fragments from the α1 chain of type-I collagen, one helical segment from α1 or α2 chain of collagen, and a cross-linked peptide (pyridinoline, PYD, or deoxypyridinoline, DPD). Its molecular weight is approximately 9000 Da. ICTP is released into the circulation after the degradation of mature collagen molecules of the bone matrix. To note, although they are both, two C-terminal telopeptides, ICTP and CTX, they are released after two different enzymatic processes. The hydrolysis by cathepsin K totally abolishes ICTP, whereas CTX is unaffected.[76] In addition, ICTP and CTX respond differently in clinical situations. While serum CTX levels showed markedly response to anti-resorptive therapies, such as bisphosphonates, hormone replacement, and SERMs, ICTP did not.[76]

As for β-CrossLaps, the current assays of plasma ICTP utilizes polyclonal antibodies against a small group of cross-linked peptides harboring the amino acid sequence (EKAHDGGR) of the human α1 chain of type-I collagen.[73] Several observations have demonstrated a good correlation between plasma ICTP levels and bone histomorphometric parameters of bone resorption in patients with a diversity of bone metabolic diseases.[73,77] However, other clinical studies did not support this dosage as a specific indicator of bone resorption rate.[78] In the case of patients with CKD-MBD, ICTP tends to accumulate in the serum with the decrease in renal function, and even further in hemodialysis patients. The few studies performed in hemodialysis patients did not support its use as a useful biomarker of bone resorption.[56,76,78]

Type I collagen N-terminal cross-link telopeptide

Type I collagen N-terminal cross-link telopeptide (NTX) also originates directly from the osteoclast-mediated proteolytic cleavage of bone type I collagen. Few studies have assessed the utility of serum NTX measurement in the evaluation of CKD-MBD. Nevertheless, it appears that serum NTX is well correlated with serum concentrations of PTH, BSAP, β-CrossLaps, PYD, DPD, and intact OC in hemodialysis patients.[79]

Interestingly, serum NTX levels are negatively correlated with bone mineral density at the distal radius in these patients. Together with β-CrossLaps, they also predicted the annual bone loss at the distal radius.[79] Therefore, serum NTX, in addition to other biomarkers, may be a useful tool for assessing CKD-MBD.

Pyridinium cross-links (pyridinoline and deoxypyridinoline)

Eighty-five to ninety per cent of bone protein matrix consists of type I collagen.[80,81] It is this molecule, in fact, which mostly provides the mechanical force of bone tissue because of its particular intramolecular and intermolecular cross-links, which are responsible for the tensile strength of collagen fibres.[80,81] To date, only two main collagen intermolecular cross-link molecules have been thoroughly studied, pyridinoline (PYD, hydroxylysylpyridinium or HP), which is formed from the condensation, ring closure, and oxidation of one hydrolysine and two hydrolysine-derived aldehyde molecules, and deoxypyridinoline (DPD, lysylpyridinium or LP) from one lysine and two hydrolysine-derived aldehydes.[80,81] Both, PYD and DPD are present in bone and cartilage; however, most of the pyridinium cross-links found in the cartilage is in form of PYD, by contrast with DPD, which is predominant in bone. Metabolically, these molecules are non-reducible and cannot be reutilized during new collagen synthesis.[82] Furthermore, diet-derived cross-links molecules are not absorbed from the intestine. Following bone resorption and bone collagen degradation by specific osteoclast-related enzymes, PYD and DPD are released into the circulation and because of their low molecular weight (429–591Da) they are normally excreted into the urine, with as much as 40% in their free forms.[82] Usually, serum PYD and DPD are extremely low, and even undetectable in normal individuals; therefore, their measurement is commonly performed in urine. The renal clearance is different for free and conjugated forms. The free form has a fractional clearance higher than one, suggesting some tubular secretion, whereas the conjugated one has a clearance less than one.[83] Based on these properties, it has been suggested that quantitative analysis of PYD and DPD in the serum, as well as in the urine could provide valuable information about bone resorption rate.

Specific polyclonal and monoclonal antibodies have recently been developed for the direct measurement of PYD and DPD.[84] The concentrations of PYD and DPD measured by ELISA methods are usually 4–10 times lower than the values obtained previously by HPLC. Nevertheless, the values obtained with either method are excellently correlated. Measurement of PYD and DPD, released after hydrolysis of the urine sample, either by HPLC or ELISA, have been shown to serve as excellent markers of bone resorption rate in malnourished children, osteoporotic and post-menopausal women, primary and secondary hyperparathyroidism, rheumatoid arthritis, and osteoarthritis, Paget's disease, acromegaly, hyperthyroidism, in patients with tumor-associated hypercalcemia, and in CKD patients.[77]

Serum PYD and DPD have been found increased in patients with severe renal failure, with levels 50–100 times higher than in control subjects, the levels decreased after dialysis and PYD and DPD were ultrafilterable, and could be measured in the dialysate fluid.

Using a competitive ELISA method (Metra Biosystems, Inc., CA, USA), it was found that hemodialysis patients had markedly increased (10–30 fold) serum PYD levels compared with normal individuals and were associated with high bone turnover, and were positively correlated with bone resorption and bone formation parameters. These correlations were comparable with those found between serum BSAP and bone histomorphometric parameters., Serum PYD correlated however significantly better with bone histology than both PTH and osteocalcin. The type of dialysis membrane did not have a major influence on serum PYD levels.[56]

In another study, using a serum DPD radioimmunoassay from Nichols, it was found that serum levels higher than 21 nmol/l had a sensitivity of 88% and a specificity of 93% in the diagnosis of high turnover bone disease[85] and that DPD levels were associated with the annual bone loss in distal radius of hemodialysis patients.[79]

From these studies, it can be argued that serum PYD and DPD may be useful biomarkers of bone resorption in CKD-MBD. Hopefully, more sensitive measurement of collagen cross-linked molecules and other bone resorption associated proteins will be developed and will become common tests in clinical practice.

Bone sialoprotein

Bone sialoprotein (BSP) is a glycoprotein of the bone matrix with a molecular weight of 70–80 kDa, produced by osteoblasts, osteoclasts, and hypertrophic chondrocytes. It is almost exclusively found in mineralized tissues and, therefore, considered as a potential marker of bone resorption. It has been suggested that BSP may function at several steps in bone modeling and remodeling. In addition to its ability to nucleate hydroxyapatite crystal formation and promote mineralization, BSP can also induce cell adhesion and increase osteoclastogenesis and bone resorption.[86] Furthermore, although BSP expression is coincident with *de novo* bone formation and ectopic calcification, namely, cardiovascular calcifications,[60] high BSP level in serum has been associated with excessive bone resorption, as shown in patients with Crohn's disease, cancer, and in post-menopausal women.[87] Serum BSP decreased after different anti-resorptive treatments in parallel with a decrease of bone resorption markers and an increase of bone mineral density.[87] Based on these data, circulating BSP appears to be a valuable marker of bone resorption and monitoring bone-focused therapies, it has, however, not so far been evaluated in patients with CKD-MBD.

Galactosyl hydroxylysine

Similar to DPD, galactosyl hydroxylysine (Gal-Hyl) has been proposed as a substitute of hydroxyproline for the evaluation of bone resorption because it is a more specific marker of bone tissue than hydroxyproline.[88] The measurement of Gal-Hyl in the urine has been used as a simple and non-invasive method for the evaluation of bone resorption rate in children, normal adult subjects, post-menopausal women, Paget's disease, and other metabolic bone disorders.[88] However, to the best of our knowledge there has not been any study evaluating serum or urinary Gal-Hyl in patients with CKD-MBD.

Summary

In the absence of bone biopsy, there is no ideal marker of bone remodeling in CKD patients. Recent studies have shown that PTH alone is not necessarily a good biomarker for bone turnover in the setting of CKD, particularly when the levels are modestly increased (3–9 times the upper limit of normal). As such, increased plasma PTH levels are not always synonymous of high turnover bone disease and vice versa. Other bone biomarkers discussed in this chapter provide useful information at the extremes but each one alone is not more valuable that PTH, particularly at distinguishing low from normal bone turnover. The combined use of PTH with some of the more accessible biomarkers of bone remodeling have the potential to improve the diagnosis, monitoring, and treatment monitoring of CKD-MBD in the future. However, further studies are clearly required to examine the utility of these biomarkers and their correlations with bone histology in the current era.

References

1. Yajima A, Inaba M, Tominaga Y, et al. Bone formation by minimodeling is more active than remodeling after parathyroidectomy. *Kidney Int* 2008;**74**:775–81.

2. Moe S, Drueke T, Cunningham J, et al. Definition, evaluation, and classification of renal osteodystrophy: a position statement from Kidney Disease: Improving Global Outcomes (KDIGO). *Kidney Int* 2006;**69**:1945–53.

3. Houillier P, Froissart M, Maruani G, et al. What serum calcium can tell us and what it can't. *Nephrol Dial Transplant* 2006;**21**:29–32.

4. Gauci C, Moranne O, Fouqueray B, et al. Pitfalls of measuring total blood calcium in patients with CKD. *J Am Soc Nephrol* 2008;**19**:1592–8.

5. Payne RB, Little AJ, Williams RB, et al. Interpretation of serum calcium in patients with abnormal serum proteins. *Br Med J* 1973;**4**:643–6.

6. Block GA, Klassen PS, Lazarus JM, et al. Mineral metabolism, mortality, and morbidity in maintenance hemodialysis. *J Am Soc Nephrol* 2004;**15**:2208–18.

7. Stevens LA, Djurdjev O, Cardew S, et al. Calcium, phosphate, and parathyroid hormone levels in combination and as a function of dialysis duration predict mortality: evidence for the complexity of the association between mineral metabolism and outcomes. *J Am Soc Nephrol* 2004;**15**:770–9.

8. Tentori F, Blayney MJ, Albert JM, et al. Mortality risk for dialysis patients with different levels of serum calcium, phosphorus, and PTH: the Dialysis Outcomes and Practice Patterns Study (DOPPS). *Am J Kidney Dis* 2008;**52**:519–30.

9. Wald R, Sarnak MJ, Tighiouart H, et al. Disordered mineral metabolism in hemodialysis patients: an analysis of cumulative effects in the Hemodialysis (HEMO) Study. *Am J Kidney Dis* 2008;**52**:531–40.

10. Young EW, Albert JM, Satayathum S, et al. Predictors and consequences of altered mineral metabolism: the Dialysis Outcomes and Practice Patterns Study. *Kidney Int* 2005;**67**:1179–87.

11. Eknoyan G, Levin N. NKF-K/DOQI Clinical Practice Guidelines: Update 2000. Foreword. *Am J Kidney Dis* 2001;**37**:S5–6.

12. de Boer IH, Rue TC, Kestenbaum B. Serum phosphorus concentrations in the third National Health and Nutrition Examination Survey (NHANES III). *Am J Kidney Dis* 2009;**53**:399–407.

13. Block GA, Hulbert-Shearon TE, Levin NW, et al. Association of serum phosphorus and calcium x phosphate product with mortality risk in chronic hemodialysis patients: a national study. *Am J Kidney Dis* 1998;**31**:607–17.

14. D'Amour P, Rakel A, Brossard JH, et al. Acute regulation of circulating parathyroid hormone (PTH) molecular forms by calcium: utility of PTH fragments/PTH(1–84) ratios derived from three generations of PTH assays. *J Clin Endocrinol Metab* 2006;**91**:283–9.

15. Murray TM, Rao LG, Divieti P, et al. Parathyroid hormone secretion and action: evidence for discrete receptors for the carboxyl-terminal region and related biological actions of carboxyl- terminal ligands. *Endocr Rev* 2005;**26**:78–113.

16. Couttenye MM, D'Haese PC, VanHoof VO, et al. Bone alkaline phosphatase (BAP) compared to PTH in the diagnosis of adynamic bone disease (ABD). *Nephrol Dial Transplant* 1994;**9**:905 (Abst.).

17. Torres A, Lorenzo V, Hernandez D, et al. Bone disease in predialysis, hemodialysis, and CAPD patients: evidence of a better bone response to PTH. *Kidney Int* 1995;**47**: 1434–42.

18. Urena P, Hruby M, Ferreira A, et al. Plasma total versus bone alkaline phosphatase as markers of bone turnover in hemodialysis patients. *J Am Soc Nephrol* 1996;**7**:506–12.

19. Urena P. The need for a reliable serum parathyroid hormone measurements. *Kidney Int* 2006;**70**:240–3.

20. Joly D, Drueke TB, Alberti C, et al. Variation in serum and plasma PTH levels in second-generation assays in hemodialysis patients: a cross-sectional study. *Am J Kidney Dis* 2008;**51**:987–95.

21. Souberbielle JC, Boutten A, Carlier MC, et al. Inter-method variability in PTH measurement: implication for the care of CKD patients. *Kidney Int* 2006;**70**:345–50.

22. Berson SA, Yalow RS. Immunochemical heterogeneity of parathyroid hormone in plasma. *J Clin Endocrinol Metab* 1968;**28**:1037–47.

23. Nussbaum S, Zahradnik R, JR, et al. Highly sensitive two-site immunoradiometric assay of parathyrin, and its clinical utility in evaluating patients with hypercalcemia. *Clin Chem* 1987;**33**:1364–7.

24. Brossard JH, Cloutier M, Roy L, et al. Accumulation of a non-(1-84) molecular form of parathyroid hormone (PTH) detected by intact PTH assay in renal failure: importance in the interpretation of PTH values. *J Clin Endocrinol Metab* 1996;**81**:3923–9.

25. Gao P, Scheibel S, D'Amour P, et al. Development of a novel immunoradiometric assay exclusively for biologically active whole parathyroid hormone 1–84: implications for improvement of accurate assessment of parathyroid function. *J Bone Miner Res* 2001;**16**:605–14.

26. John M, Goodman W, Gao P, et al. A novel immunoradiometric assay detects full-length human PTH but not amino-terminally truncated fragments: Implications for PTH measurements in renal failure. *J Clin Endocrinol Metab* 1999;**84**:4287–90.

27. Brandi L, Egfjord M, Olgaard K. Comparison between 1alpha(OH)D3 and 1,25(OH)2D3 on the suppression of plasma PTH levels in uremic patients, evaluated by the 'whole' and 'intact' PTH assays. *Nephron Clin Pract* 2005;**99**:c128–37.

28. Weiss MJ, Junal R, Henthorn PS, et al. Structure of the human liver/bone/kidney-type alkaline phosphatase gene. *J Biol Chem* 1988;**263**:12002–10.

29. Fedde K, Michell M, Henthorn P, et al. Aberrant properties of alkaline phosphatase in patient fibroblasts correlate with clinical expressivity in severe forms of hypophosphatasia. *J Clin Endocrinol Metab* 1996;**81**:2587–94.

30. Garrido JC, Aguayo FJ, Moreno CA. Comparison of three bone alkaline phosphatase quantification methods in patients with increased alkaline phosphatase activities. *Clin Chem* 1992;**38**:1165–6.

31. Gomez B, Ardakani S, Ju J, et al. Monoclonal antibody assay for measuring bone-specific alkaline phosphatase activity in serum. *Clin Chem* 1995;**41**:1560–6.

32. Couttenye MM, D'Haese PC, VanHoof VO, et al. Low serum levels of alkaline phosphatase of bone origin: a good marker of adynamic bone disease in hemodialysis patients. *Nephrol Dial Transplant* 1996;**11**:1065–72.

33. Urena P, De Vernejoul MC. Circulating biochemical markers of bone remodeling in uremic patients. *Kidney Int* 1999;**55**:2141–56.

34. Woitge H, Seibel M, Ziegler R. Comparison of total and bone-specific alkaline phosphatase in patients with nonskeletal disorders or metabolic bone diseases. *Clin Chem* 1996;**42**:1796–804.

35. Behnke B, Kemper M, Kruse H-P, et al. Bone alkaline phosphatase in children with chronic renal failure. *Nephrol Dial Transplant* 1998;**13**:662–7.

36. Urena P, Bernard-Poenaru O, Cohen-Solal M, et al. Plasma bone-specific alkaline phosphatase changes in hemodialysis patients treated by alfacalcidol. *Clin Nephrol* 2002;**57**:261–73.

37. Whyte M, Landt M, Ryan L, et al. Alkaline phosphatase: placental and tissue-nonspecific isoenzymes hydrolyze phosphoethanolamine, inorganic pyrophosphate, and pyridoxal 5'-phosphate. *J Clin Invest* 1995;**95**:1440–5.

38. Marie P, Lomri A, DeVernejoul M, et al. Relationship between histomorphometric features of bone formation and bone cell characterisation *in vitro* in renal osteodystrophy. *J Clin Endocrinol Metab* 1989;**69**:1166–73.

39. Urena P, Ferreira A, Morieux C, et al. PTH/PTHrP receptor mRNA is down-regulated in epiphyseal cartilage growth plate of uremic rats. *Nephrol Dial Transplant* 1996;**11**:2008–16.

40. Lepage R, Roy L, Brossard JH, et al. A non-(1-84) circulating parathyroid hormone (PTH) fragment interferes significantly with intact PTH commercial assay measurements in uremic samples. *Clin Chem* 1998;**44**:805–9.

41. Withold W, Friedrich W, Degenhardt S. Serum bone alkaline phosphatase is superior to plasma levels of bone matrix proteins for assessment of bone metabolism in patients receiving renal transplants. *Clin Chim Acta* 1997;**261**:105–15.

42. Ureña P, Prieur P, Pétrover M. Calcitriol may directly suppress bone turnover. *Nephron* 1996;**75**:116–17.

43. Belozeroff V, Goodman WG, Ren L, et al. Cinacalcet lowers serum alkaline phosphatase in maintenance hemodialysis patients. *Clin J Am Soc Nephrol* 2009;**4**:673–9.

44. Blayney MJ, Pisoni RL, Bragg-Gresham JL, et al. High alkaline phosphatase levels in hemodialysis patients are associated with higher risk of hospitalisation and death. *Kidney Int* 2008;**74**:655–63.

45. Regidor DL, Kovesdy CP, Mehrotra R, et al. Serum alkaline phosphatase predicts mortality among maintenance hemodialysis patients. *J Am Soc Nephrol* 2008;**19**:2193–203.

46. Fahrleitner-Pammer A, Herberth J, Browning SR, et al. Bone markers predict cardiovascular events in chronic kidney disease. *J Bone Miner Res* 2008;**23**:1850–8.

47. Deftos LJ. Bone protein and peptide assays in the diagnosis and management of skeletal disease. *Clin Chem* 1991;**37**:1143–8.

48. Koshihara Y, Hoshi K. Vitamin K2 enhances osteocalcin accumulation in the extracellular matrix of human osteoblasts *in vitro*. *J Bone Miner Res* 1997;**12**:431–8.

49. Kohlmeier M, Saupe J, Schaefer K, et al. Bone fracture history and prospective bone fracture risk of hemodialysis patients are related to apolipoprotein E genotype. *Calcif Tissue Int* 1998;**62:**278–81.

50. Zhang R, Ducy P, Karsenty G. 1,25-dihydroxyvitamin D3 inhibits osteocalcin expression in mouse through an indirect mechanism. *J Biol Chem* 1997;**272:**110–16.

51. Novak JF, Hayes JD, Nishimoto SK. Plasmin-mediated proteolysis of osteocalcin. *J Bone Miner Res* 1997;**12:**1035–42.

52. Ducy P, Desbois C, Boyce B, et al. Increased bone formation in osteocalcin-deficient mice. *Nature* 1996;**382:**448–52.

53. Lee NK, Sowa H, Hinoi E, et al. Endocrine regulation of energy metabolism by the skeleton. *Cell* 2007;**130:**456–69.

54. Tracy RP, Andrianorivo A, Riggs BL, et al. Comparison of monoclonal and polyclonal antibody-based immunoassays for osteocalcin: a study of sources of variation in assay results. *J Bone Miner Res* 1990;**5:**451–61.

55. Diaz Diego EM, Guerrero R, de la Piedra C. Six osteocalcin assays compared. *Clin Chem* 1994;**40:**2071–7.

56. Urena P, Ferreira A, Kung VT, et al. Serum pyridinoline as a specific marker of collagen breakdown and bone metabolism in hemodialysis patients. *J Bone Miner Res* 1995;**10:** 932–9.

57. Rix M, Andreassen H, Eskildsen P, et al. Bone mineral density and biochemical markers of bone turnover in patients with predialysis chronic renal failure. *Kidney Int* 1999;**56:**1084–93.

58. Luo G, Ducy P, McKee MD, et al. Spontaneous calcification of arteries and cartilage in mice lacking matrix Gla protein. *Nature* 1997;**386:**78–81.

59. Price PA, Nguyen TM, Williamson MK. Biochemical characterisation of the serum fetuin-mineral complex. *J Biol Chem* 2003;**278:**22153–60.

60. Moe SM, Reslerova M, Ketteler M, et al. Role of calcification inhibitors in the pathogenesis of vascular calcification in chronic kidney disease (CKD). *Kidney Int* 2005;**67:**2295–304.

61. Coen G, Ballanti P, Balducci A, et al. Renal osteodystrophy: alpha-Heremans Schmid glycoprotein/fetuin-A, matrix Gla protein serum levels, and bone histomorphometry. *Am J Kidney Dis* 2006;**48:**106–13.

62. Hamdy NA, Risteli J, Risteli L, et al. Serum type I procollagen peptide: a non-invasive index of bone formation in patients on hemodialysis? *Nephrol Dial Transplant* 1994; **9:**511–16.

63. Coen G, Mazzaferro S, Ballanti P, et al. Procollagen type I C-terminal extension peptide in predialysis chronic renal failure. *Am J Nephrol* 1992;**12:**246–51.

64. Coen G, Mazzaferro S, Ballanti P, et al. PTH and bone markers of renal osteodystrophy in predialysis chronic renal failure. *J Endocrinol Invest* 1992;**15:**129–33.

65. Orum O, Hansen M, Jensen CH, et al. Procollagen type I N-terminal propeptide (PINP) as an indicator of type I collagen metabolism: ELISA development, reference interval, and hypovitaminosis D induced hyperparathyroidism. *Bone* 1996;**19:**157–63.

66. Ueda M, Inaba M, Okuno S, et al. Clinical usefulness of the serum N-terminal propeptide of type I collagen as a marker of bone formation in hemodialysis patients. *Am J Kidney Dis* 2002;**40:**802–9.

67. Halleen J, Hentunen TA, Hellman J, et al. Tartrate-resistant acid phosphatase from human bone: purification and development of an immunoassay. *J Bone Miner Res* 1996;**11:**1444–52.

68. Andersson G, Ek-Rylander B, Hollberg K, et al. TRACP as an osteopontin phosphatase. *J Bone Miner Res* 2003;**18**:1912–15.

69. Zenger S, Hollberg K, Ljusberg J, et al. Proteolytic processing and polarised secretion of tartrate-resistant acid phosphatase is altered in a subpopulation of metaphyseal osteoclasts in cathepsin K-deficient mice. *Bone* 2007;**41**:820–32.

70. Hayman AR, Jones SJ, Boyde A, et al. Mice lacking tartrate-resistant acid phosphatase (Acp 5) have disrupted endochondral ossification and mild osteopetrosis. *Development* 1996;**122**:3151–62.

71. Halleen JM, Hentunen TA, Karp M, et al. Characterisation of serum tartrate-resistant acid phosphatase and development of a direct two-site immunoassay. *J Bone Miner Res* 1998;**13**:683–7.

72. Shidara K, Inaba M, Okuno S, et al. Serum levels of TRAP5b, a new bone resorption marker unaffected by renal dysfunction, as a useful marker of cortical bone loss in hemodialysis patients. *Calcif Tissue Int* 2008;**82**:278–87.

73. Bonde M, Garnero P, Fledelius C, et al. Measurement of bone degradation products in serum using antibodies reactive with an isomerised form of an 8 amino acid sequence of the C-telopeptide of type I collagen. *J Bone Miner Res* 1997;**12**:1028–34.

74. Urena Torres P, Friedlander G, de Vernejoul MC, et al. Bone mass does not correlate with the serum fibroblast growth factor 23 in hemodialysis patients. *Kidney Int* 2008;**73**:102–7.

75. Urena P, Bernard-Poenaru O, Ostertag A, et al. Bone mineral density, biochemical markers and skeletal fractures in hemodialysis patients. *Nephrol Dial Transplant* 2003;**18**:2325–31.

76. Sassi ML, Eriksen H, Risteli L, et al. Immunochemical characterisation of assay for carboxyterminal telopeptide of human type I collagen: loss of antigenicity by treatment with cathepsin K. *Bone* 2000;**26**:367–73.

77. Garnero P, Gineyts E, Riou JP, et al. Assessment of bone resorption with a new marker of collagen degradation in patients with metabolic bone disease. *J Clin Endocrinol Metab* 1994;**79**:780–5.

78. Garnero P, Shih WJ, Gineyts E, et al. Comparison of new biochemical markers of bone turnover in late postmenopausal osteoporotic women in response to alendronate treatment. *J Clin Endocrinol Metab* 1994;**79**:1693–700.

79. Maeno Y, Inaba M, Okuno S, et al. Serum concentrations of cross-linked N-telopeptides of type I collagen: new marker for bone resorption in hemodialysis patients. *Clin Chem* 2005;**51**:2312–7.

80. Prockop DJ, Kivirikko KI, Tuderman L, et al. The biosynthesis of collagen and its disorders (second of two parts). *N Engl J Med* 1979;**301**:77–85.

81. Prockop DJ, Kivirikko KI, Tuderman L, et al. The biosynthesis of collagen and its disorders (first of two parts). *N Engl J Med* 1979;**301**:13–23.

82. Robins SP, Stead DA, Duncan A. Precautions in using an internal standard to measure pyridinoline and deoxypyridinoline in urine. *Clin Chem* 1994;**40**:2322–3.

83. Black D, Duncan A, Robins SP. Quantitative analysis of the pyridinium cross-links of collagen in urine using ion-paired reversed-phase high-performance liquid chromatography. *Anal Biochem* 1988;**169**:197–203.

84. Robins SP, Woitge H, Hesley R, et al. Direct, enzyme-linked immunoassay for urinary deoxypyridinoline as a specific marker for measuring bone resorption. *J Bone Miner Res* 1994;**9**:1643–9.

85. Coen G, Ballanti P, Bonucci E, et al. Bone markers in the diagnosis of low turnover osteodystrophy in hemodialysis patients. *Nephrol Dial Transplant* 1998;**13:**2294–302.

86. Valverde P, Zhang J, Fix A, et al. Overexpression of bone sialoprotein leads to an uncoupling of bone formation and bone resorption in mice. *J Bone Miner Res* 2008;**23:**1775–88.

87. Shaarawy M, Hasan M. Serum bone sialoprotein: a marker of bone resorption in postmenopausal osteoporosis. *Scand J Clin Lab Invest* 2001;**61:**513–21.

88. Al-Dehaimi AW, Blumsohn A, Eastell R. Serum galactosyl hydroxylysine as a biochemical marker of bone resorption. *Clin Chem* 1999;**45:**676–81.

Chapter 12

Imaging of the skeleton and the joints in CKD

Yaakov H. Applbaum

Introduction

Imaging by X-ray, computed tomography (CT), magnetic resonance imaging (MRI), and ultrasound (US) of the musculoskeletal system in patients with chronic kidney disease has many goals. These include the diagnosis of the effects of the metabolic changes on the skeleton, joints, and other soft tissues, detection of complications of therapy, and the assessment and monitoring of these changes. While all imaging modalities play a role in renal osteodystrophy, radiography often remains the only imaging examination that is used. Other imaging modalities, such as CT, MRI, and US, contribute to the diagnosis of specific abnormalities especially complications of treatment. While the KDIGO initiative has reserved the term 'renal osteodystrophy' for histologically proven bone changes,[1] these changes are sometimes evident on imaging studies, making bone biopsy unnecessary in these cases.[2] In recent years, improved understanding and subsequent advances in therapy have changed the presentation of bone and joint disease in chronic renal failure. In the past, secondary hyperparathyroidism (2HPT) was most common with osteomalacia second in importance. Recently, adynamic bone disease appears earlier and in a greater percentage of cases. This may be due to changing patterns of therapy. As there are no specific imaging findings in this condition and the changes of 2HPT and osteomalacia are less prominent, imaging plays a minor role in the diagnosis of the bone disorders and is more important in diagnosing the effects of these disorders.

Renal osteodystrophy

Renal osteodystrophy is a general term for abnormalities of the musculoskeletal system in patients with chronic renal insufficiency. There is a spectrum of metabolic abnormalities that include 2HPT, osteomalacia and rickets, and adynamic bone disease.[3-5]

Secondary hyperparathyroidism

Early in chronic renal failure, there is often evidence of increased levels of parathyroid hormone and typical changes can be seen in the bones on X-ray examination. These changes have collectively been dubbed 'osteitis fibrosa cystica'. There are three major types of bone disturbances: bone resorption, sclerosis and brown tumours.[3] In addition, high levels of parathyroid hormone (PTH) play a role in the deposition of calcium crystals in joints and soft tissues.

Bone resorption

PTH causes increased osteoclastic activity with bone resorption. This is evident at numerous locations that can be categorised as subperiosteal, intracortical, endosteal, subchondral, and trabecular. To recognise bone resorption on imaging studies it is necessary to be aware of the common target sites, as well as the typical appearance.

Subperiosteal bone resorption is the most specific finding in hyperparathyroid bone disease and in certain locations is virtually diagnostic. The most frequent location in which subperiosteal bone resorption is seen is on the radial side of the carpal phalanges, especially in the middle phalanx of the second and third fingers. The resorption appears at first lace-like, and progresses to a spiculated border and eventually to complete cortical destruction. An early location in which subperiosteal resorption can be seen is in the tuft of the distal phalanx in the finger with loss of the cortical line. However, as there is much variation in the normal appearance of the tufts, only experienced observers should depend on changes in this location when considering a diagnosis of hyperparathyroidism. Other locations include the medial aspect of the proximal humerus, femur, and tibia, the superior and inferior rib margins, and the lamina dura of the teeth. However, the combination of early findings with consistent locations makes hand radiographs the single most important imaging study in the radiological diagnosis of hyperparathyroidism. Subperiosteal bone resorption may occur at the margins of joints. When this occurs in the hand or foot these changes may be confused for rheumatoid arthritis or other inflammatory joint diseases (Fig. 12.2).

Intracortical bone resorption occurs within cortical Haversian canals. These appear as linear striations and lucent tunnels in the cortex of bone. They may combine with subperiosteal resorption in the destruction of the cortex. These findings are not specific and can be seen in other conditions with high turnover of bone.

Endosteal bone resorption occurs along the inner edge of the cortex with a scalloped appearance or thinning of the cortex similar to changes common in multiple myeloma.

Subchondral bone resorption is most commonly seen in the axial skeleton especially the sacroiliac, sternoclavicular, and acromioclavicular joints and in the symphysis pubis. Less commonly, large and small joints in the limbs may be involved. As with the marginal erosions seen in subperiosteal bone resorption, subchondral resorption may mimic other joint diseases, such as ankylosing spondylitis in the sacroiliac joint or rheumatoid arthritis in the acromioclavicular joints (Fig. 12.2).

Trabecular bone resorption is evident as a loss of distinct trabecular edges. This is most often noticed on radiography in the skull as the typical 'salt and pepper' appearance with small areas of interspersed lucency and increased density.

Brown tumors

Brown tumors or osteoclastomas are foci of fibrous tissue and giant cells that replace bone. These lesions may undergo necrosis and appear cystic (Fig. 12.3a). They may expand the cortex of the bone and have sharp borders. Brown tumors usually occur with other typical findings of 2HPT especially subperiosteal resorption, and may be solitary

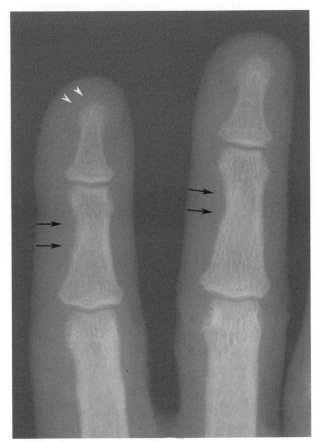

Fig. 12.1 Secondary hyperparathyroidism. Subperiosteal resorption of bone on the radial side of the middle phalanx of the second and third fingers (black arrows). Resorption of the distal tuft is also seen (white arrowheads).

or multiple. While this has traditionally been considered typical of primary hyperparathyroidism, many brown tumors are seen in patients with chronic renal failure.

The MRI appearance of brown tumors has been described in the literature as hypointense on T1-weighted images (Fig. 12.3b), strongly enhancing following administration of gadolinium-based intravenous contrast injection, and hyper- or hypointense on T2-weighted images. Brown tumors with blood-fluid levels have also been described. These findings, however, are not specific. On MRI hemosiderin within tissues results in loss of signal due to magnetic susceptibility, an effect most pronounced on gradient echo images. While this finding may be more specific and, therefore, guide diagnosis, it has only rarely been reported.[6]

Bone sclerosis

Bone sclerosis or increased bone density is seen more commonly in 2HPT than in primary HPT. The increase in bone density may be generalised, but is more usually

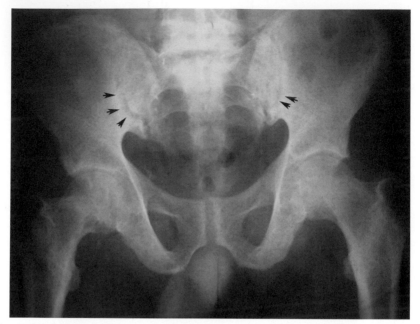

Fig. 12.2 Secondary hyperparathyroidism. Widening of the sacroiliac joints due to subchondral resorption in secondary hyperparathyroidism (black arrows) with generalised sclerosis.

located in the axial skeleton. The deposition of subchondral bone in vertebral bodies appears as dense thick bands in the end plates. This finding is known as 'rugger jersey spine' due to the stripes seen on shirts, often worn by players of rugby football (Fig. 12.4). The exact mechanism of bone sclerosis is not known.

Soft tissue calcification (uremic tumoral calcinosis)

While vascular calcifications are treated elsewhere in this book, calcification of other soft tissues has clinical significance in its own right. Calcification of soft tissues is seen in primary HPT, but is much more common in patients with chronic kidney failure. Soft issue deposits occur in myriad locations, from the skin and eyes to the heart, lungs, kidneys, and stomach, and may not always be evident with imaging. When the calcifications are peri-articular in location, they may lead to symptoms and signs that mimic joint disease or even tumors. This, as well as the large size of the masses of mineral deposits that may enlarge rapidly, may be the reason for some of the confusing and alarming names that this condition has received: 'tumoral calcinosis' (Fig. 12.5) and 'metastatic calcification'. Peri-articular deposits may be large and numerous. They are typically seen around the hips, knees, shoulders, elbows, and the wrists. Multiple locations may be involved as well. The calcifications may be bilateral and symmetrical. Ligaments and tendons may also calcify. The masses may liquefy over time and a fluid/fluid level may be seen on erect films.

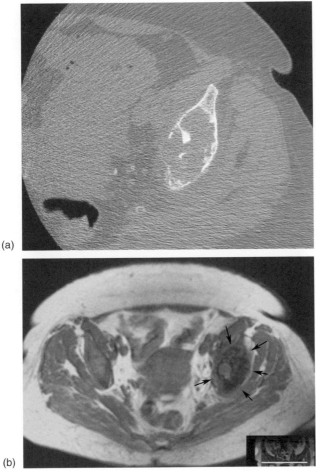

Fig. 12.3 (a) Brown tumor. Axial CT of the pelvis. A lytic lesion is seen in the roof of the acetabulum. (b) Brown tumor. Axial T1-weighted MRI of the pelvis. Signal voids are seen in the left acetabulum as evidence of hemosiderin deposit with a small lytic area (black arrows).

Osteomalacia

Osteomalacia is defined as the delayed or incomplete mineralization of osteoid in cortical and spongy bone.[7] In the immature skeleton there may also be disruption of normal mineralization at the growth plate and this is known as 'rickets' in children. The radiographic manifestations of osteomalacia are not always obvious in chronic renal failure. The other forms of bone disease may overshadow the changes due to osteomalacia. For example, decreased bone density is a sign of osteomalacia, but is not specific. A more pathognomonic finding is Looser's zones or pseudofractures, also known as Milkman's fractures (Fig. 12.6). These are radiolucent lines in the cortex and underlying medulla that are seen perpendicular to the bone surface. They are due to unmineralized

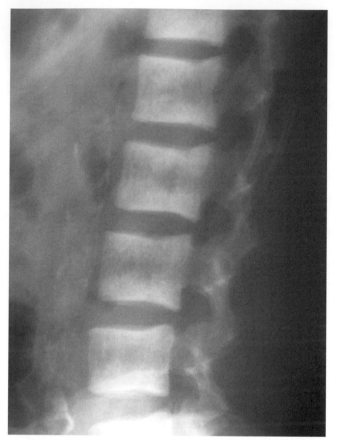

Fig. 12.4 Secondary hyperparathyroidism—osteosclerosis. Lateral radiograph of the lumbar spine demonstrates alternating bands of sclerosis and lucency known as 'rugger jersey' sign.

seams of osteoid. These may be bilateral and symmetrical. Looser's zones are most often seen in the pubic ramus, iliac bone, rib, neck of femur, body of scapula, and long bones. The prevalence of Looser's zones is low having been seen in only 1% of patients with chronic renal failure. Looser's zones must be differentiated from fatigue fractures that may be seen in the same locations.[8] Looser's zones usually do not appear to heal over time. They appear as broad radiolucent bands, perpendicular to the cortex with mild to moderate sclerosis. It must be noted that patients with what appears on imaging as typical pseudofractures, but with no evidence of osteomalacia on bone biopsy have been reported.

In children, the changes of rickets are seen in the metaphyses, which are thickened, cupped, frayed, and of lower density. The growth plate is wide. As rickets is a disorder of the growth plate it is most evident at sites of rapid growth, particularly around the knees, wrists, and anterior ribs. In addition, in the growing skeleton the bones are soft and deformed. Common deformities are seen in the knees (genu varum and genu

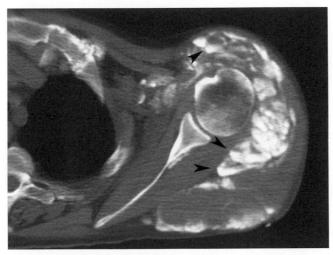

Fig. 12.5 Tumoral calcinosis. Axial CT exam of the left shoulder. Widespread calcifications are seen in the bursae surrounding the shoulder with fluid-fluid levels as evidence of liquification (black arrowheads).

valgum), hips (coxa vara and coxa valga), as well as rib and pelvis deformities (Harrison's groove, protrusion acetabuli; Fig. 12.7).

ß2-Microglobulin amyloidosis

Amyloidosis develops in patients with long-term uremia on hemodialysis.

ß2-microglobulin is a major component of hemodialysis-associated amyloidosis. The most common complaint is carpal tunnel syndrome due to amyloid accumulation in soft tissues. Amyloid accumulates in joints and adjacent bones. The shoulder, hip, femur, and knee are often involved.[9] Another site of disease is the spine. Amyloid deposition occurs in synovial fluid first, and progresses to the synovial membrane, then to the adjacent bone. Radiolucent lesions are seen, and may be multiple and bilateral (Fig. 12.8a). They have sharp well-defined borders and may have sclerotic borders and internal septi. Pathological fractures often occur.

On MRI, bone lesions show decreased signal intensity on T1-weighted images. On T2-weighted images, bone lesions have varied signal intensity. On contrast-enhanced MR images, bone lesions enhance moderately (Fig. 12.8b,c). Contrast-enhanced MR images also demonstrate enhancement of thickened synovial membrane in involved joints.[10]

US can be used for detecting amyloid deposits along tendons and ligaments and has an important role in diagnosing amyloidosis as the cause of carpal tunnel syndrome in end stage renal patients.

Aluminum toxicity

Aluminum intoxication was prevalent in the past in chronic renal failure patients undergoing hemodialysis due to high levels of aluminum in the water. Later, aluminum intoxication was seen due to its use in phosphate chelating agents. In addition to

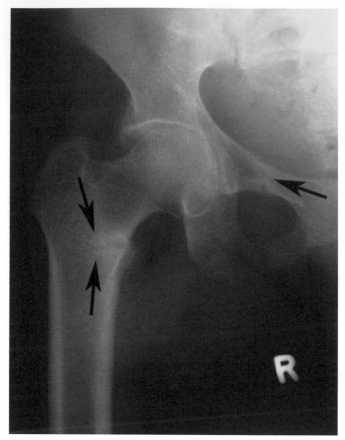

Fig. 12.6 Osteomalacia. AP Radiograph of right hip joint. Typical Looser's zones in the femur and pubis (black arrows).

neurological symptoms, patients with high levels of aluminum complain of bone pain and suffer a high rate of fractures. Fractures of the ribs and proximal femur are typical. Radiographic findings are non-specific although some authors have suggested that fractures of the second, third, and fourth ribs, as well as non-traumatic fractures of the dens and long bones without healing are typical, and must raise the possibility of aluminum toxicity.[11,12] Definite diagnosis can only be made with bone biopsy. Biopsy specimens show increased, normal, or reduced amounts of osteoid with aluminum accumulation at the bone-osteoid junction. With elimination of the source of contamination, the symptoms reside. At present, aluminum intoxication appears to be uncommon in the developed world, although it is still be a problem in many countries.

Adynamic bone disease

Even without evidence of hyperparathyroidism or osteomalacia, patients with chronic renal failure are at a greater risk for fractures than the population at large. This may be due to adynamic bone disease in which there is low turnover of bone without evidence

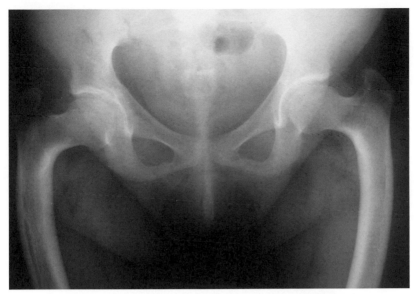

Fig. 12.7 AP radiograph of proximal thighs demonstrates coxa vara and bowing of the femur in a 27-year-old patient who had chronic renal failure in childhood.

of osteomalacia, although this is in dispute.[13,14] It is characterized histopathologically by an overall paucity of bone cells. The numbers of osteoblasts and osteoclasts are diminished, and bone formation and turnover are reduced when measured by quantitative histomorphometry. The histological features of adynamic bone do not differ from those of several other skeletal disorders in which bone remodeling rates are low. These include diabetes, osteoporosis after treatment with corticosteroids, hypoparathyroidism whether idiopathic or surgically-induced, immobilisation, and either post-menopausal or age-related osteoporosis. Adynamic bone is thus not unique to patients with CKD and is also found in renal transplant patients who also have an increased risk of fractures (Fig. 12.9). Fractures, especially of the proximal femur are a major cause of morbidity and contribute to mortality, especially in elderly patients (who are already at a high risk for hip fractures).

Fluorosis

Fluorine intoxication is endemic to certain geographic locations, particularly in India and China, and is sporadic in the rest of the world, often due to occupational exposure.

Fluorine intoxication may be aggravated by renal failure. The skeletal manifestations of fluorosis are most evident in the axial skeleton. Osteosclerosis is the first sign to be seen on radiographs in the spine, pelvis, and ribs. Osteophytes thicken and new ones form at the sites of ligament attachments especially around the pelvis. Paraspinal ligaments may calcify. In the appendicular skeleton, osteopenia is seen with thick periosteal reaction and osteophytes form at ligament and muscle attachments. These changes may lead to limitations in the range of motion in the spine, chest and

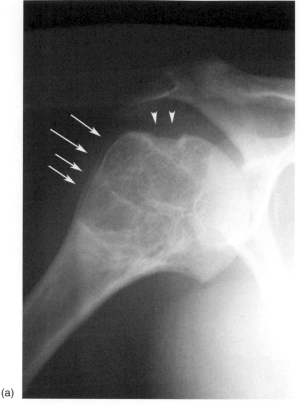

(a)

Fig. 12.8 (a) β2 microglobulin amyloidosis. AP radiograph of the shoulder demonstrates erosions (white arrowheads) and 'cystic' lesions (white arrows) in the head of the humerus.

other joints. Deformities such as kyphosis may occur. There may be encroachment of neural foraminae.

The bone in fluorosis appears thickened and dense, but it is not clear if it is stronger. Fractures have been reported in the spine and in long bones. With cessation of fluoride ingestion and continued renal secretion, the bone changes may be reversible on imaging. As other causes of osteosclerosis, osteopenia, and calcifications of ligaments and tendons are common in end-stage kidney disease, fluorosis may be overlooked until it reaches a late stage.

Oxalosis

In patients with primary oxalosis oxalic acid combines with calcium to produce oxalate crystals. Hyperoxaluria causes renal failure and there is a rapid accumulation of oxalate in other tissues including bones. As the kidneys are the only route of excretion of oxalate, chronic renal failure without may theoretically cause a slow accretion of oxalate crystals in different tissues causing 'secondary oxalosis'. This is rarely clinically

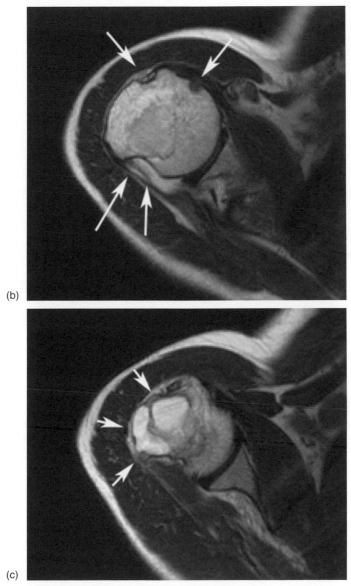

Fig. 12.8 (b) β2 microglobulin amyloidosis. T2-weighted MRI exam of right shoulder demonstrates erosions in the humeral head (arrows). (c) β2 microglobulin amyloidosis. T2-weighted MRI exam of right shoulder demonstrates amyloid deposits in the proximal humerus (arrows).

significant and the bone changes are rarely seen on radiographs. Crystal deposition may cause an inflammatory reaction causing bone erosions and cyst formation.

Oxalate accumulation in bones can appear as sclerosis with trabecular thickening or with lytic 'cystic' areas mimicking hyperparathyroidism. Oxalate deposits in soft tissues may involve tendons, joint capsules cartilage and synovium. The deposits may

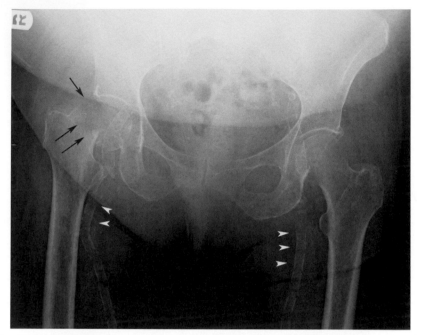

Fig. 12.9 AP radiograph of the pelvis and proximal thighs. Displaced right femoral neck fracture (black arrows). Note prominent vascular calcifications (white arrowheads), cortical thinning and loss of trabeculae.

cause bone erosions and appear similar to gout or amyloid. They may calcify and be seen on radiographs in joint capsules and cartilage. These are often confused with CPPDD (calcium pyrophosphate dihydrate deposition disease). The radiological diagnosis of oxalosis in renal failure is therefore very difficult.

Joint complications

Many patients with CKD develop symptoms and signs of joint disease. Single or multiple joints may be involved with different clinical presentations. This is due to the many possible etiologies involved which may often be mixed and may not be directly due to the metabolic abnormalities of impaired renal function. The underlying etiology of the kidney disease may by itself also affect joints, as well the treatments undertaken to treat any underlying disease. Therapy for the renal failure may also have an impact on the joints, and cause arthropathies or bone and soft tissue abnormalities that affect joints. For instance, diabetes may cause both kidney disease, as well as peripheral neuropathy that in turn may cause neuropathic arthropathy (Charcot Joint) or lead to infection. In addition, joint diseases are common, especially in the elderly population and this may be mistaken for a disease caused by renal failure. There is often overlap of clinical, laboratory, and imaging findings between the different joint diseases, making the task of elucidating the particular effects of chronic kidney disease on joints in a particular patient a daunting one.

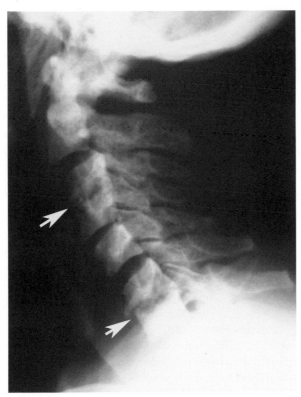

Fig. 12.10 Destructive spondyloarthropathy. Lateral radiograph of the cervical spine. Disc space irregularity and narrowing with bone erosions at the C3–C4 and C6–C7 levels (white arrows).

Destructive spondyloarthropathy

Patients undergoing chronic hemodialysis have been reported to suffer from a rapidly progressive disease of the spine characterized by loss of intervertebral disk space, erosion of subchondral bone in the adjacent vertebral bodies, and new bone formation.[15] The most common site involved is the lower portion of the cervical spine, although the craniocervical junction, and occasionally the thoracic and lumbar spine may also be affected. The disease usually is seen at multiple spinal levels with rapidly progressive destructive lesions (Fig. 12.10).

The precise pathogenesis of this condition is unclear and may be multifactorial although ß2-microglobulin amyloidosis is clearly involved. Infection has not been shown to be a cause of destructive spondyloarthropathy. This is important because the imaging findings may be similar to those seen in vertebral infection and spinal infection must be diagnosed early in order to facilitate therapy and improve outcomes. Radiography features consist of:

- narrowing or obliteration of the intervertebral disk space;
- erosion or resorption of subchondral bone in the opposing superior and inferior endplates of vertebral bodies, with or without cystic lesions;

+ subchondral bone sclerosis;

+ minimal osteophyte formation.

CT is useful in revealing small lesions earlier than X-ray and, therefore, detecting multiple levels earlier than on radiography. CT aids in the prevention of complications by earlier detection of spinal instability. In addition, CT can help diagnose infection by detecting abscesses. MRI is even more sensitive in detecting fluid collections, as well as spinal cord compromise. However, there are conflicting reports as to the appearance of the soft tissue findings and these may be identical or similar to the findings in infection. MRI should therefore be performed and interpreted in light of other imaging findings.

Crystal-induced arthritis

We have already seen that calcium crystals deposit in soft tissues around joints in patients with renal failure. In joints there may be an accumulation of calcium pyrophosphate in fibrocartilage in the wrist, knee, and symphysis pubis. This rarely manifests itself clinically as pseudogout with an acute inflammatory process. More commonly, the patient is asymptomatic or has a more chronic joint disease similar to osteoarthritis. It may be impossible to prove that calcium pyrophosphate deposition is the cause of the disease as calcium deposits in joints are very common in the older population. Calcium pyrophosphate deposition disease (CPPDD) is recognised on radiographs and CT as calcifications in the joint most commonly in fibrocartilage. This can be seen in the wrist in the triangular fibrocartilage, in the knees in the meniscus, in the hips and shoulder in the labrum, as well as in the joint capsule and along tendons and ligaments. CPPDD causes joint space narrowing in a pattern that is often different than the typical pattern in osteoarthritis and this may aid in diagnosis.

Similar to CPPD, in gout patients with chronic renal failure are hyperuricemic (before dialysis) and may develop secondary gouty arthritis. The frequency of acute arthritis is not high. Radiographically, the disease resembles primary gout with soft tissue swelling (to phi), as well as eccentric osseous erosions in an asymmetric distribution. These findings may take years and even decades to be evident on radiographs. In secondary gout these findings may be in atypical locations.

Other skeletal complications

Osteonecrosis

Osteonecrosis is often seen after renal transplantation. Although corticosteroid therapy is assumed to be the etiology, osteonecrosis is seen, albeit less commonly, in patients who have not received steroid therapy.[16] In addition, some diseases that lead to renal failure have also been associated with osteonecrosis. Osteonecrosis has been reported in 1.4–40% of renal transplants. The most common site of osteonecrosis is the femoral head. Other locations include the distal femur, proximal humerus, talar dome, distal humerus, and cuboid and carpal bones. There may be multiple sites. Early radiographic findings include a linear subchondral lucency with sclerosis developing around the lucency. Later findings include fragmentation, collapse, sclerosis, and the formation of cysts. Cartilage loss with joint space narrowing is often delayed.

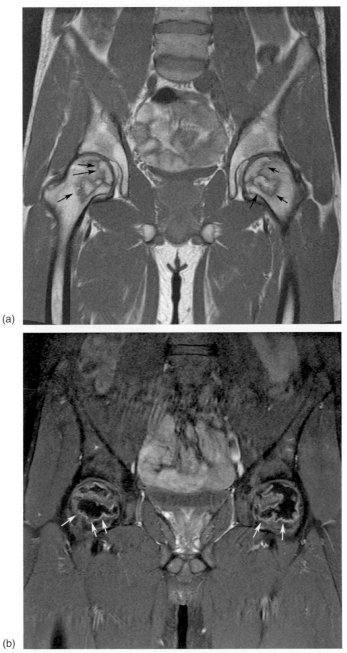

Fig. 12.11 (a) Osteonecrosis. Coronal T1-weighted MRI scan of the hip joints. Bilateral osteonecrosis of the head of the femur is seen. The serpiginous lines following the border of the necrotic are (a) (black arrows) (b) Osteonecrosis. Coronal T1-weighted fat suppressed MRI scan after IV gadolinium injection. The darker areas inside the bright border demonstrates lack of perfusion in the necrotic bone (white arrows).

In non-weight-bearing bone, significant collapse of bone may be absent. CT demonstrates similar changes as well as changes in the trabecular architecture. However, both radiographs and CT are unremarkable in the early stages of the disease.

Early diagnosis of osteonecrosis requires either radionuclide bone scan or MRI. Bone scintigraphy is a sensitive technique, but may not be able to differentiate osteonecrosis from insufficiency fractures and bone marrow edema syndromes. Single-photon emission computed tomography (SPECT) may be more accurate. Overall, MRI appears to be the most accurate technique for diagnosing hip pain and osteonecrosis in post-transplant patients.[17] Not only is it sensitive, it also can accurately measure the area of bone involved in osteonecrosis. This is important for prognosis and in planning treatment.

MRI findings of osteonecrosis in the femoral head include, in T1-weighted images, a peripheral band of low signal in the superior portion of the femoral head outlining a central area of bone marrow (Fig. 12.11). On T2-weighted images the inner border of the peripheral band demonstrates high signal. This is termed the 'double-line' sign and is pathognomonic for osteonecrosis. It is present in 80% of cases. Contrast enhancement is useful for distinguishing viable from non-viable marrow. Non-viable tissue does not enhance after contrast administration. Care should however clearly be taken when choosing the contrast material, as some, such as gadolinium, should not be used in CKD patients.

Post-transplant distal limb syndrome

Post-transplant distal limb syndrome manifests as episodes of bone and joint pain exclusively in the distal lower limbs.[18] The pain typically presents bilaterally and symmetrically within the first year after renal transplantation, and may lead to significant morbidity because of pain-induced immobilisation. The pain eases on rest and worsens on physical stress, sometimes leading to morbidity because of immobilisation. The etiology of post-transplant distal limb syndrome has not been determined definitely so far. As the syndrome varies in severity and presentation, and as different etiologies have been suggested, different names have so far been proposed, e.g. post-renal transplant distal limb bone pain, reflex sympathetic dystrophy syndrome, calcineurin-inhibitor induced pain syndrome or post-transplant distal-limb bone marrow edema.

On fat-suppressed T2-weigthed MRI scans, a typical bilateral bone marrow edema around affected knees and or feet can be demonstrated. Another typical feature is that the hip regions are spared. This, as well as the lack of long-term sequelae, helps distinguish post-transplant distal limb syndrome from steroid-induced aseptic osteonecrosis.

Tendon and ligament abnormalities

Tendinosis, spontaneous rupture of tendons, subtendinous and subligamentous bone resorption and avulsion fractures are often seen in chronic renal failure patients. This may occur with or without evidence of calcification. The Achilles tendon, rotator cuff, and quadriceps tendon are most commonly involved. High-resolution US is a useful tool for evaluating superficial tendons and ligaments. Loss of normal fibrillar appearance, fluid pockets, calcifications, thinning, thickening and frank tears are well imaged

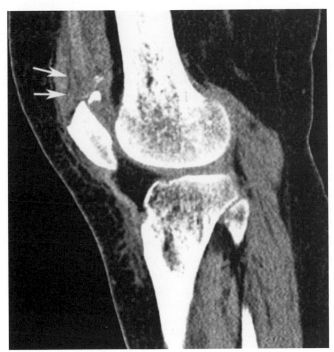

Fig. 12.12 Reformatted sagittal image from CT scan of left knee. The distal quadriceps tendon is avulsed from the patella with fracture fragments, thickening and swelling of the tendon (white arrows).

with ultrasound. With MRI, tendon and ligament injury, as well as fractures can be accurately diagnosed in superficial and deep structures. CT allows accurate diagnosis of small calcifications and avulsion fragments that may not be well seen on MRI (Fig. 12.12).[19]

Musculoskeletal infection

Hemodialysis increases the risk for infection due to central venous access and arteriovenous fistulae. In kidney transplant patients, immunosuppression is necessary. Osteomyelitis and septic arthritis may occur at any site and myriad organisms have been involved, including mycobacteriae and fungi. Three stage bone scintigraphy and MRI allow for early diagnosis, although MRI is more specific and allows evaluation of soft tissue involvement and complications, especially in the spine. Antigranulocyte scintigraphy with radiolabel monoclonal antibodies, leukocyte tagging, or gallium citrate scans increase specificity when added to bone scintigraphy.

Summary

The musculoskeletal manifestations of chronic renal failure are myriad. Loss of renal function itself and metabolic effects are not the only causes of these changes. The etiology of the kidney failure, the patient's general health, as well as the treatment that the patient receives all influence the bones, joints, and soft tissues in ways that we understand only in part.

The role of imaging in all of its aspects is changing. Radiography is no longer as crucial as before for the diagnosis of renal osteodystrophy. Imaging is important in recognising the complications of renal bone disease, as well as in the early diagnosis of complications of therapy and in guiding treatment.

References

1. Moe S, Drueke T, Cunningham J, et al. Definition, evaluation, and classification of renal osteodystrophy: a position statement from Kidney Disease: Improving Global Outcomes (KDIGO). *Kidney Int* 2006;**69:**1945–53.

2. Pecovnik Balon B, Bren A. Bone histomorphometry is still the golden standard for diagnosing renal osteodystrophy. *Clin Nephrol* 2000;**54:**463–9.

3. Resnick D, Niwayama G. Parathyroid disorders and renal osteodystrophy. In: D. Resnick (ed.), *Diagnosis of bone and joint disorders*. Philadelphia: W.B. Saunders, 1995:2012–75.

4. Adams JE: Renal bone disease: radiological investigation. *Kidney Int* 1991;**56:**S38–41.

5. Jevtic V, Imaging of renal osteodystrophy. *Eur J Rad* 2003;**46:**85–95.

6. Knowles NG, Smith DL, Eric K. Outwater EK. MRI diagnosis of brown tumor based on magnetic susceptibility. *J Magn Reson Imag* 2008;**28:**759–61.

7. Pitt MJ: Rickets and osteomalacia. In: D. Resnick (ed.), *Diagnosis of bone and joint disorders*. Philadelphia: W.B. Saunders, 1995:1885–920.

8. McKenna MJ, Kleerekoper M, Ellis BI, Rao DS, Parfitt AM, Frame B. Atypical insufficiency fractures confused with Looser's zones of osteomalacia *Bone* 1987;**8:**71–8.

9. Kiss E, Keusch G, Zanetti M, et al. Dialysis-related amyloidosis revisited. *Am J Roentgenol* 2005;**185:**1460–7.

10. Otake S, Tsuruta Y, Yamana D, et al. Amyloid arthropathy of the hip joint: MR demonstration of presumed amyloid lesions in 152 patients with long-term hemodialysis. *Eur Radiol* 1998;**8:**1352–6.

11. Kriegshauser JS, Swee RG, McCarthy JT, et al. Aluminum toxicity in patients undergoing dialysis: radiologic features. *Radiology* 1987;**164:**399–403.

12. Sundaram M, Dessner D, Balal S. Solitary spontaneous cervical and large bone fracture in aluminium osteodystrophy. *Skeletal Radiol* 1991;**20:**91–4.

13. Brandenburg VM, Floege J. Adynamic bone disease—bone and beyond. *NDT Plus* 2008;**3:**135–47.

14. Heaf J. Causes and consequences of adynamic bone disease. *Nephron* 2001;**88:**97–106.

15. Theodorou DJ, Theodorou SJ, Resnick D. Imaging in dialysis spondyloarthropathy. *Semin Dialysis* 2002;**15:**290–6.

16. S. Tang, T.M. Chan and S.L. Lui et al. Risk factors for avascular bone necrosis after renal transplantation. *Transplant Proc* 2000;**32:**1873–5.

17. Malizos KN, Karantanas AH, Varitimidis SE, et al. Osteonecrosis of the femoral head: etiology, imaging and treatment. *Eur J Rad* 2007;**63:**16–28.

18. Tillmann FP, Jaeger M, Blondin D, et al. Post-transplant distal limb syndrome: clinical diagnosis and long-term outcome in 37 renal transplant recipients. *Transplant Int* 2008;**21:**547–53.

19. Murphey MD, Sartoris DJ, Quale JL, Pathria MN, Martin NL. Musculoskeletal manifestations of chronic renal insufficiency. *Radiographics* 1993;**13:**357–79.

Chapter 13

Non-invasive assessment of vascular calcification and arterial stiffness

Paolo Raggi and Gérard M. London

Introduction

Patients suffering from advanced renal failure have extensive calcification of the cardiovascular system, which poses an increased risk of adverse events in advanced phases of chronic kidney disease (CKD).[1-3] Diffuse calcification of large conduit arteries promotes arterial stiffening with deleterious hemodynamic consequences.[4] The systolic blood pressure increases in conjunction with a decrease in diastolic blood pressure and widening of the pulse pressure; in the long-term these pressure changes induce left ventricular hypertrophy.[5] Ultimately, reduced coronary perfusion and myocardial ischemia can occur even in the absence of obstructive disease of the epicardial coronary arteries. Since the publication of the most recent guidelines, that recommended considering the CKD syndrome as inclusive of bone, mineral, and cardiovascular disease,[6] detection, and quantification of vascular calcification has assumed a more relevant role than ever before. Additionally, progression of vascular calcification appears to be slowed by some therapies, while others facilitate it. Plane X-rays of abdomen and extremities, 2D-ultrasound and echocardiography can be used to identify vascular calcifications in various blood vessels, such as carotid arteries, femoral arteries, and aorta, as well as the cardiac valves. More sophisticated and expensive imaging technologies, such as electron beam computed tomography (EBCT) and multi-slice computed tomography (MSCT) have emerged as tools to evaluate and accurately quantify cardiovascular calcification. These modalities allow not only detection, but also accurate quantification and monitoring of calcification progression. One of the most deleterious consequences of vascular calcification, arterial stiffening, can be assessed non-invasively by measuring pulse wave velocity and indirect indices of wave reflection from the periphery.

A clinical approach based on application of some of these techniques may provide helpful information that may improve the outcome of CKD patients. In this chapter we review the strengths and limitations of the most commonly employed non-invasive techniques for assessment of vascular calcification and some of the clinical evidence developed with them.

Plane roentgenography

Plane radiography is a low cost and low radiation imaging tool for identification of vascular calcification (VC), tested both in the general population[7] and in CKD patients.[8] Calcification patterns seen on plane radiographs help distinguish intimal from media arterial calcification. Medial calcification is typically considered present when linear tram-track radio-opaque lesions are visible along the course of an artery, while intimal calcification is more characteristically identified by patchy and irregular radio-opaque lesion.[8] Both types of calcifications have been associated with adverse clinical outcomes. In fact, despite the absence of luminal obstruction the loss of arterial compliance ultimately reduces end-organ perfusion while it increases myocardial after-load with an attendant increase in cardiovascular morbidity and mortality. Published clinical evidence supports this notion. In a cross-sectional study of 202 hemodialysis patients, medial and intimal calcification was detected in 27 and 37% of the X-ray films of the pelvis and thighs. In that study, both medial and intimal calcifications were independently associated with all-cause mortality [RR 15.7 (95% CI: 4.8–51.4; $p < 0.00001$) and 4.85 (1.68–14.1; $p = 0.0036$).[8]

Adragao et al. used plain X-rays of the pelvis and hands in a second cross-sectional study of 123 hemodialysis patients to generate a simple VC score.[9] The score was devised by assigning a point each for the presence of calcification in the iliac, femoral, digital, and radial arteries of either limb (score 0 for no calcification to 8 if all four vessels were calcified bilaterally). VC was detected in 75% of the study patients and almost half of the patients had a score≥3. During 37 months of follow-up, the mortality rate was approximately 5-fold higher in patients with a baseline score ≥3 compared with patients with a score< 3 (23% versus 5%; $p=0.01$). Even after adjustment for confounding variables, this simple VC score was predictive of mortality (hazard ratio for score ≥3: 3.9 [95% CI 1.1–12.4; $p=0.03$]). Similarly, Schwaiger et al. demonstrated a 2-fold increased risk of cardiovascular events in CKD patients with pelvic and/or lower legs calcification on plane X-rays.[10]

Other approaches utilizing plane X-rays have also given fruitful results. Kauppila et al.[11] originally suggested that a lateral X-ray of the lumbar spine can be used to semi-quantitatively assess the presence of abdominal aorta calcification (Fig. 13.1). The score is based on the number of segments of aorta showing evidence of calcification in front of the first four lumbar vertebrae and also the extent of the calcification process (a small calcification extending for less than a 1/3 of the width of a vertebral body receives a score of 1; a long calcification extending over ½ the width of the vertebral body gets a score of 3). The score has been associated with incident myocardial infarction and congestive heart failure.[7,12] In a 25-year follow-up of the Framingham study population an increase in aorta score obtained with this technique was linked with a reduction in metacarpal bone density.[13] Furthermore, a loss of metacarpal bone density was associated with a long term increase in cardiovascular morbidity and mortality.[14] An X-ray of the lumbar spine to visualize abdominal aorta calcification was therefore suggested by a group of experts[6] as a reliable method to show prognostically relevant VC, and was subsequently shown to have a good correlation with CT derived calcium scores.[15] In a recent publication, this semi-quantitative method was shown to

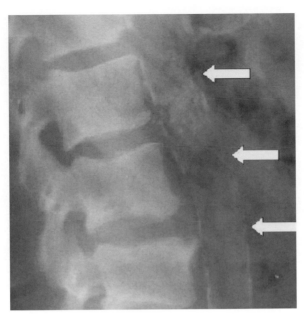

Fig. 13.1 Plane radiographs of the abdomen of a 54-year-old African American patient with diabetes mellitus and hypertension on maintenance hemodialysis for 3 years showing calcification along the length of the abdominal aorta (arrows).

be predictive of all-cause death and cardiovascular events in a cohort of 515 hemodialysis patients.[16]

Plane radiographs are qualitative and do not allow an accurate assessment of temporal changes of VC. Nonetheless, in a small study Izumi et al. recently showed that plane thoracic X-rays can be used to semi-quantitatively follow progression of aortic calcification in patients exposed to different phosphate binding therapies.[17]

Plane X-ray screening for VC can therefore provide helpful prognostic information. Given the low cost and risk to the patient it may be worth implementing as an in-office tool to risk stratify CKD patients and make informed choices regarding the best drugs to treat mineral metabolism abnormalities.

Ultrasonography

Vascular ultrasound studies are relatively easy to perform given the universal availability of the tool, the low cost of the test and the ease of identification of superficial vessels such as the carotid and femoral arteries. The pathognomonic finding of VC on ultrasound imaging is a dark shadow projected beyond the calcified plaque that blocks the ultrasound (US) beam from penetrating the diseased area (Fig. 13.2). This method, like plane radiography, provides mostly a qualitative assessment of VC. Nonetheless, there is good evidence that VC identified by means of ultrasonographically holds prognostic utility. Blacher et al. used a combination of vascular ultrasound and plane

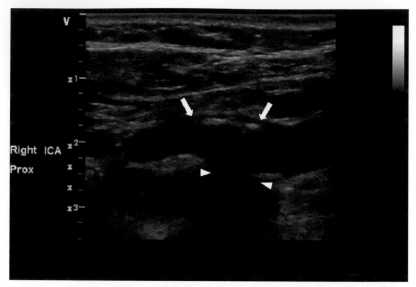

Fig. 13.2 Ultrasound study of the right internal carotid artery showing dense calcification of the near wall (arrows) causing shadowing (image disappearance included between the 2 arrowheads) of the far wall of the carotid artery.

radiographs to detect VC of the common carotid arteries, the abdominal aorta and femorotibial axes.[1] They prospectively followed 110 patients on maintenance hemodialysis for an average of 53 ±21 months after having stratified them according to a score generated by the combination of US and X-ray findings. These investigators showed that the mere presence of VC and the number of affected sites were associated with all-cause, as well as cardiovascular mortality. The adjusted hazard ratios for all-cause and cardiovascular mortality for each point increase in calcification severity were 1.9 (95% CI: 1.4–2.6) and 2.6 (95% CI: 1.2–2.4), respectively ($p < 0.01$ for both).[1]

The portability, safety, and low cost of US imaging make it very desirable for in-office applications.

Echocardiography

Echocardiography is the gold standard for assessment of cardiac valve morphology and function; it is non-invasive, does not expose the patient to radiation, and is only moderately expensive. A bright hyperechoic signal is the pathognomonic finding of valvular calcification on echocardiography (Fig. 13.3). Calcification of the cardiac valves is found in dialysis patients with a prevalence four-to five times higher than in the general population.[18] Although a less frequent finding than VC, valvular calcification shares common risk factors and pathogenic features with VC.[19] It appears that calcification of valves and vessels follows similar pathophysiological pathways, as inflammatory cells, lipoproteins and bone matrix proteins have been found in both structures.[19]

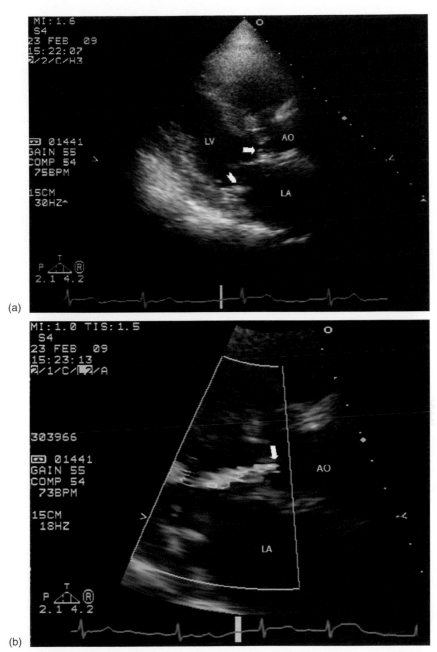

Fig. 13.3 (a) Echocardiography: parasternal long axis view of the heart showing dense calcification of the posterior leaflet of the mitral valve (arrow head) and aortic valve (arrow). AO: aorta; LA: left atrium; LV: left ventricle. (b) Color flow Doppler shows aortic valve regurgitation starting at the point of poor coaptation of the aortic leaflets (arrow).

There is mounting clinical evidence that calcification of the mitral and the aortic valve, even in the absence of hemodynamically significant stenoses, is associated with poor prognosis in the general population,[20] as well as CKD patients.[21] In an earlier publication, Riberio et al.[18] noted that valvular calcification is more prevalent in hemodialysis patients than in patients with normal renal function (mitral calcification 44.5% versus 10%, $p=0.02$; aortic calcification 52% versus 4.3%, $p=0.01$). In that study mitral and aortic calcification were significantly associated with peripheral arterial calcification ($p=0.009$) and alterations of mineral metabolism.[18] During a mean follow-up of 18 months, Wang et al.,[21] showed a marked increase in all-cause, as well as cardiovascular mortality in 192 peritoneal dialysis patients with no (15%), one (40%), or two (57%) calcified valves. All-cause and cardiovascular mortality did not differ significantly between patients having either valvular calcification or atherosclerotic vascular disease, reinforcing the hypothesis that valvular calcification represents a marker of systemic atherosclerosis and/or cardiovascular disease. In a subsequent publication, the same authors demonstrated that there is an interaction between serum fetuin-A levels, malnutrition, inflammation, atherosclerosis, valvular calcification and an adverse outcome in peritoneal dialysis (238 patients).[22] The serum fetuin-A level was inversely related to the presence of valvular calcification and cardiovascular outcome of these patients. Valvular calcification has also been demonstrated to relate well to another marker of atherosclerosis, such as carotid intima-media thickness (CIMT).[22] In a cohort of 92 continuous ambulatory peritoneal dialysis patients the investigators demonstrated a 6.5-fold higher risk of valvular calcification for each 1-mm increase in CIMT (95% CI 1.58–26.73; $p=0.009$). Furthermore, the presence of carotid calcification and carotid plaques was associated with a 7.2-fold (95% CI, 2.39–21.51; $p=0.001$) and 5.0-fold (95% CI, 1.77–14.13; $p=0.002$) increased risk of valvular calcification, respectively.[22] Of interest, attenuation of valvular calcification progression has been demonstrated in the general population with statins[23] and in CKD-5 patients with sevelamer treatment.[24] However, Panuccio et al.[25] reported a significant association between valvular calcification, and all-cause and cardiovascular mortality in 202 chronic hemodialysis patients that disappeared after adjusting for traditional risk factors and left ventricular hypertrophy. These findings would suggest that the presence of valvular calcification is a marker of other underlying pathologies and not an independent predictor of risk.

Nonetheless, given the ease of acquisition and the low cost, it is possible that in the near future identification of valvular calcification may be advocated as a method to assess risk in CKD patients and lead to changes in patient management.

Computed tomography techniques

Electron beam computed tomography (EBCT) and multi-slice computed tomography (MSCT) represent the gold standard for assessing the extent of coronary artery (CAC), aortic and valvular calcification (Figs 13.4 and 13.5). The technical advantage that the older EBCT technology offered was a superior temporal resolution, with diagnostic images obtainable at heart rates as high as 100 bpm. Despite the fact that the more recent MSCT scanners are slower (lower temporal resolution) they have a substantially

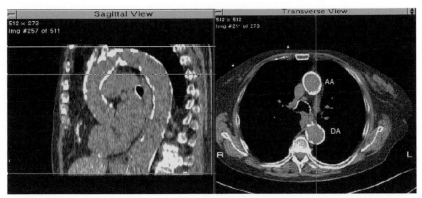

Fig. 13.4 Computed tomography image of the aorta. The sagittal view on the left shows multiple calcification sites of the ascending aorta, arch, and descending thoracic aorta. Calcified areas are highlighted in yellow. The axial view on the right corresponds to a transverse cut at the level of the lower white line seen in the sagittal view on the left. Note the almost circumferential distribution of calcium in the ascending (AA) and descending (DA) aorta.

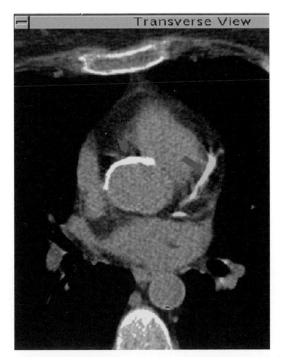

Fig. 13.5 Axial computed tomography image of the heart showing calcification of the aortic root (arrow head) and left anterior descending coronary artery (arrow).

better spatial resolution (greater image quality) than EBCT. In fact, with MSCT it is possible to acquire images with 0.4–0.5mm spatial resolution while EBCT permitted at best 1.5mm slicing. In direct comparisons[26] the two technologies have been found to be equivalent as far as quantification of calcification, especially when considering the most recent MSCT scanners (16 sections or greater).[26–28] The multislice CT technology has advanced very rapidly and in just a few years the manufacturers modified the design of CT scanners in a rather dramatic way: from 4-slice CTs produced in 2004 we quickly moved to 320-slice CT scanners in 2008, with a variety of other options, such as 128- or 256-slice and single (X-ray) source or dual-source. The increase in number of slices acquired during a single rotation of the X-ray tube brought about a substantial improvement in image quality, but also, in most cases, a substantial increase in radiation dose. The radiation exposure provided by an EBCT scanner for the quantification of CAC is about 0.6mSv, while a typical 64-slice CT scanner can provide as much as 1.5–2.5 mSv (40–200 chest X-rays). This radiation dose should be viewed in the context of the average yearly radiation exposure due to natural causes for a subject living in North America this dose amounts to about 3.5mSv. It is estimated that an additional 10mSv of radiation may cause one extra case of cancer per 1000 subjects exposed, although the fatality rate is obviously smaller. The risk of cancer is strictly linked to the age of the patient at the time of exposure (the younger the patient the greater the risk) and the risk of death connected with it should be weighted against the background risk of the patient exposed.[29] Therefore, if one considers that the average age of a patient entering dialysis in the US is about 55 years and that this individual often carries several serious comorbidities besides suffering from advanced renal failure, the additional risk posed by a screening CT for CAC is minor. Nonetheless, it is appropriate to minimize exposure in all patients and most manufacturers have implemented imaging algorithms to reduce radiation exposure with MSCT. The most frequently used one is 'dose modulation': with this approach the X-ray tube current is decreased during systole (when due to more severe motion the images are often non diagnostic) and increased during diastole. Typically, at the time of image reconstruction only the images obtained during diastole are then utilized to calculate the calcium score. In fact, with CT imaging it is possible to precisely quantify the extent of CAC by means of scores such as the Agatston[30] and the volume score.[31] The Agatston score is calculated as the product of area (total calcified plaque surface) by the peak density of the plaque (measured in Hounsfield units). Hence, it incorporates information relative to the size as well as the calcium content of the plaque. The volume score, on the contrary, takes into consideration all voxels in the context of a plaque with a minimum density of 130 Hounsfield units.[31] This is a direct evaluation of the size of a plaque not influenced by the peak density of the plaque that may vary according the calcium content. Despite the availability of both scores on most workstations, to date most studies have reported results based on the Agatston score.

Computed tomography (CT) technologies have been employed to investigate the natural history of VC and the impact of different therapeutic strategies in CKD. Using CT, the prevalence of coronary artery calcification was reported to be 40% in 85 CKD-4 patients[32] and approximately 85% in 205 maintenance hemodialysis patients.[33] On the contrary, VC was found only in 13% of controls with normal renal function.[32]

Consistent with these findings, Sigrist et al.[34] reported a prevalence of coronary calcification of 46% in 46 CKD-4 patients compared with 70% and 73%, respectively, in 60 hemodialysis and 28 peritoneal dialysis patients ($p = 0.02$). It is, therefore, obvious that the prevalence of VC increases dramatically after initiation of dialysis.

Extensive coronary artery calcium can be found not only in adult but also in pediatric and young hemodialysis patients (aged 19–39 years)[35] and in both groups a strong trend for rapid progression of VC has been reported.

Several factors seem to affect progression of VC in dialysis patients. Among others age, baseline calcium score, dialysis vintage, diabetes mellitus, abnormalities of mineral metabolism,[35,36] as well as use and dose of calcium based phosphate binders.[37,38] Russo et al.[39] recently demonstrated ~60% increase in coronary calcium scores measured with MSCT over 24 months in 53 CKD 3–5 patients not yet requiring dialysis. The single best predictor of progression was serum phosphorus. Similarly, Adeney et al.[40] found a close association between serum phosphate levels with valvular and vascular calcification in patients enrolled in the Multi Ethnic Study of Atherosclerosis (MESA) suffering from moderate CKD (average eGFR= 50ml/min/1.73m^2).

Given the impact of phosphorus on the presence and progression of vascular calcification several studies were conducted to assess the effect of various therapies to slow VC progression. Sevelamer and calcium-based phosphate binders were compared in a randomized clinical trial of 200 maintenance hemodialysis patients to slow the progression of VC.[37] The subjects were randomized to 1 year of open label treatment with either sevelamer or calcium salts. Throughout the study both drugs provided comparable phosphate control ($p = 0.33$). However, patients treated with calcium salts had a significantly higher serum calcium concentration ($p = 0.002$), a greater incidence of hypercalcemic episodes (16 vs. 5%; $p = 0.04$), and lower PTH level (138pg/mL versus 224pg/mL) compared with sevelamer treated subjects. At study completion, patients treated with calcium salts showed a significant progression of coronary calcium score (CCS), while sevelamer treated subjects did not (median percent progression of CCS 25% versus 6%, $p = 0.02$, with calcium and sevelamer, respectively).[37] A similar protocol was adopted in a second study of 129 incident hemodialysis patients.[41] Subjects treated with calcium containing phosphate binders showed a more rapid and more severe increase in CCS compared with those receiving sevelamer ($p = 0.01$ at 18 months follow-up).[41] Russo et al.[42] further demonstrated that VC progression can be halted with sevelamer treatment compared with calcium salts even in CKD-4 patients. An isolated study[43] concluded that calcium salts and sevelamer allow VC to progress by the same extent. However, the authors administered statins to 100% of the calcium treated and 80% of the sevelamer treated patients, and these drugs have been shown to not slow and even promote progression of VC in randomized trials in the general population.[44–46] Additionally, the mean PTH was very elevated throughout the study in both groups, and significantly more so in the sevelamer than calcium salts treated patients (434pg/mL versus 316pg/mL, $p < 0.05$). These shortcomings limit the validity of the conclusions of the study.

Other therapeutic agents have been utilized in small studies to attempt to inhibit VC progression. The effect of cyclic etidronate therapy to slow progression of VC was assessed in a study of 35 hemodialysis patients using MSCT.[47] Patients were left untreated for 1 year and were then treated with etidronate. Twenty-six of 35 hemodialysis patients showed a significant decrease in CCS progression with etidronate treatment (median absolute increase in CCS with and without treatment 195 versus 490mm^3; $p < 0.01$).[47] Interestingly, bone mineral density measured by DEXA did not change significantly with and without etidronate. On the contrary, using quantitative CT technology Raggi et al. demonstrated an increase in vertebral bone density in patients treated with sevelamer, while calcium salts treated patients showed a progressive loss in density.[48] Finally, a randomized trial is ongoing to assess the effect of treatment of secondary hyperparathyroidism with the calcimimetic cinecalcet on progression of VC, but at the time of this writing there are no available data to present.

There are only two small studies to support the notion that CT-generated CCS have an important prognostic value in dialysis patients. Matsuoka et al.,[2] followed 104 chronic hemodialysis patients for an average of 43months after a screening EBCT. Patients with a baseline CCS above the median (CCS = 200) had a significantly greater (all-cause) mortality than patients with a score below the median (32.1% versus 15.8%, $p = 0.0003$). In the long-term follow-up of the RIND study,[49] the risk of all-cause death increased as the baseline CCS increased from 0 ($\sim 10\%$ mortality at 4 years) to >400 ($\sim 75\%$ mortality, $p = 0.0035$).

In summary, modern cardiac CT techniques allow accurate assessment of VC and quantification of its progression. While assessment of coronary artery calcium is an accepted and established technique to assess risk of events in the general population, similar data are just emerging in CKD populations. There are, however, some limitations to the technology. Sub-intimal (atherosclerotic) calcification and medial calcification in the arterial wall cannot be differentiated with the current CT methodologies. This approach is further limited by the cost of CT and the substantial radiation exposure. Thus, other non-invasive imaging techniques may be preferable to screen for the presence of VC, while CT may be reserved for more conceptual research projects.

Measurement of arterial stiffness

An indirect effect of calcification of the vessel wall is an increase in vessel stiffness that has long-term substantial prognostic implications. One of the main roles of arteries is to dampen the pressure and flow oscillations resulting from intermittent ventricular ejection of blood, and to transform the pulsatile flow and pressure of arteries into the steady flow required in peripheral tissues and organs. The large arteries can instantaneously accommodate a large part of the stroke volume by distending their walls, with part of the energy produced by the heart diverted to this distension and 'stored' in the walls. During diastole, most of that stored energy causes recoil of the aorta and large conductance vessels, squeezing the stored blood forward into the peripheral tissues, thereby ensuring continuous perfusion of organs and tissues. This dampening function is most efficient when the diverted energy is minimized (increasing the energy for direct perfusion). The physical principle behind this phenomenon can be best described in terms of *stiffness*, which expresses the transmural pressure as a function of the volume contained in the vasculature (total or segmental) over the physiological range of pressures. In physiology, stiffness or elastance (E) is defined as the change in pressure (ΔP) due to a change in volume (ΔV), that is $E = \Delta P / \Delta V$. The pressure–volume relationship is non-linear and E represents the instantaneous slope of that relationship. In contrast to stiffness, which provides information about the 'elasticity' of the artery as a hollow structure, the elastic incremental modulus (Einc; Young's modulus) provides information on the intrinsic elastic properties of the biomaterials that compose the arterial wall independent of vessel geometry.[50] Arterial stiffening is characterized by an increased systolic (SBP) and decreased diastolic blood pressure (DBP) with resulting high pulse pressure. Systolic BP depends on the interaction between left ventricular (LV) ejection and the physical properties of the arterial tree that influence SBP via two mechanisms. The first direct mechanism involves the generation of a higher pressure wave (*incident or forward–traveling wave*) by the LV ejecting its stroke volume into a stiff arterial system, and decreased diastolic recoil resulting in lowered DBP. The forward–traveling pressure wave, propagates at a velocity that increases with stiffening of the artery and is also known as pulse wave velocity (PWV); it is reflected at any point of structural and functional discontinuity in the arterial tree, generating a reflected wave traveling retrograde toward the ascending aorta and LV. The timing of incident and reflected pressure waves depends on the duration of LV ejection (heart rate) and the transit time of pressure waves to and back from reflecting sites is strictly dependent on stiffness. In subjects with low arterial stiffness (low pulse wave velocity – PWV), the reflected waves affect central artery pressure after the LV ejection phase has ended. The resultant increase in pressure within the ascending aorta during early diastole has a boosting effect on coronary perfusion without increasing LV after load. With stiffening and higher PWV, the reflected waves return earlier in central arteries, during systole rather than diastole, thereby amplifying aortic and LV pressures during systole while reducing aortic pressure during diastole. This increases the aortic peak- and end-systolic pressures, raising the left ventricular pressure load and increasing myocardial oxygen consumption inducing LV hypertrophy while decreasing the diastolic BP and coronary blood flow.[50]

Arterial stiffness can be measured with several methodological approaches depending on the clinical use or experimental situation. In clinical practice the non-invasive estimation of arterial stiffness can be done by three principal methodologies:

- pulse transit time for evaluation of pulse wave velocity (PWV);

- analysis of the arterial pressure wave contour;

- direct stiffness estimation using measurements of diameter or arterial luminal cross-sectional area and distending pressure measured at the site of diameter changes.

Two most frequently used methods are measurement of PWV (Fig. 13.6) and central pulse wave analysis (Fig. 13.7), recorded directly at the carotid artery or indirectly in the ascending aorta; the latter is computed from the radial artery pulse wave using a transfer function. The measurement of carotid-femoral ('aortic') PWV is generally considered the gold standard. PWV measured along the aortic and aorto-iliac pathway (carotid-femoral PWV) is the most relevant, because the aorta is the principal capacitative artery and is responsible for the pathophysiological effects of arterial stiffening and its association with cardiovascular events.[51]

Carotid-femoral pulse wave velocity

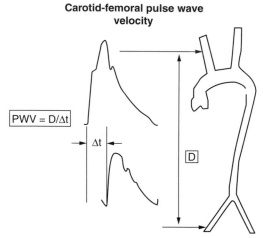

Fig. 13.6 Measurement of carotid-femoral pulse wave velocity. D, distance from recording point at the carotid artery to femoral artery; ΔT, transit time of pressure wave from the recording sites. PWV, pulse wave velocity.

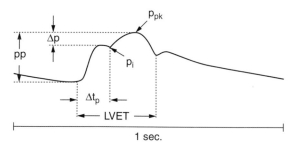

Fig. 13.7 Central artery pressure wave contour: PP, pulse pressure; Pi, incident pressure wave and early systolic shoulder; Δp, late systolic peak amplitude; Ppk, peak of the systolic pressure; LVET, left ventricular ejection time; Δtp, travel time of the reflected wave; sec, second. The Augmentation Index is the ratio Δp/PP; on this schema, it appears clearly determined by the amplitude of waves and their timing. It is also clearly influenced by the heart rate and height (index of reflection sites) of the patient.

Pulse wave velocity analysis

PWV is an assessment of stiffness of an artery as a hollow structure and it depends on the geometry of the artery (thickness, h; radius, r), as well as the intrinsic elastic properties of the arterial wall (i.e. elastic incremental modulus, E) and blood density (ρ). According to the Moens and Korteweg's formula: $PWV^2 = Eh/2r.\rho$. Bramwell and Hill described the relationship in terms of relative change in volume ($\Delta V/V$) and pressure (ΔP) during *ex vivo* experiments: $PWV^2 = \Delta P.V/\Delta V.\rho$. The assessment of PWV involves measurement of two parameters (Fig. 13.6): transit time of the arterial pulse along the analyzed arterial segment (t), and distance between recording sites (D) measured over the body surface: PWV = D/t . The carotid-femoral ('aortic') PWV is considered the gold standard. To measure aortic PWV the recording sites are the arterial pulse over the common carotid artery and femoral artery in the groin. For the measurement of the transit time different automatic methods have been developed to give instantaneous values of PWV. Different devices are commercially available and used worldwide. The Complior System® (Artech, Les Lilas, France) permits simultaneous recording of carotid and femoral arterial pulses, through mechano-transducer probes. SphygmoCor® system (ArtCor, Sydney, Australia) uses the Millar® probe and requires sequential recordings of the carotid and femoral pulses timed to a simultaneously acquired surface ECG. The SphygmoCor® system can also perform central aortic pulse wave analysis through a validated transfer function. Other devices are commercially available such as the Pulse pen® device (Diatecne, Milano, Italy), and Omron (Japan) based on the brachial-ankle pulse wave velocity (baPWV) with several assumptions; one of them being that the baPWV is the primary independent correlate of aortic PWV. Doppler based methods have been used to assess PWV between the aorta (suprasternal notch) and femoral artery or aortic bifurcation after echographic localization.[52]

The distance between recording sites is measured on the body surface. Several assumptions are made regarding the reference for recording points for transit time estimation. The general agreement is to measure distance as a simple subtraction formula: the distance between the carotid artery pulse and the suprasternal notch is subtracted from the distance between the carotid artery and the femoral artery pulses. Several alternatives could be used, such as the simple distance from the carotid artery to femoral artery sites without any other calculation, or the distance between the supra sternal notch and the femoral pulse. The principles are simple but the methodology must be strictly followed and blood pressure must be accurately measured within minutes during the PWV recording time (since arterial stiffness is influenced by systolic or mean blood pressure). Measurement of PVW should be performed before a meal and should not be preceded by the ingestion of coffee, alcohol or tobacco use.

Central pulse wave analysis

Analysis of central pressure waveform (Fig. 13.7) and amplitude (in the carotid artery or proximal aorta) represents an important advance in the assessment of large artery properties. Central pressure differs markedly from peripheral blood pressure (i.e. measured at the brachial artery level), mostly because of wave reflection, and its analysis provides information on the role of different arterial trees on the ventricular-vascular coupling. The aortic pressure waveform can be estimated from the radial artery waveform, using a transfer function (SphygmoCor device, AtCor Medical, West Ryde, Australia). Radial artery tonometry is widely used because of its simplicity. Carotid tonometry is more difficult and requires greater expertise, but because aortic and carotid pressure waveforms are very similar it is a direct measure not requiring the implementation of a transfer function. The principal parameters analyzed are central systolic pressure (and pulse pressure), and the effect of reflected waves on pressure shape and amplitude. This effect could be estimated in absolute terms, i.e. augmented pressure in mmHg, or in relative terms, i.e. Augmentation index (Aix %), the ratio between the amplitude of the reflected wave and pulse pressure. The Aix is frequently considered to be a stiffness index, but this is only partially true. Aix changes can be dissociated from changes in stiffness and PWV. The relationship between Aix and arterial stiffness per se are complex. Aix depends on several parameters including: the speed of travel, i.e. PWV stiffness, pressure waves traveling distance to the reflectance point (body length), duration, and pattern of LV ejection (determining the overlap between forward and reflected waves), and reflection intensity (reflection coefficient).[53] As an integrator of different parts of the cardiovascular system, its clinical interest is clearly linked to epidemiological insights and its predictive value for cardiovascular events. However, it is not a specific method for arterial stiffness measurement.

Clinical relevance of arterial stiffness in chronic kidney disease

Worsening renal function as well as aging and multiple cardiovascular risk factors contribute to the development of vascular stiffness. Wang et al. demonstrated that arterial stiffness increases as the estimated GFR declines.[54] Ix et al.[55] showed that arterial stiffness increases in association with serum phosphorus levels in the general population with normal kidney function or only moderate CKD (eGFR 65–70mL/min/1.73m^2). Haydar et al.[56] demonstrated that aortic PWV was significantly and strongly correlated with EBCT-generated coronary artery calcium scores in a cohort of 82 CKD patients ($r = 0.65$; $p = 0.0001$) even after adjustment for confounding variables. Guerin et al.[38] also showed that PWV increased as the daily dose of calcium carbonate increased and the level of iPTH decreased in a cohort of 120 hemodialysis patients. In the same cohort, increased PWV was associated with a simple calcification score obtained with a combination of carotid ultrasound and plain radiographs of the abdominal aorta and the femorotibial axes.[38] A significant increase in PWV was noted across different VC groups (from 9.14m/s in the group with no evidence of VC to 13.02m/s in the group with all arterial regions calcified; $p = 0.001$; Guerin, 2000).[30] More importantly, an increased aortic PWV was shown to be an independent predictor of all-cause and CV mortality.[57]

Hence, reduced arterial compliance and VC appear closely related, and both are markers of increased mortality risk. Prospective studies will be required to investigate whether changes in VC will also result in changes in arterial stiffness, as well as a reduction in adverse outcomes.

Conclusions

Increasing awareness of the negative prognostic impact of VC in CKD patients has generated great interest in the natural history and pathogenesis of this condition. The identification of factors associated with VC, as well as its progression sparked a wave of research into methods to assess VC and to inhibit its progression. Although quantitatively accurate, CT technologies are expensive, deliver a substantial dose of radiation and cannot be utilized in an ambulatory setting. Hence, Goodman et al.[58] proposed a simplified approach to identify and semi-quantitatively assess the extent of

VC in CKD patients. This approach includes a combination of echocardiography to detect valvular calcification, plain X-rays for peripheral and abdominal aorta calcification, as well as measurement of arterial pulse pressure as an indirect index of arterial stiffness. The long-term impact of this approach will need to be further elucidated, although preliminary evidence indicates that it may improve the risk stratification of CKD patients.

References

1. Blacher J, Guerin AP, Pannier B, Marchais SJ, London GM. Arterial calcifications, arterial stiffness, and cardiovascular risk in end-stage renal disease. *Hypertension* 2001;**38**:938–42.

2. Matsuoka M, Iseki K, Tamashiro M, et al. Impact of high coronary artery calcification score (CACS) on survival in patients on chronic hemodialysis. *Clin Exp Nephrol* 2004;**8**:54–8.

3. Shaw LJ, Raggi P, Schisterman E, Berman DS, Callister TQ. Prognostic value of cardiac risk factors and coronary artery calcium screening for all-cause mortality. *Radiology* 2003;**228**:826–33.

4. London GM, Guerin AP, Marchais SJ, et al. Cardiac and arterial interactions in end-stage renal disease. *Kidney Int* 1996;**50**:600–8.

5. London GM, Guerin AP, Marchais SJ. Pathophysiology of left ventricular hypertrophy in dialysis patients. *Blood Purif* 1994;**12**:277–83.

6. Moe S, Drueke T, Cunningham J, et al. Definition, evaluation, and classification of renal osteodystrophy: a position statement from Kidney Disease: Improving Global Outcomes (KDIGO). *Kidney Int* 2006;**69**:1945–53.

7. Wilson PW, Kauppila LI, O'Donnell CJ, et al. Abdominal aortic calcific deposits are an important predictor of vascular morbidity and mortality. *Circulation* 2001;**103**:1529–34.

8. London GM, Guerin AP, Marchais SJ, Metivier F, Pannier B, Adda H. Arterial media calcification in end-stage renal disease: impact on all-cause and cardiovascular mortality. *Nephrol Dial Transplant* 2003;**18**:1731–40.

9. Adragao T, Pires A, Lucas C, et al. A simple vascular calcification score predicts cardiovascular risk in hemodialysis patients. *Nephrol Dial Transplant* 2004;**19**:1480–8.

10. Schwaiger JP, Neyer U, Sprenger-Mahr H, et al. A simple score predicts future cardiovascular events in an inception cohort of dialysis patients. *Kidney Int* 2006;**70**:543–8.

11. Kauppila LI, Polak JF, Cupples LA, Hannan MT, Kiel DP, Wilson PW. New indices to classify location, severity and progression of calcific lesions in the abdominal aorta: a 25-year follow-up study. *Atherosclerosis* 1997;**132**:245–50.

12. Walsh CR, Cupples LA, Levy D, et al. Abdominal aortic calcific deposits are associated with increased risk for congestive heart failure: the Framingham Heart Study. *Am Heart J* 2002;**144**:733–9.

13. Kiel DP, Kauppila LI, Cupples LA, Hannan MT, O'Donnell CJ, Wilson PW. Bone loss and the progression of abdominal aortic calcification over a 25 year period: the Framingham Heart Study. *Calcif Tissue Int* 2001;**68**:271–6.

14. Samelson EJ, Kiel DP, Broe KE, et al. Metacarpal cortical area and risk of coronary heart disease: the Framingham Study. *Am J Epidemiol* 2004;**159**:589–95.

15. Bellasi A, Ferramosca E, Muntner P, et al. Correlation of simple imaging tests and coronary artery calcium measured by computed tomography in hemodialysis patients. *Kidney Int*, 2006;**70**(9):1623–8. Epub 6 September 2006.

16. Okuno S, Ishimura E, Kitatani K, et al. Presence of abdominal aortic calcification is significantly associated with all-cause and cardiovascular mortality in maintenance hemodialysis patients. *Am J Kidney Dis* 2007;**49:**417–25.

17. Izumi M, Morita S, Nishian Y, et al. Switching from calcium carbonate to sevelamer hydrochloride has suppressive effects on the progression of aortic calcification in hemodialysis patients: assessment using plain chest X-ray films. *Ren Fail* 2008;**30:**952–8.

18. Ribeiro S, Ramos A, Brandao A, et al. Cardiac valve calcification in hemodialysis patients: role of calcium-phosphate metabolism. *Nephrol Dial Transplant* 1998;**13:**2037–40.

19. Mohler ER, 3rd, Gannon F, Reynolds C, Zimmerman R, Keane MG, Kaplan FS. Bone formation and inflammation in cardiac valves. *Circulation* 2001;**103:**1522–8.

20. Otto CM, Lind BK, Kitzman DW, Gersh BJ, Siscovick DS. Association of aortic-valve sclerosis with cardiovascular mortality and morbidity in the elderly. *N Engl J Med* 1999;**341:**142–7.

21. Wang AY, Wang M, Woo J, et al. Cardiac valve calcification as an important predictor for all-cause mortality and cardiovascular mortality in long-term peritoneal dialysis patients: a prospective study. *J Am Soc Nephrol* 2003;**14:**159–68.

22. Wang AY, Woo J, Lam CW, et al. Associations of serum fetuin-A with malnutrition, inflammation, atherosclerosis and valvular calcification syndrome and outcome in peritoneal dialysis patients. *Nephrol Dial Transplant* 2005;**20:**1676–85.

23. Pohle K, Maffert R, Ropers D, et al. Progression of aortic valve calcification: association with coronary atherosclerosis and cardiovascular risk factors. *Circulation* **104:** 1927–32.

24. Raggi P, Bommer J, Chertow GM. Valvular calcification in hemodialysis patients randomised to calcium-based phosphorus binders or sevelamer. *J Heart Valve Dis* 2004;**13:**134–41.

25. Panuccio V, Tripepi R, Tripepi G, et al. Heart valve calcifications, survival, and cardiovascular risk in hemodialysis patients. *Am J Kidney Dis* 2004;**43:**479–84.

26. Stanford W, Thompson BH, Burns TL, Heery SD, Burr MC. Coronary artery calcium quantification at multi-detector row helical CT versus electron-beam CT. *Radiology* 2004;**230:**397–402.

27. Moe SM, O'Neill KD, Fineberg N, et al. Assessment of vascular calcification in ESRD patients using spiral CT. *Nephrol Dial Transplant* 2003;**18:** 1152–8.

28. Nitta K, Akiba T, Suzuki K, et al. Assessment of coronary artery calcification in hemodialysis patients using multi-detector spiral CT scan. *Hypertens Res* 2004;**27:**527–33.

29. Einstein AJ, Henzlova MJ, Rajagopalan S. Estimating risk of cancer associated with radiation exposure from 64-slice computed tomography coronary angiography. *J Am Med Ass* 2007;**298:**317–23.

30. Agatston AS, Janowitz WR, Hildner FJ, Zusmer NR, Viamonte M, Jr, Detrano R. Quantification of coronary artery calcium using ultrafast computed tomography. *J Am Coll Cardiol* 1990;**15:**827–32.

31. Callister TQ, Cooil B, Raya SP, Lippolis NJ, Russo DJ, Raggi P. Coronary artery disease: improved reproducibility of calcium scoring with an electron-beam CT volumetric method. *Radiology* 1998;**208:**807–14.

32. Russo D, Palmiero G, De Blasio AP, Balletta MM, Andreucci VE. Coronary artery calcification in patients with CRF not undergoing dialysis. *Am J Kidney Dis* 2004;**44:**1024–30.

33. Raggi P, Boulay A, Chasan-Taber S, et al. Cardiac calcification in adult hemodialysis patients. A link between end-stage renal disease and cardiovascular disease? *J Am Coll Cardiol* 2002;**39:**695–701.

34. Sigrist M, Bungay P, Taal MW, McIntyre CW. Vascular calcification and cardiovascular function in chronic kidney disease. *Nephrol Dial Transplant* 2006;**21**:707–14.

35. Oh J, Wunsch R, Turzer M, et al. Advanced coronary and carotid arteriopathy in young adults with childhood-onset chronic renal failure. *Circulation* 2002;**106**:100–5.

36. Chertow GM, Raggi P, Chasan-Taber S, Bommer J, Holzer H, Burke SK Determinants of progressive vascular calcification in hemodialysis patients. *Nephrol Dial Transplant* 2004;**19**:1489–96.

37. Chertow GM, Burke SK, Raggi P. Sevelamer attenuates the progression of coronary and aortic calcification in hemodialysis patients. *Kidney Int* 2002;**62**:245–52.

38. Guerin AP, London GM, Marchais SJ, Metivier F. Arterial stiffening and vascular calcifications in end-stage renal disease. *Nephrol Dial Transplant* 2000;**15**:1014–21.

39. Russo D, Corrao S, Miranda I, et al. Progression of coronary artery calcification in predialysis patients. *Am J Nephrol* 2007;**27**:152–8.

40. Adeney KL, Siscovick DS, Ix JH, et al. Association of serum phosphate with vascular and valvular calcification in moderate CKD. *J Am Soc Nephrol* 2009;**20**:381–7.

41. Block GA, Spiegel DM, Ehrlich J, et al. Effects of sevelamer and calcium on coronary artery calcification in patients new to hemodialysis. *Kidney Int* 2005;**68**:1815–24.

42. Russo D, Miranda I, Ruocco C, et al. The progression of coronary artery calcification in predialysis patients on calcium carbonate or sevelamer. *Kidney Int* 2007;**72**:1255–61.

43. Quinibi W, Moustafa M, Muenz LR, et al. A 1-year randomised trial of calcium acetate versus sevelamer on progression of coronary artery calcification in hemodialysis patients with comparable lipid control: the Calcium Acetate Renagel Evaluation-2 (CARE-2) Study. *Am J Kidney Dis* 2008;**51**:952–65.

44. Arad Y, Spadaro LA, Roth M, Newstein D, Guerci AD. Treatment of asymptomatic adults with elevated coronary calcium scores with atorvastatin, vitamin C, and vitamin E: the St. Francis Heart Study randomised clinical trial. *J Am Coll Cardiol* 2005;**46**:166–72.

45. Raggi P, Davidson M, Callister TQ, et al. Aggressive versus moderate lipid-lowering therapy in hypercholesterolemic postmenopausal women: beyond endorsed lipid lowering with EBT scanning (BELLES). *Circulation* 2005;**112**:563–71.

46. Schmermund A, Achenbach S, Budde T, et al. Effect of intensive versus standard lipid-lowering treatment with atorvastatin on the progression of calcified coronary atherosclerosis over 12 months: a multicenter, randomised, double-blind trial. *Circulation* 2006;**113**:427–37.

47. Nitta K, Akiba T, Suzuki K, et al. Effects of cyclic intermittent etidronate therapy on coronary artery calcification in patients receiving long-term hemodialysis. *Am J Kidney Dis* 2004;**44**:680–8.

48. Raggi P, James G, Burke SK, et al. Decrease in thoracic vertebral bone attenuation with calcium-based phosphate binders in hemodialysis. *J Bone Miner Res* 2005;**20**:764–72.

49. Block GA, Raggi P, Bellasi A, Kooienga L, Spiegel DM. Mortality effect of coronary calcification and phosphate binder choice in incident hemodialysis patients. *Kidney Int* 2007;**71**(5):438–41. Epub 3 January 2007.

50. O'Rourke M. *Handbook of Hypertension. Arterial Stiffness in Hypertension.* M E Safar & M F O'Rourke (eds), Vol. **23**. Philadelphia: Elsevier, 2006:3–20.

51. Pannier BM, Avolio AP, Hoeks A, Mancia G, Takazawa K. Methods and devices for measuring arterial compliance in humans. *Am J Hypertens* 2002;**15**:743–53.

52. Cruickshank K, Riste L, Anderson SG, Wright JS, Dunn G, Gosling RG. Aortic pulse-wave velocity and its relationship to mortality in diabetes and glucose intolerance: an integrated index of vascular function? *Circulation* 2002;**106**:2085–90.

53. London G, Yaginuma, T. Wave reflections: clinical and therapeutic aspects. In: M E Safar & M F O'Rourke (eds), *The Arterial System in Hypertension*. Dordrecht: Kluwer Academic Publishers 2003;221–37.

54. Wang MC, Tsai WC, Chen JY, Huang JJ. Stepwise increase in arterial stiffness corresponding with the stages of chronic kidney disease. *Am J Kidney Dis* 2005;**45**:494–501.

55. Ix JH, De Boer IH, Peralta CA, et al. Serum phosphorus concentrations and arterial stiffness among individuals with normal kidney function to moderate kidney disease in MESA. *Clin J Am Soc Nephrol*. 2009;**4**(3):609–15. Epub 11 February 2009.

56. Haydar AA, Covic A, Colhoun H, Rubens M, Goldsmith DJ. Coronary artery calcification and aortic pulse wave velocity in chronic kidney disease patients. *Kidney Int* 2004;**65**: 1790–4.

57. Guerin AP, Blacher J, Pannier B, Marchais SJ, Safar ME, London GM. Impact of aortic stiffness attenuation on survival of patients in end-stage renal failure. *Circulation* 2001;**103**:987–92.

58. Goodman WG, London G, Amann K, et al. Vascular calcification in chronic kidney disease. *Am J Kidney Dis* 2004;**43**:572–9.

Chapter 14

Osteopenia in uremia

Ezequiel Bellorin-Font, Judith Adams, and
John Cunningham

Introduction

The progressive loss of kidney function results in a series of disorders of mineral metabolism that ultimately lead to bone alterations, cardiovascular and other soft tissue calcifications. In addition the treatment given to many patients with chronic kidney disease (CKD) may increase the risks of bone and mineral disorders. Recent studies indicate that a strong association exists between alterations of bone and mineral metabolism, fractures, and cardiovascular disease, the leading cause of mortality in patients with CKD.[1,2]

The bone changes in CKD have been reported mainly in patients with end-stage kidney disease (CKD 5 and CKD 5D), while relatively few articles address bone health in patients at earlier stages of CKD. This is surprising since derangements in mineral metabolism initiate early in the course of CKD as a means to maintain body homeostasis; consequently, one should expect that relatively early disturbances of bone structure may result from these changes in mineral homeostasis.

Recently, the 'KDIGO Controversy Conference on Definition, Evaluation and Classification of Renal Osteodystrophy' recommended that the term renal osteodystrophy be reserved exclusively to the bone alterations found in patients with CKD.[3] However, it is reasonable to think that many patients that reach CKD may carry other disorders of bone that may contribute to the final picture of renal osteodystrophy. Indeed, osteoporosis is the most prevalent bone disorder in the general population, but relatively little attention has been paid to its possible contribution to the bone alterations observed in patients with CKD, particularly in the increasing population of middle and older age groups that account for more than half of the patients on dialysis.

Definition of osteoporosis and osteopenia

The term osteoporosis (porous bone) arises from the appearance of the bone interior walls after fracture. However, this definition is vague and does not provide a relationship between clinical findings, bone fragility and the need for treatment. The World Health Organisation (WHO) has defined osteoporosis as a condition of skeletal fragility characterized by reduced bone mass and micro-architectural deterioration.[4]

From the clinical point of view, this term identifies the clinical syndrome of a reduction in bone mass, evidenced by radiological rarification of calcified bone, occurrence of vertebral, wrist or hip fractures, and bone pain resulting in impairment of physical activity.[5] The term has evolved after the development of bone mineral densitometry methodologies, especially central dual energy X-ray absorptiometry (DXA), which has allowed the diagnosis of osteoporosis before clinical manifestation such as fragility fractures occur.

Diagnosis of osteoporosis and bone densitometry

If fractures or specific radiographic features (thinned cortex, trabeculae which are thinned and reduced in number) are not present, then judging bone density from radiographs is not a precise science. However, radiographic osteopenia is a strong predictor of osteoporosis and an indication for DXA bone densitometry.

Dual energy X-ray absorptiometry

Dual energy X-ray absorptiometry was introduced in the late 1980s, and is the most widely used and available bone densitometry technique.[6] Dual-energy X-ray beams are required to correct bone density measurements for overlying soft tissue, and are produced by a variety of techniques by different manufacturers, and the energies are selected to optimize separation of mineralized and soft tissue components of the skeletal site scanned.

DXA can be applied to sites of the skeleton at which osteoporotic fractures occur; in the central skeleton this includes the lumbar spine (L1–4) and proximal femur (total hip, femoral neck, trochanter, and Ward's area). DXA can also be applied to peripheral skeletal sites (forearm, calcaneus). DXA provides an 'areal' bone mineral density (BMD_a; g/cm^2) of integral (cortical and trabecular) bone. The measurement sites generally used in clinical diagnosis (in contrast to research) are mean BMD_a for lumbar spine (L1–4), femoral neck and total hip. If hyperparathyroidism (primary or secondary, as occurs in chronic kidney disease) is suspected a distal forearm measurement should be performed, since cortical bone is lost preferentially from this site. Cortical/trabecular ratios vary in different sites [50/50 postero-anterior (PA) lumbar spine; 60/40 total hip; 95/5 in distal radius]. As a result of the variable composition of bones and rates of change, measurements in different skeletal sites in the same individual will not give the same results. In research studies, BMD measurements in different anatomical sites, and by various bone density methods [DXA, quantitative computed tomography (QCT), quantitative ultrasound (QUS)] may be complementary. With appropriate software whole-body DXA scanning can also be performed, from which can be extracted whole-body and regional bone mineral content (BMC in g, which would include the extra-skeletal soft tissue metastatic calcification which can occur in CKD) and whole-body and regional body composition [lean (muscle) and fat mass].

With skilled and trained technical staff performing DXA precision (reproducibility; CV%) for DXA total hip and lumbar spine is 1%; femoral neck 2.5% and distal forearm 1%. The accuracy of DXA lies between 3 and 8%; inaccuracies are related to marrow fat and DXA taking soft tissue as a reference. Inaccuracies may occur with excessive under- or overweight subjects, and with large changes in weight between scans, but exactly how this can be corrected for in adults is uncertain. Artefacts can cause inaccuracies in DXA measurements and are most common in the lumbar spine in the elderly population. All the calcium in the path of the X-ray beam will contribute to the BMD_a measured [degenerative disc disease, osteophytes, osteoarthritis with hyperostosis of facet joints; vertebral fracture (same amount of calcium as before fracture, but in reduced area)] and cause false elevation. In treatment with strontium ranelate some of the apparent increase in BMD_a is artefactual, related to the high atomic number strontium, which accumulates in bone and contributes to the X-ray attenuation.

For interpretation of BMD_a results it is essential that age-, gender-, and ethnically matched reference data are available—these are generally provided by the scanner manufacturer. There is a paucity of appropriate reference ranges for children and certain ethnic minorities. A patient's results can be interpreted in terms of the SD from the mean of either gender-matched peak bone mass (PBM, T-score) or age-matched BMD (Z-score).

The WHO has defined osteoporosis in terms of bone densitometry as a T-score at, or below, −2.5 in the lumbar spine, femoral neck, total femur, and distal forearm.[7] This definition is now also applied to males, but importantly is not appropriate in children or adolescents who have not yet reached peak bone mass. The diagnosis of osteoporosis in children should not be made on the basis of densitometric criteria alone. Terminology such as 'low bone density for chronological age' may be used if the Z-score is below −2.0. The WHO T-score definition does not apply to other techniques (e.g. QCT, QUS) or other anatomical sites (e.g. calcaneus), nor is it yet confirmed to be applicable to younger women and men. Until PBM has been reached (i.e. in children and young adults up to approximately 20 years) interpretation can be made only by comparison to the age-matched mean (Z-score). For DXA hip, use of the NHANES reference database is preferred. In patients with CKD who may lack $1,25(OH)_2D$ with osteomalacic bone changes it is important to note that DXA BMD_a cannot differentiate low calcium content of bone being due to osteoporosis (reduced bone mass) or osteomalacia (reduced calcium/osteoid ratio).

Although there is consensus on the definition of osteoporosis in terms of bone mineral densitometry (WHO T-score less than −2.5), there is as yet no consensus on levels of BMD_a, which justify cost-effective therapeutic interventions. This is not surprising, since it is the individual patient that is being treated, not the bone density result, and age is such a strong independent predictor of fracture. Other factors in addition to age including previous low trauma fracture over age 50, parental hip fracture, oral glucocorticoid therapy (for more than 3 months at a dose 5mg daily or more), rheumatoid arthritis, current smoking, alcohol consumption (more than 3 units per day), secondary causes of osteoporosis, including type I (insulin dependent) diabetes, osteogenesis imperfecta in adults, untreated long-standing hyperthyroidism, hypogonadism or premature menopause (<45 years), chronic malnutrition, or malabsorption and chronic liver disease contribute to prediction of fracture risk.[8] In 2008 the WHO published a tool to calculate 10-year fracture risk for individual patients aged between

40 and 90 years using these clinical risk factors (with or without femoral neck BMD_a; http://www.shef.ac.uk/FRAX/index.htm).

Subsequently, national guidelines for appropriate treatment interventions were launched in several countries (http://www.shef.ac.uk/NOGG).[9,10] Chronic kidney disease is not yet included in the secondary causes of osteoporosis in the WHO calculator, presumably as there is an inadequate database for fracture prediction.

Change in BMD_a is calculated from the difference in g/cm^2 between scans at two time points. Significant change in BMD_a is 2.77 multiplied by precision (CV) at the site of measurement. As changes in bone density are generally small it is essential in an individual patient to leave an adequate time interval between DXA measures, usually 18–24 months, unless large changes in BMD_a are anticipated (e.g. following organ transplantation together with large doses of glucocorticoids). Scanner manufacturers use different edge detection algorithms and regions of interest (ROIs) in hip analyses, so results from different scanners are not interchangeable. In longitudinal studies it is essential to use the same scanner and software program. DXA involves very low radiation doses (1–6μSv), similar to those of natural background radiation (NBR = 2400μSv per annum; about 7μSv per day).

Bone strength depends upon several factors that include bone volume, architecture, micro-architecture, turnover, and mineralization.[11] In osteoporosis bone structure is abnormal due to a reduced quantity of normal mineralized bone, cortical thinning and porosity, and reduced and disconnected trabeculae, resulting from an imbalance between resorption and formation.

In contrast, osteopenia, which defines the histological finding of decreased bone mass below the normal range for the age and gender of the patient[5] has been defined by the WHO as a BMD T-score between −1.0 SD and −2.5 SD below the bone density of a normal young adult.[7] In general, osteopenia and osteoporosis may be caused by the resorption of bone at a rate that exceeds formation. The term osteopenia does not imply disease, but rather an increase in the risk of developing the more advanced state of osteoporosis.

The prevalence of osteopenia in the general population is high. Thus, about half of post-menopausal women have a T-score at the femoral neck between −1.0 and −2.5 SD.[12] A much lesser proportion of male patients of middle and older age suffer this condition.

Fracture prediction

Since whether a patient suffers a fracture depends on factors in addition to BMD_a (age, falls, nature of fall, and response to a fall), it is impossible for bone densitometry techniques to completely discriminate between those with and without fractures. However, the lower the DXA BMD_a the more at risk the patient is of suffering a fracture. DXA BMD_a measurements made in any skeletal site (central and peripheral) are predictive of fracture, with the risk of fracture increased in individuals with the lower BMD_a. The relative risk (RR) of fracture per 1 SD decrease in BMD below age-adjusted mean varies between 1.4 and 2.6.[13] This reduction in BMD_a in predicting fracture is as good as a rise of 1 SD in blood pressure is in predicting stroke, and a 1 SD rise in cholesterol is in predicting myocardial infarction. Site-specific measurements are best in predicting fracture in that particular anatomical place.

DXA in children

As DXA provides an 'areal' density in g/cm^2, it is size dependent, under-estimating BMD_a in small or slender bones, and over-estimating in large bones.[14] This is a particular problem in children and much of the change in DXA BMD_a in normally growing children during growth is due to increase in size of bones. This size dependency is pertinent to children with CKD and it has been suggested that DXA is not an appropriate bone density method to apply in these children.[15] To overcome this limitation to some extent, a 'calculated volumetric BMD' [bone mineral apparent density (BMAD g/cm^3)] can be made in the spine (assuming the vertebrae are cubes or cylinders) and femoral neck (cylinder). Other methods for size correction have been made, but to date there is no consensus on whether size correction should be applied and which method is optimum. Measurement sites for DXA in children are typically the lumbar spine (L1–4) and total body, where precision is similar to that achieved in adults (CV = 1%). The forearm and proximal femur have been used in some studies, as has the lateral distal femur where deformity and contracture (e.g. cerebral palsy) preclude use of DXA in the normal measurement sites. Normative reference data are available for spine, femoral neck, total body and lateral distal femur. Because the hip shape in young children (10 years and under) is very different from that in the adult analysis is unreliable. The International Society of Clinical Densitometry (ISCD). Published guidelines on the appropriate use of DXA in both adults and children are available at http://www.iscd.org/Visitors/positions/OfficialPositionsText.cfm.[16,17]

Other bone densitometry techniques

Quantitative computed tomography

Quantitative computed tomography (QCT) has advantages over DXA in that it provides not only bone density, but also information of size and shape of the bone, which also contribute to bone strength. However, currently QCT remains largely a research tool, with few data on its ability to predict fracture.[18,19] QCT uniquely allows for the separate estimation of trabecular and cortical BMD, and provides a true volumetric density in g/L (mg/cm^3), rather than the 'areal' (g/cm^2) BMD_a of DXA. QCT is therefore not size dependent, and is of particular relevance in children and in diseases that result in small stature.

QCT is performed with a solid hydroxy-apatite calibration reference phantom to transform HU in to bone mineral equivalent units. Original CT scanners used rotate-translate technology, which permitted only single 2D sections. The recent technical developments in CT (spiral rotation of the X-ray tube; multiple rows of detectors) enable rapid 3D volume scanning. As a consequence, precision has improved (better than CV = 1%), and the method is applicable to measure bone size and density in the hip. The WHO definition of osteoporosis (T-score below –2.5) is not applicable to QCT; a Z-score of –2.0 and below is abnormal. Some use the definition of a QCT of

$100mg/cm^3$ or below as 'osteopenia', and $80mg/cm^3$ or below as 'osteoporosis'. Although usually applied to the vertebral trabecular bone, more recently dedicated, small CT scanners (peripheral pQCT) have been developed, which allow separate analysis of cortical and trabecular bone in the non-dominant forearm and the tibia. Measurement of cross-sectional bone and muscle area, and certain biomechanical parameters (moment of inertia, stress strain index) can also be made from these scans.

Other research methods

Quantitative ultrasound

Quantitative ultrasound (QUS) measures broadband ultrasound attenuation (BUA) and speed of sound (SOS), and shows potential in fracture prediction. It is predominantly applied to the calcaneus, where it predicts hip fracture risk in elderly females. However, it cannot be used to diagnose osteoporosis, as defined by the WHO. It is temperature sensitive, is a poor monitoring tool that has been applied to numerous other skeletal sites (e.g. phalanges), and it is not clear how it should be used in clinical practice in other patient groups (men, young women, and children).

Imaging trabecular bone structure

Quantitative magnetic resonance (QMR) has been applied in research to assessing bone density and trabecular bone structure. The diameter of bone trabeculae range from about 50–200 μm, and can be demonstrated on conventional radiographs, particularly in the appendicular skeleton (hands), where visualization can be enhanced by magnification techniques. More recently, there has been increase in the research application of high resolution computed tomography (HRCT; in plane resolution 82μ) and high resolution magnetic resonance imaging (HRMRI) to examining trabecular structure *in vivo* in peripheral skeletal sites.[20] They also can identify and quantitate cortical porosity, which may be particularly relevant in CKD. The strengths and potentials of these techniques, which are technically challenging, are to extend knowledge and understanding of how disease and treatment affect the different components of bone, rather than in the clinical diagnosis of osteoporosis. These research contributions may be particularly pertinent to the study of bone disease in CKD.[21,22] Micro-CT systems have been developed with increased spatial resolution, but these are generally only applicable to examine small tissue samples *in vitro* because of the large radiation doses required.

Conclusions

Reasonably accurate and precise methods of non-invasive bone density assessments are now available and have been applied to the study of bone disorders in patients with CKD. However, more research is required to know how best to apply these various techniques in clinical practice. DXA, the most widely available and utilized technique has short comings, particularly in children. The bone disease associated with CKD is complex and multifactorial [1,25(OH)$_2$D deficiency; secondary hyperparpathyroidism, phosphate retention with metastatic soft tissue calcification, adynamic bone disease] and BMD_a measurements alone may not be adequate to characterize the bone disorder, and other diagnostic tools (bone turnover markers, bone biopsy) may be required to determine appropriate treatment.[23]

Definition of osteoporosis and osteopenia in CKD

The definition of osteoporosis and osteopenia in CKD is more complex than in the general population. Patients with advanced CKD (stages 4, 5, and 5D) have a high risk of bone fractures that exceeds the prevalence in the general population, but it does not necessarily results from osteoporosis itself since, at least by the current methods of measuring BMD, there is no clear correlation between BMD and fractures in these patients.[24] Furthermore, as shown in Table 14.1, in addition to CKD-MBD, patients with CKD share similar risk factors with the general population for osteoporosis, making it very difficult to ascertain the relative weight of osteoporosis on the possible mechanisms of bone mass loss, particularly in earlier stages of CKD when overt renal osteodystrophy is not established.

Table 14.1 Risk factors for osteoporosis

Demography	Ethnicity
	Gender
	Family history
	Age
Habits	Nutrition
	Physical activity
	Cigarette smoking
	Alcohol consumption
Hormones	Estrogen deficiency
	Androgen deficiency
Comorbidity	Chronic disease
	Low body mass index
	Immobilization
Bone conditions	BMD
	Size and geometry
	Micro-architecture
	Low BMD peak
Drugs	Glucocorticoids
	Warfarin and heparin
	Anticonvulsants
CKD related	Time on dialysis
	Low PTH
	Metabolic bone disease
	Amyloidosis β2 microglobulin
	Chronic acidosis
	Aluminum

An important limitation for the diagnosis of osteoporosis in CKD patients is the increasing prevalence of adynamic bone disease.[25] As mentioned above, in the general population the diagnosis of osteoporosis relays particularly on determinations of BMD. However, patients with adynamic bone disease may also have low BMD.[26,27] Therefore, the differentiation between the bone alterations is very difficult in CKD, unless bone histology and histomorphometry are examined.

Prevalence and risk factors of osteoporosis and fractures in uremic patients

Decreased bone mineral density (BMD) has been well described among patients with advanced CKD. A cross-sectional study in Japanese dialysis patients showed vertebral fracture in close to 20.9% of them and suggested that low lumbar-spine BMD might be a sensitive predictor of vertebral fracture in HD patients.[28] Alem et al., using data from the USRDS, showed that the overall incidence of hip fractures among patients who had undergone dialysis between 1989 and 1996 was 7.45 per 1000 person/year for males and 13.63 per 1000 person/year for females, 4-fold higher than that expected in the general population.[29] In another study by the same group, the multivariate analysis showed that age, female gender, race (blacks compared with whites), body mass index (BMI), and the presence of peripheral vascular disease were independently associated with hip fracture, whereas serum intact parathyroid hormone (iPTH), aluminum, diabetes, and bicarbonate levels did not appreciably influence the risk of hip fracture, indicating that factors that predict risk of hip fracture in the population at large also do so in end-stage kidney disease patients. These results suggest a major role of osteoporosis as a cause of fracture in dialysis patients.

Recently, Nickolas et al.,[30] in a cross-sectional analysis of the NHANES III study, showed that moderate to severe kidney disease was independently associated with more than 2-fold increase in the incidence of hip fracture; an association stronger than traditional risk features for fracture, such as age, gender, race, body weight, and BMD.

According to the 2002 United States Renal Data System (USRDS) report,[31] 38.5% of the prevalent dialysis population in the US is in the age range 45–65 years. Similarly, in the European countries reporting to the European Renal Association–European Dialysis and Transplant Association registry,[32] and the registry of the Latin American Society of Nephrology,[33] the prevalence of patients in dialysis in those age groups ranges between 35–43% and 37–44.8%, respectively. Furthermore, almost half of these patients are female, suggesting that in these CKD populations there may be an increase in the risk factors for osteoporotic bone fractures as occurs in the general population. In fact, in a recent review, several of the studies analyzed indicate an increased risk for hip and vertebral fractures in both patients with CKD stages 3 and 5, and CKD stage 5D, compared with the general population.[21] However, there are some limitations in the interpretation of studies referred to patients with CKD 3 and 4 since in most of them the patient population examined was female and older than 50 years, a group with a natural increased risk for osteoporosis. In addition, the prevalence of CKD in this age group is also higher compared with younger people.

Nonetheless, there seems to be no doubt that in CKD 3 and 4, the odds ratio for bone fracture (hip predominantly) is increased between 1.5- and 3-fold.

In patients with CKD stage 5D, several studies have shown a prevalence of hip fracture range between 10 and 40%. About half of these patients were older than 50 years. Interestingly, the incidence rate of hip fractures in all patients who started dialysis in the US from 1989 to 1996 was 4.4 times higher than the general population used as control. Younger patients showed a higher relative risk. The incidence rate in women doubled that in men (1.36 versus 0.74% per year for men and for women, respectively).[29,34] Similar rates were reported by Coco et al.[35] in a single dialysis unit, and an incidence rate of 0.89% per year was found in a large international study. Fractures occur more commonly in elderly patients, in women, in diabetic patients, in those using glucocorticoids, and in those with longer exposure to dialysis.

In summary, there seems to be no doubt that patients with CKD of moderate to severe degree have an increase risk for fracture. Although it has been proposed that factors such as renal osteodystrophy and metabolic acidosis may determine the increased risk for fractures observed in these patients, it is possible that the relatively high incidence and prevalence of CKD stage 5 in the middle-aged and older population may also play an important role. In fact, as discussed below, a great proportion of women with CKD have an increased risk for osteoporosis due to age prevalence, and alterations of estrogen and other sexual hormone metabolism. It should be clear, however, that the pathophysiology of osteoporosis largely differs from that of the complex syndrome of renal osteodystrophy. Thus, the bone may be affected not only of decrease mineral content, but also from a wide spectrum of abnormalities resulting directly from disorders of mineral metabolism that occur as a consequence of the progressive loss of renal function. These considerations have prompted KDIGO to avoid osteoporosis per se as a part of the syndrome of CKD-MBD and particularly from the definition of renal osteodystrophy.[3]

Pathogenesis and bone histology of osteoporosis in uremic patients

As discussed above, the pathophysiology of osteoporosis and osteopenia in patients with progressive renal failure is difficult to define. In CKD patients, the bone may be affected not only by decrease mineral content, but also from a wide spectrum of abnormalities that range from low bone turnover to high turnover, as well as maturation defects.

As mentioned previously, the differentiation between osteoporosis and adynamic bone disease based on BMD is difficult in CKD, unless bone histology and histomorphometry are examined. In patients with advanced CKD, such as those on dialysis, it is practically impossible to describe the typical histological changes of osteoporosis since the normal bone structure is substituted by florid manifestations of renal osteodystrophy. In these cases, some of the manifestations of osteoporosis may be indistinguishable from those of the predominant form of renal osteodystrophy.[36,37] In a recent study, Lobão et al.[38] examined bone histology in a group of pre-dialysis patients with a median creatinine clearance of 29mL/min and with low BMD by DXA. The risk of low bone mineral density was higher for patients with alkaline phosphatase levels above 190 U/L and low iPTH (below 70pg/mL). Post-menopausal women comprised 65 and 50% of the low BMD group. In patients with low bone density, bone histomorphometry revealed adynamic bone disease (52.5%), osteomalacia (42.5%), and mixed uremic bone disease (5%). Trabecular bone volume was lower in patients with adynamic bone or osteomalacia. No correlation was observed between trabecular bone volume and bone mineral density. They concluded that low bone mineral density is frequent in pre-dialysis CKD patients and in low turnover bone disease, manifesting as adynamic bone disease and osteomalacia.

In a preliminary report, Rojas et al.[39] examined the spectrum of renal osteodystrophy in 47 patients with CKD stages 3–5 prior to dialysis. The mean age was 54.3 ± 13 years and a mean creatinine clearance of 25.8 ±12.5mL/min (8–57mL/min). Secondary hyperparathyroidism was the most frequent finding, corresponding to 30% of all cases, all with CKD 4 and 5; whereas osteoporosis, the second most prevalent finding, was observed in 25% of cases, particularly in stages 3 and 4. Adynamic bone disease, the second most prevalent disorder in stage 3 was also observed in CKD stages 4 and 5. Mixed bone disease (12.5%) occurred in all CKD stages. Patients with osteoporosis were mainly post-menopausal women (70%), who had better renal function (creatinine clearance 28.5 ± 13mL/min), and relatively normal iPTH (59 ± 49pg/mL). It was concluded that renal osteodystrophy varies with progression of CKD and that osteoporosis is frequent in earlier stages. However, progression to stages 4 and 5 is associated with decreased prevalence of osteoporosis and an increase in secondary hyperparathyroidism, which may overcome the possible contribution of osteoporosis.

Conclusions

So far, we may conclude that given the high prevalence of CKD, osteopenia, and osteoporosis in the increasing population of middle and older age people it is plausible that osteoporosis plays an important role in the final picture of the CKD-related bone disease. This is particularly during the earlier stages of the disease when the consequences of CKD-dependent deranged mineral metabolism are not so evident. However, with progression of CKD, bone histology will be more an expression of the predominant status of bone turnover, which may mask earlier alterations of bone, such as those determined by age or hormonal related osteoporosis. Unfortunately, the results of the very few studies in which correlation of bone histology and BMD have been examined suggest that with the available methodology it is still very unlikely to differentiate between osteoporosis and the bone loss that follows the mineral and bone metabolic alterations induced by CKD.

Treatment and prevention of osteoporosis and fractures in uremic patients

The approach to the management of the CKD patient, who may have MBD-CKD, osteoporosis/osteopenia, or both, is far from straightforward. The physician must handle both conceptual complexity and practical uncertainty, and often needs to make therapeutic decisions based on remarkably thin evidence.

Certain general points apply to all patients.

- *Osteoporosis/MBD-CKD* is not a condition that may be considered and treated in isolation—there are many important links between MBD-CKD and other components of the clinical syndromes that accompany CKD, in particular cardiovascular disease, and the high morbidity and mortality resulting from this. These links appear to operate at the level of causation and it is possible that therapeutic choices in the treatment of MBD-CKD will show significant outcome implications for the cardiovascular components of the CKD syndrome.

- *Patient level outcomes* following the available therapeutic interventions are poorly documented, and in most cases not established at all. There is, therefore, heavy reliance on various surrogates for hard endpoints, as well as an understandable tendency to base therapies on the underlying pathogenesis and the predicted response of this to specific interventions. The detachment that exists between effects of treatment on surrogate markers and those on hard endpoints is considerable in the case of skeletal outcomes and, at the time of writing, universal in the case of cardiovascular and survival outcomes.

- *Patients who have CKD* are not excluded from developing other important causes of secondary osteoporosis. Prominent amongst these are drug-induced bone disease, in particular glucocorticoid and calcineurin inhibitor-related side effects. Vitamin D deficiency, thyroid disease, diabetes mellitus, endogenous Cushing's disease and sex hormone deficiency (androgen and estrogen) are all potential contributors to osteoporosis in the non-renal population and it is likely that they contribute in the CKD population as well. Those conditions require treatment on their merits.

Two further general observations should be made. First, there is good evidence that some potentially relevant surrogates can be improved considerably by appropriate therapies. Examples are hyperphosphatemia, hypo- or hypercalcemia, and hyperparathyroidism. A number of these interventions have favorable effects on disordered bone metabolism at the ultra structural level. For example, therapies used to treat severe hyperparathyroidism dramatically improve abnormally increased bone turnover. The problem is that, impressive though these responses may be, they have not been shown convincingly to translate to any beneficial patient level outcome.

Osteoporosis/osteopenia is conventionally diagnosed by measurements of BMD judged against population criteria published by the WHO. This approach has proved very effective in non renal populations, amongst whom BMD is a good surrogate for fracture risk, and treatment related improvements to BMD correlate reasonably well with reduction of fracture risk. Because there is moderately good evidence that these relationships exist in the early stages of CKD, it is reasonable to hope that the application of demonstrably effective treatments in the non CKD population will also reap benefits for the early CKD population as well. 'Early' in this context implies CKD up to and including stage 3. However, at CKD stage 4 and above, these associations break down with important implications both for diagnosis and treatment—in these groups there remains a complete lack of outcome-based data to establish efficacy of standard therapies for osteoporosis/osteopenia.

Specific therapies

Anti-resorptive agents

Bisphosphonates

There is now quite good prospective evidence demonstrating the efficacy of bisphosphonates given to patients with GFR down to 30mL/min. In most of these patients the reduction of GFR was attributable to age rather than to identify intrinsic nephropathies. In these patient groups, bisphosphonate treatment is associated with improvement of both bone mineral density and fracture rates.[40,41] These encouraging findings are supported by the excellent safety record of these agents in general, and also in patients with moderate levels of age related renal impairment. Whether these encouraging safety profiles apply to patients with CKD stage 2 and 3 resulting from underlying nephropathies is less clear, although significant numbers of patients with diabetes have been included within the studies and some of these would undoubtedly have had underlying diabetic nephropathy.[42,43] In patients with CKD stage 4 and 5 the position is much less clear. There are no hard data in support of bisphosphonates leading to reduction in fracture rate at CKD stage 5. At stage 4, *post hoc* analyses of two large studies point to efficacy of risedronate[44] and alendronate[45] with acceptable safety up to 3 years. Furthermore, there are credible theoretical concerns regarding skeletal safety—a substantial proportion of these patients will manifest abnormally low bone turnover or even full blown adynamic bone disease. It is implausible to think that bisphosphonates would enhance bone metabolism in these patients and conversely it is quite likely that these agents would further reduce low bone turnover, potentially making the lesion more intractable. Based on available data there is, therefore, no real justification for using bisphosphonates in patients with CKD 4 or worse, notwithstanding that given in these groups bisphosphonates are likely to be 'off label' in many countries. Some authors have suggested reducing the dose in patients with CKD. The initial clearance of an administered dose is skeletal and renal at a ratio of roughly 50:50 with some variation between the different bisphosphonates. It is likely, although not established, that this ratio moves in favor of bone as the GFR falls. If so, dose reduction is logical, though no data exist to support maintenance of efficacy at lower doses in CKD patients.

Raloxifene

A similar approach has been used in the case of raloxifene, a selective estrogen receptor modulator (SERM) used extensively as treatment for osteoporosis.[46] *Post hoc* subgroup analyses of the large amount of raloxifene data suggest that this treatment is effective, although efficacy is less convincing. In another study, Hernandez et al.[47] showed that after 1 year on raloxifene, post-menopausal women on hemodialysis had a significant increase in trabecular BMD, decrease in bone resorption markers, suggesting that SERMs could constitute a therapeutic alternative to improve bone metabolism. However, the possible long-term effects of raloxifene in CKD patients remain to be determined.

Estrogens

No studies on the effects of estrogen specifically examining the CKD population have been published, or at least no studies of sufficient size exist. The very large studies of estrogen therapy in non-renal post-menopausal women with osteoporosis were conducted over two decades ago. Subgroup analyses of those enrolees with moderate renal insufficiency could extract relevant data applicable to patients with kidney disease up to stage 3. In the absence of such data there remains doubt as to the utility of estrogen in any patient group manifesting significant reduction of GFR.

RANKL antagonists and osteoprotegerin

These new therapies offer the prospect of potent and selective inhibition of osteoclastogenesis. Emerging data in the non renal population attest to their efficacy and safety.[48] The participants in this study were women aged 60–90 years and, although not explicitly stated, it is inevitable that many would have had GFR in the CKD 4 and probably 3 range. Nevertheless, as yet there is no clear information as to their utility and safety in the CKD population.

Calcitonin

No data attest to the efficacy of calcitonin in patients with CKD. It seems unlikely that calcitonin would be any more effective than bisphosphonates in these scenarios and the reservations about anti-resorptives in patients who may have low turnover bone disease would also apply to calcitonin. It is difficult, therefore, to see a role for calcitonin in these patients.

Vitamin D

Native vitamin D

Ample evidence points to the endemic nature of vitamin D insufficiency and overt deficiency in the CKD population. Given the wide range of actions of vitamin D and its metabolites, in bone and other tissues, it seems intuitive to correct vitamin D deficiency when identified. There is, however, no outcome level evidence that this measure improves either skeletal or cardiovascular health, although many indirect lines of evidence would support this action. The doses required to achieve vitamin D sufficiency in all treated subjects are considerably higher than those generally recommended hitherto, typically in the order of 20 to 30,000 units of cholecalciferol per week.[49]

Active vitamin D compounds

These agents are highly effective for the treatment of hyperparathyroidism, serving to reduce accelerated bone turnover and improve some of the histological and radiological manifestations of hyperparathyroid bone disease. It is disappointing to note, therefore, that no study has documented a reduction of fracture rate in patients so treated. These compounds should also be considered in the wider context of their pleotrophic actions on a background of very large historical cohort studies apparently showing important associations between treatment with active vitamin D compounds and survival.[50] Although prospective data are lacking, there is a strengthening case for the administration of active vitamin D compounds to all patients in whom there is no obvious contra indication. The problem with this approach is that, with low bone turnover and adynamic bone disease highly prevalent in the CKD 5D population, this would be expected to deteriorate further under the influence of active vitamin D therapy, particularly if given at pharmacological doses. Set against this is the apparent maintenance of survival benefit across the whole range of PTH from severe hyperparathyroidism down to over suppressed PTH with underlying low turnover bone disease.

Calcimimetics

These agents are highly effective for the treatment of hyperparathyroidism in CKD. These benefits are largely confined to patients with advanced disease on dialysis while their use in patients with earlier stages of CKD has not been particularly successful, mainly as a result of exacerbating hyperphosphatemia. A very large prospective study (EVOLVE) is underway to examine the effect of cinacalcet on a composite endpoint of cardiovascular outcomes. This study will be large enough, however, for any clinically meaningful effects on fracture rate to be identified as well. There are grounds for optimism in that a post hoc analysis of four randomized prospective studies of cinacalcet versus conventional treatment for hyperparathyroidism showed a 50% reduction in fracture rate.[51] It remains to be seen whether that preliminary observation, to date the only one showing a marked effect on fracture in dialysed patients, is supported by the more robust studies now underway.

Conclusions

From the available data we can conclude that, with the possible exception of cinacalcet in patients with moderate and severe hyperparathyroidism, there is no basis for the treatment of osteoporosis/osteopenia or CKD-MBD in the expectation that fracture rates will be reduced in CKD 4–5 patients. There is, however, a fairly convincing evidence base for the use of bisphosphonates in patients with CKD stage 3 or less. In this group, fracture rates appear to fall in bisphosphonate treated patients and the therapy appears to be tolerated as well as in the non-CKD population.

There remains an urgent need for more prospective studies to fill the extensive gaps in the present evidence base. Until then the established therapeutic options will remain limited.

References

1. Moe SM. Vascular calcification and renal osteodystrophy relationship in chronic kidney disease. *Eur J Clin Invest* 2006;**36**(Suppl 2):51–62.
2. Hruska KA, Saab G, Mathew S, Lund R. Renal osteodystrophy, phosphate homeostasis, and vascular calcification. *Semin Dial* 2007;**20**:309–15.
3. Moe S, Drüeke T, Cunningham J, et al. Definition, evaluation, and classification of renal osteodystrophy: a position statement from Kidney Disease: Improving Global Outcomes (KDIGO). *Kidney Int* 2006;**69**:1945–53.

4. World Health Organisation. *Guidelines for Preclinical Evaluation and Clinical Trials in Osteoporosis.* Geneva: WHO, 1998.

5. Malluche HH, Faugere MC (eds). *Atlas of Mineralized Bone Histology.* Basel: Karger, 1986.

6. Adams JE. Dual energy X-ray absorptiometry. In: . SGrampp (ed.), *Radiology of Osteoporosis,* 2nd edn. Berlin: Springer, 2008:105–24.

7. World Health Organisation Study Group. *Assessment of fracture risk and its application to screening for postmenopausal osteoporosis, WHO Technical Report Series 843.* Geneva, WHO, 1994.

8. Kanis JA, Oden A, Johansson H, Borgström F, Ström O, McCloskey E. FRAX and its applications to clinical practice. *Bone* 2009;**44:**734–43.

9. Compston J, Cooper A, Cooper C, et al. National Osteoporosis Guideline Group (NOGG). Guidelines for the diagnosis and management of osteoporosis in postmenopausal women and men from the age of 50 years in the UK. *Maturitas* 2009;**62:**105–8.

10. Tosteson AN, Melton LJ 3rd, Dawson-Hughes B, et al. National Osteoporosis Foundation Guide Committee. Cost-effective osteoporosis treatment thresholds: the United States perspective. *Osteoporos Int* 2008;**1:**437–47.

11. Seeman E, Delmas PD. Bone quality—the material and structural basis of bone strength and fragility. *N Engl J Med* 2006;**354:**2250–61.

12. Steven R. Cummings, MD, Discussant, *J Am Med Ass* 2006;**296:**2601–10.

13. Marshall D, Johnell O, Wedel H. Meta-analysis of how well measures of bone density predict occurrence of osteoporotic fractures. *Br Med J* 1996;**312:**1254–9.

14. Adams JE, Bishop N. *Dual energy X-ray absorptiometry (DXA) in adults and children,* American Society of Bone and Mineral Research (ASBMR) Primer on the Metabolic Bone Diseases and Disorders of Mineral Metabolism. ASBMR, Philadelphia, 2009:152–8.

15. Weber LT, Mehls O. Limitations of dual x-ray absorptiometry in children with chronic kidney disease. *Pediatr Nephrol* 2009;Jul 15. [Epub ahead of print.]

16. Lewiecki EM, Gordon CM, Baim S, et al. International Society for Clinical Densitometry 2007 Adult and Pediatric Official Positions. *Bone* 2008;**43:**1115–21.

17. Bianchi ML, Baim S, Bishop NJ, et al. Official positions of the International Society for Clinical Densitometry (ISCD) on DXA evaluation in children and adolescents. *Pediatr Nephrol* 2009;Jul 15. [Epub ahead of print.]

18. Engelke K, Adams JE, Armbrecht G, et al. Clinical use of quantitative computed tomography and peripheral quantitative computed tomography in the management of osteoporosis in adults: the 2007 ISCD Official Positions. *J Clin Densitom* 2008;**11:**123–62.

19. Adams JE. Quantitative computed tomography. *Eur J Radiol* 2009;**71:**415–24.

20. Bauer JS, Link TM Advances in osteoporosis imaging. *Eur J Radiol* 2009;**71:**440–9.

21. Nickolas TL, Leonard MB, Shane E. Chronic kidney disease and bone fracture: a growing concern. *Kidney Int* 2008;**74:**721–31.

22. Leonard MB A structural approach to skeletal fragility in chronic kidney disease. *Semin Nephrol* 2009;**29:**133–43.

23. Miller PD Is there a role for bisphosphonates in chronic kidney disease? *Semin Dial* 2007;**20**(3):186–90.

24. Jamal SA, Hayden JA, Beyene J. Low bone mineral density and fractures in long-term hemodialysis patients: a meta-analysis. *Am J Kidney Dis* 2007;**49:**674–81.

25. Andress DL. Adynamic bone in patients with chronic kidney disease. *Kidney Int* 2008;**73:**1345–54.

26. Cannata Andía JB Adynamic bone and chronic renal failure: an overview. *Am J Med Sci* 2000;**320**:81–4.

27. Fletcher S, Jones RG, Rayner HC, et al. Assessment of renal osteodystrophy in dialysis patients: use of bone alkaline phosphatase, bone mineral density and parathyroid ultrasound in comparison with bone histology. *Nephron* 1997;**75**:412–19.

28. Atsumi K, Kushida K, Yamazaki K, et al. Risk factors for vertebral fractures in renal osteodystrophy. *Am J Kidney Dis* 1999;**33**:287–93.

29. Alem AM, Sherrard DJ, Gillen DL, et al. Increased risk of hip fracture among patients with end-stage renal disease. *Kidney Int* 2000;**58**:396–9.

30. Nickolas TL, MacMahon DLJ, Shane E. Relationship between moderate to severe kidney disease and hip fracture in the United States. *J Am Soc Nephrol* 2006;**17**:3223–32.

31. United States Renal Data System. *USRDS 2002 Annual Data Report.* Bethesda: National Institutes of Health, National Institute of Diabetes and Digestive and Renal Diseases, 2002.

32. Zoccali C, Kramer A, Jager K. The databases: renal replacement therapy since 1989—the European Renal Association and European Dialysis and Transplant Association (ERA-EDTA) *Clin J Am Soc Nephrol.* 2009, **4** (Supp 1):S18–22.

33. Mazzuchi N, Gonzalez-Martınez, Schwedt E, et al. Incidence and prevalence of the treatment of end stage renal disease in Latin America. *Nefrol Latinoam* 1999;**6**:154–9.

34. Crans GG, Genant HK, Krege JH. Prognostic utility of a semiquantitative spinal deformity index. *Bone* 2005;**37**:175–9.

35. Cocco M, Rush H. Increased incidence of hip fractures in dialysis patients with low serum parathyroid hormone. *Am J Kidney Dis* 2002;**36**:1115–21.

36. Cunningham J, Sprague SM, Cannata-Andia J, et al. Osteoporosis Work Group. Osteoporosis in chronic kidney disease. *Am J Kidney Dis* 2004;**43**:566–71.

37. Boling E, Primavera C, Friedman G, et al. Non-invasive measurements of bone mass in adult renal osteodystrophy. *Bone* 1993;**14**:409–13.

38. Lobão R, Carvalho AB, Cuppari L, et al. High prevalence of low bone mineral density in pre-dialysis chronic kidney disease patients: bone histomorphometric analysis. *Clin Nephrol* 2004;**62**:432–9.

39. Rojas E, Infante M, Hernández G, et al. The pattern of renal osteodystrophy in progressive chronic kidney disease (CKD): from stage 3 to stage 5 (Abstract). *ASN Renal Week*, 2008.

40. Eisman JA, Civetelli R, Adami S, et al. Efficacy and tolerability of intravenous ibandronate injections in postmenopausal osteoporosis: 2-year results from the DIVA study. *J Rheumatol* 2008;**35**:488–97.

41. Black DM, Delmas PD, Eastell RR, et al. Once yearly zoledronic acid for treatment of postmenopausal osteoporosis. *N Engl J Med* 2007;**356**:1809–22.

42. Lewiecki EM, Miller PD. Renal safety of intravenous bisphosphonates in the treatment of osteoporosis. *Expert Opin Drug Saf* 2007;**6**:663–72.

43. Perazella MA, Markowitz GS. Bisphosphonate nephrotoxicity. *Kidney Int* 2008;**74**:1385–93.

44. Miller PD, Roux C, Boonen S, Barton I, Dunlap L, Burgio D. Safety and efficacy of risedronate in patients with age-related reduced renal function as estimated by the Cockcroft and Gault method: a pooled analysis of nine clinical trials. *J Bone Miner Res* 2005;**20**:2015–115.

45. Jamal SA, Bauer DC, Ensrud KE, et al. Alendronate treatment in women with normal to severely impaired renal function: an analysis of the fracture intervention trial. *J Bone Miner Res* 2007;**22**:503–8.

46. Ishani A, Blackwell T, Jamal SA, Cummings SR, Ensrud KE. MORE Investigators. The effect of raloxifene treatment in postmenopausal women with CKD. *J Am Soc Nephrol* 2008;**19**:1430–88.

47. Hernandez E, Valera R, Alonzo E, et al. Effects of raloxifene on bone metabolism and serum lipids in postmenopausal women on chronic hemodialysis. *Kidney Int* 2003;**63**:2269–74.

48. Cummings SR, San Martin J, McClung MR, et al. The FREEDOM Trial* Denosumab for Prevention of Fractures in Postmenopausal Women with Osteoporosis. *N Engl J Med* 2009;**361**:1–10.

49. Heaney RP. Vitamin D in health and disease. *Clin J Am Soc Nephrol* 2008;**3**:1535–41.

50. Teng M, Wolf M, Ofsthun MN, et al. activated injectable vitamin D and hemodialysis survival: a historical cohort study. *J Am Soc Nephrol* 2005;**16**:1115–25.

51. Cunningham J, Danese M, Olson K, Klassen P, Chertow GM. Effects of the calcimimetic cinacalcet HCl on cardiovascular disease, fracture, and health-related quality of life in secondary hyperparathyroidism. *Kidney Int* 2005;**68**:1793–800.

Chapter 15

Acidosis and renal bone disease

David A. Bushinsky

Clinical relevance

In humans the daily cellular metabolism of dietary amino acids leads to production of ~1mmol/kg of acid (protons, H^+), so called endogenous acid production.[1] Additional endogenous acid production occurs during pathophysiological conditions including diabetic ketoacidosis and lactic acidosis. This additional acid results in a reduction of systemic pH, secondary to a reduction in blood bicarbonate concentration [HCO_3^-], which is termed metabolic acidosis. The physiological response to metabolic acidosis is to rapidly increase in extracellular fluid pH toward the physiologic neutral of 7.40 in order to maintain optimal cellular function.[1] This homeostatic response to metabolic acidosis involves first buffering of the acid, then increasing respiratory rate to lower the partial pressure of carbon dioxide (PCO_2) and finally renal excretion of the additional acid. The initial step, buffering of the additional acid, is critical to the immediate restoration toward neutral pH allowing the preservation of life. The final step, renal excretion of the acid, begins hours after the acid challenge and is complete only days later. Renal acid excretion relies upon normal kidney function; as we age our ability to excrete acid declines and humans become slightly, but significantly, more acidemic.[2]

During *in vivo* acute metabolic acidosis [HCO_3^-], ~60% of the administered hydrogen ions are buffered outside of the extracellular fluid by soft tissues and by bone.[1] The *in vivo* evidence that bone acutely buffers hydrogen ions and, in the process, releases calcium, derives principally from the loss of bone sodium and/or potassium, and carbonate, and the increase in serum calcium observed during acute metabolic acidosis.[3-5] Bone sodium (or potassium) loss implies hydrogen for sodium (or potassium) exchange and carbonate loss indicates consumption of this buffer by the administered acid. As the vast majority of body calcium is contained within the bone mineral, the increase in serum calcium almost certainly is derived from mineral stores.

Chronic metabolic acidosis, found in patients with chronic kidney disease and renal tubular acidosis, increases urinary calcium excretion secondary to a direct reduction in renal tubular calcium reabsorption.[1] There is little, if any increase in intestinal calcium absorption resulting in a net loss of body calcium.[1] The source of much of this additional urinary calcium appears to be acid-mediated dissolution and resorption of bone mineral.[1,6] Chronic metabolic acidosis decreases bone mineral content[6] and has been shown to significantly decrease bone density, formation and growth.[7] Patients with proximal renal tubular acidosis, a defect in renal acid excretion, are shorter in height and have decreased radial bone densities and thinner iliac cortices than unaffected relatives.[8] Patients with distal renal tubular acidosis have a lower bone mineral density in most areas when compared with normal controls and also had a decreased bone formation rate.[7] After treating these patients with the base $KHCO_3$ for 1 year, bone mineral density significantly improved in the trochanter, and total femur and bone formation rate normalized.[9]

During the ongoing metabolic acidosis of severe chronic kidney disease, blood pH remains stable, although substantially reduced, in spite of progressive acid retention, suggesting the availability of large stores of proton buffers.[1] During renal failure there is ample clinical evidence that acidosis adversely affects bone, which may be corrected by HCO_3^- treatment. Bone carbonate is decreased in acidic, uremic patients,[10] which may represent dissolution of bone carbonate or replacement by phosphate, resulting in the incorporation of acid into the mineral. In view of the deleterious effect of metabolic acidosis on bone, the National Kidney Foundation has published evidence-based guidelines that recommend treatment of metabolic acidosis to help prevent renal osteodystrophy.[11]

In addition to its effects on existing bone, metabolic acidosis also affects de novo bone formation. The independent effect of acidosis to suppress bone formation was elegantly demonstrated in children with renal tubular acidosis.[12] McSherry et al. found that 6 of 10 children with renal tubular acidosis were short (height < 2.5 SD), 2 were too young for it to be determined if they were short (< 2 weeks old) and 2 were previously not acidemic.[12] With alkali therapy each patient attained and maintained normal stature, the mean height increased from 1.4 to 37th percentile and the rate of growth increased 2–3-fold.

The common high protein diet of North Americans, coupled with the known effects of bone to buffer an acid load,[1] coupled to the age-related decline in renal function,[2] has led to the suggestion that excess dietary acid derived from the high protein diets may play a role in the etiology of osteoporosis.[1,13] Treatment of post-menopausal women with the base $KHCO_3$, which neutralizes endogenous acid production, leads to improved calcium retention, reduced bone resorption, and increased bone formation.[13,14] Severe, life-threatening metabolic acidosis must be treated; however, the mild metabolic acidosis present in the initial stages of chronic kidney disease and in aging, worsened in the latter case by the common acidogenic high protein diet, is rarely treated.[1]

Acute acidosis

Calcium release

Cultured calvariae exhibit acid dependent net calcium efflux (J_{Ca}) during both acute (3h)[15] and more chronic (>24–99h) incubations.[3,16–30] The mechanism of acid-mediated calcium efflux from bone during acute incubations is direct physicochemical calcium release and not cell-mediated.[16] This finding was confirmed by demonstrating calcium efflux from synthetic carbonated apatite (CAP) disks, a cell-free model of bone mineral, cultured in physiologically acid medium.[31]

The type of bone mineral in equilibrium with the medium, and thus altered by physicochemical forces might be carbonate or phosphate in association with calcium. Bone carbonate is solubilized during an acute reduction in pH leading to a release of calcium.[32,33] Further support for the role of carbonate in acid-mediated bone mineral dissolution comes from the observation that at a constant pH, whether physiologically neutral or acid, calcium flux from bone is dependent on the medium $[HCO_3^-]$; the lower the $[HCO_3^-]$, the greater the Ca efflux.[34]

Hydrogen ion buffering

The *in vitro* evidence for acid buffering by bone is derived from studies of acidosis-induced proton flux into bone,[5,15,32,35,36] ion microprobe evidence for a depletion of bone sodium and potassium during acidosis,[3–5,37–39] and from a depletion of bone carbonate and phosphate during acidosis.[5] When calvariae are cultured in medium acidified by a decrease in $[HCO_3^-]$, there is a net influx of protons into bone, decreasing medium acidity and indicating that the additional acid is being buffered by bone, ultimately leading to an increase in medium pH.[5,15,32,35,36] During acute acidosis there appear to be two principal mechanisms by which the acid is buffered: protons for sodium and/or potassium exchange,[3–5,37–39] and consumption of the buffers carbonate and phosphate.[5,15,32–34,40]

Proton for sodium and/or potassium exchange

Bone is a reservoir for sodium and potassium, and its surface has fixed negative sites, which normally complex with sodium, potassium and hydrogen.[41] A high resolution scanning ion microprobe was used to determine how protons alter the ion composition of bone mineral.[3–5,37–40,42–46] The calvarial surface is rich in sodium and potassium relative to calcium.[3–5,37–40,42–46] The excess mineral potassium is maintained through cell-mediated processes.[42] A model of metabolic acidosis causes release of bone calcium, and leads to a decrease in the surface ratio of sodium to calcium and potassium to calcium, indicating a greater relative release of mineral sodium and potassium than calcium.[38] To better understand the effects of acidosis on potassium relative to calcium, the mineral was labeled *in vivo* with the stable isotope ^{41}K and we found that mineral is indeed rich in potassium relative to calcium and that acidosis induces a fall in the ratio of $^{41}K/Ca$, indicating loss of this stable isotope from the bone mineral.[4]

Fall in bone carbonate and phosphate

Bone contains ≈80% of the total carbon dioxide in the body and acute metabolic acidosis decreases bone total carbon dioxide.[47] Bone also contains a substantial amount of the total body phosphate, estimated to be ~90%,[48] largely in the form of hydroxyapatite $[Ca_{10}(PO_4)_6(OH)_2]$ and other forms of apatite.[49] During metabolic acidosis, protonation of the phosphate in apatite will consume protons and help restore the pH toward normal.[1,50,51] Using chemical analysis we found that a model of metabolic acidosis induces the release of bone calcium and carbonate[32] leading to a progressive loss of bone carbonate.[33]

The microprobe was used to study the bone content of carbonate and phosphate in response to a model of acute metabolic acidosis.[5] There was a marked preferential loss of surface HCO_3^- and of cross-sectional phosphate. When both the *in vitro* and *in vivo* studies are considered together, there is clear evidence that bone is a proton buffer capable of maintaining the extracellular fluid pH near the physiological normal. The loss of bone sodium, potassium, carbonate, and phosphate suggests that in addition to sodium and potassium for proton exchange, bone carbonate and phosphate are lost from the mineral in response to acidosis, each of which helps to restore the pH toward normal.

Chronic acidosis

Increased bone resorption

Chronic metabolic acidosis induces the release of bone calcium, predominantly by enhanced cell–mediated bone resorption and decreased bone formation,[3,17–21,24–28, 36,40,46,52] although there continues to be a component of direct physicochemical acid-induced dissolution.[4,5,15,16,31–35,37–39,52,53] Osteoblastic collagen synthesis and alkaline phosphatase activity both are decreased after 48h incubation in a model of metabolic acidosis compared with neutral medium,[18] while the ligand for the osteoclast receptor activator of NFκB (RANKL) synthesis was increased.[26,30] Release of osteoclastic β-glucuronidase, a lysosomal enzyme whose secretion correlates with osteoclast-mediated bone resorption, is increased during culture in medium modeling metabolic acidosis. Conversely, an increase in $[HCO_3^-]$, modeling metabolic alkalosis, decreases calcium efflux from bone through an increase in osteoblastic bone formation and a decrease in osteoclastic bone resorption.[20]

Further support for a direct effect of metabolic acidosis to regulate osteoblastic function was obtained using primary cells isolated from the calvariae. These isolated cells, almost exclusively osteoblasts, synthesize collagen, and form nodules of apatitic bone.[52] Compared with cells incubated in neutral medium, cells incubated in a model of metabolic acidosis produced fewer nodules and had decreased calcium influx into the nodules.[52]

In addition to the acidosis that occurs during clinical chronic kidney disease, there is also often an increase in parathyroid hormone (PTH) secretion.[54] Acidosis and PTH independently stimulated calcium efflux from bone, inhibited osteoblastic collagen synthesis and stimulated osteoclastic β-glucuronidase secretion. In the presence of acidosis + PTH there was a greater effect on each of these parameters than either alone[21] suggesting an additive deleterious effect of PTH and acidosis on bone.

Mechanism of proton signaling

Bone responds to metabolic acidosis through a coordinated homeostatic response aimed at normalizing systemic pH, often at the cost of decreased mineral content; however, the mechanism by which extracellular pH is sensed was previously not clear. A novel class of G-protein coupled receptors that respond to both protons and lysosphingolipids has been recently characterized.[55] This family includes the ovarian G-protein coupled receptor 1 (OGR1), GPR4, T-cell death-associated gene 8 (TDAG8), and G2A, which share 40–50% homology. Activation of OGR1 and G2A by decreased pH leads to inositol phosphate (IP) accumulation, while GPR4 and TDAG8 are coupled to cAMP formation. However, the activation of G2A shows little pH dependence and H$^+$ sensing may be a minor role for this receptor.

To test the hypothesis that OGR1 acts as an H$^+$ sensing receptor in bone cells[22] we first demonstrated that OGR1 was present in cultured neonatal mouse calvariae and then investigated whether an inhibitor of OGR1 (CuCl$_2$) would diminish acidosis-induced Ca efflux from bone, whether metabolic acidosis would increase intracellular calcium in cultured bone cells, and if transfection of OGR1 into a heterologous cell type would permit cells to mimic the intracellular calcium response to acidosis of primary bone cells.[22] We found that CuCl$_2$ inhibits the acidosis-induced increase in calcium efflux from bone cells and that primary mouse calvarial bone cells respond to a decrease in extracellular pH with an increase in intracellular calcium. We then found that Chinese hamster ovary fibroblasts (CHO cells) increased intracellular calcium in response to a model of metabolic acidosis only after being transfected with murine OGR1 cDNA. These data are consistent with a primary role for OGR1 as a proton sensor in bone cells.

Role of PGE$_2$

Acidosis increases the level of prostaglandins in a variety of model systems. In both toad bladder and rat kidney, PGE$_2$ levels increase in response to chronic metabolic acidosis, leading to enhanced acid excretion. In the rat, acute metabolic acidosis increases urinary prostaglandin excretion, which may regulate renal ammonia synthesis and acid excretion. Prostaglandins, especially PGE$_2$, are potent multifunctional regulators with complex effects on both bone resorption and formation. Prostaglandins have been shown to promote new bone formation *in vivo* and in isolated osteoblasts. However, in bone organ culture PGE$_2$, the most abundant eicosanoid in bone, has been shown to directly stimulate bone resorption and to stimulate RANKL expression in calvarial osteoblasts. The relative effects of prostaglandins on bone may be dependent on timing or magnitude of dose,[56] as has been found for PTH or dependent on stage of osteoblast differentiation. Thus, on the cellular and molecular level, regulation of PGE$_2$ remains important to understand the intracellular mechanisms of action of acidosis in the osteoblast.

Incubation of neonatal mouse calvariae in acidic medium increases medium PGE$_2$ in parallel with an increase in net calcium efflux.[27] Inhibition of PGE$_2$ production by indomethacin strongly limited this acidosis-induced bone calcium release, as well as acid stimulation of RANKL.[26] Culture of calvariae in neutral pH medium with an amount of exogenous PGE$_2$ similar to that found in medium of calvariae incubated in medium modeling metabolic acidosis induces net Ca efflux from bone.[27] Incubation of primary mouse calvarial bone cells, which consist mostly of osteoblasts,[57] in a model of metabolic acidosis led to a marked increase in medium PGE$_2$ levels, which was again completely suppressed by indomethacin.[27] The magnitude of this acid-induced increase in medium PGE_2 levels was comparable with that observed in cultured calvariae incubated in acid medium. Cortisol inhibits acid-induced bone resorption through a decrease in osteoblastic PGE_2 production. These results suggest that acid-induced, cell-mediated calcium efflux from bone is regulated, at least in part, by an increase in endogenous PGE_2 production in the osteoblast leading to an increase in RANKL.

Prostaglandin synthesis is regulated by the release of arachidonic acid from membrane phospholipids. The rate limiting step converting arachidonic acid to specific prostanoids is catalysed by prostaglandin G/H synthase, also called cyclo oxygenase (COX). There are two forms of COX: COX1, which is constitutively expressed, and COX2, which is the inducible form of the enzyme. Both forms of COX are expressed in osteoblasts. COX2 expression is regulated by several bone-resorbing factors, including interleukin-1, PTH, interleukin-6, TGF-α and TNF-α, and basic fibroblast growth factor. NS-398, a specific COX2 inhibitor, significantly inhibits H^+-induced Ca release from calvariae, which supports the hypothesis that this enzyme is stimulated by acidosis.[27–29] We tested the effects of COX2 knockout using calvariae from the offspring of matings of COX2 +/– mice and correlating genotype and phenotype. We found that in neutral medium, bones from –/– pups (knockouts) released less calcium than did bones from +/+ (wild type) mice. A model of metabolic acidosis stimulated calcium efflux from bones from +/+ and +/– (heterozygotes), but did not stimulate calcium efflux from –/– bones. The extent of calcium release in a model of metabolic acidosis was less from +/– and –/– bones than from +/+ bones and release from –/– bones was less than release from +/– bones. Thus, COX2 is necessary for acid-induced bone calcium release and it appears that the gene dosage of COX2 sets the level of basal and of H^+-induced bone resorption. Using northern analysis, as well as real-time PCR, incubation of primary bone cells in Met causes greater stimulation of COX2 RNA levels than in Ntl, with no change in COX1.[29]

Regulation of gene expression

External pH modulates gene expression in several cell types. Metabolic acidosis induces rat renal cells to increase ammonia production, increases the RNA expression of the sodium/citrate cotransporter NaDC-1, and the Na/H exchangers NHE3 and NHE2 in renal cells. To determine if metabolic acidosis would alter specific gene expression in osteoblasts we examined several immediate early response genes in primary neonatal mouse calvarial cells, including egr-1, junB, c-jun, junD, and c-fos. In response to incubation in acidic medium, only the magnitude of egr-1 stimulation was dependent on medium pH.[23] Osteoblasts express type 1 collagen as the major component of the bone extracellular matrix, which subsequently becomes mineralized. Similarly to egr-1, type I collagen RNA synthesis was decreased by acidosis and increased by alkalosis.[23]

Primary mouse calvarial cells differentiate in culture to form bone nodules. These osteoblastic cells express a number of bone specific matrix proteins, including bone sialoprotein, osteocalcin, osteonectin (ON), osteopontin (OPN), and matrix Gla protein (MGP).[58] Since acidic medium decreases bone nodule number, size, and calcium content,[52] we hypothesized that acidosis would alter the pattern of matrix gene expression in these long term cell cultures. After 3–4 weeks in neutral medium OPN RNA levels increased, while incubation in acid medium completely inhibited this increase.[24] The RNA levels of two other proteins, ON and transforming growth factor β_1, as well as the housekeeping gene, GAPDH, did not vary with pH. RNA for MGP was also induced by incubation in neutral differentiation medium while acidic medium almost totally prevented the increase in MGP RNA levels. The inhibition of MGP and OPN RNA levels by acidosis was found to be reversible.[24]

We hypothesized that the acidosis-induced bone resorption was a result of alterations in osteoblastic expression of osteoclastogenic factors. Such factors include macrophage colony-stimulating factor (M-CSF), a growth factor for osteoclast precursor cells; RANKL, the ligand for the osteoclast receptor activator of NFκB (RANK); and osteoprotegerin (OPG), a decoy receptor for RANKL that prevents the RANK/RANKL interaction. Activation of RANK by RANKL initiates a differentiation cascade that culminates in mature, bone-resorbing osteoclasts, as well as stimulation of mature osteoclast activity and inhibition of apoptosis. Analysis of RNA extracted from calvariae incubated for 24 or 48h in neutral or acidic medium by RT-PCR indicated that expression of RANKL RNA was up-regulated by acidosis, while expression of M-CSF, OPG, and β-actin were not altered.[26] Quantitation by northern blotting confirmed that acidic medium induced an increase in RANKL RNA expression. Analysis of culture supernatants by ELISA demonstrated that calvariae in acidic medium produced greater amounts of soluble RANKL protein than calvariae cultured at neutral pH; production of OPG was not affected.[30]

To examine the role of PGE$_2$ synthesis in RANKL expression, calvariae were incubated in the absence or presence of indomethacin to inhibit COX activity; calcium flux was determined, as well as RANKL RNA content by northern analysis. Indomethacin significantly inhibited acid-induced calcium flux and completely suppressed the induction of RANKL RNA by Met.[26] Thus, acidosis-induced synthesis of PGE$_2$ causes an autocrine or paracrine stimulation of osteoblastic prostaglandin receptors. Activation of these receptors consequently induces an increase in RANKL RNA expression, which in turn increases osteoclastogenesis and activation of mature osteoclasts.

Changes in bone ion composition

Bone mineral contains approximately 4–6% carbonate which increases the reactivity of the mineral to acid. The acid-labile nature of carbonate in apatite may provide part of the explanation for the acid-mediated effects. Carbonate-containing mineral has been shown to dissolve preferentially from dental enamel (a carbonated-apatite similar to bone mineral) during the early stages of acid challenge. To better understand the chronic effects of acid on bone we established an *in vivo* model of metabolic acidosis. We utilized the ion microprobe to determine the mass spectra of important ion groups from femurs of mice acidified by drinking NH$_4$Cl for 1 week compared with mice given only dH$_2$O.[40] NH$_4$Cl is metabolized to HCl resulting in a reduction in serum [HCO$_3^-$]. We found that compared with mice given only dH$_2$O, the addition of NH$_4$Cl led to a marked change in the positive ion spectrum.[40] In control femurs there is more potassium and sodium than calcium. However, after oral NH$_4$Cl, there is a fall in the ratios of potassium and sodium relative to calcium, as in acute acidosis. With respect to the negative ions we found that there was almost as much phosphate as carbon:carbon (C_2) and carbon:nitrogen (CN) bonds in the mid-cortex of the control femurs. However, 1 week of NH_4Cl led to a fall in the ratios of phosphate to C_2 and phosphate to CN and a marked decrease in the ratio of HCO_3^- to C_2 and HCO_3^- to CN [40]. We next found that chronic acidosis induced a fall in both cross-sectional HCO_3^- and a greater fall in phosphate with no change in surface HCO_3^- and phosphate.[46]

Thus, after 7 days of *in vivo* metabolic acidosis there was an overall reduction of bone HCO_3^- and phosphate, both of which would serve to buffer the additional acid during metabolic acidosis and return the system pH toward normal. We found that over the first 3h there was a reduction in surface HCO_3^- and cross-section phosphate, while with more prolonged incubations there was a fall in cross-section HCO_3^- and phosphate, with the fall in phosphate predominating over the fall in HCO_3^-. A clear pattern of proton buffering by bone has emerged, based on our microprobe studies, in which the surface HCO_3^- and cross-section phosphates are important for acute acid buffering, while the cross-section phosphate predominates in more chronic acidosis.

Comparison of the effects of respiratory and metabolic acidosis on bone

Most *in vivo* and *in vitro* studies have utilized NH_4Cl and HCl (respectively) to decrease $[HCO_3^-]$ as a model of metabolic acidosis. This non-anion gap acidosis mimics the clinical disorders of RTA, moderate to severe diarrhea and early renal failure. pH is a function of $[HCO_3^-]$ and the partial pressure of carbon dioxide (PCO_2), as predicted by the Henderson–Hasselbalch equation. Thus, pH can be also lowered by an increase in PCO_2, to model respiratory acidosis.

There is a clear distinction between the effects of metabolic and respiratory acidosis on net bone calcium release and proton buffering. There is far greater calcium release when the medium pH is lowered by a reduction in $[HCO_3^-]$, a model of metabolic acidosis, than when there is an isohydric reduction of medium pH achieved by increasing the PCO_2, a model of respiratory acidosis.[15,17,19,25,28,32–35,37,52,53,59] We have shown that the decreased net calcium efflux in a model of respiratory, compared with metabolic, acidosis is due to decreased unidirectional calcium efflux from the mineral coupled to deposition of medium calcium on the bone surface during hypercapnia.[53] We also found decreased bone carbonate in response to a model of metabolic, but not respiratory, acidosis.[33] These results suggest that over this short time period acidosis affects the physicochemical driving forces for mineral formation and dissolution.[16,31,32,34,39] During metabolic acidosis the decreased $[HCO_3^-]$ favors dissolution, while during respiratory acidosis the increased Pco_2 and $[HCO_3^-]$ favors deposition of carbonated apatite. Indeed there is no net proton influx into bone during respiratory acidosis.[35] Extending these studies to compensated metabolic and respiratory acidosis we found that at a constant pH, whether physiologically neutral or acidic, net calcium efflux from bone is dependent on decreased $[HCO_3^-]$; the lower the medium $[HCO_3^-]$ the greater the calcium efflux from bone.[34]

During more chronic incubations, there is cell-mediated net calcium efflux from bone during metabolic, but not respiratory, acidosis.[17,19] In addition, there is increased osteoblastic PGE$_2$ and decreased osteoblastic collagen synthesis in response to metabolic, but not respiratory, acidosis.[19] Respiratory acidosis does not appreciably alter the surface ion composition of bone,[37] as does metabolic acidosis.[3,4,37–39] Respiratory acidosis also does not increase PGE$_2$ levels in calvariae, which could account for the increased cell-mediated bone resorption observed in response to metabolic, but not respiratory, acidosis.[28] Thus, in most parameters there is a fundamental difference between an isohydric lowering of pH by decreasing the [HCO$_3^-$] compared with increasing the PCO$_2$. Perhaps the newly discovered H$^+$ receptor is modified by [HCO$_3^-$]?

Overview of the response of bone to acid

Our studies have shown that metabolic acidosis induces changes in the bone mineral, which are consistent with its purported role as a proton buffer (Fig. 15.1). Initially, over the first few hours, there is buffering of the acidic medium pH[5,15,35,36] through physicochemical dissolution of bone mineral,[32,39] releasing calcium, as well as the acid buffers, carbonate, and phosphate,[5,15,33,34,40] and exchange of bone sodium and potassium for hydrogen.[3–5,37–39] Hours later, cellular mechanisms increase bone resorption and decrease bone formation, both of which help normalize systemic pH.[3,16–21] Increased bone resorption further liberates carbonate and phosphate from the mineral,[40,46] and decreased bone formation lessens the amount of acid produced during bone mineralization. The acidic pH is sensed by the proton receptor OGR1[22] and acidosis alters expression of a number of genes in osteoblasts.[23–26] Acidosis increases osteoblastic prostaglandin E$_2$ (PGE$_2$) synthesis[27–29] leading to an increase in receptor activator of NFκB-ligand (RANKL) expression and osteoclastic bone resorption.[26,30]

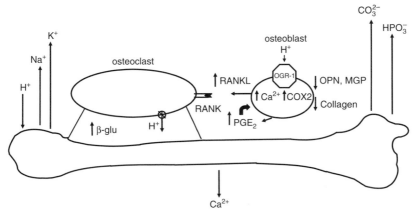

Fig. 15.1 Model of the effects of acidosis on bone. Abbreviations: H$^+$, hydrogen; Na$^+$, sodium; K$^+$, potassium; β-glu, β-glucuronidase; RANK, receptor activator of NFκB; RANKL, receptor activator of NFκB-ligand; PGE2, prostaglandin E2; Ca^{2+}, calcium; COX2, cyclo-oxygenase 2; OPN, osteopontin, MGP, matrix Gla protein; CO2, carbonate; HPO3$^-$, phosphate.

Acknowledgements

Supported by grants RO1 DK 75462 and RO1 AR 46289 from the National Institutes of Health.

References

1. Lemann J, Jr., Bushinsky DA, Hamm LL. Bone buffering of acid and base in humans. *Am J Physiol Renal Physiol* 2003;**285**:F811–32.

2. Frassetto LA, Morris RC, Jr., Sebastian A. Effect of age on blood acid-base composition in adult humans: role of age-related renal functional decline. *Am J Physiol (Renal Fluid Electrolyte Physiol 40)* 1996;**271**:F1114–22.

3. Bushinsky DA, Gavrilov K, Stathopoulos VM, Krieger NS, Chabala JM, Levi-Setti R. Effects of osteoclastic resorption on bone surface ion composition. *Am J Physiol (Cell Physiol 40)* 1996;**271**:C1025–31.

4. Bushinsky DA, Gavrilov K, Chabala JM. Featherstone JDB, Levi-Setti R. Effect of metabolic acidosis on the potassium content of bone. *J Bone Min Res* 1997;**12**:1664–71.

5. Bushinsky DA, Smith SB, Gavrilov KL, Gavrilov LF, Li J, Levi-Setti R. Acute acidosis-induced alteration in bone bicarbonate and phosphate. *Am J Physiol Renal Physiol* 2002;**283**:F1091–7.

6. Barzel US. The skeleton as an ion exchange system: Implications for the role of acid-base imbalance in the genesis of osteoporosis. *J Bone Min Res* 1995;**10**:1431–6.

7. Domrongkitchaiporn S, Pongsakul C, Stitchantrakul W, et al. Bone mineral density and histology in distal renal tubular acidosis. *Kidney Int* 2001;**59**:1086–93.

8. Lemann JJr, Adams ND, Wilz DR, Brenes LG. Acid and mineral balances and bone in familial proximal renal tubular acidosis. *Kidney Int* 2000;**58**:1267–77.

9. Domrongkitchaiporn S, Pongskul C, Sirikulchayanonta V, et al. Bone histology and bone mineral density after correction of acidosis in distal renal tubular acidosis. *Kidney Int* 2002;**62**:2160–6.

10. Pellegrino ED, Blitz RM. The composition of human bone in uremia. *Medicine* 1965;**44**:397–418.

11. National Kidney Foundation. K/DOQI clinical practice guidelines for bone metabolism and disease in chronic kidney disease. *Am J Kidney Dis* 2003;**42**:S1–201.

12. McSherry E. Acidosis and growth in nonuremic renal disease. *Kidney Int* 1978;**14**:349–54.

13. Frassetto L, Morris RC, Jr., Sebastian A. Long-term persistence of the urine calcium-lowering effect of potassium bicarbonate in postmenopausal women. *J Clin Endocrinol Metab* 2005;**90**:831–4.

14. Jehle S, Zanetti A, Muser J, Hulter HN, Krapf R. Partial neutralisation of the acidogenic western diet with potassium citrate increases bone mass in postmenopausal women with osteopenia. *J Am Soc Nephrol* 2006;**17**:3213–22.

15. Bushinsky DA, Krieger NS, Geisser DI, Grossman EB, Coe FL. Effects of pH on bone calcium and proton fluxes in vitro. *Am J Physiol (Renal Fluid Electrolyte Physiol 14)* 1983;**245**:F204–9.

16. Bushinsky DA, Goldring JM, Coe FL. Cellular contribution to pH-mediated calcium flux in neonatal mouse calvariae. *Am J Physiol (Renal Fluid Electrolyte Physiol 17)* 1985;**248**:F785–9.

17. Bushinsky DA. Net calcium efflux from live bone during chronic metabolic, but not respiratory, acidosis. *Am J Physiol (Renal Fluid Electrolyte Physiol 25)* 1989;**256**:F836–42.

18. Krieger NS, Sessler NE, Bushinsky DA. Acidosis inhibits osteoblastic and stimulates osteoclastic activity in vitro. *Am J Physiol (Renal Fluid Electrolyte Physiol 31)* 1992;**262**:F442–8.

19. Bushinsky DA. Stimulated osteoclastic and suppressed osteoblastic activity in metabolic but not respiratory acidosis. *Am J Physiol (Cell Physiol 37)* 1995;**268**:C80–8.

20. Bushinsky DA. Metabolic alkalosis decreases bone calcium efflux by suppressing osteoclasts and stimulating osteoblasts. *Am J Physiol (Renal Fluid Electrolyte Physiol 40)* 1996;**271**:F216–22.

21. Bushinsky DA, Nilsson EL. Additive effects of acidosis and parathyroid hormone on mouse osteoblastic and osteoclastic function. *Am J Physiol (Cell Physiol 38)* 1995;**269**:C1364–70.

22. Frick KK, Krieger NS, Nehrke K, Bushinsky DA. Metabolic acidosis increases intracellular calcium in bone cells through activation of the proton receptor OGR1. *J Bone Min Res* 2009;**24**:305–13.

23. Frick KK, Jiang L, Bushinsky DA. Acute metabolic acidosis inhibits the induction of osteoblastic egr-1 and type 1 collagen. *Am J Physiol (Cell Physiol 41)* 1997;**272**:C1450–6.

24. Frick KK, Bushinsky DA. Chronic metabolic acidosis reversibly inhibits extracellular matrix gene expression in mouse osteoblasts. *Am J Physiol (Renal Physiol 44)* 1998;**275**:F840–7.

25. Frick KK, Bushinsky DA. In vitro metabolic and respiratory acidosis selectively inhibit osteoblastic matrix gene expression. *Am J Physiol (Renal Physiol 46)* 1999;**277**:F750–5.

26. Frick KK, Bushinsky DA. Metabolic acidosis stimulates RANK ligand RNA expression in bone through a cyclooxygenase dependent mechanism. *J Bone Miner Res* 2003;**18**:1317–25.

27. Krieger NS, Parker WR, Alexander KM, Bushinsky DA. Prostaglandins regulate acid-induced cell-mediated bone resorption. *Am J Physiol Renal Physiol* 2000;**279**:F1077–82.

28. Bushinsky DA, Parker WR, Alexander KM, Krieger NS. Metabolic, but not respiratory, acidosis increases bone PGE_2 levels and calcium release. *Am J Physiol (Renal Fluid Electrolyte Physiol)* 2001;**281**:F1058–66.

29. Krieger NS, Frick KK, LaPlante Strutz K, Michalenka A, Bushinsky DA. Regulation of COX-2 mediates acid-induced bone calcium efflux in vitro. *J Bone Min Res* 2007;**22**:907–17.

30. Frick KK, LaPlante K, Bushinsky DA. RANK Ligand and TNF-α mediate acid-induced bone calcium efflux in vitro. *Am J Physiol Renal Physiol* 2005;**289**:F1005–11.

31. Bushinsky DA, Sessler NE, Glena RE, Featherstone JDB. Proton-induced physicochemical calcium release from ceramic apatite disks. *J Bone Miner Res* 1994;**9**:213–20.

32. Bushinsky DA, Lechleider RJ. Mechanism of proton-induced bone calcium release: calcium carbonate-dissolution. *Am J Physiol (Renal Fluid Electrolyte Physiol 22)* 1987;**253**:F998–1005.

33. Bushinsky DA, Lam BC, Nespeca R, Sessler NE, Grynpas MD. Decreased bone carbonate content in response to metabolic, but not respiratory, acidosis. *Am J Physiol (Renal Fluid Electrolyte Physiol 34)* 1993;**265**:F530–6.

34. Bushinsky DA, Sessler NE. Critical role of bicarbonate in calcium release from bone. *Am J Physiol (Renal Fluid Electrolyte Physiol 32)* 1992;**263**:F510–15.

35. Bushinsky DA. Net proton influx into bone during metabolic, but not respiratory, acidosis. *Am J Physiol (Renal Fluid Electrolyte Physiol 23)* 1988;**254**:F306–10.

36. Bushinsky DA. Effects of parathyroid hormone on net proton flux from neonatal mouse calvariae. *Am J Physiol (Renal Fluid Electrolyte Physiol 21)* 1987;**252**:F585–9.

37. Chabala JM, Levi-Setti R, Bushinsky DA. Alteration in surface ion composition of cultured bone during metabolic, but not respiratory, acidosis. *Am J Physiol (Renal Fluid Electrolyte Physiol 30)* 1991;**261**:F76–84.

38. Bushinsky DA, Levi-Setti R, Coe FL. Ion microprobe determination of bone surface elements: Effects of reduced medium pH. *Am J Physiol (Renal Fluid Electrolyte Physiol 19)* 1986;**250**: F1090–7.

39. Bushinsky DA, Wolbach W, Sessler NE, Mogilevsky R, Levi-Setti R. Physicochemical effects of acidosis on bone calcium flux and surface ion composition. *J Bone Miner Res* 1993;**8**:93–102.

40. Bushinsky DA, Chabala JM, Gavrilov KL, Levi-Setti R. Effects of in vivo metabolic acidosis on midcortical bone ion composition. *Am J Physiol (Renal Physiol 46)* 1999;**277**:F813–19.

41. Widdowson EM, Dickerson JWT. Chemical composition of the body. In: Comar CL, Bronner F (eds) *Mineral Metabolism*. New York: Academic Press, Inc., New York, 1964: 1–247.

42. Bushinsky DA, Chabala JM, Levi-Setti R. Ion microprobe analysis of mouse calvariae in vitro: evidence for a 'bone membrane'. *Am J Physiol (Endocrinol Metab 19)* 1989;**256**:E152–8.

43. Bushinsky DA, Chabala JM, Levi-Setti R. Ion microprobe analysis of bone surface elements: effects of 1,25(OH)$_2$D$_3$. *Am J Physiol (Endocrinol Met Physiol 20)* 1989;**257**:E815–22.

44. Bushinsky DA, Chabala JM, Levi-Setti R. Comparison of in vitro and in vivo [44]Ca labeling of bone by scanning ion microprobe. *Am J Physiol (Endocrinol Metab 22)* 1990;**259**:E586–92.

45. Bushinsky DA, Gavrilov KL, Chabala JM, Levi-Setti R. Contribution of organic material to the ion composition of bone. *J Bone Min Res* 2000;**15**:2026–32.

46. Bushinsky DA, Smith SB, Gavrilov KL, Gavrilov LF, Levi-Setti R. Chronic acidosis-induced alteration in bone bicarbonate and phosphate. *Am J Physiol Renal Physiol* 2003;**285**:F532–9.

47. Bettice JA. Skeletal carbon dioxide stores during metabolic acidosis. *Am J Physiol (Renal Fluid Electrolyte Physiol 16)* 1984;**247**:F326–30.

48. Bushinsky DA. Disorders of calcium and phosphorus homeostasis. In: Greenberg A (ed.), *Primer on Kidney Diseases*. San Diego: Academic Press, 2005:120–30.

49. Neuman WF, Neuman MW. *The Chemical Dynamics of Bone Mineral*. Chicago: University Chicago Press, 1958.

50. Bushinsky DA. Acid-base imbalance and the skeleton. *Eur J Nutrition* 2001;**40**:238–44.

51. Krieger NS, Frick KK, Bushinsky DA. Mechanism of acid-induced bone resorption. *Curr Opin Nephrol Hypertens* 2004;**13**:423–36.

52. Sprague SM, Krieger NS, Bushinsky DA. Greater inhibition of in vitro bone mineralization with metabolic than respiratory acidosis. *Kidney Int* 1994;**46**:1199–206.

53. Bushinsky DA, Sessler NE, Krieger NS. Greater unidirectional calcium efflux from bone during metabolic, compared with respiratory, acidosis. *Am J Physiol (Renal Fluid Electrolyte Physiol 31)* 1992;**262**:F425–31.

54. Levin A, Bakris GL, Molitch M, et al. Prevalence of abnormal serum vitamin D, PTH, calcium, and phosphorus in patients with chronic kidney disease: results of the study to evaluate early kidney disease. *Kidney Int* 2006;**71**:31–8.

55. Tomura H, Mogi C, Sato K, Okajima F. Proton-sensing and lysolipid-sensitive G-protein-coupled receptors: A novel type of multi-functional receptors. *Cell Signal* 2005;**17**:1466–76.

56. Raisz LG, Fall PM, Petersen DN, Lichtler A, Kream BE. Prostaglandin E2 inhibits alpha 1(1) procollagen gene transcription and promoter activity in the immortalised rat osteoblastic clonal cell line Py1a. *Mol Endocrin* 1993;**7**:17–22.

57. Krieger NS, Hefley TJ. Differential effects of parathyroid hormone on protein phosphorylation in two osteoblast-like cell populations isolated from neonatal mouse calvaria. *Calc Tiss Int* 1989;**44**:192–9.

58. Stein GS, Lian JB, Stein JL, van Wijnen AJ, Montecino M. Transcriptional control of osteoblast growth and differentiation (Review). *Physiol Rev* 1996;**76**:593–629.

59. Ori Y, Lee SG, Krieger NS, Bushinsky DA. Osteoblastic intracellular pH and calcium in metabolic and respiratory acidosis. *Kidney Int* 1995;**47**:1790–6.

Chapter 16

Dialysis-associated amyloidosis

T. Bardin

In 1978, Kenzora reported for the first time the identification of amyloid deposition in a carpal tunnel biopsy specimen from a patient undergoing hemodialysis.[1] From this time, dialysis-associated amyloidosis has been recognized as an increasingly significant problem in renal failure patients maintained on long-term dialysis therapies.[1,2,3] Deposits involve mainly articular and peri-articular tissues resulting in a disabling arthropathy, the frequency of which increases with length of survival upon dialysis. Amyloid arthropathy is at present considered as one of the main factors limiting the quality of life of long-term survivors. Moreover, systemic deposition and neurological compromise following destructive involvement of spine are rare, but life-threatening complications. This review will attempt to picture the features of the disease and to differentiate them from articular symptoms of other etiologies in dialysis patients.

Pathophysiology

In 1985, two groups of investigators demonstrated that ß2 microglobulin was the main component of dialysis associated amyloidosis.[4,5] Since this discovery, and even though deposits were later shown to also contain small amounts of other proteins, such as amyloid P component, proteoglycans and protease inhibitors, the accumulation of ß2 microglobulin in dialysis patients has been held to play a key role in the pathogenesis of the disease. Schematically, three factors explain ß2 microglobulin accumulation and serum concentration raise in dialysis patients:

- the normal renal catabolism of the molecule is deficient;
- elimination during dialysis sessions is not or insufficiently achieved;
- synthesis is increased following the release of cytokines from circulating monocytes in contact with dialysis membranes, the extent of this increase depending on the type of membrane and dialysate used.[6]

In vitro, ß2 microglobulin, which has a ß pleated structure, can form amyloid fibrils, at a very high concentration and acidic pH. Such acidic pH is present in the lysosomes of macrophages, but monomeric ß2 microglobulin has been shown to be extensively degraded by lysosomal enzymes, so that macrophages are very unlikely to play a role in fibril formation.[7] In contrast, macrophage enzymes appear to be inactive on ß2 microglobulin amyloid fibrils so that these cells are believed to be unable to clear amyloid deposits. The mechanism of amyloid fibril formation at neutral pH remains incompletely understood and appears, in vitro, as a two step phenomenon: a nucleation step, followed by an extension phase during which ß2 microglobulin polymerizes more rapidly into amyloid fibrils. Presently proposed mechanisms for the nucleation step include a seeding effect of truncated ß2 microglobulin fragments, which have been shown to be present in the amyloid deposits or blood of dialysis patients and could promote ß2 microglobulin fibril generation at pHs encountered in human joints.[8,9] Partial proteolysis allows unfolding of the molecule, a step which appears important in initial fibril formation. In the presence of these first fibrils full length ß2 microglobulin can form further fibrils at neutral pH, leading to amyloid deposits. *In vitro*, Cu^{2+} has also been shown partially to unfold ß2 microglobulin and enhance fibril formation.[10] This could have medical implications as some ultrafiltration membranes contain copper, which could link out to the plasma. Interestingly, collagen[11] and specific glycosaminoglycans[12] appear to promote ß2 microglobulin fibril formation at neutral pH and this could explain why amyloid deposits localize in the joints. Although not promoting fibril formation, Procollagen C-proteinase enhancer 1 (PCPE-1), which is a component of synovial tissue, has been shown to bind ß2 microglobulin and could be involved in the initial accumulation of ß2 microglobulin in joints.[13]

In 1993 Miyata et al. demonstrated that a large part of serum and amyloid deposit ß2 microglobulin in dialysis patients was modified by advanced glycation end products (AGE). Moreover, AGE modified ß2 microglobulin was latter shown in vitro to stimulate monocytes through specific receptors (RAGEs), thereby enhancing the release of inflammatory and bone resorbing cytokines.[14] The *in vitro* affinity of ß2 microglobulin has also been shown to be increased by AGE modifications of type I and IV collagen and this could contribute to the localization of amyloid in the joint.[15]

Epidemiology

Effect of duration of dialysis treatment

Clinical manifestations of ß2 microglobulin amyloid usually occur late during the course of dialysis therapy even though asymptomatic deposits may antedate the onset of symptoms and be observed early after dialysis onset[16] or even in long standing uremia, before the start of dialysis therapy.[17] Histological prevalence of amyloid deposits increases with duration of survival under dialysis treatment and was found to be 100% at 13 years of hemodialysis in one post-mortem study,[16] where most deposits appeared asymptomatic. In most of the patients with clinical features of ß2 microglobulin amyloid described in the literature, the average duration of hemodialysis was 8–12 years.[1,2,3] In our experience, up to 65% of patients hemodialysed for more than 10 years were affected by symptomatic ß2 microglobulin amyloid, and even higher percentages were observed after 15 years of treatment.[18]

Effect of patients' age

Clinical features of dialysis associated amyloidosis have not been described in children. Their frequency increases with age, independently of duration of survival under dialysis.[18]

Effect of dialysis treatment

The condition has initially been described in patients dialysed with cuprophan membranes. Since then, amyloid arthropathy and carpal tunnel syndrome have been observed in patients treated with all available techniques of dialysis, including long-term intermittent hemofiltration or peritoneal dialysis.[19] However, retrospective studies have indicated that the prevalence of carpal tunnel syndrome and amyloid arthropathy may depend on the dialysis membrane used. Use of highly permeable membranes has been associated with lower frequency of arthropathy in most centres,[18] but not in others.[20] The addition of ß2 microglobulin adsorption column to the dialysis device has recently been reported further to decrease the incidence of the disease.[21]

Bacteriological contamination of the dialysate has also been suspected to play an important part in stimulating the inflammatory response and increasing the production of ß2 microglobulin.[6] Therefore, not only the type of membrane used, but also dialysate purity could influence the development of amyloid arthropathy. Retrospective studies support the view that ultrapure dialysate and synthetic dialyser membranes may reduce the incidence and severity of dialysis-associated amyloidosis and explain why the disease may have decreased in frequency,[6] or why its onset may have been delayed.[22]

Clinical features of dialysis-associated amyloidosis

Carpal tunnel syndrome

The first report of dialysis patients developing carpal tunnel syndrome was from Warren and Otieno in 1975. These authors followed by others insisted on the etiological role of the vascular access. In 1980 Assénat et al. first identified amyloid deposits in carpal tunnel tissues of patients treated by hemodialysis for non-amyloid nephropathies and requiring surgery for carpal tunnel syndrome. Their observation has been widely confirmed and ß2 microglobulin amyloid deposits in the transverse carpal ligament or finger flexor synovium are now considered a prominent finding in long-term dialysis patients undergoing surgery for carpal tunnel syndrome, where they are identified in 60 to more than 70% of dialysis patients requiring surgery for carpal tunnel syndrome.[1]

Carpal tunnel syndrome is an early and prominent feature of ß2 microglobulin amyloid and appears as almost constant during the course of the disease.

The amyloid carpal tunnel syndrome of dialysis patients is most frequently bilateral. Females and males are roughly equally affected. It is typically revealed by paraesthesia of the affected hand in the medial nerve distribution. Symptoms have an insidious onset. Their severity usually steadily increases over time. Entrapment of the ulnar nerve in the wrist or elbow may be associated and explain involvement of the 5th finger. EMG confirmation of the medial nerve entrapment in the wrist may be necessary to rule out uremic neuropathy or cervical root compression, when destructive spondylarthropathy of the cervical spine is associated.

There are other causes than amyloid of carpal tunnel syndrome in dialysis patients, especially in those treated for a short time. These non-amyloid etiologies include vascular factors and edema in relation with vascular access (which should be suspected when paraesthesias involve the side of the fistula and worsen during dialysis sessions) and fluid retention (suggested by symptoms starting on the nights before the most espaced dialysis session). Uremic neuropathy and vitamin B6 deficiency can also favor the development of carpal tunnel syndrome in dialysis patient. Calcium phosphate crystal deposition is a potential cause of nerve compression either acute during crystal-induced acute inflammatory flares or chronic due to progressive growth of deposits within the carpal tunnel. The amyloid nature of the compression can only be securely diagnosed by pathological examination of carpal tunnel tissues removed during surgery. However, it can be suspected when dialysis duration exceeds 8–10 years, especially if other features of ß2 microglobulin amyloid, such as finger flexor tenosynovitis, shoulder involvement or radiological erosions of subchondral bones are present.

Amyloid arthropathy

Several reports have stressed the high frequency of chronic arthropathy in HD patients. Most of the late reports insisted on the prominent role of ß2 amyloid deposition in the development of these arthropathies.[1] Amyloid deposits are not responsible for all the articular features of dialysis patients; in other words, dialysis arthropathy and ß2 microglobulin amyloid arthropathy are not synonymous. However, a large number of studies of dialysis patients with proven ß2 microglobulin amyloid allow to identify a pattern of articular involvement associated with carpal tunnel syndrome and reminiscent of the arthropathy of primary (AL) amyloidosis.[1,2,22,23]

The onset of symptoms of ß-2 microglobulin amyloid arthropathy is usually insidious and the disease follows a chronic and progressive course, even though acute exacerbations may be observed. Chronic arthralgias are a prominent feature. They are typically bilateral. The shoulders are frequently involved. In clinical practice, shoulder arthralgia must be carefully differentiated from the pain sometimes caused by C5 root involvement by a destructive spondylarthropathy (see below). Arthralgias of the shoulders begins approximately at the same time as symptoms of medial nerve entrapment and are frequently associated with amyloid CTS. They are the first symptom in 25–50 % of patients. Exacerbation of pain during dialysis sessions is noted in approximately one-third of patients. The pathophysiology of this striking feature remains unexplained. Spontaneous remissions are not uncommon, but are usually of short duration. Shoulders swelling is not constantly observed and true shoulder pad sign is rare. Joint mobility, which may be normal at the onset of arthralgias, usually becomes restricted during the course of the disease. Shoulder involvement by ß-2 microglobulin amyloid is complex, as best demonstrated by magnetic resonance imaging.[24] MRI indeed allows to identify two main factors of shoulder pain in dialysis arthropathy:

- ♦ a major thickening of rotator tendons and/or subacromial bursa by amyloid deposits leading to subacromial impingement, which could be treated by decompressive surgery;

- ◆ synovitis of the shoulder joint or subacromial bursitis which can be treated by radiation synovectomy.

Other joints, and particularly the knees, wrists, and small joints of the hands, may be the site of chronic arthralgias. Involvement is roughly bilateral and symmetrical. Loss of motion is commonly associated, especially of the wrists and finger joints. Symptoms are frequently incompletely relieved by rest. Patients commonly complain of stiffness of short duration in the morning or after rest.

Chronic tenosynovitides of the finger flexors are frequently observed in long-term dialysis patients. They are responsible for pain, palmar swelling, and loss of extension and flexion of the involved fingers, related to amyloid infiltration of the synovium and tendon tethering. A similar clinical picture has been described in amyloid AL. Acute inflammatory flares can occur, and are associated with exacerbation of swelling and pain leading to insomnia. Trigger fingers are commonly associated and may be due to nodular amyloid deposits or additional degenerative changes of the tendons.

Chronic joint swelling is also an important feature of the disease. The knees, shoulders, wrists, finger joints, elbows, and ankles may be affected. Knee involvement may lead to the development of popliteal cyst. The sternoclavicular joint can be swollen, but its amyloid involvement is most commonly asymptomatic[25] and infection should be carefully ruled out. Joint infusions are usually paucicellular. In our experience, white blood cell concentration in dialysis amyloid synovial fluid does not exceeded 1100/ml. Synovial fluid examination may allow to demonstrate amyloid in small fragments of synovium, which can be characterized by Congo red staining and immunohistology.[26] Amyloid synovitis may also be demonstrated by synovial biopsy. Some patients develop a grossly symmetrical polyarthritis associated with multiple bone cysts and medial nerve entrapment, a presentation similar to what is observed in the amyloid arthropathy associated with multiple myeloma.

Recurrent hemarthrosis may be observed in ß2 microglobulin amyloid arthropathy and may be responsible for the iron deposits frequently observed in synovium. Repeated blood anticoagulation during dialysis procedure is likely to play an important role in the genesis of articular bleeding. Synovial amyloidosis affects mainly the interstitium and seldom blood vessels.[16]

Destructive arthropathies

Destructive arthropathies are defined by the association of disk or joint cartilage wearing with subchondral bone erosions. Those involving large peripheral joints and the spine are part of the clinical spectrum of ß2 microglobulin amyloidosis, as amyloid deposits are usually (but not constantly in spinal lesions) present in involved joints, even though their pathogenesis is certainly multifactorial. Destructive arthropathies of large joints of the limbs affected 16% of patients treated by hemodialysis for more than 10 years in two dialysis centers in Paris.[27] One or more joints can be involved, sometimes bilaterally. Pain, swelling, and loss of motion of affected joints are common. Cell count in synovial fluid is usually low (less than 2000 cells/mm^3). The first radiological findings are subchondral bone lucencies, followed, after 2–4 years, by joint space narrowing and collapse of subchondral bone. Articular destruction is often very rapid, more than 50% of the joint space disappearing within 3–12 months. Epiphyseal sclerosis may develop tardily, but no osteophytosis is observed. Two types of cartilage loss can be seen in affected hips: concentric and superolateral. Destructive arthropathies of the knee can affect the whole femorotibial joint space or one of the femorotibial compartments, including the lateral one, which is rarely affected by common osteoarthritis. When destructive arthropathies affect weight-bearing joints, they lead to severe disability and may require surgery for prosthetic joints replacements. As a rule, pathological study at this stage allows to identify massive deposits of amyloid in the synovium, capsule or subchondral bone of affected joints.[28]

In 1984, Kuntz et al. described erosive lesions of the spine in 10 dialysis patients, and named this syndrome destructive spondylarthropathy.[29] Since then, many reports of similar findings have been published. The frequency of destructive spondylarthropathy increases with duration of survival. In patients treated for more than 10 years by hemodialysis, prevalence estimates vary according to centers between 12 and 48%. These discrepancies may be explained by differences in ages, dialysis durations, associated putative etiological factors (i.e. aluminum intoxication and secondary hyperparathyroidism) and reading of radiographs in particular for early lesions. Destructive spondylarthropathies have also been described in patients treated by peritoneal dialysis.[19] Clinically, destructive spondylarthropathies are frequently asymptomatic and may remain undiagnosed if lateral views of the spine are not systematically performed. This was the case in 84% of affected patients in a systematic study.[30] These lesions can also be responsible for cervical pain most frequently of mild intensity and relieved by standard analgesics, or, in a few cases, for cervicobrachialgia or lumbar nerve root pain, and/or even spinal cord or cauda equina compression. Therefore, the clinical severity of these spinal lesions ranges from asymptomatic lesions to severe neurological involvement, which may be lethal. The diagnosis of destructive spondylarthropathy is based on the following radiological features:

- severe intervertebral space narrowing;
- erosions and cysts of the adjacent vertebral plates;
- absence of significant osteophytosis.[29]

Osteosclerosis of the affected vertebral plate may also develop lately. Sequential radiographs may show a rapid progression of lesions, often within less than one year, some times in a few months. Destructive spondylarthropathies are usually multiple and generally located in the cervical spine. In the series of 35 dialysis patients with destructive spondylarthropathy that we studied in 1988, 43 of 57 lesions involved the cervical spine. The C4–C5 and C5–C6 disks were the most affected. The thoracic and lumbar spine may also be involved, usually later than cervical involvement. In the initial description, no increased uptake of the isotope was noted at the site of destructive spondylarthropathies. However, this appears variable and hyperfixation of some of these lesions has been observed,[30] possibly in association with the occurrence of vertebral plate osteosclerosis. CT scan demonstrates numerous erosions and cavitations of vertebral plates, frequently filled with gas, a finding very important to rule out infectious discitis. MRI characteristically shows normal disk signals in T1 and T2 sequences,[30] in contrast with infectious discitis characterized by low T1 and high T2 signal intensities. Most importantly, CT scan and MRI demonstrate the lack of soft tissue mass or abscess, and allow study the consequences of lesions on neurological tissues. The posterior arch may also be involved. Bone lucencies can be discerned by regular radiographs or even more frequently by CT scan views. Involvement of the interapophyseal joints can be demonstrated by CT scan, which shows joint space narrowing and frequent subchondral erosions. Alternatively, a paradoxical widening of joint space can be observed in severe involvement of interapophyseal joints, due to major subchondral bone destruction. The involvement of interapophyseal joints and spinal ligaments may lead to major instability of the affected vertebrae, diagnosed upon the appearance of a spondylolisthesis on lateral views, generally worsened on dynamic (forced flexion and extension) views. These radiological features are of great predictive value of the neurological tolerance of destructive spondylarthropathies. Radicular encroachment and/or spinal cord compression are usually associated with unstable spondylolisthesis.

The etiology of destructive spondylarthropathies is still debated and this syndrome is most probably of multifactorial origin. Dialysis therapy is not necessary for their development since destructive spondylarthropathies have also been observed in non dialysed uremic patients, with or without amyloid deposits. Pathological studies most commonly demonstrate amyloid deposits in the intervertebal disc and adjacent ligaments and the vast majority of affected patients have other features of amyloid arthropathy.[30] Moreover, post-mortem studies of dialysis patients have shown that spinal amyloid deposits are frequently seen in short-term dialysis patients and that cervical disk involvement is extremely common in long-term survivors.[31] The deposition of ß2 microglobulin amyloidosis in the spinal disks can therefore be hypothesized to favor the development of destructive lesions. AGE modified ß2 microglobulin stimulates release of inflammatory cytokines by monocytes *in vitro* and a pathological study has shown macrophage infiltration around amyloid deposits in cervical discs, together with the presence of IL1 and TNF alpha in the lesions. These cytokines could mediate discovertebral destruction. Moreover, amyloid involvement of spinal ligaments may be a factor of spinal instability. However, some of these lesions are not associated with amyloid deposits and destructive spondylarthropathy cannot be used as a criterion of ß2 microglobulin in dialysis patients. Other factors including age and mechanical stress play a part since the frequency of these lesions increases with age and they affect the same hypermobile segments of the spine as does osteoarthritis. Secondary hyperparathyroidism is known to cause subperiostal and subchondral resorption of bone, leading to an erosive arthropathy, and has therefore been proposed to intervene in the genesis of these lesions. It is also a source of tendinous hyperlaxity and, which could worsen the instability of spinal lesions. Secondary hyperparathyroidism is also a factor of apatite crystal deposition, which has initially been proposed to play a role in the pathogenesis of these lesions.[29]

ß2ß2 amyloidosis may also involve the atlanto-occipital joint.[32] This involvement is responsible for a pseudotumor of the craniocervical junction best demonstrated by MRI, frequently associated with erosions of lateral masses of the atlas and odontoid process. Such lesions are usually asymptomatic, but may result in neurological symptoms, such as great occipital nerve neuralgia, hypoglosseal nerve palsy, or quadriparesis. They are frequent in long-term dialysis patients and should be searched for before general anesthesia for surgical procedures since forced neck movements required by intubation may result in a fracture of the weakened dens and serious neurological compromise. Finally, amyloid deposits in the ligamentum flavum or extradural space may also be responsible for or worsen[33] nerve root or spinal cord compression.

Pathological fractures of bone

Amyloid bone cysts may lead to pathological fractures in long-term hemodialysis patients[1] as in patient suffering from AL amyloidosis associated with multiple myeloma. Pathological fractures of weight bearing bones such as the femoral neck are serious complications which require surgical repair. Such fractures were observed in six of our first 50 patients with dialysis amyloidosis. They occurred at the site of large cysts or multiple small radiolucencies. AL intoxication was commonly associated and could have enhanced the fragility of bone. Fractures can also be favored by amyloid cysts in other locations, such as the scaphoid bone at the wrist, the supra-acetabular area, or vertebral body or posterior arch.

Systemic deposits

ß2 microglobulin amyloidosis has a strong affinity for joint tissues. Systemic deposits are rare, but may be observed in patients who usually developed amyloid arthropathy.[1] Most of the systemic deposits are asymptomatic. However, linear vascular deposits replace the muscular layer of small vessels, and may result in:

- vascular fragility and bleeding;
- nodular vascular deposits may occlude vascular lumen and lead to necrosis and perforation of viscera;
- massive interstitial deposits rarely cause malabsorption or muscle dysfunction.

The gastrointestinal tract is the less rarely affected organ. Enlargement of the tongue, gastric or intestinal hemorrhage, intestinal pseudo-obstruction, and intestinal infarction and perforation have been reported in a few cases each. Myocardial deposits can be suspected by echocardiography and may result in muscle dysfunction or arrhythmia. Involvement of the pleurae, external auditory canals, and pelvis have been recently described. Deposits in heart and lung vessels are generally asymptomatic, but have caused pulmonary hypertension and low cardiac output. Cutaneous amyloidomas have been reported in a few long-term (>10 years) dialysis patients, and may involve the buttocks in a bilateral and symmetrical way. Biopsies of clinically uninvolved skin are negative.

Diagnosis of ß2 microglobulin amyloid

The gold standard for diagnosis is the demonstration of ß2 amyloid deposits in a tissue or synovial fluid sample. Amyloid of all types has a strong affinity for Congo red, which gives to deposits a characteristic dichroidism, when viewed under compensated polarized light microscopy. When sections are pretreated with sodium permanganate, ß2 microglobulin amyloid no longer display this affinity and dichroidism. Typing of the amyloid can be further achieved by immunohistology, as anti-ß2 microglobulin antibodies strongly bind to deposits.[34]

ß2 microglobulin amyloid arthropathy can be strongly suspected when radiographs disclose, multiple, large (>4mm in diameter) subchondral bone cysts or erosions, which increase in size and number over time, and have a roughly symmetrical distribution, particularly in the wrists and hips (see chapter on X-rays). These subchondral bone cysts have a excellent diagnostic value even in patients with severe secondary hyperparathyroidism.[17] Peri-articular soft tissue enlargement can be evidenced by radiographs and ultrasonography. Finally, serum amyloid P component scintigraphy or more specifically ^{131}I or [111]In ß2 microglobulin scintigraphy can be used for the diagnosis of ß2 microglobulin amyloid.[35]

Differential diagnosis of amyloid arthropathy

There are numerous other causes of joint pain in dialysis patients than amyloid arthropathy.[1] which may require specific management and may co-exist with amyloid arthropathy. Bone and joint infections are well documented complications of hemodialysis and require urgent management with appropriate antibiotics. Immune defenses of patients treated with hemodialysis are impaired, and the arteriovenous fistula is a potential source of hematogenous spread. Intra- or peri-articular steroid injections are also an important source of infection and should be avoided in dialysis patients. Pre-existing articular disease is a well known predisposing factor of septic arthritis. In dialysis patients, amyloid synovitis can favor superinfection. Infectious arthritis in dialysis patients is frequently atypical: the involvement may be polyarticular, inflammation may be subacute, fever may be missing or when present may be explained by other causes. Physicians should be aware of this high incidence of septic arthritis when facing a dialysis patient with swollen joint(s). Needle aspiration of the synovial fluid allows appropriate diagnosis by cell count (a high cell count in this setting is highly suggestive of infection) and bacteriological studies that should be performed before starting antibiotics. In difficult cases, a synovial biopsy may help to rule out infection. Microorganisms may be atypical, including listeriosis associated with secondary iron overload after transfusions and synovial fluid should be cultured over a large set of bacteriological media.

Infectious discitis is similarly an important differential diagnosis of destructive spondylarthropathies. Its clinical presentation is usually more acute and includes fever and high erythrocyte sedimentation rate. Stiffness of the involved spinal segment is usually prominent. In doubtful instances, MRI presently appears as the best imaging technique to diagnose infectious discitis, as previously mentioned. Bone scan may be useful as it shows almost constantly increased fixation of the isotope at the site of the infectious lesion. CT scan allows to study the adjacent soft tissues in search of an abscess, but this is even better achieved by MRI. CT scan of aseptic destructive spondylarthropathy lesions may also detect the presence of small erosions of vertebral plates filled with very low density gas. Such vacuum phenomenon very strongly argues against the diagnosis of infection. Radioguided biopsy allows to diagnose infectious discitis with certainty and to identify the responsible agent.

Arthralgias and articular erosions are known to occur in primary hyperparathy-roidism, and before the wide recognition of amyloid arthropathy in dialysis patients, chronic arthralgias were frequently considered as an indication for subtotal parathy-roidectomy. Small articular erosions, which affect mainly the hands have been observed in 16–38% of hemodialysis patients and have been reported to correlate with secondary hyperparathyroidism and/or para-articular calcifications. These erosions appear to be rarely associated with joint symptoms and several investigators have pointed out the lack of correlation of dialysis arthropathy with secondary hyperpara-thyroidism. However, physicians should be aware that secondary hyperparathyroidism remains as a possible etiology of chronic bone and joint pain in dialysis patients, which can be observed in severe parathyroid dysfunction and may then be relieved by subto-tal parathyroidectomy. The erosive osteopathy, which can develop in severe hyperpara-thyroidism is a source of arthralgias and heel pain, and bears a high risk of tendinous rupture. This is an indication for prompt management of hyperparathyroidism, which is usually followed by articular pain relief.

An erosive arthropathy of small finger joints is frequently observed in dialysis patients.[36] The radiographical picture can suggest erosive osteoarthritis or be even more destructive with prominent lysis of subchondral bone. This condition usually causes little pain, but may lead to deviation and instability of (mostly distal) inter-phalangeal joints. An erosive arthropathy of the trapeziometacarpal joint may be associated. There is no strong female predominance (in contrast to osteoarthritis) and the arthropathy can be observed early after the start of dialysis therapy, even though its frequency increases with duration of survival. Hyperparathyroidism may be an etiological factor, although the small joint erosions observed in overt hyparparathy-roidism are usually not associated with joint space loss, and the condition did not correlate with serum levels of parathyroid hormone. Even when the lesions occurred in the clinical setting of amyloid arthropathy, no local amyloid deposits were discernable by pathological examination.[36]

Tendon rupture is not a feature of amyloid arthropathy. In addition to severe secondary hyperparathyroidism, it can be favored by the use of steroids, even in low dosage, and/or of fluoroquinolones.

Calcium phosphate (predominantly apatite) crystals can deposit around joints of dialysis patients and can be the source of acute inflammatory flares, sometime accom-panied by fever. These self-limited episodes are distinct from the chronic arthralgias of amyloid arthropathy. In our experience, para-articular calcifications are very rarely the source of long-lasting articular pain.[27]

Finally, any rheumatic disease may be observed in dialysis patients, including rheumatoid arthritis, which must be differentiated from polyarticular amyloid arthopathy.

Management of amyloid carpal tunnel syndrome and arthropathy in dialysis patients

The most appropriate treatment of carpal tunnel syndrome in dialysis patients is early surgical release of medial nerve, which should be performed before the appearance of neurological deficiencies. Extension splints of the wrists may relieve incipient symptoms during the night. Local injections of steroids are only temporarily effective and carry a risk of serious infectious complications in dialysis patients. Surgery usually dramatically relieves the paraesthesia, but is less effective on established neurological defects. Recurrences usually associated with further amyloid deposition can be observed following surgery.

Management of the amyloid arthropathy of dialysis patients remains difficult. Preliminary reports have indicated that replacement of the cuprophane membrane by polyacrylonitrile membranes or switching to peritoneal dialysis may rapidly relieve joint pain but placebo effect has not been ruled out. Addition of a ß2 microglobulin adsorption column to the dialysis circuit was also reported to improve clinical features of dialysis-related amyloidosis,[21] but cost issues as well as some concerns about the specificity of ß2 microglobulin adsorption have prevented large use of these devices. Standard analgesics (paracetamol) are widely used because of their excellent efficacy/tolerance ratio. In contrast, non-steroidal anti-inflammatory drugs (NSAIDs) should be used with great caution when prescribed by a systemic route, because they can compromise useful residual diuresis and carry a high risk of life-threatening gastroduodenal complications. Their prescription should be restricted to short periods of time for the treatment of acute articular flares (more commonly crystal- than amyloid-induced). The lowest efficient dose should be used, since toxicity correlates with daily dosage. Topical NSAIDs or lidocain can be helpful and are better tolerated, although they can cause skin rashes. Colchicine may appear as a logical treatment of ß2 microglobulin amyloid since this drug has inhibitory effects on amyloid fibril formation in experimental amyloidosis and is useful in human amyloids of other types. However, the effects of colchicine on ß2 microglobulin amyloidosis have not been studied in the long run and toxicity restrains long-term use in dialysis patients. Intra- or peri-articular steroid injections are widely used for symptomatic management of numerous rheumatic diseases in non uremic patients. In dialysis patients we believe that such injections that are, as a rule, only transiently efficient, should be avoided because of their risk of infectious complications.

We perform medical synovectomies by injecting radionuclides into amyloid joints or subacromial bursae affected by long lasting and/or recurrent effusions. These procedures have been widely used in Europe for the management of inflammatory arthritides, CPPD crystal-induced effusions, hemarthrosis, and have been proposed for the management of amyloid AL arthropathy. They carry less septic risk and have a longer effect than steroid injections.

Corticosteroids can be proposed to dialysis patients affected by severe arthropathy. They are widely used for the symptomatic treatment of various inflammatory arthropathies in non uremic patients and are thought to be far less toxic than non-steroidal anti-inflammatory drugs for the gastrointestinal tract, when used in moderate doses. Low dose (0.1mg/kg/day) prednisone usually allows dramatic improvement of amyloid arthropathy although symptoms rapidly recur after steroid discontinuation.[37] However, the potential risk of corticosteroid-induced atherosclerosis limit the indication of steroids to patients whose amyloid arthropathy remains disabling despite other forms of therapy.

Orthopedic surgery of various sorts can be proposed to patients suffering from dialysis arthropathy. In dialysis patients with painful shoulders, many operative techniques have been used, including arthroscopic or surgical synovectomy, bursectomy, curettage and filling with hydroxyapatite ceramic of humeral cysts, resection of the hypertrophied sheath of the long head tendon of the biceps or plain resection of this tendon, resection of coracoacromial ligament by arthroscopy or open surgery, cuff tear suture. It is difficult to assess which technique is the most effective, as all their performers reported good results. We use MRI examination of the shoulder to decide what strategy to apply to painful dialysis shoulders.[24] When this procedure discloses large effusions in the shoulder joint or in the subacromial bursa, a radionuclide synovectomy or bursectomy is first offered to the patient, whereas when thickening of the rotator cuff is the main MRI finding, resection of coracoacromial ligament and acromioplasty appears the preferable technique. We had this later operation performed in five patients with fair immediate results, which were unfortunately not favorable in the long run. Prescription of low dose prednisone now appears to improve shoulder pain to such an extent that shoulder surgery is rarely necessary.

Total prosthetic joint replacements are indicated in destructive arthropathies of the shoulder, the hip or the knee causing important disability in the absence of major contraindication. These procedures expose to the risk of infection and have been reported to be followed by loosening in a high proportion of patients.

Destructive spondylarthropathies do not require any specific treatment when they are (as frequently) asymptomatic. Medical management, including standard analgesics, immobilization of the affected segment by a rigid collar or corset can be sufficient in painful lesions without or with mild neurological involvement. Operative treatment must be considered for lesions leading to major neurological symptoms. As spinal instability appears to be the main factor of neurological compromise, we favor fusions of the unstable vertebrae rather than decompressive surgery, which carry a higher mortality and may worsen spinal instability.[38]

Pathological fractures must be treated according to standard surgical procedures.

Finally, kidney transplantation usually dramatically improves joint symptoms and appears to halt the disease progression,[39] even though this procedure does not allow dissolution of amyloid deposits, as judged on the persistence of unchanged radiological erosions and of histologically proven amyloid deposits as long as 10 years after kidney transplantation.[39] Kidney transplantation must therefore be considered as a potential treatment of dialysis arthropathy. Most importantly, this procedure presently appears as the best technique available for prevention of ß2 microglobulin amyloidosis. The frequency of dialysis arthropy in patients hemodialysed for more than 10 years and its potential severity favors early kidney transplantation.

References

1. Kay J, Bardin T. Osteoarticular disorders of renal origin: disease-related and iatrogenic. *Baillieres Best Pract Res Clin Rheumatol* 2000;**14**:285–305.
2. Floege J, Ketteler M. Beta2-microglobulin-derived amyloidosis: an update. *Kidney Int* 2001;**78**(Suppl):S164–71.

3. Winchester JF, Salsberg JA, Levin NW. Beta-2 microglobulin in ESRD: an in-depth review. *Adv Ren Replace Ther* 2003;**10**:279–309.

4. Gejyo F, Yamada T, Odani S, et al. A new form of amyloid protein associated with chronic hemodialysis was identified as beta 2-microglobulin, *Biochem Biophys Res Comm* 1985;**129**:701–6.

5. Gorevic PD, Casey TT, Stone WJ, DiRaimondo CR, Prelli FC, Frangione B. Beta-2 microglobulin is an amyloidogenic protein in man. *J Clin Invest* 1985;**76**:2425–9.

6. Lonnemann G, Koch KM. Beta(2)-microglobulin amyloidosis: effects of ultrapure dialysate and type of dialyzer membrane. *J Am Soc Nephrol* 2002;**13**(Suppl 1):S72–7.

7. Morten IJ, Gosal WS, Radford SE, Hewitt EW. Investigation into the role of macrophages in the formation and degradation of beta2-microglobulin amyloid fibrils. *J Biol Chem* 2007;**282**:29691–700.

8. Corlin DB, Johnsen CK, Nissen MH, Heegaard NH. A beta2-microglobulin cleavage variant fibrillates at near-physiological pH. *Biochem Biophys Res Comm* 2009;**381**:187–91.

9. Monti M, Amoresano A, Giorgetti S, Bellotti V, Pucci P. Limited proteolysis in the investigation of beta2-microglobulin amyloidogenic and fibrillar states. *Biochim Biophys Acta* 2005;**1753**:44–50.

10. Villanueva J, Villegas V, Querol E, Aviles FX, Serrano L. Monitoring disappearance of monomers and generation of resistance to proteolysis during the formation of the activation domain of human procarboxypeptidase A2 (ADA2h) amyloid fibrils by matrix-assisted laser-desorption ionisation-time-of-flight-MS. *Biochem J* 2003;**374**:489–95.

11. Relini A, Canale C, De Stefano S, et al. Collagen plays an active role in the aggregation of beta2-microglobulin under physiopathological conditions of dialysis-related amyloidosis, *J Biol Chem* 2006;**281**:16521–9.

12. Borysik AJ, Morten IJ, Radford SE, Hewitt EW. Specific glycosaminoglycans promote unseeded amyloid formation from beta2-microglobulin under physiological conditions. *Kidney Int* 2007;**72**:174–81.

13. Morimoto H, Wada J, Font B, et al. Procollagen C-proteinase enhancer-1 (PCPE-1) interacts with beta2-microglobulin (beta2-m) and may help initiate beta2-m amyloid fibril formation in connective tissues. *Matrix Biol* 2007;**27**:211–19.

14. Miyata T, Inagi R, Iida Y, et al. Involvement of beta-microglobulin modified with advanced glycation end products in the pathogenesis of hemdialysis-associated amyloidosis. Induction of human monocyte chemotaxis and macrophage secretion of tumor necrosis factor and interleukin-1. *J Clin Invest* 1994;**93**:521–8.

15. Hou FF, Chertow GM, Kay J, et al. Interaction between beta-2 microglobulin and advanced glycation end products in the development of dialysis-related amyloidosis, *Kidney Int* 1997;**51**:1514–9.

16. Jadoul M, Garbar C, Noel H, et al. Histological prevalence of beta 2-microglobulin amyloidosis in hemodialysis: a prospective post-mortem study, *Kidney Int* 1997;**51**:1928–32.

17. Zingraff J, Noel LH, Bardin T, Kuntz D, Dubost C, Drueke T. Beta 2-microglobulin amyloidosis: a sternoclavicular joint biopsy study in hemodialysis patients. *Clin Nephrol* 1990;**33**:94–7.

18. van Ypersele de Strihou C, Jadoul M, Malghem J, Maldague B, Jamart J. Effect of dialysis membrane and patient's age on signs of dialysis-related amyloidosis. The Working Party on Dialysis Amyloidosis. *Kidney Int* 1991;**39**:1012–19.

19. Cornelis F, Bardin T, Faller B, et al. Rheumatic syndromes and beta 2-microglobulin amyloidosis in patients receiving long-term peritoneal dialysis. *Arthritis Rheum* 1989;**32**:785–8.

20. Kessler M, Netter P, Maheut H, et al. Highly permeable and biocompatible membranes and prevalence of dialysis-associated arthropathy. *Lancet* 1991;**337**:1092–3.

21. Gejyo F, Kawaguchi Y, Hara S, et al. Arresting dialysis-related amyloidosis: a prospective multicenter controlled trial of direct hemoperfusion with a beta2-microglobulin adsorption column. *Artif Organs* 2004;**28**:371–80.

22. Otsubo S, Kimata N, Okutsu I, et al. Characteristics of dialysis-related amyloidosis in patients on hemodialysis therapy for more than 30 years. *Nephrol Dial Transplant* 2004;**24**:1593–8.

23. Yamamoto S, Kazama JJ, Maruyama H, Nishi S, Narita I, Gejyo F. Patients undergoing dialysis therapy for 30 years or more survive with serious osteoarticular disorders, *Clin Nephrol* 2004;**70**:496–502.

24. Bernageau J, Bardin T, Goutallier D, Voisin MC, Bard M. Magnetic resonance imaging findings in shoulders of hemodialyzed patients. *Clin Orthop Relat Res* 1994;**304**:91–6.

25. Zingraff J, Drueke T, Bardin T. Dialysis-related amyloidosis in the sternoclavicular joint. *Nephron* 1989;**52**:367.

26. Munoz-Gomez J, Gomez-Perez R, Sole-Arques M, Llopart-Buisan E. Synovial fluid examination for the diagnosis of synovial amyloidosis in patients with chronic renal failure undergoing hemodialysis. *Ann Rheum Dis* 1987;**46**:324–6.

27. Bardin T, Vasseur M, de Vernejoul MC, et al. [Prospective study of articular involvement in patients on hemodialysis for 10 years], *Rev Rhum Mal Osteoartic* 1988;**55**:131–3.

28. Bardin T, Kuntz D, Zingraff J, Voisin MC, Zelmar A, Lansaman J. Synovial amyloidosis in patients undergoing long-term hemodialysis. *Arthritis Rheum* 1985;**28**:1052–8.

29. Kuntz D, Naveau B, Bardin T, Drueke T, Treves R, Dryll A. Destructive spondylarthropathy in hemodialyzed patients. A new syndrome. *Arthritis Rheum* 1984;**27**:369–75.

30. Maruyama H, Gejyo F, Arakawa M. Clinical studies of destructive spondyloarthropathy in long-term hemodialysis patients. *Nephron* 1992;**61**:37–44.

31. Ohashi K, Hara M, Kawai R, et al. Cervical discs are most susceptible to beta 2-microglobulin amyloid deposition in the vertebral column. *Kidney Int* 1992;**41**:1646–52.

32. Rousselin B, Helenon O, Zingraff J, et al. Pseudotumor of the craniocervical junction during long-term hemodialysis. *Arthritis Rheum* 1990;**33**:1567–73.

33. Marcelli C, Perennou D, Cyteval C, et al. Amyloidosis-related cauda equina compression in long-term hemodialysis patients. Three case reports. *Spine (Phila Pa 1976)* 1996;**21**:381–5.

34. Bardin T, Zingraff J, Shirahama T, et al. Hemodialysis-associated amyloidosis and beta-2 microglobulin. Clinical and immunohistochemical study. *Am J Med* 1987;**83**:419–24.

35. Floege J, Schaffer J, Koch KM. Scintigraphic methods to detect beta2-microglobulin associated amyloidosis (Abeta2-microglobulin amyloidosis). *Nephrol Dial Transplant* 2001;**16**(Suppl 4):12–16.

36. Flipo RM, Le Loet X, Siame JL, et al. Destructive arthropathy of the hands in chronic hemodialysis patients. A report of seven cases with pathological documentation. *Rev Rhum Engl Ed* 1995;**62**:241–7.

37. Bardin T. Low dose prednisone in dialysis arthropathy. *Rev rhumat (Engl edn)*, 1994;**61**:97S–100S.

38. Van Driessche S, Goutallier D, Odent T, et al. Surgical treatment of destructive cervical spondyloarthropathy with neurologic impairment in hemodialysis patients. *Spine (Phila Pa 1976)* 2006;**31**:705–11.

39. Bardin T, Lebail-Darne JL, Zingraff J, et al. Dialysis arthropathy: outcome after renal transplantation. *Am J Med* 1995;**99**:243–8.

Chapter 17

Pathogenesis of vascular calcification: experimental studies

Rukshana C. Shroff and Catherine M. Shanahan

Introduction

Cardiovascular disease is increasingly recognized as a life-limiting problem in patients with chronic kidney disease (CKD). Cardiovascular dysfunction begins early in the course of renal decline and results in a significantly higher cardiovascular mortality and morbidity, even in children on dialysis, when compared with the age matched normal population. A seminal paper by Foley et al. in 1998 awakened the nephrology community to the very high cardiovascular mortality even in young CKD patients. Further studies showed that the increased burden of cardiovascular disease was due, at least in part, to calcification of the vessel wall. For many years vascular calcification was thought to be an unregulated physicochemical 'dumping' of calcium (Ca)–phosphate (P) in tissues, and to represent an end-stage degenerative process of dead or dying cells. Thus, in the context of elevated circulating levels of Ca and P in CKD patients this 'dumping' was extreme. However, calcification can occur in the absence of elevated Ca–P levels as seen in old age, diabetes, atherosclerosis, and certain human genetic diseases.[1] Moreover, in recent years, converging evidence from in vitro studies, molecular genetic techniques and human single-gene defects has shown that vascular calcification involves a complex interplay between promoters and inhibitors of calcification.[2] Indeed, proteins involved in bone mineralization are up-regulated in the calcifying vessel wall, such that calcification in the vasculature has many similarities to bone formation and is now regarded as an actively regulated process. The uremic milieu provides a 'perfect storm' for accelerated calcification—mineral dysregulation, vascular smooth muscle cell (VSMC) damage, perturbation of circulating and cellular inhibitors of Ca and P precipitation, inflammatory insults and co-existing pro-atherosclerotic risk factors all converge in advanced CKD.[2–4]

This chapter discusses our current understanding of the process of vascular calcification focusing specifically on risk factors in CKD patients, and linking clinical and basic research experimental findings into a working theoretical model to explain the pathway of development of vascular calcification in CKD. Given that vascular calcification is a highly regulated cell mediated process, opportunities to inhibit the progression or even induce regression of vascular calcification are now emerging.[4]

Identification of the promoters and inhibitors of calcification will lead the way for future therapeutics to identify and modulate these agents, thereby reducing cardiovascular morbidity and mortality in CKD patients.

Calcification occurs at distinct sites in CKD patients

Four distinct, but sometimes overlapping, sites of calcification have been described in CKD patients—arterial intimal calcification, arterial medial calcification, calcific uremic arteriolopathy, and calcification within the cardiac valves. Intimal calcification is seen with advancing age, hypertension, dyslipidemia, and smoking, and takes the form of atherosclerotic vascular disease.[5] It is a patchy and discontinuous process that involves inflammatory macrophages and VSMCs in lipid-rich regions of the atherosclerotic plaque. In contrast, calcification in the tunica media, also known as Mönckeberg's sclerosis, is organized along the elastic lamellae and is almost exclusively associated with VSMCs.[6] Mönckeberg's sclerosis, as first described in 1903, was used to describe the histological picture of sheet-like calcification of the tunica media, without involvement of the intima, and was assumed to be a degenerative age-related problem. Medial calcification is now well characterized in diabetes and CKD, and, at least in adolescents and young adults with CKD, can occur independently of intimal calcification. However, as a number of 'traditional' Framingham risk factors for atherosclerosis are also present in CKD patients, varying combinations of intimal and medial calcification may co-exist. Importantly, as described in the next chapter, the anatomical site of calcification within the vessel wall determines the nature of its clinical manifestations, but even the most sophisticated imaging modalities cannot differentiate clearly between intimal and medial calcification.

Dialysis patients also develop a distinct form of medial calcification of the cutaneous vessels known as calcific uremic arteriolopathy that results in necrotizing skin lesions and is associated with an extremely high mortality. Finally, calcification of the cardiac valve leaflets is a major cause of failure of both native and bioprosthetic valves. Although this form of calcification is not covered in detail in this chapter it is clear that many of the basic mechanisms and risk factors leading to vascular calcification are also causal in valve calcification.

The differences between intimal and medial calcification imply different etiologies. However evidence from a large number of *in vitro* and *in vivo* studies have now clearly defined common pathogenic mechanisms leading to calcification in both the media and intima. The cell type that is central to all vessel wall calcification is the VSMC (Fig. 17.1).

Vascular smooth muscle cell phenotypic change in response to injury

VSMCs within the normal tunica media are responsible for maintaining vascular tone and express a number of unique contractile proteins including α-smooth muscle actin (α-SM actin), SM-MHC, SM22α, and calponin, agonist receptors and signal transduction molecules that are required to regulate their contractile phenotype. In contrast,

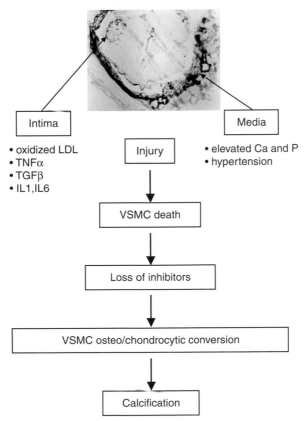

Fig. 17.1 Factors inducing vascular injury in the vessel media and intima.

VSMCs associated with the diseased vessel wall show altered properties and exhibit a gene expression profile that differs from that of contractile VSMCs. This is because unlike skeletal and cardiac muscle, VSMCs do not terminally differentiate, but retain the capacity to dedifferentiate and proliferate to repair the vessel wall. However, in so doing, VSMCs display an extraordinary capacity to undergo phenotypic change and to acquire the characteristics of a diverse range of mesenchymal lineages, such as osteo-blastic, chondrocytic, or adipocytic cell types.[7,8] Thus, the first step in the process of calcification is VSMC injury. In atherosclerosis, lipid-induced inflammation is the most prevalent injury, while in CKD, VSMC injury is induced by a mineral imbalance.[9,10] As a consequence of injury VSMCs die and/or release membrane debris that act as a nidus for mineralization. In addition, VSMC injury and death reduces their capacity to express inhibitors of mineralization locally.[4] In parallel with the loss of local inhibitors of calcification, systemic changes such as inflammation, contribute to the loss of circulating inhibitors of calcification. In addition, deranged levels of hormones, minerals, and other factors also contribute to ongoing VSMC damage and so, eventually, calcification ensues. Concomitant with the development of calcification,

VSMCs undergo osteo/chondrocytic conversion and begin to express mineralization-regulating proteins normally restricted to bone and cartilage.[6,11] This conversion of VSMCs, which can be induced by both lipids and a mineral imbalance, acts to further orchestrate and regulate the process of extracellular matrix mineralization in the vessel wall. The complex details of how these processes are initiated and finely regulated have been gleaned by a multitude of histological and experimental studies that are summarized below.

Physiological versus pathological calcification: similarities between bone ossification and ectopic calcification— *in vivo* evidence

Mineralization of the extracellular matrix in skeletal and dental tissues is a cell-mediated process that is required for the normal development of bones and teeth. In such tissues where calcification is required, resident cells have developed specific mechanisms to enable mineral nucleation and crystal growth under normal physiological conditions.[6,7] A variety of factors are required to create this unique environment. First, mesenchymal precursors of chondrocytes and osteoblasts are induced to express transcription factors Runx2, Osterix, Msx2, and Sox9 that act sequentially and in concert to induce differentiation.[7] Once differentiated, chondrocytes and osteoblasts express a number of proteins that are constituents of an extracellular matrix that is permissive for calcification. These proteins include collagens I, II, and IX, as well as proteoglycans. Differentiated chondrocytes and osteoblasts also express a number of mineralization regulating proteins, including alkaline phosphatase (AP), bone sialoprotein (BSP), and osteocalcin (OC), which act to induce and/or regulate crystal growth.[6] However, expression of these proteins alone is generally not sufficient for mineralization. Specialized structures termed 'matrix vesicles' are required to create a microenvironment permissive for mineral nucleation. Matrix vesicles are specialized small membrane bound structures that act to concentrate Ca and P to enable mineral nucleation.[9] They were first described in chondrocytes and osteoblasts during developmental osteogenesis, and form a micro-environment capable of concentrating Ca and P, thus allowing crystal nucleation to occur. Once a crystal is nucleated it will continue to grow within the extracellular matrix to mineralize the tissue. To enable Ca and P to be concentrated vesicles contain AP, which creates a P source by processing pyrophosphate, as well as annexins and other components that bind calcium. Importantly, these same processes of mineralization have been shown to occur during calcification of the vessel wall. However, the major difference between bone and the vasculature is that in bone, the cellular changes are normal physiological responses, while in the vasculature, the changes are pathological and induced by VSMC response to injury (Fig. 17.2).

Studies of human vessel samples have provided evidence for vascular mineralization as a regulated process similar to bone mineralization. Firstly, X-ray crystallography and electron microprobe analysis have shown that the mineral deposited in the vessel wall is basic Ca–P in apatitic form, some of which is hydroxyapatite [$Ca_{10}(PO_4)_6(OH)_2$], the same crystal found in bone. Moreover, electron microscope

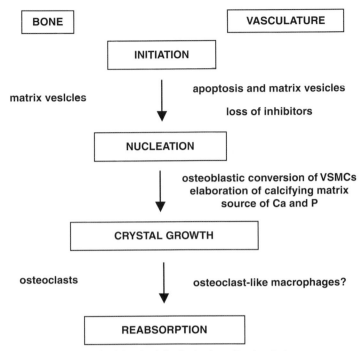

Fig. 17.2 Mechanisms involved in physiological mineralization in bone versus pathological mineralization in the vessel wall.

analyses of VSMCs *in vivo* have shown that matrix vesicles can bud from the plasma membrane. Secondly, studies using RT-PCR and immunohistochemical analysis of gene expression in normal and calcified arteries, including arteries from CKD patients, have shown that VSMCs express Runx2 and Sox 9, obligate transcription factors for osteoblastic and chondrocytic differentiation, as well as their target genes, AP, BSP, OC, and collagen II, at sites of calcification *in vivo*. Analysis of the temporal pattern of protein expression in relation to the onset of calcification has demonstrated that, in the normal vessel wall, VSMCs express constitutive inhibitors of calcification, such as MGP, but these inhibitors are down-regulated in calcified vessels and concurrently VSMCs up-regulate expression of mineralization regulators normally expressed in bone.[12] Finally, in advanced atherosclerotic lesions and the peripheral arteries of diabetic patients osteoid has been observed that mineralizes to form mature bone tissue.

The cellular origin of this ossification, as opposed to calcification, is unknown. It is possible that resident VSMCs transdifferentiate or that stem cells from the circulation or derived locally from the vessel wall media or adventitia are recruited to the calcified area. Within the calcified environment these cells are exposed to signals that lead to the initiation of a developmental osteogenic differentiation program rather than a reparative VSMC program.[7]

Model systems to study vascular calcification

Experimental studies have begun to unravel the mechanisms and factors that can act to accelerate calcification and a number of model systems have been utilized including:

- ◆ Animal knock-out models.[2,3,13–15]
- ◆ Human VSMC explant cultures.[6,9–11,16–18]
- ◆ Organ culture of vessel rings.[12,19]

Each of these model systems has advantages and disadvantages. Animal knock-out models have provided insights into the effects of single gene defects and the crucial role of calcification inhibitors in preventing ectopic calcification. Major mechanistic insights into the process of vascular calcification have come from *in vitro* studies, in particular, studies utilizing human VSMCs in culture. When human VSMCs are cultured *in vitro* they spontaneously convert to an osteo/chondrocytic phenotype, mimicking the phenotypic changes observed in calcified arteries.[11] The cells also form multicellular nodules, a feature only observed in osteoblasts and chondrocytes in culture. These nodules spontaneously calcify, due to apoptosis/death and vesicle release by the resident nodular VSMCs.[9] In addition, monolayer VSMCs also release vesicles very similar in structure to chondrocyte matrix vesicles. These membrane vesicles and debris form the initial nidus for mineral nucleation and subsequent calcification.[9] However, VSMCs cultured from explants lack the matrix and architecture of a normal vessel wall, and rapidly lose their contractile properties *in vitro*. In contrast, vessel rings have an intact matrix structure including elastic lamellae, the initial site of calcification in the vessel wall, and VSMC can maintain a normal contractile phenotype for a prolonged period. In addition, vessels derived from CKD patients can be experimentally manipulated *in vitro* using this model system (Fig. 17.3). Insights gained from these 3 model systems are discussed in detail below.

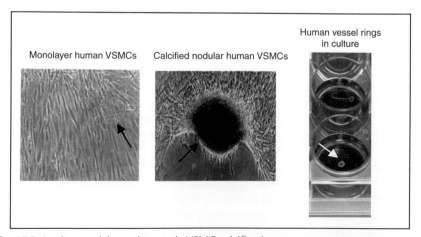

Fig. 17.3 *In vitro* models used to study VSMC calcification.

Mouse gene knock-outs develop ectopic soft-tissue and vascular calcification

Until the advent of animal knock-out models, evidence for a regulated calcification process was only circumstantial and based on the observation that VSMCs both *in vitro* and *in vivo* displayed some phenotypic features of bone cells. Animal studies were able to reveal more fully the complexity of the mechanisms that have evolved to prevent soft tissue calcification and maintain tissue homeostasis. In addition, they focused attention on proteins involved in the regulation of both vascular calcification and bone mineralization, and suggested that these processes may in some way be mechanistically linked.

Marix Gla protein (MGP)

The first and most dramatic of these animal models was the matrix Gla protein (MGP) knock-out. MGP is a small protein highly expressed in the aorta and in cartilage. Homozygous mice deficient in MGP developed rampant calcification as well as cartilaginous metaplasia of the aorta and its branches, and typically died of aortic rupture 4 weeks after birth, as a direct consequence of vascular calcification.[14] Thus, knock-out of this single gene demonstrated for the first time that VSMCs constitutively express proteins that act as local inhibitors of vessel wall calcification. This model also implied that VSMCs are in a constant, active state of inhibiting mineralization, even under normal physiological conditions, and that if these inhibitors are missing or dysfunctional calcification will occur.[20]

Fetuin-A

The second model that extended our understanding of how vascular calcification is regulated was the fetuin-A knock-out. Fetuin-A is produced in the liver and is present in the circulation. When it is missing, animals develop calcification in almost all their soft tissues, demonstrating for the first time that systemic inhibitors, produced at remote sites, play a key role in preventing soft tissue calcification.[15,21] This study indicated that all soft tissues are in a 'hostile environment', even when circulating Ca and P are at physiological levels, in terms of their propensity to calcify. Indeed, as described in detail below, fetuin-A is a key protein in the circulation that acts to encapsulate Ca and P to ensure that tissues are not exposed to high levels of these ions.[22] Importantly, fetuin A knock-out mice developed increased calcification when fed on mineral and vitamin D-rich diets and on a high-fat diet. These studies indicated a role for fetuin-A not only in inhibiting calcification in association with a mineral imbalance, but also in damaged blood vessels where VSMCs have undergone phenotypic modulation.[15]

Osteoprotegerin

Knock-out of osteoprotegerin was the third model to highlight an important aspect of vascular calcification as it clearly linked, for the first time, bone and vascular mineralization. Animals deficient for this protein developed both medial arterial calcification and osteoporosis.[13] Osteoprotegerin is present in the circulation, but is also produced locally in bone and the vasculature. In bone, it blocks osteoclast activity preventing bone resorption and, hence, its absence promotes osteoporosis. In the vasculature its function is unclear. Importantly, this study suggested that common mechanisms regulate both bone and vascular calcification.[3] However, factors that influence one tissue bed to induce calcification may have an opposing effect on another, complicating any attempts to therapeutically manipulate the calcification process in patients. Moreover, it highlighted the importance of a balance in both the local production of inhibitors, as well as their circulating levels as important for both vascular and bone health.

In addition to these 3 key studies, each introducing a new paradigm into the field of vascular calcification, a plethora of other knock-out models have highlighted further the multiple levels of regulation that have evolved to protect the vasculature from calcification (Table 17.1).[2,3] In many of these knock-out animal models vascular calcification was induced by the absence of a single protein. These include genes involved in matrix synthesis (fibrillin), regulation of tissue pH (carbonic anhydrase), and the production of key local inhibitors of crystal growth such as pyrophosphate: Inactivation of the enzyme ecto-nucleotide pyrophosphatase/phosphodiesterase 1 (ENPP1) led to ossification of the aorta. In addition, TGFβ-superfamily signaling was identified as essential in maintaining VSMC differentiation: Loss of SMAD6, a bone morphogenetic protein (BMP) inhibitor led to ossification of the aorta during embryonic development. Other knock-out models have further demonstrated the link between bone and vascular calcification as well as defining a central role for mineral metabolism in maintaining both vascular and bone homeostasis. These include the Klotho/FGF23 knock-out models that are examined in detail in other chapters.

There is also evidence from single gene defects in man that the phenotypes observed in animal knock-outs are relevant to human physiology.[2,3] Mutations in MGP, leading to absent or non-functional MGP, cause Keutel Syndrome, which is characterized by abnormal calcification of cartilage in the ears, nose, larynx, trachea, and ribs. These patients on post-mortem show extensive medial vascular calcification at an early age. Idiopathic arterial calcification in infancy, characterized by extreme and rapid medial calcification is caused by mutations in the gene encoding enzyme ecto-nucleotide pyrophosphatase/phosphodiesterase 1 (ENPP1), an essential step in the production of pyrophosphate. Taken together these studies emphasize a key feature of vascular calcification; that multiple inhibitory mechanisms need to be overcome for calcification to occur.

The role of mineral imbalance in ectopic calcification—clinical and experimental studies

The susceptibility of CKD patients to the development of vascular calcification and increased mortality is highly correlated with dysregulated mineral metabolism. Block et al. first reported that elevated P levels are an independent risk factor for increased mortality in adult dialysis patients. P is also an independent risk factor for death in the pre-dialysis population. Large observational studies have also correlated serum Ca levels with increased mortality in hemodialysis patients and have shown that the greatest mortality risk is seen when high Ca and P levels co-exist. Studies in children with CKD have shown that mineral dysregulation leads to VSMC damage and phenotypic

Table 17.1 Calcification inhibitors: outcome of gene disruption studies.

Inhibitors	Gene disruption studies in mice	Human single gene studies and genetic polymorphisms
Fetuin-A	Ectopic calcification of small blood vessels, most organs (e.g. myocardium, lung, kidney, skin)	Polymorphisms may predispose patients to vascular calcification
Matrix-Gla protein	Medial calcification of arteries, aortic valves (not arterioles, capillaries, or veins), cartilaginous metaplasia within the vessel wall	Keutel syndrome—extensive vascular calcification and abnormal calcification of cartilage. Polymorphisms may be prognostic for vascular calcification
Osteoprotegerin	Medial and subintimal calcification of the aorta and renal arteries, presence of multinuclear osteoclast-like cells within the vascular wall	Juvenile Paget's disease—an autosomal recessive osteopathy, but no clear association with vascular disease. Polymorphisms in the promoter region of OPG are associated with atherosclerosis
Klotho/FGF23	All calibers of arteries affected, intimal thickening of medium-sized arteries	Polymorphism may be a genetic risk factor for coronary artery disease
Nucleotide Pyrophosphatase/ phosphodiesterase 1	Aortic medial calcification, intra-aortic cartilaginous differentiation of VSMC	Infantile idiopathic arterial calcification— calcification of the internal elastic laminae of large vessels, often with death in the first year of life
Carbonic anhydrase	Age-dependent medial calcification of small arteries in a number of organs,with the most extensive arterial alcinosis in the male genital tract	Autosomal recessive disorder characterized by osteopetrosis, renal tubular acidosis, and cerebral calcification
Fibrillin	Mice defective in fibrillin, an important microfibril associated with elastin,develop medial aortic calcification	Variations in the fibrillin-1 genotype in humans cause Marfan's syndrome, which is associated with aortic stiffness and an increased risk of cardiovascular disease

modulation *in vivo*.[12] Arteries harvested from children after different exposure times to dysregulated mineral metabolism in CKD showed an increased Ca load that correlated with the patients' mean serum Ca × P product. Calcification was significantly greater in vessels exposed for longer periods during dialysis and correlated with all the indicators of VSMC damage and phenotypic modulation identified in *in vitro* studies including VSMC apoptosis and vesicle release, loss of inhibitors, and osteo/chondrocytic differentiation.[12] Taken together these studies point to a role for dysregulated mineral metabolism as a major driving factor in accelerated calcification in CKD. However, they do not inform of its mechanisms of action. Importantly, *in vitro* studies have confirmed that calcification is induced because elevated Ca and P directly impinge on VSMC function.[9,10,17]

VSMC death and vesicle release—*in vitro* studies

One of the earliest events in the induction of calcification is VSMC death and apoptotic body release.[9] Using human aortic VSMC cultures it was demonstrated that apoptosis occurs before the onset of calcification in VSMC nodules. Experimental evidence showed that inhibition of apoptosis with the caspase inhibitor ZVAD.fmk reduced calcification while stimulation of apoptosis caused a 10-fold increase in calcification. Importantly, apoptotic bodies derived from dying VSMCs have been shown to have the ability to act as nucleating structures for calcium crystal formation.[23] Under normal circumstances apoptotic bodies should be phagocytosed by local VSMCs and, therefore, be rapidly cleared before calcification can occur. However, *in vitro* and animal studies have shown that in the damaged vessel wall phagocytosis is impaired, apoptotic bodies are left uncleared and calcification ensues. Factors such as fetuin-A enhance phagocytosis, while lipids block phagocytosis.[4;18] Thus, is CKD as well as in atherosclerosis there is limited phagocytosis and calcification of deposited membrane debris is likely to occur.

Exposure of VSMCs to media containing elevated levels of Ca and/or P, within the range observed in patients with CKD, rapidly induces calcification[10]. In addition, elevation of both ions simultaneously has synergistic effects on calcification. Experimental studies have revealed that the addition of increased levels of extracellular Ca and/or P cultures rapidly induces VSMC apoptosis while the inhibition of apoptosis with ZVAD.fmk ameliorated calcification.[10] Moreover, after exposure to Ca and P the apoptotic bodies released by VSMC showed an increased ability to accumulate Ca, amplifying their calcification effects.[9,10] However, apoptosis was shown to account for only part of the accelerated calcification observed after exposure to Ca and P.

In response to extracellular Ca viable/living VSMCs were also induced to release matrix vesicles in a manner analogous to growth plate chondrocytes. These vesicles were shown to be 'mineralization competent' in that they contained preformed Ca – P apatite accounting for a dramatically increased calcification capacity *in vitro*.[9] The mechanisms that induce the release of vesicles have not been determined, however, Ca is the most potent factor in initiating this process. This has led to the suggestion that vesicle release is an adaptation that enables VSMCs to release large amounts of unwanted Ca thus protecting the cell from Ca overload and cell death. This idea has been tested in animal models of vitamin D overload, but has not been tested in VSMCs *in vitro* due to the lack of inhibitors available to block vesicle release. However, studies have confirmed a role for apoptosis and vesicle release in calcification *in vivo*.

However, not all matrix vesicles released by VSMCs are mineralization competent, indeed the majority may not be. This is because under conditions of health VSMC vesicles are loaded with mineralization inhibitors including the constitutive inhibitor MGP and the circulating inhibitor fetuin-A.[18,20,24] These proteins act to limit the calcification potential of vesicles thus providing indirect evidence that vesicle release is a protective mechanism in response to Ca overload and that under normal conditions calcification will not occur. Experimental studies have shown that vesicles released in the presence of high P and Ca will not calcify if functional inhibitors are present. However, if MGP function is compromised or, Ca and P are added to VSMC cultures in the absence of serum (and therefore in the absence of fetuin-A), VSMCs died by apoptosis and calcified more.[18] Moreover, the vesicles released by VSMCs in the absence of these inhibitors showed the greatest calcification potential (Fig. 17.4).

Apoptosis may not be the only form of cell death that promotes calcification. Numerous studies have linked necrotic cell death with calcification of soft tissues. Calcification in atherosclerosis is associated with the necrotic core of the plaque, although in medial calcification in CKD so far, there is no direct evidence for necrosis

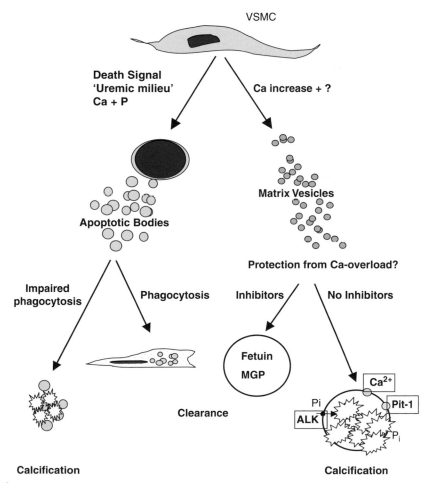

Fig. 17.4 Role for apoptosis, phagocytosis, and matrix vesicle release in VSMC calcification.

of the vessel wall. However, *ex vivo* studies using cultured rat aortic rings have highlighted the role of vascular injury in the induction of calcification.[19] When rat aortic rings from normal vessels were incubated in medium with elevated P no calcification occurred. However, mechanical injury of the vessel, which is likely to result in extensive necrotic cell death, resulted in medial calcification. Importantly, aortic rings taken from rats exposed to experimental renal failure were able to calcify spontaneously *ex vivo* when exposed to elevated Ca and/or P. Thus, suggests that vessels are pre-injured *in vivo* by exposure to dysregulated mineral metabolism and this injury contributes to calcification. In these studies the nature of the injury was not studied in detail, however, it is likely to include VSMC loss. In the future, this model may enable investigators to directly study the mechanisms of damage and death over a defined time course.

In vitro studies have also confirmed that there are a multitude of factors, in addition to dysregulated mineral metabolism, that contribute to VSMC damage in CKD (Table 17.2). These studies have also identified key VSMC survival factors, including Gas6, that are dysfunctional in response to elevated P but further studies are required to clearly define the signaling pathways responsible for cell loss in CKD. In addition, it is not clear by what mechanisms many of the factors investigated act to enhance calcification. Some may also induce VSMC apoptosis and/or enhance the apoptotic effects of elevated Ca and P. Others may alter the expression of inhibitors or impact on VSMC differentiation as described below.

Table 17.2 Factors dysregulated in CKD that induce calcification of VSMCs *in vitro*

Factor	Effect *in vitro*	Levels in CKD and potential effects
Bone morphogenetic protein-2 (BMP2)	Inducer?	Increased in CKD?
Bone morphogenetic protein-7 (BMP7)	Inhibitor?	?
Calcium (Ca)	Inducer	Increased in CKD, risk factor for cardiovascular events in dialysed patients1
Phosphate (P)	Inducer	Increased in CKD and vascular calcification
Magnesium (Mg)	Inhibitor	Inverse relationship between serum magnesium and vascular calcification in CKD
Parathyroid hormone (PTH)	Inducer/ Inhibitor	Increases Ca absorption and influences bone turnover, direct effect on VSMCs?
Vitamin D	Inducer/ Inhibitor	Promotes increased Ca and P absorption, increases Ca uptake by VSMCs, reduces VSMC migration and differentiation.
Vitamin K	Inhibitor	Promotes γ-carboxylation of MGP and reduces calcification

Phenotypic transformation of VSMCs to osteoblast-like cells: *in vitro* studies

Osteo/chondrocytic conversion of VSMCs, is characterized by the expression of Cbfa1/Runx2. Runx2 is a transcription factor essential for osteoblast differentiation that regulates the expression of multiple genes expressed in osteoblasts including the early marker AP, BSP, the late marker OC and osteopontin (OPN).[6,8,11] VSMCs also express other important osteo/chondrocytic transcription factors including osterix, which acts downstream of Runx2, and Sox9, which mediates expression of chondrocytic markers including collagen II and proteoglycans. There is also evidence that other transcriptional pathways including Msx2 and Wnt signaling may also be involved;[7] however these have not been studied in any detail in CKD models.

It remains unclear whether expression of this plethora of mineralization-regulating proteins by VSMCs represents an adaptation of the cells to regulate the calcification process or a direct transdifferentiation in response to pathological stimuli that directly acts to enhance and orchestrate calcification. This is because while some of the proteins expressed, such as BSP are involved in the nucleation of apatite crystals others, such as OPN and OC, directly block crystal growth. Also, it remains unclear whether calcification precedes osteogenic conversion, although recent studies suggest these processes may be concomitant. However, what is clear is that osteogenic conversion of VSMCs is almost invariably associated with calcification (Fig. 17.5).

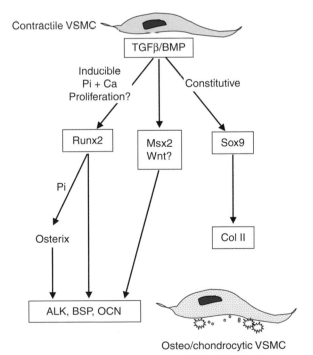

Fig. 17.5 Potential pathways for osteo/chondrocytic differentiation of VSMCs.

In vitro studies have shown that the factors that regulate VSMC phenotypic hetero-geneity and initiate phenotypic change are multiple. One of the key pathways that act to induce osteo/chondrocytic differentiation of VSMCs *in vitro* is the TGF β/BMP signaling cascade,[8,11] although details of how this pathway is dysregulated *in vivo* remain elusive. However, a second mechanism whereby Ca and P directly impinge on VSMC calcification is by interfering with their normal differentiation and enhancing osteogenic differentiation. Studies by Giachelli et al. have shown that in the presence of increased intracellular P the sodium-dependent phosphate co-transporter, Pit-1, signals through Runx2 to induce osteoblastic differentiation of VSMCs.[17] Thus, P can act as a signaling molecule and induce phenotypic changes in the VSMCs, as well as directly contribute to the mineralization process. Likewise, elevated Ca levels in the culture media enhance mineralization and phenotypic transformation of VSMCs, also via the sodium-dependent phosphate co-transporter. Prolonged exposure of VSMCs to elevated Ca induced Pit-1 mRNA levels, suggesting that elevated Ca regulates the P sensitivity of VSMCs.[25]

P may also play a role in the upregulation of AP independently of Runx2 activation. Vessel ring studies suggest that AP may be up-regulated by vessel injury and P before Runx2 expression and osteo/chondrocytic differentiation occurs.[12] If this is proven correct, then inactivation of pyrophosphate by AP, maybe an early priming event for calcification in the vessel wall.

Inhibitors of calcification: deficiency of systemic or local calcification inhibitors

As highlighted throughout this chapter, a major event in the calcification cascade in the vasculature is the loss of local or circulating calcification inhibitors. This section examines how experimental studies have unravelled the mechanisms whereby the absence or dysregulation of these inhibitors impinges on VSMC calcification. Importantly, key inhibitors, such as MGP and fetuin-A have been shown to be reduced or dysfunctional in CKD patients, and aspects of the CKD milieu that impact on expression and function of these inhibitors are also explored.[3,20] Ways of overcoming these failures in inhibition maybe important for arresting calcification in the context of a mineral imbalance.

MGP: a local calcification inhibitor

Matrix Gla (γ-carboxyglutamic acid) protein (MGP) is an extracellular matrix protein synthesized by chondrocytes and VSMCs that belongs to a family of proteins that contain γ-carboxyglutamic acid residues. These proteins require a vitamin K dependent γ-carboxylation to convert their inactive undercarboxylated form (uc-MGP or Glu-MGP) into the active γ-carboxylated form (Gla-MGP).[20] The γ-carboxyglutamic acid residues in MGP can bind calcium and transgenic studies have suggested that impaired γ-carboxylation of MGP and not MGP levels *per se* are associated with vascular calcification. In healthy arteries functional Gla-MGP is deposited in association with elastic fibres in the media, with no undercarboxylated or dysfunctional Glu-MGP present. In contrast, in vessels with intimal and/or medial calcification, undercarboxy-lated Glu-MGP is localized around all areas of calcification, suggesting that impaired carboxylation of MGP is a factor in calcification *in vivo*. Experimental studies in rats have shown that treatment with the vitamin K antagonist, warfarin, at doses that inhibit the vitamin K-dependent γ-carboxylation of MGP, induces rapid calcification of elastic lamellae of the arterial media with increased MGP mRNA expression, perhaps in a feed back mechanism to block further calcification. In humans, small observational studies have suggested that the use of warfarin is associated with increasing coronary artery and valvular calcification.

MGP acts as a regulator of both calcification and cell differentiation in the vasculature. Its ability to bind Ca, via its Gla residues, accounts for its capacity to inhibit calcification in matrix vesicles released by VSMCs. Together with fetuin-A MGP can form a complex with hydroxyapatite and block further mineral growth. In addition, MGP is also a regulatory protein for BMP-2 and can inhibit the activity of this potent morphogen of the TGF-β superfamily. It is possible that in MGP-deficient mice, the unopposed action of BMP-2 allows local VSMC to develop into chondrocytes. Like many mineralization regulating proteins MGP is also present in the circulation, but the role of circulating MGP, if any, remains largely unknown and the influence of circulating MGP levels on vascular calcification is unclear.

Fetuin-A: a systemic calcification inhibitor

All extracellular fluids, even under normal circumstances, are saturated with respect to Ca and P suggesting that potent inhibitors of vascular calcification are normally circulating to prevent ectopic soft tissue calcification. The addition of normal human serum to VSMCs *in vitro* in the presence of elevated Ca and P significantly inhibits the time-course and extent of calcification when compared to VSMCs treated in the absence of serum.[18] Experimental studies have identified fetuin-A as the key component of serum that acts to limit calcification. Fetuin-A is a member of the cystatin superfamily of cysteine protease inhibitors. It is a circulating glycoprotein that is produced by the liver and contributes to almost 50% of the calcification inhibitory capacity of human plasma.[18,22] Fetuin-A is unique in that it acts both systemically and in a cell specific manner.

Fetuin-A acts systemically by binding excess mineral and inhibiting basic Ca–P precipitation in serum and extracellular fluids. It can form a stable complex with Ca–P and prevent the growth, aggregation and precipitation of hydroxyapatite.[22] Fetuin-A can also modulate the calcification processes locally. At sites of vascular damage fetuin-A is taken up by VSMCs, incorporated into intracellular vesicles, and then released within matrix vesicles where it potently inhibits mineral nucleation. In addition, fetuin-A inhibits VSMC apoptosis and aids in phagocytosis of extracellular vesicles, thus further limiting mineralization.[18]

In addition to these calcification inhibitory effects, fetuin-A is a negative acute phase reactant; various interleukins, particularly interleukin-1α, decrease its synthesis.[21,24] Circulating fetuin-A levels are significantly lower in dialysis patients than in healthy controls[24] and this has been linked with cardiovascular mortality, presumably as a result of accelerated vascular calcification.[21] However, it may also be that patients with calcification have genetically lower levels or perturbations in the fetuin-A functional activity that predisposes them to calcify.[21,24] Polymorphisms in the fetuin-A gene may determine the magnitude of decrease in fetuin-A production in the face of inflammation and influence an individual's susceptibility to calcify. Further studies to determine the factors that regulate the production of fetuin-A are now required as increasing the levels of this protein may provide protection from calcification in CKD patients.

Osteoprotegerin – maintains both bone and vessel wall homeostasis

Osteoprotegerin (OPG) is a member of the tumor necrosis factor receptor superfamily and acts as a decoy receptor for receptor activator of nuclear factor-κB ligand (RANKL), which stimulates all aspects of osteoclast function, including differentiation, activation, fusion and survival, which together mediate bone resorption. By blocking RANKL, OPG inhibits osteoclastic bone resorption, but OPG is produced by a number of tissues, including arterial VSMCs. Mice deficient in OPG develop medial calcification of the great arteries and early-onset osteoporosis as a result of unopposed stimulation of RANKL receptors leading to increased osteoclastic activity.[13] Calcification in these mice could be rescued by introduction of an *opg* transgene from mid-gestation, but not by parenteral application of OPG after mineralized lesions were established. This is in contrast to osteoporosis, which could be efficiently treated by a parenteral OPG regimen. This implies that while circulating OPG has a direct action on bone it is the local production of OPG in the vessel wall that is important in inhibiting calcification.[2,3]

The precise role of OPG in the vascular wall and its possible interaction with VSMCs has yet to be determined. OPG inhibits warfarin-induced vascular calcification in rats, but its mechanisms of action are unknown. OPG is deposited at sites of calcification and globally down-regulated in the diseased vasculature; however, the factors that regulate OPG expression in VSMCs have not been determined. Given that OPG is produced by a variety of cell types, the source of elevated OPG remains elusive and it is unclear whether increased systemic OPG levels reflect the cause or consequence of vascular calcification or are unrelated.[3] However, given that circulating OPG could not ameliorate calcification in animal models it is interesting to speculate that high levels of circulating OPG may be damaging for VSMCs in a manner analogous to glucose in diabetes and PTH in CKD. Table 17.3 summarizes the actions of these inhibitors, and they are discussed at length in other chapters.

Summary

Experimental studies have elucidated many of the mechanisms that lead to calcification of the vessel wall in CKD. VSMC injury and death, loss of inhibitors and osteo/chondrocytic differentiation have been identified as key events in the calcification cascade. In addition experimental studies have identified many of the factors that contribute to VSMC damage and dysfunction in CKD and demonstrated how these factors impinge on one or more aspects of the calcification cascade. Importantly, dysregulated mineral metabolism appears to have a major impact on VSMC function and detailed studies aimed at further interrogating the molecular mechanisms, whereby dysregulated mineral metabolism impacts on VSMC function are now required. An issue that is now increasingly important to address is the relationship

Table 17.3 Actions of mineralization inhibitors locally and in the circulation

Factor	Role in circulation	Levels in circulation	Human single gene defects or genetic polymorphisms
Fetuin-A (α2 Heremans-Schmid glycoprotein)	Inhibitor	Reduced in CKD	Polymorphisms may predispose patients to vascular calcification
Matrix Gla protein (MGP)	No effect?	Changes in ucMGP serum levels in vascular Calcification	Keutel syndrome -extensive vascular calcification and abnormal calcification of cartilage MGP gene polymorphisms may be prognostic for vascular calcification
Osteoprotegerin (OPG)	?	Increased in CKD and patients with vascular Calcification	Juvenile Paget's disease—an autosomal recessive osteopathy, but no clear association with vascular Disease. Polymorphisms in the promoter region of OPG are associated with atherosclerosis
Klotho	?	Decline with age	Polymorphism may be a genetic risk factor for coronary artery disease
Fibroblast growth factor-23 (FGF23)	?	Increased in CKD	?
Inorganic pyro-phosphate (PPi)	? Inhibitor	Reduced in CKD, and also removed by hemodialysis	Infantile idiopathic arterial calcification—calcification of the internal elastic laminae of large vessels, often with death in the first year of life

between vascular and bone health as potential therapies and interventions may impact on both these tissues. These studies cannot be performed *in vitro* and require a more complex physiological model system. Importantly, a number of animal models have now been developed that model CKD (Table 17.4). In addition, animal models of calcification specifically in the vasculature will be important in dissecting vessel and

Table 17.4 Animal models for studying calcification in CKD

Animal model	Phenotype	Pathology
Adenine feeding	CKD	Renal failure
4/5 Nephrectomy	CKD	Renal failure
Phosphate feeding	In combination with CKD	Medial calcification
Vitamin D feeding	Dose dependent effects	Medial calcification
Warfarin feeding	Inactivation of MGP	Medial calcification
LDLR KO	Atherosclerosis, diabetes	Intimal and medial calcification
ApoE KO	Atherosclerosis	Intimal calcification

bone relationships. Also it should be remembered that vessel wall calcification occurs in the context of other disease states including atherosclerosis and diabetes and animal models superimposing these features on CKD have already proved informative and will provide important test systems for potential therapeutics.

Although we are still a long way from being able to inhibit the relentless progression of calcification in CKD, experimental studies have provided important insights and have identified targets for normalization as well as for therapeutic intervention and we await new experimental insights.

References

1. Goldsmith D, Ritz E, Covic A. Vascular calcification: a stiff challenge for the nephrologist: does preventing bone disease cause arterial disease? *Kidney Int* 2004;**66:**1315–33.
2. Shroff RC, Shanahan CM. The vascular biology of calcification. *Semin Dial* 2007;**20:**103–9.
3. Schoppet M, Shroff RC, Hofbauer LC, Shanahan CM. Exploring the biology of vascular calcification in chronic kidney disease: what's circulating? *Kidney Int* 2008;**73:**384–90.
4. Shanahan CM. Vascular calcification—a matter of damage limitation? *Nephrol Dial Transplant* 2006;**21:**1166–9.
5. Demer LL, Tintut Y. Vascular calcification: pathobiology of a multifaceted disease. *Circulation* 2008;**117:**2938–48.
6. Shanahan CM, Cary NR, Salisbury JR, Proudfoot D, Weissberg PL, Edmonds ME. Medial localisation of mineralisation-regulating proteins in association with Monckeberg's sclerosis: evidence for smooth muscle cell-mediated vascular calcification. *Circulation* 1999;**100:**2168–76.
7. Iyemere VP, Proudfoot D, Weissberg PL, Shanahan CM. Vascular smooth muscle cell phenotypic plasticity and the regulation of vascular calcification. *J Intern Med* 2006;**260:**192–210.
8. Shanahan CM, Proudfoot D, Tyson KL, Cary NR, Edmonds M, Weissberg PL: Expression of mineralisation-regulating proteins in association with human vascular calcification. *Z Kardiol*;2000:**89** Suppl 2:63-68.
9. Proudfoot D, Skepper JN, Hegyi L, Bennett MR, Shanahan CM, Weissberg PL. Apoptosis regulates human vascular calcification *in vitro*: evidence for initiation of vascular calcification by apoptotic bodies. *Circ Res* 2000;**87:**1055–62.
10. Reynolds JL, Joannides AJ, Skepper JN, et al. Human vascular smooth muscle cells undergo vesicle-mediated calcification in response to changes in extracellular calcium and phosphate concentrations: a potential mechanism for accelerated vascular calcification in ESRD. *J Am Soc Nephrol* 2004;**15:**2857–67.
11. Tyson KL, Reynolds JL, McNair R, Zhang Q, Weissberg PL, Shanahan CM. Osteo/chondrocytic transcription factors and their target genes exhibit distinct patterns of expression in human arterial calcification. *Arterioscler Thromb Vasc Biol* 2003;**23:**489–94.
12. Shroff RC, McNair R, Figg N, et al. Dialysis accelerates medial vascular calcification in part by triggering smooth muscle cell apoptosis. *Circulation* 2008;**118:**1748–57.
13. Bucay N, Sarosi I, Dunstan CR, et al. Osteoprotegerin-deficient mice develop early onset osteoporosis and arterial calcification. *Genes Dev* 1998;**12:**1260–8.
14. Luo G, Ducy P, McKee MD, Pinero GJ, Loyer E, Behringer RR, Karsenty G. Spontaneous calcification of arteries and cartilage in mice lacking matrix Gla protein. *Nature* 1997;**386:**78–81.

15. Schinke T, Amendt C, Trindl A, Poschke O, Muller-Esterl W, Jahnen-Dechent W. The serum protein alpha2-HS glycoprotein/fetuin inhibits apatite formation in vitro and in mineralising calvaria cells. A possible role in mineralisation and calcium homeostasis. *J Biol Chem* 1996;**271:**20789–96.

16. Demer LL, Tintut Y. Pitting phosphate transport inhibitors against vascular calcification. *Circ Res* 2006;**98:**857–9.

17. Giachelli CM: Vascular calcification: in vitro evidence for the role of inorganic phosphate. *J Am Soc Nephrol* 2003;**14:**S300–4.

18. Reynolds JL, Skepper JN, McNair R, et al. Multifunctional roles for serum protein fetuin-a in inhibition of human vascular smooth muscle cell calcification. *J Am Soc Nephrol* 2005;**16:**2920–30.

19. Lomashvili KA, Cobbs S, Hennigar RA, Hardcastle KI, O'Neill WC. Phosphate-induced vascular calcification: role of pyrophosphate and osteopontin. *J Am Soc Nephrol* 2004;**15:**1392–401.

20. Proudfoot D, Shanahan CM. Molecular mechanisms mediating vascular calcification: role of matrix Gla protein. *Nephrol (Carlton)* 2006;**11:**455–61.

21. Ketteler M, Wanner C, Metzger T, et al. Deficiencies of calcium-regulatory proteins in dialysis patients: a novel concept of cardiovascular calcification in uremia. *Kidney Int* 2003;**Suppl:**S84–7.

22. Price PA, Lim JE. The inhibition of calcium phosphate precipitation by fetuin is accompanied by the formation of a fetuin-mineral complex. *J Biol Chem* 2003;**278:**22144–52.

23. Proudfoot D, Skepper J, Hegyi L, Bennett MR, Shanahan CM, Weissberg PL. Apoptosis regulates human vascular calcification *in vitro*—evidence for initiation of vascular calcification by apoptotic bodies. *Circ Res* 2000;**87:**1055–62.

24. Ketteler M, Giachelli C. Novel insights into vascular calcification. *Kidney Int* 2006;**Suppl:**S5–9.

25. Giachelli CM, Speer MY, Li X, Rajachar RM, Yang H. Regulation of vascular calcification: roles of phosphate and osteopontin. *Circ Res* 2005;**96:**717–22.

Chapter 18

Clinical consequences of arterial calcifications and soft-tissue calcifications in chronic kidney disease

Gérard M. London, Bruno Pannier, Alain P. Guerin, and Sylvain J. Marchais

Introduction

Damaged large arteries represent a major contributory factor to the cardiovascular complications that are the leading cause of mortality in chronic kidney disease (CKD) and end-stage renal disease (ESRD).[1,2] This risk for the development of cardiovascular complications is associated with numerous deleterious changes in the structure and function of the cardiovascular system, including the arterial system. The structural and functional changes are, in many aspects, similar to those occurring with aging, with this age-related process being accelerated and intensified in ESRD patients.[3] Although atherosclerosis and plaque-associated occlusive lesions are the frequent underlying causes of these complications, the spectrum of arterial alterations in ESRD is broader, including non-atheromatous remodeling, characterized by outward remodeling of large arteries and stiffening of arterial walls, with consequences that differ from those due to atherosclerotic plaques.[2] The frequency of traditional risk factors does not fully explain the extension and severity of arterial disease, and other factors associated with CKD and ESRD must also be involved.[4] Arterial calcification (AC) is a common complication of CKD and ESRD,[5–7] and the extents of AC in general populations and kidney patients are predictive of subsequent cardiovascular mortality beyond established conventional risk factors.[8–10]

Methods for assessing arterial calcification

Several non-invasive methods enable AC to be detected and quantified. The most widely used methods enabling quantitative analyses are electron-beam computed tomography (EBCT) and multi-slice computed tomography.[5,11] Both techniques can assess AC quantity and progression. The results are typically reported using the Agatson score, which is calculated as the product of the calcified plaque area and density coefficient.[11] However, these two imaging techniques are limited by their inabilities to distinguish between the two predominant AC sites, i.e. the intima and the media.

Ultrasonography and plain radiographs are semi-quantitative techniques that can be used to detect AC.[7,12] They are good initial screening tools for detecting the presence of AC, but they have relatively low sensitivity and are less useful for the quantification of AC progression over time. With plain radiographs, it is sometimes possible to discriminate between intima and media calcification in peripheral arteries.[10] The abdominal aortic calcification score (AoCS) using lateral spine radiographs at the level of the first four (L1–L4) lumbar vertebrae is a simple method.[8] Indeed, it has been shown that this score is an important predictor of vascular morbidity and mortality,[8] and the results of a recent study demonstrated very good correlation between AoCS and coronary calcification scores using EBCT.[12]

The AC score should be completed by the evaluation of its impact on arterial function. Functional assessment could be done by evaluating angiographically the extent and degree of stenotic lesions, or the presence of atherosclerotic occlusive lesions.[13,14]

In addition, arterial stiffness can be measured. Stiffness is a term describing the ability of arteries to accommodate the volume ejected by the left ventricle (LV), and expresses the given transmural pressure as a function of contained volume of the vasculature over the physiological range of pressure. In physiology, stiffness or elastance (E) is defined as the pressure change (ΔP) due to a volume change (ΔV) that is, $E=\Delta P/\Delta V$. The reciprocal value of stiffness is compliance ($C=\Delta V/\Delta P$). Stiffness/elastance represents the instantaneous slope of the pressure–volume relationship. Artery rigidity is characterized by an increased slope of the pressure–volume relationship. Carotid–femoral ('aortic') pulse wave velocity (PWV) determination is generally considered the gold standard. According the Moens–Koerteweg equation: $PWV^2=/2\rho r$, where E is Young's elastic modulus, h is the arterial wall thickness, r the radius of the vessel, and ρ the tissue density; PWV integrates the parameters of intrinsic wall properties (E) and its geometry ($h/2r$). The technique is simple, robust, and reproducible with several commercially available devices.[15,16]

Mechanisms of arterial calcification

The precise pathophysiology of AC is not fully understood. For a long time it was thought that these calcifications resulted from passive deposition of calcium salts as the consequence of extracellular fluid volume oversaturation with a high calcium–phosphate product. Experimental and clinical studies have shown that AC is a process akin to bone formation, regulated by equilibrium between factors promoting or inhibiting calcification, with proteins involved in bone metabolism being expressed in arterial tissues, reflecting changes of the phenotype of vascular smooth-muscle cells (VSMC).[17–19] Emerging evidence indicates that diabetes, inflammation, dyslipidemia, oxidative stress, estrogen deficiency, and vitamin D and K deficiencies could provide stimuli for osteogenic phenotype expression, and also decrease the efficiency of mechanisms preventing calcium deposition.[20–23]

In vitro, VSMC transformation into osteoblast-like cells, with subsequent mineralization, is induced or regulated by the balance between a variety of factors inducing or inhibiting calcification, including calcium and phosphate. Calcium and phosphate act synergistically and independently on VSMC calcification. This process was inhibited by phosphonoformic acid, an antagonist of the sodium–phosphate cotransporter (Pit-1). Phosphate may initiate calcification by enhancing the activation of Runx2/ Cbfa1, a factor that stimulates the differentiation of mesenchymal cells into the osteoblastic lineage, including the formation of matrix vesicles, nodules and apoptotic bodies, which serve as initiation sites for apatite crystallization.[19–23] Moreover, VSMC synthesize bone-associated proteins, including alkaline phosphatase, osteocalcin, osteopontin, and a coat of collagen–rich extracellular matrix.

However, in the presence of normal serum, VSMC do not become calcified and are able to inhibit spontaneous calcium and phosphate precipitation in solution, indicating that systemic calcification inhibitors are present serum and VSMC.[24] VSMC constitutively express potent local inhibitors of calcification, such as matrix Gla protein,[25] which may limit AC by binding to bone morphogenic proteins (BMP-2), a potent osteogenic differentiation factor.[26] Osteopontin is another inhibitor of AC *in vivo*, and inactivation of its gene enhances the calcification process.[27] Osteoprotegerin is a decoy receptor for RANKL, and acts as an AC inhibitor and osteoprotegerin-deficient animals develop severe AC of the media of aorta and renal arteries, and osteoporosis.[28] Fetuin-A (AHSG or α_2.HS glycoprotein) is a potential circulating AC inhibitor that is abundant in plasma.[29] *In vitro*, the phosphate-stimulated apatite production can be completely inhibited by adding pyrophosphates that antagonize the cellular sodium–phosphate cotransport system.[30]

AC develop in two distinct sites: the intima and media layers of the large and medium-sized arterial wall.[31] Intima calcification occurs when minerals are deposited within atherosclerotic plaque in the arterial wall intima. This process is a progressive feature of common atherosclerosis found in the general population and is not specific to CKD, except for its higher frequency in ESRD patients. Calcium accumulation in the media of arteries is observed with high frequency in diabetes and CKD. These two forms are frequently associated, as common atherosclerosis is also common in diabetic and renal disease patients. AC is tightly associated with aging and arterial remodeling, including intima–media thickening, but also changes of the geometry and function of aortic valves, e.g. decreased aortic valve surface area and smaller valve opening (Fig. 18.1). The calcification process in the intima and media shares several common osteogenic mechanisms, but also differs in several aspects. Intima atherosclerotic calcifications are typical for advanced common atherosclerosis – generated at the blood–endothelium–intima interface.[31] The location of intima calcification/ plaque principally concerns the aorta, large elastic arteries and coronary arteries. The location is influenced by several factors including the embryonic origin of VSMC[32] and the mechanical stresses, like tensile stress and shear stress patterns.[20,21,33] These stresses and strains are important stimuli that regulate the VSMC phenotype and maintain the contractile phenotype. Nikolovski et al.[33] demonstrated that expression of bone-associated genes was down-regulated in tissue exposed to cyclic strain, and that cyclic strain inhibited the switching of VSMC to an osteoblast-like phenotype. Low shear stress and oscillatory shear stresses are 'atherogenic' and observed principally in areas such as inner curvatures of coronary arteries, the aortic arch or arterial bifurcations.[20,21] In contrast, plaques are not observed in straight arteries with predominant laminar flow, like the upper arm arteries. Osteogenic signals for media

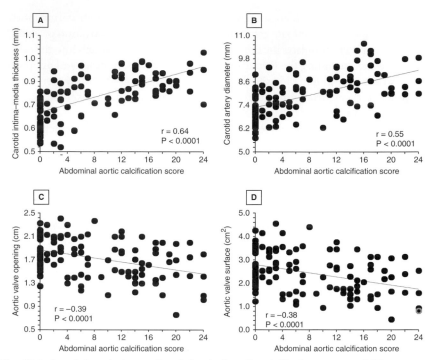

Fig. 18.1 Correlations between the abdominal aortic calcification score and (A) common carotid artery intima-media thickness, (B) common carotid artery internal diameter, (C) aortic valve opening, or (D) aortic valve surface area. All correlations are adjusted for age and body surface area (personal data).

calcification are initiated by adventitial BMP-2-Msx2-Wnt signaling conveyed to the arterial tunica media via the vasa vasorum.[22] Media calcifications could be observed in muscular-type arteries, including those characterized by laminar shear stress. As for intima calcifications, mineralization-regulating proteins are also expressed in media calcifications.[23] In uremic patients, Runx2/Cbfa1 and osteopontin are expressed in intima and media calcifications, and pooled uremic serum induced expression of Runx2/Cbfa 1 in bovine VSMC, thereby supporting the view that this key regulatory factor is up-regulated in response to 'uremic toxins', independently of the proper role of serum phosphates.[34]

Numerous population-based longitudinal studies in general populations[35,36] and ESRD patients[5,37–40] have demonstrated associations between AC or arterial stiffness, and osteoporosis, bone mineral density or bone activity. That relationship, considered to be a consequence of the aging process, remains significant after adjustment for age as demonstrated in several studies. Osteoporosis and AC are influenced by several common risk factors, such as aging, inflammation, dyslipidemia, oxidative stress, estrogen deficiency, vitamin D and K deficiencies, and involvement of the RANKL/ RANK/osteoprotegerin (OPG) system.[28,41–43]

The association between bone and vascular disorders was also observed in patients with CKD or ESRD.[5,37–39] While the osteoporosis–AC associations could be observed in general populations in the absence of overt mineral metabolism disorders, in CKD or ESRD patients, the relationships between AC and bone disorders were associated with deterioration of mineral and bone metabolism caused by changes of serum phosphate and calcium concentrations, and disruption of endocrine and humoral pathways, including parathyroid hormone (PTH), calcitriol, fibroblast growth factor-23(FGF23)–Klotho axis, and others.[17,18]

In patients with CKD or ESRD, the bone–AC association concerns two aspects of bone disorders, i.e. high bone turnover (secondary hyperparathyroidism, 2HPT) and adynamic bone disease (ABD). The increased bone resorption seen in 2HPT is frequently associated with AC. In addition to the possible role of regulatory factors secreted by the bone matrix, the release of endogenous phosphate and calcium from bone probably plays an important role. The possible direct intervention of PTH is less clear. Chronically elevated PTH up-regulates RANKL and down-regulates *OPG* gene expression and raises the RANKL/OPG ratio.[44] In 2HPT, endogenous release of phosphate and calcium could play a pivotal role in the induction of AC. Experimental *in vitro* studies showed that PTH-related peptide and PTH act as local regulators, limiting calcification, and that 1,25-dihydroxyvitamin D_3 increases *in vitro* AC by modulating/decreasing PTH-related peptide.[45] Active bone plays an important role in calcium and phosphate metabolism, as these elements are incorporated into the bone matrix. Hyperphosphatemia in the case of ABD is also of exogenous origin (nutritional) and could be an important factor inducing VSMC transdifferentiation. The ABD–AC process is more pronounced in patients with PTH over-suppressed by positive calcium balances, whether due to high calcium intake, high doses of active vitamin D or high dialysate calcium concentration,[6,7] with decreased PTH levels participating in ABD pathogenesis. Intoxication with vitamin D or its analogues could be associated with AC, but the results of several studies conducted in general populations and ESRD patients indicate that serum concentrations of calcium, 1,25-dihydroxy vitamin D_3 and PTH were not correlated with coronary calcifications.[37,46]

A third form of vascular calcifications concerns the arteriolar media calcifications of subcutaneous and dermal vessels—calcific uremic arteriolopathy (calciphylaxis). The characteristic lesions consist of narrowing of small arterioles with intravascular calcium deposits within the media, endovascular fibrosis, inflammatory reaction, and frequent thrombotic occlusions. Clinically, it is characterized by painful purple skin lesions with purpura and livedo reticularis, progressing to ischemic skin lesions and necrotic ulcerations. The pathogenesis is not well understood, but, like classical intima and media calcifications, calciphylaxis is a regulated process associated with *in situ* expressions of molecular regulators of skeletal and extraskeletal mineralization. Clinically, it is characterized by high morbidity and mortality and some 'specific' risk factors, such as female sex, obesity, and/or diabetes.[53]

AC are frequently associated with extra-osseous calcifications, like subcutaneous nodules, peri-articular temporal calcinosis, and conjunctival and corneal calcifications. Whether the pathogenesis of these calcifications is similar or shares common mechanisms with arterial calcifications is not known.

Clinical impact of arterial calcifications

While intima and media calcifications are associated with morbidity and mortality, they have different impacts on arterial functions and different pathological mechanisms.[8,10] The arterial system has two distinct, interrelated hemodynamic functions:

- conduit function, whose role is to deliver an adequate supply of blood from the heart to peripheral tissues, as dictated by metabolic activity;

- dampening/cushioning function whose role is to dampen blood pressure oscillations caused by intermittent ventricular ejection and transform the pulsatile flow in the aorta and large arteries into continuous flow, and perfusion of peripheral organs and tissues.

Conduit dysfunctions result from the narrowing of the arterial lumen with ischemia affecting the tissues and organs downstream, while dampening dysfunctions reflect alterations of arterial wall visco-elastic properties and have deleterious effects upstream on the heart and the arteries themselves. Because the two forms of AC are frequently associated the conduit and cushioning abnormalities could be associated.

Intima plaque calcification occurs in the context of common atherosclerosis, and progresses in parallel with the plaque evolution. The imaging techniques for quantification of AC are unable to distinguish between intima and media calcifications, but have shown that coronary calcification scores are associated with the extent and degree of stenosis evaluated by coronary angiography, and are predictive of cardiovascular events.[13] Usually, atherosclerotic plaque has an impact on the arterial lumen, producing eccentric narrowing. The principal long-term alterations occur through narrowing or occlusion of arteries, with restriction of blood flow, resulting in ischemia or infarction of downstream tissues. The clinical consequences depend on the progression of lumen obstruction. In the case of chronic progression with stable plaque, basal blood flow remains unchanged until the lumen diameter is narrowed by 50–60%. Beyond 70–80% reduction of the lumen diameter (critical stenosis), basal blood flow is reduced, as is the ability to increase flow during increased demand. Plaque rupture is associated with acute coronary and arterial events. Advanced atherosclerosis is not limited to the intimal layer and expands to media. Advanced atherosclerosis also impacts on the cushioning function and combines the adverse effects of both dysfunctions.

Because calcification advances with the progression of the atherosclerosis, it is uncertain if, by itself it represents a risk factor or is just a surrogate marker of plaque burden and marker of extent of the disease. The acute coronary events and infarction are more related to biomechanical stability of atherosclerotic plaques and the rupture of the plaque's fibrous cap. Although a higher coronary AC score is associated with a poorer cardiovascular prognosis, the influence of calcification on plaque stability is controversial. The results of several studies indicated that AC does not increase plaque vulnerability, which seems more attributable to a large lipid pool, thin fibrous cap and intensity of local inflammation.[48,49]

Media calcification (Mönckeberg's sclerosis or media calcinosis) is characterized by diffuse mineral deposits within the arterial tunica media. While media calcification is frequently observed with aging in the general population, it is significantly more pronounced in patients with metabolic disorders, such as metabolic syndrome, diabetes, or CKD. Media calcification is concentric, not extending into arterial lumen in its typical pure form and is associated with abnormal cushioning function of blood vessels (arteriosclerosis – arterial hardening) by promoting arterial stiffness (Fig. 18.2). The principal consequences of arterial stiffening are an abnormal arterial pressure wave, (characterized by increased systolic and decreased diastolic pressures, resulting in high pulse pressure) and increased aortic characteristic impedance (Fig. 18.2), i.e. the appropriate term to define the intrinsic aortic factor opposing left ventricular (LV) ejection. Arterial impedance, a measure of the opposition of the aorta to oscillatory input (i.e., stroke volume), determines the amplitude and time course of the pressure wave generated in the aorta throughout the cardiac cycle.

Systolic pressure depends on the interaction between LV ejection (stroke volume and duration of systole) and the physical properties of the arterial system that influence systolic pressure by two mechanisms. The first, *direct mechanism* involves the generation of a higher pressure wave (incident or forward-travelling wave) by LV ejection into a stiff arterial system. The second *indirect* mechanism operates through the effect of arterial stiffening on propagation velocity of pressure wave (PWV) which rises with stiffness.

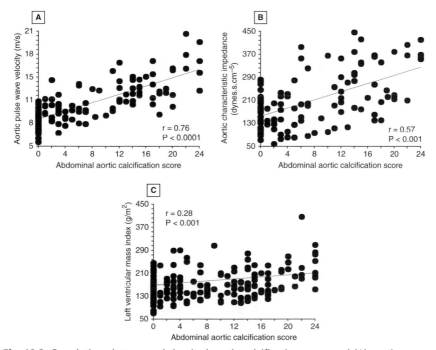

Fig. 18.2 Correlations between abdominal aortic calcification score and (A) aortic (carotid-femoral) pulse wave velocity, (B) aortic characteristic impedance, and (C) left ventricular mass index. All correlations are adjusted for age, mean blood pressure (personal data).

The consequence of higher PWV is the earlier return of reflected pressure waves from peripheral reflective sites to central arteries and aorta. The ascending aorta and central arteries are distant from reflecting sites and, depending on the PWV and artery length, the return of the reflected wave is variably delayed and, therefore, the incident and reflected waves are not in phase. The timing of incident and reflected pressure waves also depends on the duration of LV ejection (heart rate) and transit time of forward pressure waves to and reflected wave returning from reflecting sites, i.e. on PWV and travelling distance. In subjects with distensible arteries and low PWV, the reflected waves affect central arteries during diastole after LV ejection has ceased. This timing is desirable, since the reflected wave causes ascending aortic pressure to rise during early diastole, resulting in lower aortic systolic and pulse pressures. That situation is physiologically advantageous, because the increase of early diastolic pressure has a boosting effect on coronary perfusion without increasing LV after load.

The desirable timing is disrupted by increased PWV due to arterial stiffening. With increased PWV, the reflecting sites appear 'closer' to the ascending aorta and the reflected waves occur earlier, being more closely in phase with incident waves in this region. The earlier return means that the reflected wave affect the central arteries during systole, rather than diastole, thereby amplifying aortic and LV pressures during systole, and reducing aortic pressure during diastole. Increased stiffness and a steep pressure–volume relationship also have a direct effect on diastolic pressure, which declines abruptly during diastolic run-off. The decline of pressure during diastole increases with high stiffness and low resistance. By favoring early wave reflections, arterial stiffening increases peak- and end-systolic pressures in the ascending aorta, increasing myocardial pressure load leading to LV hypertrophy, and increased oxygen consumption, with a parallel reduction of diastolic blood pressure and subendocardial blood–flow (Fig. 18.3).[50–52] AC are tightly associated with arterial stiffness and PWV which is an independent predictor of all-cause and CV mortality in the general population and ESRD patients.[53,54]

Management and prevention

Once present, AC rarely regress, therefore, the primary goals are prevention and stabilization of existing calcifications. Because high proportion of AC are related to atherosclerosis, the general approach is non-specific as advocated for patients with atherosclerosis: control of blood lipids (but no evidence of a benefit with statins), use of aspirin, treatment of obesity and hypertension, physical activity, smoking cessation, and control of diabetes. More specific preventive measures for patients with CKD or ESRD include controlling serum calcium and phosphate levels, thereby avoiding over suppression of parathyroid activity and adynamic bone disease (ABD).[55] Disturbances in calcium and phosphate metabolism are associated with uremic bone disease, and the results of several studies indicated that calcium overload is associated with AC development and progression, suggesting that the over-use of high doses of calcium-based phosphate binders, pharmacological doses of vitamin D, and high calcium concentration in the dialysate should be avoided.[5–7,38,55] Several endogenous calcification inhibitors, e.g. BMP-7[56] and osteopontin,[57] are in early developmental stages and

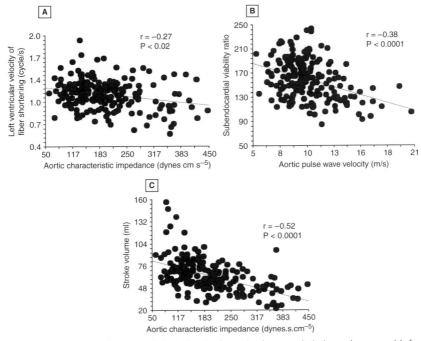

Fig. 18.3 Correlations between (A) abdominal aortic characteristic impedance and left ventricular velocity shortening, (B) aortic pulse wave velocity and subendocardial viability ratio (Buckberg index), and (C) abdominal aortic characteristic impedance and left ventricular stroke volume. All correlations are adjusted for age, and mean blood pressure (personal data).

may be of clinical benefit in treating ectopic calcification. Teriparatide (PTH 1–34) is an anabolic bone-stimulating agent, but it is not approved for the treatment of ABD. The restoration of pulsatile PTH secretion in patients with calcimimetics could be considered in the presence of ABD.[58]

Summary

The arterial calcifications from an active process implicating the interaction of promoters and inhibitors of calcifications that are responsible for phenotype transdifferentiation of vascular smooth muscle cells into ostoblast-like osteogenic cells. This process is influenced by mechanical factors including pulsatile and shear stresses. The two types of calcifications, i.e. intimal and medial have a different impact on arterial functions. The intimal calcification as a part of advanced atherosclerosis results in the development of plaques, arterial lumen decrease or occlusion, and ischemic lesions downstream. Medial calcifications result in the stiffening of arterial walls with an increased systolic and decreased diastolic pressures. This leads to cardiac pressure overload, left ventricular hypertrophy and decreased myocardial perfusion. The two types of calcifications are associated with increased mortality.

References

1. Lindner A, Charra B, Sherrard D, Scribner BM. Accelerated atherosclerosis in prolonged maintenance hemodialysis. *N Engl J Med* 1974;**290**:697–702.

2. London GM, Drüeke TB. Atherosclerosis and arteriosclerosis in chronic renal failure. *Kidney Int* 1997;**51**:1678–95.

3. Pannier B, Guérin AP, Marchais SJ, et al. Arterial structure and function in end-stage renal disease. *Artery Research*, 2007;**1**:79–88.

4. Longenecker JC, Coresh J, Powe NR, et al. Traditional cardiovascular disease risk factors in dialysis patients compared with the general population: the CHOICE Study. *J Am Soc Nephrol* 2002;**13**:1918–27.

5. Braun J, Oldendorf M, Moshage W, et al. Electron beam computed tomography in the evaluation of cardiac calcifications in chronic dialysis patients. *Am J Kidney Dis* 1996;**27**:394–401.

6. Goodman WG, Goldin J, Kuizon BD, et al. Coronary artery calcification in young adults with end-stage renal disease who are undergoing dialysis. *New Engl J Med*, 2000;**342**: 1478–83.

7. Guérin AP, London GM, Marchais SJ, Métivier F. Arterial stiffening and vascular calcifications in end-stage renal disease. *Nephrol Dial Transplant* 2000;**15**:1014–21.

8. Wilson PWF, Kauppila LI, O'Donnell CJ, et al. Abdominal aortic calcific deposits are an important predictor of vascular morbidity and mortality. *Circulation* 2001;**103**:1529–34.

9. Blacher J, Guérin AP, Pannier B, et al. Arterial calcifications, arterial stiffness, and cardiovascular risk in end-stage renal disease. *Hypertension* 2001;**38**:938–42.

10. London GM, Guérin AP, Marchais SJ, et al. Arterial media calcification in end-stage renal disease: impact on all-cause and cardiovascular mortality. *Nephrol Dial Transplant* 2003;**18**:1731–40.

11. Agatston AS, Janowitz WR, Hildner FJ, et al. Quantification of coronary artery calcium using ultrafast computed tomography. *J Am Coll Cardiol* 1990;**15**:827–32.

12. Bellasi A, Ferramosca E, Muntner P, et al. Correlation of simple imaging tests and coronary artery calcium measurement by computed tomography in hemodialysis patients. *Kidney Int* 2006;**70**:1623–8.

13. Sangiorgi G, Rumberger JA, Severson A, et al. Arterial calcification and not lumen stenosis is highly correlated with atherosclerotic plaque burden in humans: a histologic study of 723 coronary artery segments using nondecalcifying methodology. *J Am Coll Cardiol*, 1998;**31**:126–33.

14. Detrano R, Hsiai T, Wang S, et al. Prognostic value of coronary calcification and angiographic stenoses in patients undergoing coronary angiography. *J Am Coll Cardiol* 1996;**27**:285–90.

15. Laurent S, Cockcroft J, Van Bortel L, et al. Expert consensus document on arterial stiffness: methodological issues and clinical applications. *Eur Heart J* 2008;**27**:2588–605.

16. DeLoach SS, Townsend RR. Vascular stiffness: its measurement and significance for epidemiologic and outcome studies. *Clin J Am Soc Nephrol* 2008;**3**:184–92.

17. Schoppet M, Shroff RC, Hofbauer LC, Shanahan CM. Exploring the biology of vascular calcification in chronic kidney disease: what's circulating? *Kidney Int* 2008;**73**:384–90.

18. Demer LL, Tintut Y. Vascular calcification: pathobiology of multifaceted disease. *Circulation* 2008;**117**:2938–48.

19. Steitz SA, Speer ME, Curinga G, et al. Smooth muscle cell phenotypic transition associated with calcification. Upregulation of Cbfa1 and downregulation of smooth muscle lineage markers. *Circ Res*, 2001;**89**:1147–54.

20. Cheng C, Tempel D, van Haperen R, et al. Atherosclerotic lesion size and vulnerability are determined by patterns of fluid shear stress. *Circulation*, 2006;**113**:2744–53.

21. Cunningham KS, Gotlieb AI. The role of shear stress in the pathogenesis of atherosclerosis. *Lab Invest* 2005;**85**:9–23.

22. Shao J-S, Cai J, Towler DA. Molecular mechanisms of vascular calcification: lessons learned from the aorta. *Arterioscler Thromb Vasc Biol* 2006;**26**:1423–30.

23. Moe SM, O' KD, Duan D, et al. Medial artery calcification in ESRD patients is associated with deposition of bone matrix protein. *Kidney Int*, 2002;**61**:638–47.

24. Reynolds JL, Joannides AJ, Skepper JN, et al. Human vascular smooth muscle cells undergo vesicle-mediated calcification in response to changes in extracellular calcium and phosphate concentrations: a potential mechanism for accelerated vascular calcification in ESRD. *J Am Soc Nephrol* 2004;**15**:2857–67.

25. Luo G, Ducy P, McKee MD, et al. Spontaneous calcification of arteries and cartilage in mice lacking matrix Gla protein. *Nature* 1997;**386**:78–81.

26. Sweatt A, Sane DC, Hutson SM, Wallin R. Matrix Gla protein (MGP) and bone morphogenetic protein-2 in aortic calcified lesions of aging rats. *J Thromb Hemost* 2003;**1**:178–85.

27. Speer MY, McKee MD, Guldberg RE, et al. Inactivation of osteopontin gene enhances vascular calcification of matrix Gla protein-deficient mice: evidence for osteopontin as an inductible inhibitor of vascular calcification in vivo. *J Exp Med*, 2002;**196:** 1047–55.

28. Bucay N, Sarosi I, Dunstan CR, et al. Osteoprotegerin-deficient mice develop early onset osteoporosis and arterial calcification. *Genes Dev* 1998;**12**:1260–8.

29. Schafer C, Heiss A, Schwarz A, et al. The serum protein alpha 2-Heremans–Schmid glycoprotein/fetuin-A is a systemically acting inhibitor of ectopic calcification. *J Clin Invest* 2003;**112**:357–66.

30. Lomashvili K, Cobbs S, Hennigar RA, et al. Phosphate-induced vascular calcification: role of pyrophosphate and osteopontin. *J Am Soc Nephrol* 2004;**15**:1392–401.

31. Amann K. Media calcification and intima calcification are distinct entities in chronic kidney disease. *Clin J Am Soc Nephrol*, 2008;**3**:1599–605.

32. Majesky MW. Developmental basis of vascular smooth muscle diversity. *Arterioscler Thromb Vasc Biol*, 2007;**27**,1248–58.

33. Nikolovski J, Kim B-S, Mooney DJ. Cyclic strain inhibits switching of smooth muscle cells to an osteoblast-like phenotype. *FASEB J*, 2003;**17**:455–7.

34. Moe SM, Duan D, Doehle BP, et al. Uremia induces the osteoblast differentiation factor Cbfa1 in human blood vessels. *Kidney Int*, 2003;**63**:1003–11.

35. Hak AE, Pols HA, van Hemert AM, et al. Progression of aortic calcification is associated with metacarpal bone loss during menopause: a population-based longitudinal study. *Arterioscler Thromb Vasc Biol* 2000;**20**:1926–31.

36. Schulz E, Arfai K, Liu X, et al. Aortic calcification and the risk of osteoporosis and fractures. *J Clin Endocrin Metab*, 2004;**89**:4246–53.

37. London GM, Marty C, Marchais SJ, et al. Arterial calcifications and bone histomorphometry in end-stage renal disease. *J Am Soc Nephrol*, 2004;**15**:1943–51.

38. London GM, Marchais SJ, Guérin AP, et al. Association of bone activity, calcium load, aortic stiffness, and calcifications in ESRD. *J Am Soc Nephrol* 2008;**19**:1827–35.

39. Raggi P, Bellasi A, Ferramosca E, et al. Pulse wave velocity is inversely related to vertebral bone density in hemodialysis patients. *Hypertension*, 2007;**49**:1278–84.

40. Toussaint ND, Lau KK, Strauss BJ, et al. Association between vascular calcification, arterial stiffness and bone mineral density in chronic kidney disease. *Nephrol Dial Transplant* 2008;**23**:586–93.

41. Parhami F, Garfinkel A, Demer LL. Role of lipids in osteoporosis. *Arterioscler Thromb Vasc Biol* 2000;**20**:2346–8.

42. Braam LA, Hoeks APG, Brouns F, et al. Beneficial effects of vitamins D and K on the elastic properties of the vessel wall in postmenopausal women: A follow-up study. *Thromb Hemost*, 2004;**91**:373–380.

43. Hofbauer LC, Schoppet M. Clinical implications of the osteoprotegerin/RANKL/RANK system for bone and vascular diseases. *J Am Med Ass* 2004;**292**:490–5.

44. Huang JC, Sakata T, Pfleger LL, et al. PTH differentially regulates expression of RANKL and OPG. *J Bone Miner Res* 2004;**19**:234–44.

45. Jono S, Nishizawa Y, Shioi A, Morii H. 1,25-Dihydroxyvitamin D3 increases *in vitro* vascular calcification by modulating secretion of endogenous parathyroid-hormone-related peptide. *Circulation* 1998;**98**:1302–6.

46. Arad Y, Spadaro LA, Roth M, et al. Serum concentrations of calcium, 1,25-vitamin D and parathyroid hormone are not correlated with coronary calcifications. An electron beam computed tomography study. *Coron Artery Dis* 1998;**9**:513–18.

47. Weening RH. Pathogenesis of calciphylaxis. Hans Selye to nuclear factor κ-B. *J Am Acad Dermatol*, 2008;**58**:458–71.

48. Huang H, Virmani R, Younis H, et al. The impact of calcification on the biomechanical stability of atherosclerotic plaques. *Circulation*, 2001;**103**:1051–6.

49. Lin TC, Tintut Y, Lyman A, et al. Mechanical response of a calcified plaque model to fluid shear force. *Ann Biomed Eng*, 2006;**34**:1535–41.

50. London GM, Blacher J, Pannier B, et al. Arterial wave reflections and survival in end-stage renal failure. *Hypertension*, 2001;**38**:434–8.

51. Latham RD, Westerhof N, Sipkema P, et al. Regional wave travel and reflections along the human aorta: a study with six simultaneous micromanometric pressures. *Circulation*, 1985;**72**: 1257–69.

52. London GM, Yaginuma T. Wave reflections: clinical and therapeutic aspects. In: M.E. Safar and M.F. O'Rourke (eds), *The Arterial System in Hypertension*. Dordrecht: Kluwer Academic Publishers, 1993:221–37.

53. Laurent S, Boutouyrie P, Asmar R, et al. Aortic stiffness is an independent predictor of all-cause and cardiovascular mortality in hypertensive patients. *Hypertension*, 2001;**37**:1236–41.

54. Brandenburg VM, Floege J. Adynamic bone disease—bone and beyond. *NDT Plus* 2008;**3**:135–47.

55. Davies MR, Lund RJ, Hruska KA. BMP-7 is an efficacious treatment of vascular calcification in a murine model of atherosclerosis and chronic renal failure. *J Am Soc Nephrol* 2003;**14**:1559–67.

56. Li T, Surendran K, Zawaideh MA, et al. Bone morphogenetic protein 7: a novel treatment for chronic renal and bone disease. *Curr Opin Nephrol Hypertens* 2004;**13**:417–22.

57. Steitz SA, Speer MY, McKee MD, et al. Osteopontin inhibits mineral deposition and promotes regression of ectopic calcification. *Am J Pathol* 2002;**161**:2035–46.

58. Chertow GM, Burke SK, Raggi P, et al. Sevelamer attenuates the progression of coronary and aortic calcification in hemodialysis patient. *Kidney Int* 2002;**62**:245–52.

Chapter 19

Clinical management of vascular and soft tissue calcifications in chronic kidney disease patients

Markus Ketteler and Jürgen Floege

Calcification in patients with ESRD can result in a range of pathologies including vascular and valvular calcification, extra-osseous soft-tissue and solid organ calcification, corneal and conjunctival calcification, peritoneal calcification, as well as calcific uremic arteriolopathy (CUA; formerly termed 'calciphylaxis'). There is almost no restriction to sites that can calcify in CKD. Apart from more common sites of soft-tissue calcification such as hips or the shoulder region (Teutschländer's disease; Fig. 19.1), tumorous calcifications have been described in hands, feet, the nose, and within the spinal canal. In contrast to cardiovascular calcifications, very little systematic data are available on the prevalence and clinical relevance of soft tissue calcification in CKD patients and this chapter will therefore focus to a large extent on the former.

Cardiovascular and soft-tissue calcification is part of the definition of chronic kidney disease – mineral and bone disorder (CKD-MBD). Vascular calcification is not a homogenous entity, but a rather complex systemic manifestation influenced by derangements of calcium and phosphate homeostasis, by dysregulated calcification inhibitors and promoters, and by underlying arterial diseases (atherosclerosis or arteriosclerosis)—as outlined in a number of other chapters in this book edition. Despite the clear-cut risk association between the presence of cardiovascular calcification and mortality, it is currently not well defined, how this knowledge about calcification should be translated into active clinical management of affected patients. Based on experimental insights into the biology of calcification processes, epidemiological studies and, unfortunately very few, prospective trials, this chapter attempts to weigh the potential of the available therapeutic approaches to prevent or limit progressive cardiovascular calcification, and judge their benefits and harms.

Cardiovascular calcifications in chronic kidney disease

Accelerated calcifying athero- and arteriosclerosis, as well as valvular heart disease, are central characteristics of the cardiovascular disease manifestations in CKD patients. The different roles of intimal (atherosclerotic) and medial (arteriosclerotic) vascular

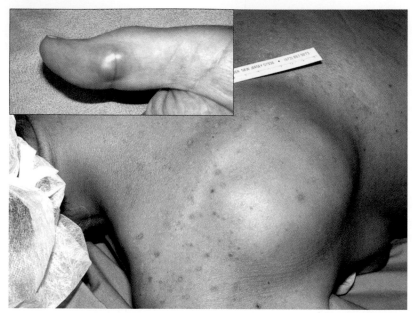

Fig. 19.1 Tumorous soft-tissue calcifications of a thumb and a shoulder joint are shown. In both patients, there was a strong association with persistent hyperphosphatemia. (Copyright: Floege J. *Kidney Int* 2004;65:2447–62).

Intimal (plaque) calcification   **Medial calcification (Mönckeberg type)**

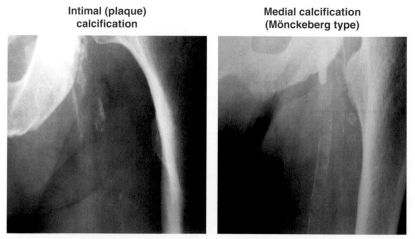

Fig. 19.2 Typical calcification patterns of atherosclerotic (left) and arteriosclerotic (right) calcifications are demonstrated on these conventional pelvic X-rays. Taken from London G, et al. *Nephrol Dial Transplant* 2003;**18**:1731–40.

pathology are well described in this population (Fig. 19.2). While plaques obstruct vessels and cause ischemic events, mediasclerosis leads to arterial stiffening contributing to increased endsystolic left ventricular (LV) pressure and the subsequent development of LV dysfunction. Different vascular beds may however show quite distinct manifestations of vascular disease and calcification which complicates the interpretation of imaging results.

While intimal plaque calcification is the key feature of genuine atherosclerosis and probably the key type of coronary artery calcification in the normal population, medial calcification seems to predominantly manifest in peripheral and small arteries. Whether larger arteries and the aorta may develop 'pure' arteriosclerosis, or whether large artery calcification may be a mixture of intimal and medial, or even mostly pure intimal calcification, is a matter of debate. The burden of cardiovascular calcification is extremely high in CKD, with diabetes and age being the most consistent exacerbating factors. However, hyperphosphatemia, hypercalcemia, or probably even more important, a positive calcium load (especially in the presence of low bone turnover) are also thought to be key factors with significant impact on cardiovascular mortality and progression of unwanted calcifications in uremia.[1] Furthermore, there is biological and some clinical evidence that deficiencies of calcification inhibitors may increase the risk of calcification and potentially mortality.

Other clinically important cardiovascular calcifications affect the valves, predominantly the aortic and mitral valve with resultant stenosis, as well as the myocardium. The latter is rarely apparent by imaging methods and its clinical relevance remains relatively speculative. However, it may contribute to the very high incidence of sudden cardiac death in the dialysis population, since myocardial microcalcifications may well result in disturbances of electric conductivity.

A rare, but generally very severe manifestation of vascular calcification is CUA. It is a life-threatening syndrome characterized by progressive and painful skin ulcerations associated with medial calcification of medium-size and small cutaneous arterial vessels (Fig. 19.3). Calciphylaxis primarily affects patients on dialysis or after renal transplantation, however, rare cases have been reported in patients with normal renal function and in association with chronic-inflammatory disease, malignancy or primary hyperparathyroidism.[2] The clinical manifestation of calciphylaxis is associated with high mortality of up to 80%, largely due to superinfection of necrotic skin lesions with subsequent sepsis and/or concomitant cardiovascular events.

Most of the available imaging studies on the prevalence and natural history of cardiovascular calcification in CKD used CT-based techniques (EBCT, MSCT). EBCT and MSCT are currently regarded as the Gold standard among imaging techniques, because they yield quantitative results and appear to be reproducible. However, reasonable correlations between CT-based coronary artery calcification (CAC) scores and plain lateral abdominal radiographs as well as echocardiography (valvular calcification) may exist.[3] The majority of the calcification imaging data were obtained in CKD stage 5D population, while some studies including patients in earlier CKD stages are available showing similar patterns, but somewhat lower frequencies of calcification manifestations when compared with the dialysis population.

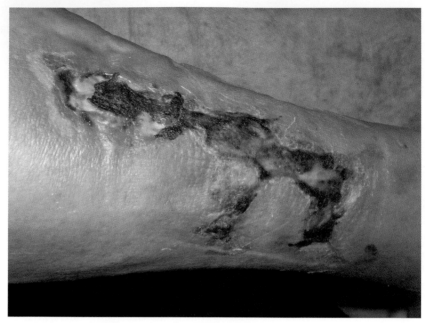

Fig. 19.3 Typical presentation of lower limb calciphylaxis (CUA) is shown. The clinical picture is completed by extreme painfulness of the necrotic lesion.

Data on calcification prevalence in more than 4.000 CKD patients are currently reported in the literature. In prevalent patients in CKD stage 5D, CAC is found in up to 90% of this population. In incident dialysis patients and patients in CKD stages 4–5, significant vascular calcification can be detected in about 50–60%. Risk associations between the development and progression of calcification, and epidemiological and biochemical parameters were analyzed in most of these studies. The prevalence of CKD-related cardiovascular calcification is dependent on age and time on dialysis, but in general quite variable. Male gender, high serum iPTH, and/or alkaline phosphatase levels, inflammation (CRP levels), calcium intake, hyperphosphatemia, and increased calcium × phosphate product were among the prominent, but less consistent risk factors of progressive cardiovascular calcification (Table 19.1).

General remarks on the pathophysiology of extra-osseous calcification

For a long time, the excessive nature of extra-osseous calcifications in uremia was interpreted as the result of persistent supersaturation of serum with calcium and phosphate ions leading to passive precipitation. Serum is 'metastable' concerning solubility of calcium and phosphate. That means that precipitation is controlled by a number of systemic and local calcium-regulatory factors. In general, the following

Table 19.1 Factors associated (+) or not associated (–) with vascular/valvular calcifications in dialysis patients. Floege *NDT* 2003 and KDIGO. Clinical practice guidelines for the management of CKD-MBD *KI* 2009;**113**:51–130.

Parameter	Association with cardiovascular calcifications*
Age of the patient	+
Duration of dialysis	+
Diabetes mellitus	+
Ca x PO_4 product; serum Ca^{2+} or PO_4^-	+/–
Oral calcium-containing phosphate-binder dose	+
iPTH serum level	+/–
Increased serum fibrinogen, CRP and/or low albumin	+
Dyslipidemia	–
Hyperhomocysteinemia	+/–

* +, Consistent association in most studies; +/–, variable association in studies; –, most studies fail to demonstrate a linear correlation with calcifications.

pathophysiological pathways contribute to unwanted extra-osseous calcification in CKD:

♦ Passive calcium and phosphate precipitation triggered by excessively high extracellular ion concentrations. This is particularly the case in patients with tumoral soft tissue calcinosis.

♦ Dysregulation of inducers of cellular osteogenic transformation and hydroxyapatite formation (especially in the vascular wall).

♦ Calcification inhibitor deficiencies (fetuin-A, matrix Gla protein, pyrophosphates, etc.).

Hyperphosphatemia seems to be among the most powerful inducers of cardiovascular calcification. In numerous experimental studies, it could be documented that high phosphate, by causing increases in intracellular phosphate concentrations, induced a phenotypic switch of vascular smooth muscle cells (VSMC) to osteoblast-like cells with consecutive hydroxyapatite deposition, expression of bone proteins and extracellular matrix, characterized by *de novo* upregulation of the osteoblast transcription factor Runx2 (cbfa-1),[1,4] as outlined in more detail elsewhere in this edition. Based on these findings, it appears most reasonable that the clinical control of hyperphosphatemia and systemic calcium load should be among the cornerstones of clinical management.

There are several calcium-regulatory factors which inhibit calcification processes at systemic and local levels.[1] Fetuin-A (α2-Schmid Heremans glycoprotein, AHSG) and matrix Gla protein (MGP) are among the prototypes of these factors. Deficiencies of calcification inhibitors shift the balance towards progressive unwanted calcification, which may then get triggered or exacerbated by hyperphosphatemia and high calcium loads. While fetuin-A is an inflammation-dependent negative acute-phase protein, MGP activity depends on vitamin K availability. How these features may translate into clinical practice will be outlined below.

Calcification progression and calcium × phosphate balance

No definite evidence is available to create algorithms on how to prevent or treat progressive cardiovascular calcification in CKD. The high mortality rates associated with hyperphosphatemia in epidemiological studies as well as the overwhelming biological plausibility that high phosphate induces vascular hydroxyapatite deposition in soft-tissues and blood vessels make hyperphosphatemia the prime target of treatment approaches in this regard. Hyperphosphatemia however is often coupled with a parallel calcium load, since in clinical practice calcium-containing phosphate binders play a major role in the attempt to abrogate high phosphate levels.

There are five reports which evaluated the effects of different phosphate binder therapies on the progression of coronary artery calcification (CAC) scores in the CKD population.[5–9] Four of those were performed in hemodialysis patients, one was performed in patients in CKD stages 3–5 not on dialysis. The Treat-to-Goal (TTG) study[5] investigated the progression of CAC and aortic calcification (EBCT) in prevalent hemodialysis patients comparing the impact of sevelamer-HCl to calcium-containing phosphate binders over a period of 1 year. Here, sevelamer-HCl use was shown to be associated with a lack of calcification progression (Fig. 19.4). In the Renagel in New Dialysis Patients (RIND) study,[6] a similar design was used and similar results were obtained in incident hemodialysis patients randomized within 90 days after starting dialysis treatment.

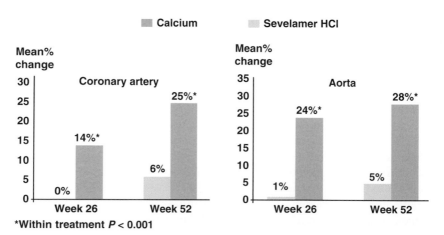

Fig. 19.4 Results from the TTG study: Over a follow-up of one year, progressive coronary artery calcification was observed with calcium-containing phosphate binder treatment versus sevelamer-HCl despite similar efficacy of phosphate lowering. Reproduced from Chertow GM, Burke SK, Raggi P. *Kidney Int* 2002;**62**:245–52. Reprinted with permission from Macmillan Publishers Ltd.

In contrast, the Calcium Acetate Renagel Evaluation-2 (CARE 2) study[7] demonstrated equal progression rates of CAC with both calcium acetate and sevelamer-HCl when atorvastatin was added to lower low density lipoprotein low density lipoprotein (LDL)-cholesterol to comparable levels in both treatment arms. However, compared with the very similar TTG study, the CARE-2 study was characterized by much more rapid progression of calcification and higher percentages of diabetics and smokers, suggesting that calcification progress was primarily driven by non-phosphate and non-calcium related factors in this study. The BRIC study[8] longitudinally investigated CAC progression and bone histomorphometry in hemodialysis patients also comparing calcium acetate versus sevelamer-HCl. The key observations in the BRIC study were that there was no difference in CAC progression or changes in bone remodeling between the two treatment groups. This study, however, had a major confounder, since high dialysate calcium concentrations (1.75mmol/l) were used in most patients. Thus, a generally positive calcium balance may have blunted or even neutralized the potential advantage of the calcium-free phosphate binder.

The study by Russo and colleagues[9] is the only current study evaluating CAC progression in CKD patients not on dialysis. Patients were stratified to treatment with low phosphate diet alone, to low phosphate diet plus calcium carbonate or to low phosphate diet plus sevelamer-HCl. CAC progression was significantly ameliorated only in the sevelamer-HCl treated group, while there was a trend towards less pronounced CAC progression in the calcium carbonate compared with the low phosphate diet alone group. Taking together the results from epidemiological trials and from these prospective studies on the surrogate outcome 'CAC progression', it appears quite possible, however, not finally proven, that a high calcium load may be an unwanted factor in the pathogenesis of CKD-related calcification in subjects with pre-existing calcification. The threshold of a tolerable versus a harmful calcium load is currently not defined and probably an individual value, and it may well depend on the co-existing magnitude of hyperphosphatemia left despite administration of calcium-containing phosphate binders, and on the actual bone turnover state.

There are a couple of studies investigating the effects of different phosphate binders on mortality. The largest study, the Dialysis Clinical Outcomes Revisited (DCOR), randomized 2103 prevalent CKD stage 5D patients to either sevelamer-HCl or to calcium-containing phosphate binders.[10] Patients were followed-up for a mean time period of 20 months. 1068 patients completed the study and there were no significant differences in all-cause or cardiovascular mortality rates when comparing both treatment arms. However, a secondary analysis of the DCOR cohort revealed a survival advantage associated with sevelamer-HCl use in patients older than 65 years (in this subgroup the majority of events occurred) and in patients treated with sevelamer-HCl for more than 2 years. Calcification progression was not recorded in the DCOR protocol.

The second study examining mortality associated with phosphate binder treatments was the RIND study.[11] One-hundred-and-twenty-seven incident dialysis patients receiving either sevelamer-HCl or calcium-containing phosphate binder were observed for a median follow-up of 44 months, so twice as long as subjects included in the DCOR trial. The difference in unadjusted mortality rates for patients randomized to calcium-containing phosphate binders was 10.6 per 100 patient-years versus 5.3 per

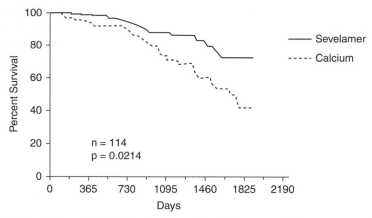

Fig. 19.5 Results from the RIND study: after extended long-term follow-up, a survival advantage for sevelamer-HCl-treated incident hemodialysis patients was demonstrated when compared with subjects treated with calcium-containing phosphate binders. Reproduced from Block GA, Raggi P, Bellas A, Kooienga L, Spiegel DM. *Kidney Int* 2007;**71**:438–41. Reprinted with permission from Macmillan Publishers Ltd.

100 patient-years for patients randomized to sevelamer-HCl, but this obvious trend failed reaching significance. However, in multivariate analysis including 10 variables, the difference between the treatment groups became statistically significant in favor of sevelamer-HCl suggesting some imbalance with respect to the covariates (Fig. 19.5). There are no reports comparing the effects of reaching different serum phosphate target levels on mortality or calcification end-points. There are also no prospective outcome studies comparing effects of lanthanum- or aluminum-based phosphate binders.

In patients with tumorous soft tissue calcification, aggressive treatment of hyper-phosphatemia and avoidance of calcium loading appear to be essential to arrest further progress. Regression of the calcifications over weeks to months is a regular observation following a successful kidney transplantation in such patients, at the cost of hypercalciuria and sometimes hypercalcemia. In contrast, available studies on the course of vascular calcification after renal transplantation consistently show an arrest, but no regression over the first 1–2 years.

Vitamin D-analogues and extra-osseous calcification

1,25-dihydroxy-vitamin D (calcitriol) and other active vitamin D analogues facilitate intestinal calcium absorption and also increase the absorbed phosphate load.[12] In experimental models with or without renal impairment, it was reproducibly shown that calcitriol treatment caused soft-tissue and vascular calcification when it was asso-ciated with increases in the calcium × phosphate product. Recent studies in rat models of secondary hyperparathyroidism and renal insufficiency were suggestive of differ-ences among the available active vitamin D-compounds, pointing to a calcification-neutral effect of paricalcitol despite similar efficacy to reduce elevated parathyroid

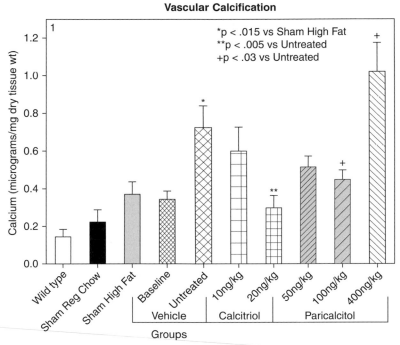

Fig. 19.6 Results from calcification-prone LDL-knockout CKD mice: Low doses of calcitriol or paricalcitol protected from vascular calcification, while high doses induced calcification. Low doses suppressed osteogenic differentiation (Runx2/cbfa-1 expression). Reproduced from Mathew S, Lund RJ, Chaudhary LR, Geurs T, Hruska KA. *J Am Soc Nephrol* 2008;**19**:1509–19.

hormone levels.[13,14] However, uncontrolled other laboratory parameters, in particular hyperphosphatemia, preclude a direct extrapolation to the dialysis patient situation. Furthermore, a study in uremic LDL-receptor knockout mice suggested that vitamin D-analogues (calcitriol, paricalcitol) may have similar differential effects on the calcification phenotype of such models depending on whether low (calcification-protective) or high (calcification-inducing) doses were administered (Fig. 19.6).[15] These protective effects may be related to the down-regulation of Runx2 (cbfa-1) in vascular smooth muscle cells, the key transcription factor of osteogenic differentiation as outlined elsewhere and above.

There are no systematic clinical observations on active vitamin D-analogues and calcification initiation or progression. Epidemiological evidence suggests that treatment with active vitamin D-analogues translates into improved survival in dialysis and CKD patients. However, low doses of active vitamin D-analogues (which are essentially steroid hormones) exert a variety of beneficial actions on cardiovascular and immune functions,[12] which may counteract any detrimental effect on calcification. It appears likely, however, that high doses of active vitamin D may be a risk factor for the development of extra-osseous hydroxyapatite deposition, by both increasing extracellular calcium and phosphate concentrations, and by potentially over-suppressing bone turnover. This assumption is in line with recent data showing that the survival benefit derived from oral calcitriol in a large dialysis population was only apparent at 0.25μ/day, but not at 1μg/day.[16]

Parathyroid hormone and bone turnover

The connection between deranged parathyroid hormone (PTH) secretion and cardio-vascular calcification is insufficiently understood. So far no clinical studies have system-atically investigated the effect of parathyroidectomy or the impact of calcimimetics on calcification progression or regression. Epidemiological data mostly point to increased mortality at extremes of serum PTH concentrations, i.e. iPTH< 100 or >800pg/mL. Experimental data *in vitro* and from *in vivo* models of renal insufficiency with second-ary hyperparathyroidism suggest that calcimimetics are calcification-neutral but actively blunted vitamin D-induced calcification (Fig. 19.7).[14,17] Our own studies observing treatment effects of calcimimetics on calcification phenotypes of fetuin-A knockout mice or adenine-induced nephropathy suggested PTH-independent, direct vascular effects by suppressing Runx2 (cbfa-1) in the vascular wall of these animals.

There are historical and incidental clinical observations in dialysis patients with severe and refractory hyperparathyroidism that vascular calcifications may disappear within weeks to months after parathyroidectomy (e.g. medial calcification of extrem-ity arteries as shown by conventional X-ray). Calcification-protective properties of calcimimetics in humans are currently tested in the prospective ADVANCE study, which evaluates the progression of CAC scores by MSCT in hemodialysis patients. The effect of cinacalcet-HCl treatment on mortality and cardiovascular event rates is currently being tested in the EVOLVE trial, which has enrolled close to 4000 patients on hemodialysis.

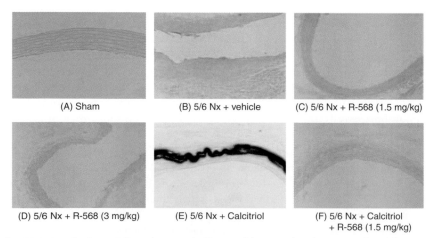

(A) Sham   (B) 5/6 Nx + vehicle   (C) 5/6 Nx + R-568 (1.5 mg/kg)

(D) 5/6 Nx + R-568 (3 mg/kg)   (E) 5/6 Nx + Calcitriol   (F) 5/6 Nx + Calcitriol + R-568 (1.5 mg/kg)

Fig. 19.7 Results from 5/6-nephrectomized rats with secondary hyperparathyroidism: calcitriol-induced medial calcifications could be abolished by co-treatment with the calcimimetic compound R-568.[17]

An important aspect linking parathyroid function and extra-osseous calcification is the impact of bone turnover, the so-called 'bone-vascular axis'. Both a high and a low bone turnover seem to be closely associated with increased cardiovascular calcification, the latter potentially being even more harmful. In 1996, Braun and colleagues were the first to demonstrate an inverse relationship between CAC scores and bone mineral density in hemodialysis patients.[18] In 2004 and 2008, London et al. demonstrated that an adynamic bone, associated with over-suppressed iPTH levels, was the key risk factor of arterial calcification.[19,20] The most powerful association was found when low bone turnover was associated with high calcium loads, e.g. by calcium-containing phosphate binder therapy. Numerous studies actually supported this scenario by employing either bone histomorphometry or CT-based imaging techniques. It seems warranted to avoid both low and high bone turnover states throughout all stages of CKD in order to protect from adverse cardiovascular outcomes.

Blood pressure and cardiovascular calcifications

While the association between arterial hypertension and mortality is quite clear both in the normal population, a connection of hypertension to progressive calcification is not established. Moreover, in patients with advanced CKD inverse relationships between hypertension and mortality were observed in some studies, the so-called phenomenon of 'reverse epidemiology' in CKD. Hypertension may indirectly favor vascular calcification by initiating endothelial damage and triggering atherosclerotic plaque development, i.e. a matrix for intimal calcification, but there are no direct study data to support such a concept. Classical rat models of arterial hypertension are not characterized by an increasing risk of vascular calcification, unless renal failure or phosphate loading are superimposed.

Vice versa, blood pressure behavior changes secondary to the magnitude of medial calcification—arterial stiffness causes widening of the gap between systolic and diastolic pressures. Increased pulse pressure develops with increasing systolic and decreasing diastolic values indicating loss of arterial compliance ('Windkessel' function). This type of hypertension accelerates left ventricular dysfunction by premature reflection of the arterial pulse wave and, thus represents, a candid morbidity risk factor, as outlined above and elsewhere in this book.

Diabetes mellitus and cardiovascular calcification

Besides age and CKD, diabetes is the third major etiology closely associated with premature, severe and progressive cardiovascular calcification (Table 19.1). Based on epidemiological data, the combination of all three factors definitely produces the highest likelihood to show unwanted extra-osseous calcification. The pathophysiology of diabetes-induced calcification is, however, less clear. One likely reason why diabetic patients are calcification-prone could be that they develop dyslipidemic patterns early on in their disease course. Dyslipidemia produces an atherosclerotic plaque burden serving as a matrix for intimal hydroxyapatite deposition. Another, however unproven hypothesis could be that glycosylation of calcification inhibitory factors, by causing subsequent inhibitory dysfunction, may produce a millieu that insufficiently antagonizes calcification processes. Independent of the underlying pathophysiology, physicians must realize the enormous cardiovascular risk burden of diabetic CKD patients, and take into account rigorous strategies to minimize hyperphosphatemia and inadequate calcium loads, in addition to the general management of metabolic control and blood pressure.

Vitamin K and cardiovascular calcification

A key factor in calcification protection is matrix Gla protein (MGP), belonging to a family of N-terminal γ-carboxylated (Gla) proteins, which require post-translational vitamin K-dependent γ-carboxylation for activation to physiologically counteract cartilage and arterial calcification. MGP gene knockout mice are characterized by severe medial calcification of the aorta leading to lethal ruptures of the bone-like aorta within a few weeks after birth.[21] Three pieces of clinical evidence connecting vitamin K deficiency to the risk of vascular calcification are currently reported. First, the Rotterdam study group identified that a low vitamin K2 (menaquinone) intake was associated with coronary artery disease-related and all-cause mortality as well with the severity of aortic calcification.[22] Secondly, long-term use of vitamin K-antagonist-based oral anticoagulation (warfarin) in patients with native aortic valve disease was found to be associated with higher coronary and valvular calcium scores as compared with a cohort without anticoagulation.[23] Finally, CUA is associated with a high coincidence of warfarin treatment. In the German Calciphylaxis Registry, 71 patients were included between November 2006 and February 2009, and more than 50% of these cases were associated with warfarin use.

Vascular calcification can be induced by warfarin in rat models. Withdrawal of warfarin and subsequent high dose vitamin K1 or K2 replacement can partially reverse such calcifications.[24] Low doses are, however, insufficient for calcification regression, once vitamin K depletion has manifested. Data from registries and prospective clinical studies (e.g. evaluation of the therapeutic impact of menaquinone on the progression of cardiovascular calcification) are urgently needed to explore the potential therapeutic impact of vitamin K replacement strategies. Importantly, even high-dose vitamin K supplementation is harmless, since it does not cause a pro-coagulant state.

Therapeutic options in calcific uremic arteriolopathy

In general, the key therapeutic strategies to limit cardiovascular calcification progression include phosphate lowering (by phosphate binders, intensified dialysis and diet), avoiding a positive calcium balance (including reduction or withdrawal of vitamin D treatment, adjustment of dialysate calcium, and oral calcium loading), aggressively treating severe hyperparathyroidism, if applicable (including cinacalcet or the option of 'emergency parathyroidectomy') and the avoidance of PTH over suppression with resultant adynamic bone disease. These mainstay approaches also represent primary treatment options in individuals developing CUA. Another basic principle of therapeutic strategies is the early initiation of broad-spectrum antibiotic administration once exulcerations become associated with a systemic pro-inflammatory state.

Based on case reports and small case-control series, there are some special approaches that may be successful to tackle individual CUA disease courses. Emergent data are available concerning the use of sodium thiosulphate and bisphosphonates. Thiosulphate is licensed as a chelating agent indicated in the treatment of cyanide intoxication. It exhibits a high affinity to calcium potentially interfering with calcium and phosphate precipitation, and producing soluble calcium thiosulphate, which is removed by dialysis. Thiosulphate may also serve as an antioxidant comparable to the glutathione-redox-system. It may be of utmost interest to evaluate the effects of thiosulphate on general cardiovascular calcification progression beyond its potential in CUA. However, there is uncertainty about potential side effects on bone histology, if thiosulphate is administered over prolonged periods.

Concerning bisphosphonates, it is currently unclear, whether this group of drugs interacts with extra-osseous calcification processes via their antiresorptive bone effects or via immediate peripheral pyrophosphate-like effects at the vascular sites. Although case reports on beneficial effects of pamidronate in CUA patients were published, caution is still advised concerning uncritical use of bisphosphonates in this patient group. A significant proportion of CUA cases may develop associated with or even caused by low bone turnover (adynamic bone disease). In these cases, bisphosphonates will further aggravate the adynamic turnover and thus potentially cause harm.

In CUA patients on warfarin treatment, warfarin withdrawal and a switch to heparin use is urgently recommended, despite a lack of clear-cut prospective clinical evidence. However, the biological plausibility that vitamin K antagonism favors vascular calcification is currently regarded as relevant and subsequent vitamin K supplementation may have to be addressed by future studies in this patient group.

Basile and colleagues reported on successful hyperbaric oxygen therapy in a small number of CUA patients.[25] This approach is based on the attempt to improve wound healing in ischemic tissues. In this study, affected areas were exposed 100% oxygen under 2.5-fold elevated atmospheric pressure in a closed chamber for 90 minutes per session. Glucocorticoid treatment in early, non-ulcerated stages of CUA may be another option, however, immunosuppression must certainly be avoided when ulcers carry the risk of superinfection.

Summary

Vascular and soft-tissue calcifications are not just a random process of passive calcium and phosphate precipitation, but involve active cellular processes influenced by the presence or absence of inhibitors and inducers. In this context, phosphate and calcium are among the key active inducers of cellular pro-calcifying pathomechanisms, especially in patients with advanced CKD. Additionally, the presence (or absence) and activity of calcification inhibitors may potently modify clinical calcification progression in CKD patients at risk. Cardiovascular calcification is amongst the strongest risk predictors of death in the CKD population, so appropriate management approaches, including phosphate lowering and avoidance of unreasonable calcium loads, are likely to improve outcomes. In the future, modifying vitamin K status, thiosulphate administration, or anti-inflammatory strategies may become additional tools in calcification-prone CKD individuals.

References

1. Ketteler M, Schlieper G, Floege J. Calcification and cardiovascular health: new insights into an old phenomenon. *Hypertension* (2006);**47:**1027–34.

2. Nigwekar SU, Wolf M, Sterns RH, Hix JK. Calciphylaxis from non-uremic causes: a systematic review. *Clin J Am Soc Nephrol* (2008);**3:**1139–43.

3. Bellasi A, Ferramosca E, Muntner P, et al. Correlation of simple imaging tests and coronary artery calcium measured by computed tomography in hemodialysis patients. *Kidney Int* (2006);**70:**1623–8.

4. Giachelli CM. Vascular calcification mechanisms. *J Am Soc Nephrol* (2004);**15:**2959–64.

5. Chertow GM, Burke SK, Raggi P. Sevelamer attenuates the progression of coronary and aortic calcification in hemodialysis patients. *Kidney Int* (2002);**62:**245–52.

6. Block GA, Spiegel DM, Ehrlich J, et al. Effects of sevelamer and calcium on coronary artery calcification in patients new to hemodialysis. *Kidney Int* (2005);**68:**1815–24.

7. Qunibi W, Moustafa M, Muenz LR, et al. CARE-2 Investigators. A 1-year randomised trial of calcium acetate versus sevelamer on progression of coronary artery calcification in hemodialysis patients with comparable lipid control: the Calcium Acetate Renagel Evaluation-2 (CARE-2) study. *Am J Kidney Dis* (2008);**51:**952–65.

8. Barreto DV, Barreto F de C, de Carvalho AB, et al. Phosphate binder impact on bone remodeling and coronary calcification–results from the BRiC study. *Nephron Clin Pract* (2008);**110:**c273–83.

9. Russo D, Miranda I, Ruocco C, et al. The progression of coronary artery calcification in predialysis patients on calcium carbonate or sevelamer. *Kidney Int* (2007);**72:**1255–61.

10. Suki WN, Zabaneh R, Cangiano JL, et al. Effects of sevelamer and calcium-based phosphate binders on mortality in hemodialysis patients. *Kidney Int* (2007);**72:**1130–7.

11. Block GA, Raggi P, Bellasi A, Kooienga L, Spiegel DM. Mortality effect of coronary calcification and phosphate binder choice in incident hemodialysis patients. *Kidney Int* (2007);**71:**438–41.

12. Holick MF. Vitamin D deficiency. *N Engl J Med* (2007);**357:**266–81.

13. Mizobuchi M, Finch JL, Martin DR, Slatopolsky E. Differential effects of vitamin D receptor activators on vascular calcification in uremic rats. *Kidney Int* (2007);**72:**709–15.

14. Lopez I, Mendoza FJ, Aguilera-Tejero E, et al. The effect of calcitriol, paricalcitol, and a calcimimetic on extra-osseous calcifications in uremic rats. *Kidney Int* (2008);**73:**300–7.

15. Mathew S, Lund RJ, Chaudhary LR, Geurs T, Hruska KA. Vitamin D receptor activators can protect against vascular calcification. *J Am Soc Nephrol* (2008);**19:**1509–19.

16. Naves-Díaz M, Alvarez-Hernández D, Passlick-Deetjen J, et al. Oral active vitamin D is associated with improved survival in hemodialysis patients. *Kidney Int* (2008);**74:**1070–8.

17. Lopez I, Aguilera-Tejero E, Mendoza FJ, et al. Calcimimetic R-568 decreases extra-osseous calcifications in uremic rats treated with calcitriol. *J Am Soc Nephrol* (2006);**17:**795–804.

18. Braun J, Oldendorf M, Moshage W, et al. Electron beam computed tomography in the evaluation of cardiac calcification in chronic dialysis patients. *Am J Kidney Dis* (1996);**27:**394–401.

19. London GM, Marty C, Marchais SJ, Guerin AP, Metivier F, de Vernejoul MC. Arterial calcifications and bone histomorphometry in end-stage renal disease. *J Am Soc Nephrol* (2004);**15:**1943–51.

20. London GM, Marchais SJ, Guérin AP, Boutouyrie P, Métivier F, de Vernejoul MC. Association of bone activity, calcium load, aortic stiffness, and calcifications in ESRD. *J Am Soc Nephrol* (2008);**19**:1827–35.

21. Luo G, Ducy P, McKee MD, et al. Spontaneous calcification of arteries and cartilage in mice lacking matrix Gla protein. *Nature* (1997);**386**:78–81.

22. Geleijnse JM, Vermeer C, Grobbee DE, et al. Dietary intake of menaquinone is associated with a reduced risk of coronary heart disease: the Rotterdam Study. *J Nutr* (2004);**134**:3100–5.

23. Koos R, Mahnken AH, Muhlenbruch G, et al. Relation of oral anticoagulation to cardiac valvular and coronary calcium assessed by multislice spiral computed tomography. *Am J Cardiol* (2005);**96**:747–9.

24. Schurgers LJ, Spronk HM, Soute BA, Schiffers PM, DeMey JG, Vermeer C. Regression of warfarin-induced medial elastocalcinosis by high intake of vitamin K in rats. *Blood* (2007);**109**:2823–31.

25. Basile C, Montanaro A, Masi M, Pati G, De Maio P, Gismondi A. Hyperbaric oxygen therapy for calcific uremic arteriolopathy: a case series. *J Nephrol* (2002);**15**:676–80.

Chapter 20

The role of the skeleton in the pathogenesis of vascular calcification in the chronic kidney disease–mineral bone disorder

Keith A. Hruska, Suresh Mathew, Yifu Fang, Imran Memon, and T. Keefe Davis

Introduction

Considerable scientific progress in the pathogenesis of vascular calcification accrued in recent years will be reviewed in this chapter with a focus on the role of the skeleton. Factors regulating mesenchymal cell differentiation and their role in the neo-intimal calcification of atherosclerosis, and the vascular media calcification observed in CKD and diabetes will be discussed, as will the role of bone regulatory proteins in bone mineralization and vascular calcification. This will include recent studies related to the discovery of new skeletal hormones involved in regulating phosphate homeostasis, sensing skeletal hydroxyapatite precipitation, regulating calcitriol production, regulating energy production and utilization, and affecting vascular calcification. Finally, the relationship between skeletal mineralization and vascular mineralization will be discussed in terms of their links, especially through the regulation of bone formation and serum phosphate concentrations.

The central issue in the background of this chapter is the excess mortality, largely cardiovascular, associated with chronic kidney disease (CKD). Cardiovascular morbidity in CKD is linked to vascular calcification, which has become a surrogate for cardiovascular mortality in CKD.[1] Vascular calcification (VC) is a process that involves the progression of atherosclerosis leading to neo-intimal calcification or the calcification of the tunica media. All of the forms of VC are stimulated by CKD. Vascular calcification occurs in all ages and stages of CKD.[2,3] However, the extent of coronary calcification appears to be more pronounced with longer time spent on dialysis, older age, male gender, white race, diabetes, and elevated serum calcium and phosphorous.[2] Coronary calcification is especially prone to be atherosclerotic.

While neo-intimal and medial calcification have similarities, it is not clear that they follow a common pathogenesis. Primary medial calcification, or Mönckeberg's sclerosis (MS), has been associated with CKD,[4] ageing,[5] and diabetes.[6] In CKD, MS was previously thought to be a passive process,[4] occurring as a direct consequence of an elevated calcium × phosphorus product. However, recent evidence indicates this is not the case. Rather, the elevated Ca × Pi product is a stimulus in an active process involving a phenotypic drift of vascular smooth muscle cells towards osteoblast-like cells secreting and mineralizing an extracellular matrix. A consensus has been reached that this mechanism is the root of atherosclerotic calcification, but the pathogenesis of MS is less clear. Nonetheless, osteoblastic differentiation and function has been demonstrated by investigators in MS.

Differentiation of mesenchymal stem cells

Osteoblasts, smooth muscle myocytes, adipocytes, fibroblasts, and chondrocytes all share a common mesenchymal progenitor stem cell. Differentiation along the osteoblast lineage requires crucial factors including the bone morphogenetic proteins (BMPs)[7] and Wnts, an amalgam of wingless (Wg) and int (Wnts).[8] The BMPs are part of the TGF-β superfamily that initiate signal transduction by binding to specific type II receptors, activating type I receptors, and affecting gene transcription through phosphorylation of regulatory Smad transcription factors. BMP-induced osteogenesis requires osteoblast lineage specific transcription factors, such as Runx2, Osx, Msx1/2 and ATF4. The transcriptomes of these factors are key and include all of the proteins involved in osteoblast mediated bone formation. Mice genetically engineered to be deficient in Runx2 or Osx show a complete lack of ossification,[9,10] while those deficient in Msx 1/2 have significant skeletal abnormalities.[11,12]

Thus, the process of osteogenic development and bone formation is critically and tightly regulated by the co-ordinated effects of the growth factors and transcription factors described above. Furthermore, the subsequent finding of these morphogens and transcription factors expressed in calcified vessel walls has led to the theory that vascular calcification is also a tightly regulated, co-ordinated, and an osteoblastic process. For example, low density lipoprotein (LDL) receptor negative (LDLR –/–) mice fed a high fat diet develop atherosclerotic plaque associated vascular calcification due to the expression of Runx2, Msx1, and Msx2.[13,14] In humans, expression of Msx2 and Runx2, together with the chondrogenic transcription factor Sox9 has been described in calcified atherosclerotic samples.[15] In addition, expression of the target genes of these factors, such as alkaline phosphatase, osteocalcin, bone sialoprotein, and type II collagen is also increased. Other bone regulatory proteins such as matrix Gla protein (MGP) and osteoprotegerin (OPG) (both discussed below) are altered in calcified vessels compared with non-calcified vessels.[15] Deposition of bone matrix proteins has also been described in medial calcification associated with CKD.[16] These findings suggest that vascular calcification is an active process that simulates matrix mineralization related to bone formation.

The vascular smooth muscle cell

Vascular smooth muscle cells (VSMCs) normally reside in the vessel wall media in a differentiated state, wherein their contractile properties regulate vascular tone. However, the VSMC phenotype is characterized by the ability to reversibly enter a synthetic state of proliferation and production of large amounts of extracellular matrix.[17]

The stimuli to change phenotype includes injury, various cytokines, growth factors, and certain components of the extracellular matrix. In the heightened synthetic state, VSMCs show decreased expression of contractile and adhesion proteins, and a concomitant increase in cytoskeletal proteins.[18] In addition to various growth factors, culture of VSMCs in medium supplemented with serum has been shown to stimulate the transition to the synthetic phenotype experimentally.[19] Transition into the synthetic state is thought to be involved in the pathogenesis of atherosclerosis and MS.

In culture during serum stimulation, proliferating VSMCs grow to form a confluent monolayer.[20] Subsequently, areas of the monolayer develop multicellular foci that form nodular aggregates consisting of non-proliferating, quiescent VSMCs. Cells from these nodules appear to re-express markers of smooth muscle cell differentiation. Proliferating osteoblasts also form condensing nodules in culture.[21] Subpopulations of human and bovine aortic VSMCs have been shown to form these nodules and then spontaneously calcify.[22]

The addition of β-glycerophosphate, a phosphate donor, or high concentrations of inorganic phosphate (4mM or greater) have been shown to induce calcification in VSMCs *in vitro*.[23] In contrast, VSMCs from atherosclerotic donors showed increased expression of Runx2, osteopontin (OPN), and alkaline phosphatase, and mineralization of the extracellular matrix with only a change in media Pi to 2mM.[14] The increase in inorganic phosphate induced the expression of osterix and bone matrix proteins.[14] Osterix knockdown in the presence of high media Pi eliminated matrix mineralization, as did the BMP inhibitor noggin. The action of Pi is stimulated through a sodium-phosphorus cotransporter in cultured VSMCs,[24,25] and thus, elevations in inorganic phosphate stimulate an osteoblastic phenotype in VSMCs *in vitro*. However, uremic serum also induces VSMCs to calcify, a process that is partly related to a factor or factors that are in addition to the serum phosphate.

The demonstration that VSMCs can be induced to calcify *in vitro* is important in the understanding of the pathogenesis of vascular calcification, since induction of CKD replicates the actions of high media phosphate, and Pi binders inhibit vascular calcification.[14] The forces driving osteogenic differentiation *in vivo* are also more than just hyperphosphatemia analogous to the uremic serum experiments *in vitro*. For instance, in addition to a higher incidence of vascular calcification, decreased bone formation is also a common finding in CKD, diabetes mellitus, and ageing. Furthermore, recent findings in animal models suggest that decreased orthotopic bone mineralization, either by decreased bone formation or increased bone resorption, leads to increased pressure towards heterotopic mineralization. We will discuss what factors are involved in this 'increased pressure', giving particular attention to phosphate and the new skeletal hormones, FGF23 and osteocalcin.

Bone metabolism and vascular calcification: a possible link

Matrix Gla protein

Matrix Gla protein (MGP) belongs to the family of mineral-binding proteins that includes coagulation factors, anticlotting factors, and osteocalcin. MGP is a vitamin K-dependent protein, requiring the vitamin for γ-carboxylation of its glutamic acid residues resulting in production of carboxyglutamic acid (Gla) residues. The Gla residues bind calcium and have been shown to inhibit hydroxyapatite precipitation.[26] The affinity of MGP binding to hydroxyapatite is enhanced by calcium, and decreased by phosphate and magnesium.[26] MGP also appears to modulate endochondral bone formation. Over expression of MGP blocks cartilage mineralization and inhibits endochondral ossification,[27] while mice genetically engineered to be deficient in MGP have inappropriate mineralization of cartilage, disorganized chondrocyte columns, and osteopenia.[28] Mice genetically engineered to be deficient in MGP also develop extensive arterial calcification and die of arterial rupture.[28] Calcified arteries from these mice show decreased expression of smooth muscle cell markers, increased expression of bone-specific markers, such as Runx2 and OPN,[29] and the presence of chrodrocytic appearing cells expressing type 2 collagen in the area of the calcifying lesions. These findings suggest that the vascular calcification associated with MGP deficiency is not solely related to an inability to inhibit hydroxyapatite precipitation, but rather involves a more active process resulting in a dramatic phenotypic change in VSMCs. Recent cell fate tracking studies demonstrate that the chondrocytic cells derived from vascular smooth muscle cell precursors in late prenatal development.[30] The function of MGP to bind BMPs in the matrix may relate to BMP activity and differentiation of neointimal cells to the osteochrondrogenic pathway.[31] Interestingly, MGP is markedly up-regulated and gamma carboxylated in VC associated with CKD.[32] This indicates that activation of defense mechanisms is appropriate and the defenses are not defective in CKD, but overwhelmed, so what is the stimulus? Furthermore, the osteoblastic differentiation of the vascular smooth muscle cells in CKD is not due to MGP deficiency.[33]

Osteoprotegerin

Osteoprotegerin (OPG), a soluble circulating ligand of receptor activator of NF-κB (RANK), is an inhibitor of osteoclast differentiation and function, and is part of the RANK/RANK ligand (RANKL)/OPG axis. Mice that are genetically engineered to be deficient in OPG (*opg–/opg–*) develop severe osteoporosis,[34] probably by uninhibited osteoclast function leading to excess bone resorption. Histomorphometric analysis of the bones of these mice reveals increased parameters of both bone resorption and bone formation, suggesting that the two processes have been coupled.[35] However, intravenous injection of recombinant OPG or transgenic over-expression of OPG can effectively reverse the osteoporotic phenotype.[36] In addition to this phenotype, OPG-deficient mice also develop extensive vascular calcification. In contrast to the osteoporosis, only the transgenic over-expression of OPG prevented vascular calcification. In other words, providing OPG to the deficient mouse did not prevent the vascular calcification. Of note, the increased bone resorption seen in these mice was not associated with an increased serum phosphate,[35] which may in part be due to the increased bone formation and mineral apposition rates seen in these mice. Furthermore, OPG-deficient mice have markedly elevated RANKL compared with wild type. Elevated RANKL may be the link between bone and vascular calcification in this model, as it has recently been shown to induce aortic myofibroblasts to form calcifying nodules with an osteogenic phenotype.[37] In addition, although RANKL is not normally expressed in the vasculature, its expression was increased in both the vessels of OPG deficient mice[36] and the aortic valves in human calcific aortic stenosis.[37]

The role of OPG in the CKD-MBD and vascular calcification is less clear. Studies correlating serum OPG levels and histomorphometric parameters of bone turnover have been inconsistent. OPG/RANKL ratios are difficult to relate to RANKL activity, and RANKL is increased in the vasculature by CKD.

Vitamin D

VSMC express the VDR and the 1 α-hydroxylase (CYP27A1).[38,39] Physiological levels of vitamin D receptor activators (VDRAs) stimulate VSMC differentiation *in vitro*, while higher doses cause VSMC apoptosis. Both physiological and pharmacological levels of VDRA stimulate osteoblastic cell functions *in vitro*. Furthermore, $1,25(OH)_2D_3$ 2D3 promotes the differentiation of osteoclasts through stimulation of RANKL in osteoblastic cells.[40]

High-dose vitamin D and VDRAs cause arterial calcification.[41–45] Vertebrae from rats treated with $1,25(OH)_2D_3$ have more osteoblasts, greater mineral appositional and bone formation rates, and more osteoclasts than untreated controls.[46] Vitamin D induced calcification in the rat is associated with a marked increase in the cross-linked N-teleopeptides, a marker of bone resorption.[43] Treatment with OPG, an inhibitor of bone resorption, prevented vascular calcification and restored serum cross-linked N-teleopeptides back to control values. Agents known to inhibit bone resorption through mechanisms other than OPG also inhibited vitamin D induced vascular calcification.[42,47] Thus, at least in these animal models, vascular calcification by vitamin D appeared to be related to bone resorption. The effects of the various metabolites of vitamin D are related to the relative dosage of the vitamin given, and this is relevant to the human clinical situation in CKD where very high doses of vitamin D analogs are used to inhibit secondary hyperparathyroidism. In the studies related to CKD, the administration of VDRAs stimulated aortic expression of Runx2 with a greater effect of doxercalciferol compared to paricalcitol.[45]

Recently, human observational studies have associated vitamin D deficiency with vascular calcification. So both deficiency and pharmacological levels of vitamin D and VDRA are associated with VC. Vitamin D receptor activation has physiological effects on the vasculature to differentiate VSMC. In CKD, low doses of paricalcitol and calcitriol, just barely able to decrease PTH levels, inhibited aortic osteoblast gene expression in the atherosclerotic high fat fed *ldlr–/–* mouse and protected against vascular calcification.[48] These doses of VDR activators are close to hormone replacement therapy, and they suggest that low doses of VDRA should be used in CKD to inhibit osteoblastic transition leading to vascular calcification. However, high doses of VDRA used to inhibit secondary hyperparathyroidism may have side effects potentially related to VC.

α2-HS glycoprotein/fetuin-A

α2-HS glycoprotein (AHSG) or fetuin-A is a bone regulatory protein that shares homologies to the fetuin superfamily, proteins present abundantly in the fetal serum.[49] Fetuins have been shown to inhibit hydroxyapatite precipitation *in vitro*[50] and to modulate the effects of the TGF-β superfamily on osteogenesis.[51] Fetuins can inhibit or stimulate osteogenesis, depending on their relative concentrations.[52] Mice that are genetically engineered to be deficient in fetuin-A are phenotypically normal, but develop more extensive ectopic calcification than control when fed a mineral and vitamin D-rich diet.[53]

A decrease in serum fetuin-A levels in hemodialysis patients is associated with an increased risk of cardiovascular mortality and an impaired *ex vivo* ability to inhibit hydroxyapatite precipitation.[54] This decrease in fetuin-A levels is in part due to inflammation, as fetuin-A has been shown to be a negative acute-phase reactant.[55] However, one must also not discount the effects of bone metabolism in this situation. The calcium-based phosphate binders and vitamin D analogues given these patients to control secondary hyperparathyroidism may also serve to deplete fetuin-A levels via increased calcium and phosphorus incorporation into the fetuin-mineral complex.

BMP-7: bone formation, phosphate, and vascular calcification

BMP-7, a member of the BMP family, is critical for renal, skeletal, and retinal development that is expressed in the adult primarily in the collecting tubule. Acute renal ischemia[56,57] and diabetic nephropathy[57,58] reduce BMP-7 expression. In CKD and renal osteodystrophy, treatment with BMP-7 restored normal bone turnover and osteoblast function[59,60] with either high or low turnover rates. BMP-7 has also been shown to significantly reduce intimal calcification in the low-density lipoprotein receptor- deficient high-fat fed atherosclerotic mouse (LDLR–/– high-fat) when CKD was induced.[61] Furthermore, LDLR–/– high-fat fed mice with CKD have low-turnover osteodystrophy,[59] and restoration of bone metabolism was associated with a significant reduction in serum phosphate.[59] That renal osteodystrophy contributes to the serum phosphorus through excess bone resorption provides a link between bone turnover and vascular calcification.

When dietary phosphorus is ingested, it enters a rapidly exchangeable pool (Fig. 20.1A). A significant portion of this pool exists along the skeletal mineralizing surfaces where phosphorus is leaving the pool to be incorporated into bone crystals. When bone formation is reduced (Fig. 20.1B), the skeletal mineralizing surface is reduced, effectively reducing the volume of distribution of phosphorus, resulting in an increase in the serum phosphate associated with intake. By restoring normal bone turnover, BMP-7 increased the volume of distribution of phosphorus, resulting in a decrease in serum phosphate. Since phosphorus has been shown to induce an osteogenic phenotype in VSMCs *in vitro*, we propose that the reduction in serum phosphate is a mechanism by which BMP-7 prevents vascular calcification. BMP-7 has also been shown to maintain the VSMC phenotype *in vitro* after stimulation into the synthetic phenotype,[62] and BMP-7 stimulates the contractile phenotype in human VSMC derived from atherosclerotic donors.[63]

Skeletal hormones, FGF23 and osteocalcin

Since phosphate homeostasis appears to be a central component of vascular calcification, understanding its regulation is essential. In addition to parathyroid hormone (PTH)

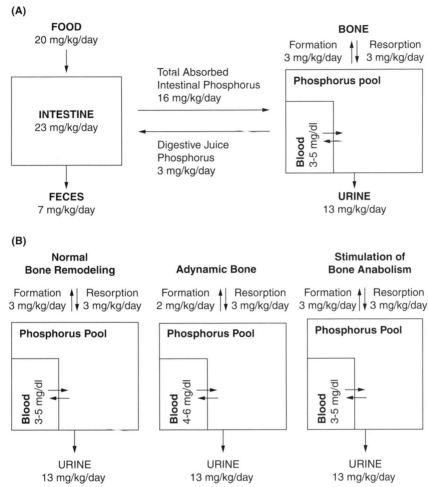

Fig. 20.1 Effects of skeletal remodeling on phosphate balance. (A) Phosphate balance diagram for a diet containing 20mg/kg body weight of elemental Pi. Absorbed Pi enters an exchangeable phosphorus pool with exits through skeletal deposition, renal excretion, and enteric secretions. (B) The adynamic bone disorder decreases the size of the exchangeable pool resulting in wider swings of the serum phosphorus due to food ingestion. Note that the adynamic bone disorder is a state of excess bone resorption and now the skeleton is a net contributor to exchangeable pool phosphorus (hyperphosphatemia). Treatment with a skeletal anabolic would produce a reversal of skeletal Pi balance such that now the skeletal reservoir function is restored and the skeleton participates in maintaining a normal serum.

and vitamin D, another hormone, fibroblast growth factor (FGF23), plays a critical role in homeostasis. FGF23 is a phosphaturic hormone involved in autosomal dominant hypophosphatemic rickets (ADHR)[64] and tumor-induced osteomalacia (TIO).[65] FGF23 also inhibits expression of renal 1α-hydroxylase, resulting in inappropriately low levels of 1,25(OH) vitamin D_3 in hypophosphatemia.[66] FGF23 levels are elevated in CKD.[67,68] Elevations in the levels of FGF23 come about secondary to osteocytic secretion and decreased clearance.[67] Interestingly, targeted deletion of the *FGF23* gene results in hyperphosphatemia, hypercalcemia, suppressed PTH, and low turnover osteopenia with accumulation of osteoid.[66] Mice homozygous for the null mutation died within 13 weeks of birth and autopsies revealed marked vascular calcification and calcification of the kidneys associated with an elevated BUN. Importantly, the vascular calcification associated with FGF23 deficiency was prevented by low dietary phosphorus or by breeding in 1 α-hydroxylase deficiency.[69]Recent human studies demonstrate that FGF23 levels are strong predictors of mortality in hemodialysis patients, probably reflecting a role as a biomarker of the phosphate pathway in vascular calcification.[70] In CKD the role of FGF23 in VC is probably indirect, since FGF23 action requires the co-receptor, Klotho, which is not expressed in the VSMC. The association of FGF23 with mortality is probably related to the actions of hyperphosphatemia due to excretion failure despite high FGF23 levels and impaired calcitriol production leading to VSMC dedifferentiation.

A second new skeletal hormone has recently, been discovered that likely plays a role in CKD stimulated VC. This hormone is osteocalcin, the long known biomarker of osteoblast activity, and a skeletal matrix Ca binding protein.[71,72] Under-carboxylated osteocalcin stimulates energy production and utilization through its actions to increase insulin sensitivity and insulin secretion. In addition, it stimulates adipocytes to secrete adiponectin a fat derived hormone that is protective against VC.[71] Osteocalcin levels are decreased in the adynamic bone disorder of CKD and in low turnover osteoporosis, both associated with increased rates of VC. Thus, bone formation rates through secretion of osteocalcin may be an important regulator of VC in CKD. These possibilities remain to be determined since osteocalcin function in CKD has not been studied.

Bone metabolism and vascular calcification: tying it all together

Evidence suggests that changes in bone remodeling, either by increased bone resorption or decreased bone formation, leads to vascular calcification. Vascular calcification occurs in both the media and the intima, possibly by different pathologic processes. Treatment with BMP-7 in the LDLR–/– high fat fed mouse model with CKD resulted in reductions in neo-intimal calcification through lowering phosphate by stimulating bone formation. Treatment of hyperphosphatemia by Pi binders decreased aortic osteoblastic gene expression and inhibited VC, CKD stimulates VSMC dedifferentiation and increases VSMC chemotaxis *in vitro*.[63] If VSMC migration did not occur as part of the pathogenesis of atherosclerosis, then perhaps neo-intimal calcification due to osteoblastic transition of the migrating VSMC would also not occur.

Primary medial calcification occurs primarily in patients with CKD or diabetes mellitus, and as a part of ageing. These three conditions also share a common characteristic of decreased bone formation. Indeed, animal models and human studies of ageing[73,74] and diabetes[75,76] have demonstrated decreased bone volume and bone formation rates. The finding of an inverse relationship between VC and bone formation rates in these experiment models is replicated by numerous human observational studies. Treatment of LDLR –/– high fat fed mice (who have the metabolic syndrome or diabetes) with another bone anabolic, PTH (1–34) fragment also results in reduced vascular calcification.[77] While it is not known what effect PTH (1–34) had on serum phosphate (presumably it would decrease it), this fragment did result in an elevation of skeletal and serum OPN, a known inhibitor of vascular calcification. While other mechanisms may be involved in this protective effect of PTH (1–34), these findings further support the link between bone remodeling and vascular calcification. They suggest the effect of CKD to inhibit bone formation may be important in the stimulation of VC.

With excess bone resorption, vascular calcification also occurs. We hypothesize that the pathogenesis involves the effects of phosphorus and reduced levels of serum

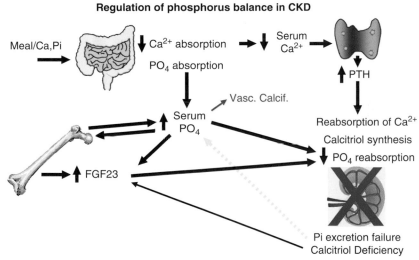

Regulation of phosphorus balance in CKD

Fig. 20.2 Regulation of phosphorus balance in CKD. Meal associated Ca^{2+} and PO_4 are absorbed. Decreased Ca^{2+} absorption and hypocalcemia stimulate parathyroid hormone secretion. Absorbed PO_4 is deposited in the skeleton through bone formation or excreted by the kidney. Skeletal osteocytes read bone formation, and when the available PO_4 exceeds skeletal deposition (bone formation), they secrete FGF23 to have the kidney excrete the excess PO_4. In CKD, renal excretion of PO_4 fails to maintain balance despite PTH and FGF23 influence and positive PO_4 balance results (yellow arrow) and the serum PO_4 begins to rise. This is a direct stimulus to heterotopic mineralization (red arrow and vascular calcification as a form of heterotopic mineralization).

fetuin-A, a known inhibitor of ectopic mineralization. However, since mice genetically engineered to be deficient in fetuin-A do not have significant ectopic calcification, reduced levels are probably not the sole factor involved in the pathogenesis. For example, high levels of serum RANKL may also be involved in vascular calcification in the OPG deficient mouse. Furthermore, serum phosphate does not appear to be elevated in these animal models of vascular calcification, perhaps due to a concomitant increase in bone formation rates in these models.

Conclusion: implications for chronic kidney disease

We have shown that prevention of secondary hyperparathyroidism results in low turnover renal osteodystrophy (adynamic bone disorder) in CKD.[78] We propose that the adynamic bone disorder develops in part due to a deficiency in Wnt and BMP activity in the skeleton and that secondary hyperparathyroidism develops as an adaptive process.[79] Furthermore, we propose that with the adynamic bone disorder (low-turnover state), there is a decreased volume of distribution for phosphorus, resulting in an increase in the serum phosphate and greater stimulation of FGF23. Inorganic phosphate has been shown to induce an osteogenic phenotype in VSMC, resulting in a more active process of mineralization. The extent of vascular calcification indeed has been shown to be associated with higher serum phosphorus in humans with CKD.[2] Thus, treatment of positive phosphate balance in CKD may be required to decrease the high rates of associated cardiovascular mortality.Clearly, vascular calcification is a significant problem for patients with CKD. In this chapter we have provided evidence that bone metabolism affects the vasculature. While vascular calcification occurs without CKD, we propose that the central mechanism in most cases is abnormal bone metabolism. Complications probably specific to CKD include chronic inflammation leading to atherosclerosis, and low serum fetuin-A levels and hyperphosphatemia from decreased excretion. Finally, one must not ignore the risk factors for atherosclerosis, such as hypertension, hyperlipidemia, diabetes, and smoking towards vascular calcification.

Given that there is such significant morbidity and mortality associated with vascular calcification, it is essential to develop treatments to prevent or slow down the progression of this process. While attempts to adjust oral calcium, calcitriol analogues, and calcium in the dialysate are keys to management of renal osteodystrophy, there is no easy way to assess for success save bone biopsy. New and improved assessment is required. We propose that bone anabolics such as BMP-7 may be novel therapeutic options for the treatment of low turnover osteopenia and the prevention of vascular calcification. Human studies must be performed to further assess this concept.

Acknowledgements

This work was supported by NIH grants (DK070790, AR41677, T32-DK062705) to KAH and research support from Shire, Genzyme, Abbott and Fresenius. We wish to thank Mat Davies, Richard Lund, and Song Wang, past fellows in the Hruska laboratory for their hard work and research contributions to this effort.

References

1. Blacher J, Safar ME, Guerin AP, Pannier B, Marchais SJ, London GM. Aortic pulse wave velocity index and mortality in end-stage renal disease. *Kidney Int* 2003;**63**:1852–60.

2. Raggi P, Boulay A, Chasan-Taber S, et al. Cardiac calcification in adult hemodialysis patients. A link between end-stage renal disease and cardiovascular disease? *J Am Coll Cardiol* 2002;**39**:695–701.

3. Goodman WG, Goldin J, Kuizon BD, et al. Coronary-artery calcification in young adults with end-stage renal disease who are undergoing dialysis. *N Engl J Med* 2000;**342**:1478–83.

4. Ejerblad S, Ericsson JLE, Eriksson I. Arterial lesions of the radial artery in uremic patients. *Acta Chir Scand* 1979;**145**:415–28.

5. Elliott RJ, McGrath LT. Calcification of the human aorta during ageing. *Calcif Tissue Int* 1994;**54**:268–73.

6. Edmonds ME. Medial arterial calcification and diabetes mellitus. *Z Kardiol* 2000;**89**:II/101–4.

7. Cheng H, Jiang W, Phillips FM, et al. Osteogenic activity of the fourteen types of human bone morphogenetic proteins (BMPs). *J Bone Joint Surg* 2003;**85**:1544–52.

8. Kato M, Patel MS, Levasseur R, et al. Cbfa1-independent decrease in osteoblast proliferation, osteopenia, and persistent embryonic eye vascularisation in mice deficient in Lrp5, a Wnt coreceptor. *J Cell Biol* 2002;**157**:303–14.

9. Komori T, Yagi H, Nomura S, et al. Targeted disruption of *Cbfa1* results in a complete lack of bone formation owing to maturational arrest of osteoblasts. *Cell* 1997;**89**:755–64.

10. Nakashima K, Zhou X, Kunkel G, et al. The novel zinc finger-containing transcription factor osterix is required for osteoblast differentiation and bone formation. *Cell* 2002;**108**:17–29.

11. Satokata I, Mass R. Msx1 deficient mice exhibit cleft palate and abnormalities of craniofacial and tooth development. *Nat Genet* 1994;**6**:348–56.

12. Satokata I, Ma L, Ohshima H, et al. Msx2 deficiency in mice causes pleiotropic defects in bone growth and ectodermal organ formation. *Nat Genet* 2004;**24**:391–5.

13. Towler DA, Bidder M, Latifi T, Coleman T, Semenkovich CF. Diet-induced diabetes activates an osteogenic gene regulatory program in the aortas of low density lipoprotein receptor-deficient mice. *J Biol Chem* 1998;**273**:30427–34.

14. Mathew S, Tustison KS, Sugatani T, Chaudhary LR, Rifas L, Hruska KA. The mechanism of phosphorus as a cardiovascular risk factor in chronic kidney disease. *J Am Soc Nephrol* 2008;**19**:1092–105.

15. Tyson KL, Reynolds JL, McNair R, Zhang Q, Weissberg PL, Shanahan CM. Osteo/chondrocytic transcription factors and their target genes exhibit distinct patterns of expression in human arterial calcification. *Arterioscler Thromb Vasc Biol* 2003;**23**:489–94.

16. Moe SM, O'Neill KD, Duan D, et al. Medial artery calcification in ESRD patients is associated with deposition of bone matrix proteins. *Kidney Int* 2002;**61**:638–47.

17. Hedin U, Roy J, Tran PK, Lundmark K, Rahman A. Control of smooth muscle cell proliferation—the role of the basement membrane. *Thromb Hemost* 1999;**82**(Suppl.):23–6.

18. Worth NF, Rolfe BE, Song J, Campbell R. Vascular smooth muscle cell phenotypic modulation in culture is associated with reorganisation of contractile and cytoskeletal proteins. *Cell Motil Cytosk* 2001;**49**:130–45.

19. Thyberg J. Differentiated properties and proliferation of arterial smooth muscle cells in culture. *Int Rev Cytol* 1996;**169**:183–265.

20. Brennan MJ, Millis AJ, Fritz KE. Fibronectin inhibits morphological changes in vascular smooth muscle cells. *J Cell Physiol* 1982;**112:**284–90.

21. Barone LM, Owen TA, Tassinari MS. Developmental expression and hormonal regulation of the rat matrix Gla protein (MGP) gene in chondrogenesis and osteogenesis. *J Cell Biochem* 1991;**46:**351–65.

22. Boström K, Watson KE, Horn S, Worthman C, Herman IM, Demer LL. Bone morphogenetic protein expression in human atherosclerotic lesions. *J Clin Invest* 1993;**91:**1800–9.

23. Shioi A, Nishizawa Y, Jono S, Koyama H, Hosoi M, Morii H. β-Glycerophosphate accelerates calcification in cultured bovine vascular smooth muscle cells. *Arterioscler Thromb Vasc Biol* 1995;**15:**2003–9.

24. Jono S, McKee MD, Murry CE, et al. Phosphate regulation of vascular smooth muscle cell calcification. *Circ Res* 2000;**87:**e10–17.

25. Chen NX, O'Neill KD, Duan D, Moe SM. Phosphorus and uremic serum up-regulate osteopontin expression in vascular smooth muscle cells. *Kidney Int* 2002;**62:**1724–31.

26. Roy ME, Nishimoto SK. Matrix Gla protein binding to hydroxyapatite is dependent on the ionic environment: calcium enhances binding affinity but phosphate and magnesium decrease affinity. *Bone* 2002;**31:**296–302.

27. Yagami K, Suh JY, Enomoto-Iwamoto M, et al. Matrix Gla protein is a developmental regulator of chondrocyte mineralization and, when constitutively expressed, blocks endochondral and intramembranous ossification in the limb. *J Cell Biol* 1999;**147:** 1097–108.

28. Luo G, Ducy P, McKee MD, et al. Spontaneous calcification of arteries and cartilage in mice lacking matrix Gla protein. *Nature* 1997;**386:**78–81.

29. Steitz SA, Speer MY, Curinga G, et al. Smooth muscle cell phenotypic transition associated with calcification. *Circ Res* 2001;**89:**1147–54.

30. Speer MY, Yang H-Y, Brabb T, et al. Smooth muscle cells give rise to osteochondrogenic precursors and chondrocytes in calcifying arteries. *Circ Res* 2009;**104:**733–41.

31. Bostrom K, Tsao D, Shen S, Wang Y, Demer LL. Matrix Gla protein modulates differentiation induced by bone morphogenetic protein-2 in C3H10T1/2 cells. *J Biol Chem* 2001;**276:**14044–52.

32. O'Neill WC. Vascular calcification: not so crystal clear. *Kidney Int* 2007;**71:**282–3.

33. Hruska KA. Vascular smooth muscle cells in the pathogenesis of vascular calcification. *Circ Res* 2009;**104:**710–11.

34. Bucay N, Sarosi I, Dunstan CR, et al. *Osteoprotegerin*-deficient mice develop early onset osteoporosis and arterial calcification. *Genes Devel* 1998;**12:**1260–8.

35. Nakamura M, Udagawa N, Matsuura S, et al. Osteoprotegerin regulates bone formation through a coupling mechanism with bone resorption. *Endocrinology* 2003;**144:**5441–9.

36. Min H, Morony S, Sarosi I, et al. Osteoprotegerin reverses osteoporosis by inhibiting endosteal osteoclasts and prevents vascular calcification by blocking a process resembling osteoclastogenesis. *J Exp Med* 2000;**192:**463–74.

37. Kaden JJ, Bickelhaupt S, Grobholz R, et al. Receptor activator of nuclear factor κB ligand and osteoprotegerin regulate aortic valve calcification*1. *J Mol Cell Cardiol* 2004;**36:**57–66.

38. Bosse Y, Maghni K, Hudson TJ. 1α,25-dihydroxy-vitamin D3 stimulation of bronchial smooth muscle cells induces autocrine, contractility, and remodeling processes. *Physiol Genom* 2007;**29:**161–8.

39. Wu-Wong JR, Nakane M, Ma J, Ruan X, Kroeger PE. Effects of vitamin D analogs on gene expression profiling in human coronary artery smooth muscle cells. *Atherosclerosis* 2006; **186**: 20–8

40. Kitazawa S, Kajimoto K, Kondo T, Kitazawa R. Vitamin D3 supports osteoclastogenesis via functional vitamin d response element of human RANKL gene promoter. *J Cell Biochem* 2003;**89**:771–7.

41. Price PA, Faus SA, Williamson MK. Warfarin-induced artery calcification is accelerated by growth and vitamin D. *Arterioscler Thromb Vasc Biol* 2000;**20**:317–27.

42. Price PA, Faus SA, Williamson MK. Bisphosphonates alendronate and ibandronate inhibit artery calcification at doses comparable to those that inhibit bone resorption. *Arterioscler Thromb Vasc Biol* 2001;**21**:817–24.

43. Price PA, June HH, Buckley JR, Williamson MK. Osteoprotegerin inhibits artery calcification induced by warfarin and by vitamin D. *Arterioscler Thromb Vasc Biol* 2001;**21**:1610–16.

44. Wu-Wong JR, Noonan W, Ma J, et al. Role of phosphorus and vitamin D analogs in the pathogenesis of vascular calcification. *J Pharmacol Exp Ther* 2006;**318**:90–8.

45. Mizobuchi M, Finch JL, Martin DR, Slatopolsky E. Differential effects of vitamin D receptor activators on vascular calcification in uremic rats. *Kidney Int* 2007;**72**:709–15.

46. Erben RG, Scutt AM, Miao D, Kollenkirchen U, Haberey M. Short-term treatment of rats with high dose 1,25-dihydroxyvitamin d3 stimulates bone formation and increases the number of osteoblast precursor cells in bone marrow. *Endocrinology* 1997;**138**:4629–35.

47. Price PA, June HH, Buckley JR, Williamson MK. SB 242784, a selective inhibitor of the osteoclastic V-H+-ATPase, inhibits arterial calcification in the rat. *Circ Res* 2002;**91**: 547–52.

48. Mathew S, Strebeck F, Hruska KA. Vascular calcification (VC) protective actions of doxercalciferol in CKD. In: Gendreau MA, Mangili A, Zavod A (eds), *Vitamin D Therapy in Dialysis Patients: Impact on Survival and Vascular Calcification*. Hampton, NH: Millennium CME Institute, Inc., 2007.

49. Elzanowski A, Barker WC, Hunt LT, Seibel-Ross E. Cystatin domains in alpha-2-HS glycoprotein and fetuin. *FEBS Lett* 1988;**227**:167–70.

50. Schinke T, Amendt C, Trindl A, Poschke O, Muller-Esterl W, Jahnen-Dechent W. The serum protein α2-HS glycoprotein/fetuin inhibits apatite formation *in vitro* and in mineralising calvaria cells. *J Biol Chem* 1996;**271**:20789–96.

51. Demetriou M, Binkert C, Sukhu B, Tenenbaum HD, Dennis JW. Fetuin/alpha2-HS glycoprotein is transforming growth factor-beta type II receptor mimic and cytokine antagonist. *J Biol Chem* 1996;**271**:12755–61.

52. Binkert C, Demetriou M, Sukhu B, Szweras M, Tennenbaum HC, Dennis JW. Regulation of osteogenesis by fetuin. *J Biol Chem* 1999;**274**:28514–20.

53. Schafer C, Heiss A, Schwarz A, et al. The serum protein {alpha}2-Heremans-Schmid glycoprotein/fetuin-A is a systemically acting inhibitor of ectopic calcification. *J Clin Invest* 2003;**112**:357–66.

54. Ketteler M, Bongartz P, Westenfeld R, et al. Association of low fetuin-A (AHSG) concentrations in serum with cardiovascular mortality in patients on dialysis: a cross-sectional study. *Lancet* 2003;**361**:827–33.

55. Lebreton JP, Joisel F, Raoult JP, Lannuzel B, Rogez JP, Humbert G. Serum concentration of human alpha 2-HS glycoprotein during the inflammatory process: evidence that alpha 2-HS glycoprotein is a negative acute-phase reactant. *J Clin Invest* 1979;**64**:1118–29.

56. Simon M, Maresh JG, Harris SE, et al. Expression of bone morphogenetic protein-7 mRNA in normal and ischemic adult rat kidney. *Am J Physiol* 1999;**276**:F382–89.

57. Wang S, Chen Q, Simon TC, et al. Bone morphogenetic protein-7 (BMP-7), a novel therapy for diabetic nephropathy. *Kidney Int* 2003;**63**:2037–49.

58. Wang S-N, Lapage J, Hirschberg R. Loss of tubular bone morphogenetic protein-7 in diabetic nephropathy. *J Am Soc Nephrol* 2001;**12**:2392–9.

59. Davies MR, Lund RJ, Mathew S, Hruska KA. Low turnover osteodystrophy and vascular calcification are amenable to skeletal anabolism in an animal model of chronic kidney disease and the metabolic syndrome. *J Am Soc Nephrol* 2005;**16**:917–28.

60. Gonzalez EA, Lund RJ, Martin KJ, et al. Treatment of a murine model of high-turnover renal osteodystrophy by exogenous BMP-7. *Kidney Int* 2002;**61**:1322–31.

61. Davies MR, Lund RJ, Hruska KA. BMP-7 is an efficacious treatment of vascular calcification in a murine model of atherosclerosis and chronic renal failure. *J Am Soc Nephrol* 2003;**14**:1559–67.

62. Dorai H, Vukicevic S, Sampath TK. Bone morphogenetic protein-7 (osteogenic protein-1) inhibits smooth muscle cell proliferation and stimulates the expression of markers that are characteristic of SMC phenotype *in vitro*. *J Cell Physiol* 2000;**184**:37–45.

63. Kokubo T, Ishikawa N, Uchida H, et al. CKD accelerates development of neo-intimal hyperplasia in arteriovenous fistulas. *J Am Soc Nephrol* 2009;**20**:1236–45.

64. White KE, Evans WE, O'Riordan JLH, et al. Autosomal dominant hypophosphatemic rickets is associated with mutations in FGF23. *Nat Genet* 2000;**26**:345–8.

65. Shimada T, Mizutani S, Muto T, et al. Cloning and characterisation of FGF23 as a causative factor of tumor-induced osteomalacia. *Proc NaH Acad Sci* 2001;**98**:6500–5.

66. Shimada T, Kakitani M, Yamazaki Y *et al.* Targeted ablation of FGF23 demonstrates an essential physiological role of FGF23 in phosphate and vitamin D metabolism. *J Clin Invest* 2004;**113**:561–8.

67. Larsson T, Nisbeth U, Ljunggren O, Juppner H, Jonsson KB. Circulating concentration of FGF23 increases as renal function declines in patients with chronic kidney disease, but does not change in response to variation in phosphate intake in healthy volunteers. *Kidney Int* 2003;**64**:2272–9.

68. Weber TJ, Liu S, Indridason OS, Quarles LD. Serum FGF23 levels in normal and disordered phosphorus homeostasis. *J Bone Miner Res* 2003;**18**:1227–34.

69. Razzaque MS, Sitara D, Taguchi T, St-Arnaud R, Lanske B. Premature ageing-like phenotype in fibroblast growth factor 23 null mice is a vitamin D-mediated process. *FASEB J* 2006;05-5432fje.

70. Gutierrez OM, Mannstadt M, Isakova T, et al. Fibroblast growth factor 23 and mortality among patients undergoing hemodialysis. *N Engl J Med* 2008;**359**:584–92.

71. Lee NK, Sowa H, Hinoi E, et al. Endocrine regulation of energy metabolism by the skeleton. *Cell* 2007;**130**:456–69.

72. Murshed M, Schinke T, McKee MD, Karsenty G. Extracellular matrix mineralization is regulated locally; different roles of two Gla-containing proteins. *J Cell Biol* 2004;**165**:625–30.

73. Wang L, Banu J, Mcmahan CA, Kalu DN. Male rodent model of age-related bone loss in men. *Bone* 2001;**29**:141–8.

74. Clarke BL, Ebeling PR, Jones JD, et al. Changes in quantitative bone histomorphometry in ageing healthy men. *J Clin Endo Metab* 1996;**81**:2264–70.

75. Suzuki K, Miyakoshi N, Tsuchida T, Kasukawa Y, Sato K, Itoi E. Effects of combined treatment of insulin and human parathyroid hormone(1–34) on cancellous bone mass and structure in streptozotocin-induced diabetic rats. *Bone* 2003;**33**:108–14.

76. Krakauer JC, McKenna MJ, Buderer NF, Rao DS, Whitehouse FW, Parfitt AM. Bone loss and bone turnover in diabetes. *Diabetes* 1995;**44**:775–82.

77. Shao JS, Cheng SL, Charlton-Kachigian N, Loewy AP, Towler DA. Teriparatide (human parathyroid hormone (1–34)) inhibits osteogenic vascular calcification in diabetic low density lipoprotein receptor-deficient mice. *J Biol Chem* 2003;**278**:50195–202.

78. Lund RJ, Davies MR, Brown AJ, Hruska KA. Successful treatment of an adynamic bone disorder with bone morphogenetic protein-7 in a renal ablation model. *J Am Soc Nephrol* 2004;**15**:359–69.

79. Hruska KA, Saab G, Chaudhary LR, Quinn CO, Lund RJ, Surendran K. Kidney-bone, bone-kidney, and cell-cell communications in renal osteodystrophy. *Semin Nephrol* 2004;**24**:25–38.

Chapter 21

Klotho: bone, kidney, vascular calcifications, and the aging process

Makoto Kuro-o

Introduction

Phosphate homeostasis is maintained by counterbalance between absorption of dietary phosphate from intestine, mobilization from bone (the major reservoir of calcium and phosphate), and excretion from kidney into urine.[1] These processes are regulated by several endocrine factors. Vitamin D and parathyroid hormone (PTH), which have been extensively studied as regulators of calcium homeostasis, play critical roles in phosphate homeostasis as well.[2,3] The active form of vitamin D (1,25-dihydroxyvitamin D_3) is secreted from renal proximal tubules, and acts on intestine to promote absorption of both calcium and phosphate. It also acts on bone to stimulate osteoclastogenesis and mobilization of calcium and phosphate from the reservoir. Thus, vitamin D can elevate not only serum calcium, but also phosphate levels. On the other hand, PTH acts on renal proximal tubules to stimulate biosynthesis of 1,25-dihydroxyvitamin D_3. However, PTH increases serum levels of calcium but not phosphate, because it has an activity that promotes renal phosphate excretion. Thus, unlike vitamin D, PTH can selectively increase serum calcium levels without concomitant increase in serum phosphate levels in subjects with normal GFR.

Although vitamin D and PTH are key endocrine regulators of phosphate metabolism, studies on a series of hereditary bone disorders associated with phosphate wasting into urine have suggested the existence of another hormone(s) that can regulate phosphate metabolism. Patients with autosomal dominant hypophosphatemic rickets (ADHR), autosomal recessive hypophosphatemic rickets (ARHR), and X-linked hypophosphatemic rickets (XHR) exhibit hypophosphatemia due to excessive phosphate excretion into urine.[4] Their serum calcium levels are within normal range. In addition, these patients have inappropriately low serum 1,25-dihydroxyvitamin D_3 levels despite the existence of hypophosphatemia. Tumor-induced osteomalacia (TIO), a rare paraneoplastic disorder, is also associated with renal phosphate wasting and low serum 1,25-dihydroxyvitamin D_3 levels, which is reminiscent of ADHR, XHR, and ARHR. It is difficult to explain the unique pathophysiology of these phosphate wasting syndromes without assuming that these patients may suffer elevated levels of a putative endocrine factor (called 'phosphatonin') that acts on kidney and induces a negative phosphate balance by suppressing renal phosphate reabsorption and/or 1,25-dihydroxyvitamin D_3 synthesis.

Recent studies have identified fibroblast growth factor-23 (FGF23) as a phosphatonin and Klotho as an indispensable component of the FGF23 receptor.[5] The purpose of this chapter is to summarize recent progress in our understanding of this novel endocrine axis mediated by FGF23 and Klotho in the regulation of phosphate and vitamin D metabolism and its impact on renal function, vascular calcification, bone metabolism, and aging.

History and effects of Klotho

In Greek mythology, three goddesses are summoned upon the ninth months of pregnancy to determine the life span of the arriving baby. They are Klotho, Lachesis, and Atropos who spin, measure, and cut the thread of life, respectively. The *klotho* gene, named after the spinner, was identified as a gene mutated in the *klotho* mouse that exhibits a shortened life span associated with multiple aging symptoms.[6] The *klotho* mouse was a serendipitous by-product during transgenic mouse experiments in which a transgene was introduced into fertilized mouse oocytes with pronuclear microinjection. In this traditional method, integration of the transgene into the mouse genome occurs randomly at any loci, and occasionally disrupts a functional mouse gene (insertional mutation). As a result, homozygotes for the transgene may develop unexpected phenotypes due to knock-out of the gene at the transgene integration site. The unexpected phenotypes in the *klotho* mouse were a premature aging syndrome, including shortened life span, hypogonadism, skin atrophy, thymic involution, sarcopenia, osteopenia, vascular calcification, pulmonary emphysema, hearing loss, and cognition impairment among others.

The gene disrupted in the *klotho* mouse (the *klotho* gene) was isolated by positional cloning using the transgene as a marker.[6] About 10 copies of the transgene were integrated in tandem at a single locus in the telomeric region of chromosome 5, which generated a deletion about 8kb. There was the first exon of a new gene around ~2kb downstream of the deletion, which later turned out to be the *klotho* gene. The *klotho* gene encodes a type-I single-pass transmembrane protein composed of 1014 amino acids with a short intracellular domain (10 amino acids) that has no known functional domains. The extracellular domain is composed of two internal repeats, termed KL1 and KL2 domains, with weak amino acid identity (21%) to each other. Each repeat has weak homology to family 1 glycosidases of bacteria, plants, and mammals (amino acid identity between 20 and 40%), rendering the *klotho* gene to this gene family. Among family 1 glycosidases Klotho protein shares the highest amino acid identity with mammalian lactose-phlorizin hydrolase (LPH), which hydrolyses lactose in milk to glucose and galactose in intestine through its β-glucosidase activity. However, Klotho protein does not have β-glucosidase activity, probably because one of the two conserved glutamate residues, which function as a proton donor and a nucleophile in the active centre, is diverged in KL1 and KL2 domains.

The *klotho* gene is expressed predominantly in the kidney.[6] Klotho mRNA and protein are detected abundantly in distal convoluted tubules and weakly in proximal tubules.

In extra-renal tissues, choroid plexus in the brain strongly expresses Klotho. In addition, several endocrine organs express Klotho, including parathyroid gland, pituitary gland, hypothalamus, ovary, testis, and mammary gland. In the *klotho* mouse, expression of the *klotho* gene is severely suppressed and undetectable by Northern blot analysis. However, more sensitive RT-PCR can detect weak expression of the *klotho* gene in the *klotho* mouse, indicating that the insertional mutation generated a severe hypomorphic allele (but not a null allele). A null allele of the *klotho* gene was later generated by conventional targeted gene disruption. The *klotho* knockout mouse exhibited phenotypes identical with those observed in the *klotho* mouse. Thus, the *klotho* mouse and the *klotho* knockout mouse have been collectively referred to as Klotho-deficient mice in this chapter.

Klotho and FGF23

The *Fgf23* gene was isolated based on the sequence similarity to the other FGF ligand family members. Although the N-terminal half of FGF23 exhibits significant homology to the other FGFs, its C-terminal half is unique to FGF23 and lacks a typical heparin-binding domain conserved in the other classical FGFs.[7] The ability of FGFs to bind to heparin and heparan sulfate is essential for their function, because (1) heparin directly participates in the physical interaction between FGFs and FGF receptors (FGFRs) by forming the heparin-FGF-FGFR ternary complex, and (2) heparin and heparan sulfate tether FGFs to the extracellular matrix and allow the FGFs to function as paracrine/autocrine factors. In fact, FGF23 that lacks the heparin-binding domain has very low affinity to any known FGFRs. In addition, FGF23 does not stay in the extracellular matrix but enters the systemic circulation to function as an endocrine factor. Among the 22 members of the FGF ligand superfamily, FGF21, FGF19, and FGF15 (the mouse ortholog of FGF19) also lack the heparin-binding domain and function as endocrine factors like FGF23. These atypical FGFs form a subfamily (the FGF19 subfamily) distinct from the other paracrine/autocrine-acting FGFs and are collectively called endocrine FGFs.[5]

Function of FGF23 was not clear until the *FGF23* gene was identified as a gene mutated in patients with ADHR, who exhibit renal phosphate wasting and low serum 1,25-dihydroxyvitamin D_3 levels.[8] ADHR patients carry mis-sense mutations in the *FGF23* gene that confers resistance to the proteolytic degeneration of FGF23 protein, resulting in high serum levels of intact FGF23. Thus, FGF23 may function as an endocrine factor that acts on kidney and induces negative phosphate balance by suppressing renal phosphate reabsorption and renal 1,25-dihydroxyvitamin D_3 synthesis. In fact, injection of recombinant FGF23 protein into rodents increases renal phosphate excretion (phosphaturia) and decreases serum 1,25-dihydroxyvitamin D_3 levels. However, the identity of FGF23 receptor remained unclear, because the affinity of FGF23 to FGFRs *in vitro* was too low ($K_D = 200 - 700$nM) to explain the potent biological activity of FGF23 at very low serum concentration *in vivo* (~1pM).[9]

Klotho and FGF23, two seemingly unrelated proteins, had been studied independently until it was realized that Klotho-deficient mice and FGF23 knockout mice developed the identical phenotypes. *Fgf23$^{-/-}$* mice display increased renal phosphate reabsorption and increased serum 1,25-dihydroxyvitamin D_3 levels as expected, which results in hyperphosphatemia, hypercalcemia, and vascular calcification.[10] In addition to these predictable phenotypes, *Fgf23*[−/−] mice unexpectedly exhibit multiple aging-like phenotypes including shortened life span, hypogonadism, skin atrophy, thymic involution, sarcopenia, osteopenia, and pulmonary emphysema. These phenotypes are reminiscent of Klotho-deficient mice, which also suffer hyperphosphatemia, hypercalcemia, and hypervitaminosis D. These observations indicate that Klotho and FGF23 may function in a common signal transduction pathway. In fact, we found that Klotho formed a binary complex with several FGFR isoforms (FGFR1c, 3c, and 4) and that binding of Klotho to these FGFRs significantly increased their affinity to FGF23.[11] Namely, Klotho functions as an obligatory co-receptor for FGF23. This finding was confirmed later in an independent study.[12] The fact that FGF23 requires Klotho for its high-affinity binding to FGFR explains why FGF23-deficient mice develop phenotypes identical with those observed in Klotho-deficient mice. It also explains why Klotho-deficient mice have extremely high levels of serum FGF23.[12] In addition, kidney-specific expression of Klotho explains why FGF23 can identify kidney as its target organ among many organs that express multiple FGFR isoforms.

Defects in the Klotho-FGF23 system result in hyperphosphatemia due to inappropriately increased renal phosphate reabsorption in both mice and humans.[5] Renal phosphate reabsorption takes place predominantly in proximal tubules.[1] Phosphate in the luminal fluid is transferred from the apical side to the basolateral side through proximal tubules primarily by transepithelial transport. Sodium-phosphate co-transporter-2a (NaPi-IIa) is expressed on the apical brush border membrane (BBM) in proximal tubular cells and functions as the major entry gate for the transepithelial phosphate transport in mice. In fact, Na+-dependent phosphate uptake in BBM vesicles from NaPi-IIa knockout mice is decreased by ~70%. In humans, another isoform of sodium-phosphate co-transporter (NaPi-IIc) is more abundant than NaPi-IIa, which explains why loss-of-function mutations in the NaPi-IIc gene cause hereditary hypophosphatemic rickets with hypercalciuria (HHRH) in humans.[13] Thus, it is likely that FGF23 suppresses renal phosphate reabsorption through reducing the expression and/or activity of sodium-phosphate co-transporters (NaPi-IIa in mice, NaPi-IIc in humans) and/or the number of these transporters inserted in the BBM of proximal tubular cells. Indeed, injection of recombinant FGF23 decreases NaPi-IIa expression in rodents.[14] In addition, inhibition of endogenous FGF23 activity by injecting FGF23 antibodies or by ablating Klotho expression increases NaPi-IIa expression as well as its insertion in the proximal tubular BBM.[15] The molecular mechanism by which FGF23 regulates expression and trafficking of NaPi-IIa and NaPi-IIc remains to be determined.

Klotho and calcitriol

Defects in the Klotho-FGF23 system cause hypervitaminosis D (high serum levels of 1,25-dihydroxyvitamin D_3). This is associated with dysregulation of expression of the enzymes involved in vitamin D activation and inactivation in the kidney. Despite high serum levels of phosphate, calcium, and vitamin D, Klotho-deficient mice and

FGF23-deficient mice show inappropriately high renal expression of the *Cyp27b1* gene that encodes 1α-hydroxylase, the enzyme that converts vitamin D from an inactive form (25-hydroxyvitamin D_3) to the active form (1,25-dihydroxyvitamin D_3). They also show inappropriately low renal expression of *Cyp24* gene that encodes 24-hydroxylase, the enzyme that inactivates 1,25-dihydroxyvitamin D_3.[9] Thus, defects in the FGF23 activity cause increased synthesis and decreased inactivation, leading to high serum levels of 1,25-dihydroxyvitamin D_3.

In contrast, over expression or injection of FGF23 reduces serum 1,25-dihydroxyvitamin D_3 levels. Mice carrying mutations that lead to increased serum FGF23 levels (such as *Hyp* mice and *Dmp-1* knockout mice) suffer low serum 1,25-dihydroxyvitamin D_3.[4] Injection of recombinant FGF23 into rodents causes reduction of serum 1,25-dihydroxyvitamin D_3 levels within hours. These are associated with decreased expression of *Cyp27b1* and increased expression of *Cyp24* in the kidney, which is opposite to the changes in FGF23-deficient or Klotho-deficient mice. Thus, all *in vivo* evidence indicate that the FGF23-Klotho system is to counter-regulate serum 1,25-dihydroxyvitamin D_3 by suppressing synthesis and promoting inactivation in the kidney. Importantly, 1,25-dihydroxyvitamin D_3 stimulates FGF23 expression in bone. In other words, FGF23 is a target gene of vitamin D.[5] 1,25-dihydroxyvitamin D_3 binds with high affinity to its nuclear vitamin D receptor (VDR). The ligand-bound VDR forms a heterodimer with retinoid X receptor (RXR), which binds to vitamin D responsive elements (VDREs) in the promoter of the FGF23 gene and transactivates its expression. In fact, administration of 1,25-dihydroxyvitamin D_3 increases expression of FGF23 in bone as well as serum FGF23 levels. The increased FGF23 suppresses synthesis and promotes inactivation of 1,25-dihydroxyvitamin D_3 and closes a negative feedback loop in vitamin D homeostasis (Fig. 21.1). FGF23 and Klotho are indispensable components of this bone-kidney endocrine axis that maintains vitamin D homeostasis, because defects in either FGF23 or Klotho disrupt this negative feedback loop and lead to hypervitaminosis D.

Because synthesis of 1,25-dihydroxyvitamin D_3 takes place in proximal tubules, it is reasonable to speculate that FGF23 binds to the Klotho-FGF receptor complex expressed on the surface of proximal tubular cells and activates the FGF signaling pathway, which eventually leads to down-regulation of the *Cyp27b1* gene and up-regulation of *Cyp24* gene. Indeed, FGF23 suppressed expression of the *Cyp27b1* gene through activating MAP kinases (ERK1/2) in cultured proximal tubular cells.[16] The inhibitory effect of FGF23 on expression and function of NaPi-IIa and NaPi-IIc may be also a result of FGF signaling activation by FGF23 in proximal tubular cells. However, it should be noted that FGF23 mainly regulates proximal tubular functions such as phosphate reabsorption and vitamin D synthesis despite the fact that expression of Klotho, the obligatory co-receptor for FGF23, is much more abundantly expressed in distal convoluted tubules than in proximal tubules.[6] This fact has raised the possibility that the primary target of FGF23 is not proximal tubules but distal convoluted tubules. If so, it is possible that activation of the Klotho-FGF receptor complex by FGF23 in distal convoluted tubules may lead to secretion of a paracrine factor(s) that instructs adjacent proximal tubules to suppress phosphate reabsorption and vitamin D synthesis. A recent study demonstrated that knockout of the *Fgfr3* gene in

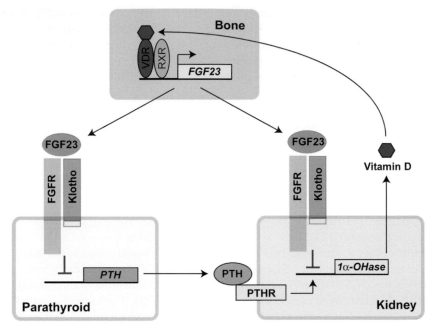

Fig. 21.1 Endocrine axes that regulate vitamin D metabolism mediated by FGF23 and Klotho. Active form of vitamin D (1,25-dihydroxyvitamin D_3) binds to vitamin D receptor (VDR) in osteocytes, which in turn forms a heterodimer with another nuclear receptor RXR and directly binds to a promoter region of the FGF23 gene to transactivate its expression. FGF23 secreted from the bone acts on the Klotho-FGFR complex in the kidney (the bone-kidney endocrine axis) and parathyroid gland (the bone-parathyroid endocrine axis). In the kidney, FGF23 suppresses expression of 1α-hydroxylase and closes a negative feedback loop for vitamin D homeostasis. In the parathyroid gland, FGF23 suppresses expression of PTH. Since PTH is a potent inducer of 1α-hydroxylase expression, suppression of PTH by FGF23 reduces 1α-hydroxylase as well as serum levels of 1,25-dihydroxyvitamin D_3, which closes another long negative feedback loop for vitamin D homeostasis. Klotho and FGF23 are indispensable for the regulation of vitamin D metabolism, because defects in either Klotho or FGF23 cause hypervitaminosis D.

Hyp mice, which have elevated serum FGF23 levels, failed to correct the phosphate-wasting syndrome.[17] Considering that proximal tubular cells primarily expresses FGFR3, but not the other FGFR isoforms, these findings suggest that the ability of FGF23 to regulate phosphate reabsorption and vitamin D synthesis is independent of FGF signaling activation in the proximal tubule. These observations are consistent with the idea that a putative paracrine factor(s) secreted from distal convoluted tubules in response to FGF23 may mediate the effects of FGF23 on proximal tubular functions. The identity of this factor(s) remains to be determined.

Since most tissues express one or more FGFR isoforms, tissue-specific expression of Klotho virtually determines which tissues can respond to FGF23. In other words, organs that express Klotho are potential target organs of FGF23. Recent studies have identified the parathyroid gland as a target organ of FGF23[18] based on the fact that the parathyroid gland is one of the few organs that express Klotho endogenously. FGF23 suppresses expression and secretion of PTH when injected into mice or directly applied to parathyroid glands *ex vivo*. The activity of FGF23 that suppresses PTH production and secretion may further potentiate the ability of FGF23 to counteract vitamin D, because PTH acts on renal proximal tubular cells to promote synthesis of 1,25-dihydroxyvitamin D$_3$. These observations suggest the existence of multiple negative feedback loops between bone, kidney, and parathyroid gland mediated by Klotho, FGF23, vitamin D, and PTH in the regulation of vitamin D metabolism (Fig. 21.1).

Klotho and vascular calcifications

Because serum vitamin D promotes absorption of dietary phosphate and calcium from intestine, elevated vitamin D levels can be a cause of hyperphosphatemia and hypercalcemia in Klotho-deficient mice and FGF23-deficient mice. Elevation of both calcium and phosphate levels in the blood leads to a significant increase in the calcium phosphate product (Ca × P), which is a predisposition to ectopic calcification of blood vessels and soft tissues. These observations suggest that increased vitamin D may be primarily responsible for vascular calcification observed in Klotho-deficient mice and FGF23-deficient mice. Several studies have addressed this possibility.[19] First, a vitamin D-deficient diet not only restored serum phosphate and calcium levels, but also rescued many aging-like phenotypes including vascular calcification in Klotho-deficient mice. Secondly, ablation of vitamin D activity in FGF23-deficient mice and Klotho-deficient mice by targeted disruption of the *Cyp27b1* gene or the vitamin D receptor (VDR) gene also rescued both hyperphosphatemia and vascular calcification. Lastly, a low phosphate diet corrected hyperphosphatemia as well as all the aging-like phenotypes including vascular calcification in FGF23-deficient mice. These studies have provided unequivocal evidence that the premature aging syndrome caused by defects in the bone-kidney endocrine axis is due to the toxicity of phosphate, calcium, and/or vitamin D. Of note, low phosphate diet rescued FGF23-deficient mice despite the fact that it further increased already elevated serum calcium and vitamin D levels, suggesting that phosphate, but not calcium or vitamin D, may be primarily responsible for the aging-like phenotypes including vascular calcification. It remains to be determined whether high serum vitamin D and/or calcium levels are a prerequisite for phosphate to induce vascular calcification. However, this may not be very likely, because patients with end-stage renal disease (ESRD) often develop hyperphosphatemia associated with low serum vitamin D and calcium levels, and still suffer vascular calcification.

Recent epidemiological studies support the notion of 'phosphate toxicity' in humans. Serum phosphate levels were shown to positively correlate all-cause mortality risk, even when serum phosphate levels are within the normal range.[20] In addition, chronic kidney disease (CKD) patients with hyperphosphatemia (> or = 6.5mg/dL) were reported to have higher risk for death resulting from several diseases including coronary artery disease than those with the lower serum phosphate levels (< 6.5mg/dL).[21] Based on these observations, controlling serum phosphate levels below 6.5mg/dL has become an important therapeutic goal for CKD. Thus, low phosphate diet and/or phosphate binders have been increasingly recognized as important therapeutic options for preventing life-threatening complications of CKD, such as vascular calcification and cardiovascular diseases.

Klotho and uremia

More than 20 million Americans, or 1 in 9 adult Americans, have CKD, which can result in renal failure and is increasingly recognized as a global public health problem in aging society. The National Kidney Foundation task force indicated that the cardiovascular mortality of a 35-year-old patient on dialysis was equivalent to that of an 80-year-old 'healthy' individual, rendering CKD to be the most potent accelerator of vascular senescence.[22] Furthermore, the American Heart Association announced in 2003 that CKD should be included in the highest risk group for cardiovascular disease.[23] Like Klotho-deficient mice, CKD patients suffer vascular calcification and have elevated serum levels of FGF23 and phosphate. Importantly, Klotho expression is decreased in CKD patients.[24] These observations suggest that Klotho deficiency may contribute to pathophysiology of CKD or CKD may be viewed as a segmental progeroid syndrome associated with Klotho-deficiency state. Consistent with this notion, recent animal studies have shown that Klotho functions as a renoprotective factor. Although the mechanism remains to be determined, over-expression of Klotho ameliorated progressive renal injury in mouse models of glomerulonephritis[25] and acute kidney injury.[26] Thus, decrease in Klotho expression potentially accelerates renal damage, leading to a deterioration spiral of Klotho expression and renal function.

Epidemiological studies have identified high serum levels of phosphate and FGF23 as independent mortality risks in CKD patients.[20,27] Importantly, serum FGF23 levels increase before serum phosphate levels increase during the progression of CKD,[28] suggesting that resistance to FGF23 may be one of the earliest changes in phosphate metabolism in CKD. Although the mechanism of FGF23 resistance is yet to be determined, it can most likely be caused by decrease in renal Klotho expression. Provided that serum FGF23 levels are a surrogate marker for renal Klotho expression levels, the fact that high serum FGF23 levels are associated with poor prognosis in patients undergoing dialysis[27] suggests that low renal Klotho expression levels may be primarily responsible for the poor prognosis. It remains to be determined whether renal Klotho expression levels reflect functional renal tubular mass that can respond to FGF23.

Provided that Klotho is a renoprotective factor, therapeutic interventions that increase renal Klotho expression may be effective in the treatment of CKD. It has been shown that 1,25-dihydroxyvitamin D_3, PPARγ agonists (thiazolidinediones), and HMG CoA reductase inhibitors (statins) increase Klotho expression, whereas angiotensin II, lipopolysaccharide, and oxidative stress decrease it.[24] Renoprotective effects of vitamin D, thiazolidinediones, statins, and ACE inhibitors may be partly attributed to their ability to up-regulate or prevent down-regulation of Klotho expression.

The extracellular domain of Klotho protein is clipped on the cell surface by a membrane-anchored protease ADAM10/17 and released into systemic circulation.[29] In fact, the Klotho ectodomain is detectable in blood, urine, and cerebrospinal fluid.[30]

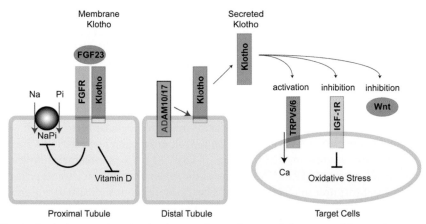

Fig. 21.2 Klotho protein exists in the membrane form and the secreted form. The membrane Klotho forms a complex with FGF receptor (FGFR) and functions as a co-receptor for FGF23 and suppresses sodium-phosphate co-transporter (NaPi) and vitamin D synthesis in renal proximal tubules. On the other hand, the membrane Klotho is clipped by membrane-anchored proteases ADAM10 and ADAM17 just above the plasma membrane. The major source of secreted Klotho is likely to be distal tubules, because Klotho expression is most abundant in distal tubules. The entire extracellular domain of Klotho is then released into blood, urine, and cerebrospinal fluid. The secreted Klotho protein has a putative sialidase activity that modifies glycans of calcium channel TRPV5 on the cell surface. A similar mechanism may explain the inhibitory effect of secreted Klotho on growth factors including insulin, IGF-1, and Wnt. The ability of secreted Klotho to inhibit IGF-1 signaling may contribute to the anti-oxidative stress.

In addition, insulin and low extracellular calcium have been reported to increase Klotho shedding,[29,31] suggesting that this is not a constitutive leak, but a regulated process. Thus, Klotho protein exists in two forms; the membrane form and the secreted form. Membrane Klotho functions as a co-receptor for FGF23. Then, what is the function of secreted Klotho? It should be noted that secreted Klotho cannot function as a soluble receptor for FGF23, because FGF23 cannot bind to Klotho protein alone with high affinity; it binds exclusively to the Klotho-FGF receptor complex.[11] Recent studies have revealed multiple functions of secreted Klotho protein. It inhibits insulin/IGF-1 receptor,[30] binds to Wnt to suppress Wnt signaling,[32] and activates calcium channels TRPV5/6.[33,34] In contrast to the specific function of membrane Klotho as a co-receptor for FGF23, function of secreted Klotho appears promiscuous. One possible explanation for the diverse activity of secreted Klotho may lie in the fact that Klotho belongs to the family 1 glycosidase. Although secreted Klotho does not exhibit any β-glucosidase activity as mentioned above, it is still possibility that secreted Klotho can function as a glycosidase that recognizes and hydrolyzes a particular sugar linkage(s). If so, secreted Klotho may exert its diverse activity through modifying particular sugar chains (glycans) of multiple glycoproteins, glycolipids, or carbohydrates on the cell surface.

More recently, it was shown that secreted Klotho indeed removed sialic acids from the glycans of calcium channel TRPV5.[34] N-linked glycans of most cell-surface glycoproteins have multiple branches whose termini are capped with sialic acids. These terminal sialic acids are attached to N-acetyllactosamine (LacNAc) through either α2,3-, or α2,6-, or α2,8-sialic linkage. Secreted Klotho has putative α2,6-sialidase activity and removes particular sialic acids from the TRPV5 glycans. Removal of terminal sialic acids by secreted Klotho exposes underlying LacNAc. LacNAc is a ligand for galectin-1, a lectin abundantly exists in the extracellular matrix. Binding of galectin-1 to the LacNAc tethers TRPV5 on the cell surface and prevents TRPV5 from internalization, leading to accumulation of TRPV5 on the plasma membrane and increase in Ca current. TRPV5 functions as the major entry gate for transepithelial calcium reabsorption in distal tubules. These observations indicate that secreted Klotho can increase renal calcium reabsorption through activating TRPV5. In fact, Klotho-deficient mice have increased calcium leak into urine despite the high serum levels of vitamin D that promotes calcium reabsorption in distal tubules. Reduced Klotho expression, as well as low serum vitamin D levels, may contribute to hypocalcemia observed in CKD patients.

Regulation of TRPV5 activity by secreted Klotho through its putative sialidase activity represents a novel mechanism by which glycoprotein function is regulated by enzymatic modification of its glycans on the cell surface. These observations have

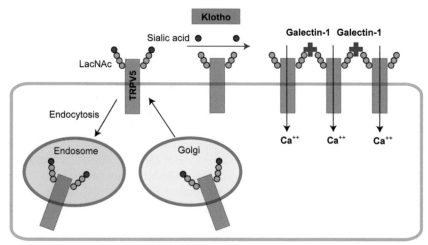

Fig. 21.3 Klotho activates calcium channel TRPV5 through its putative sialidase activity. The number of TRPV5 on the plasma membrane is determined by counterbalance between insertion from intracellular stock in Golgi and removal by endocytosis to endosomes. Terminals of N-linked glycans of cell-surface glycoproteins are capped with sialic acids (red). Secreted Klotho protein removes these sialic acids through its putative α2→6 sialidase activity and exposes underlying N-acetyllactosamine (LacNAc; green). The exposed LacNAc then binds to galectin-1 (blue) in the extracellular matrix. Galectin-1 tethers TRPV5 on the cell surface and prevents its endocytosis, resulting in accumulation of TRPV5 on the plasma membrane and increase in calcium influx.

raised the possibility that secreted Klotho potentially regulates functions of any other cell-surface glycoproteins as long as they have a particular glycan structure that can be a substrate for secreted Klotho. This may explain the seemingly promiscuous effects of secreted Klotho on ion channels and growth factor receptors.

Klotho and aging

Defects in Klotho expression cause not only impaired phosphate/vitamin D homeostasis, but also a premature aging syndrome, suggesting a potential link between aging and phosphate/vitamin D. Klotho-deficient mice are indistinguishable from their wild-type and heterozygous littermates in appearance and growth at weaning around 3 weeks of age. Thereafter, Klotho-deficient mice stop growing and hardly gain body weight until they die prematurely around 8–9 weeks of age. Although they display various disorders resembling human premature aging syndromes as described below, a cause of death has not been specified, because each disorder appears not fatal by itself.[6] The aging-like phenotypes displayed by Klotho-deficient mice include the following.

Hypogonadism

Klotho-deficient mice remain sexually immature and infertile. External and internal genital organs are severely atrophic both in males and females. Testes do not contain mature sperm, because spermatocytes do not mature beyond the pachytene stage. A vaginal opening is never observed in females. Ovaries contain only primary or secondary follicles. No Graafian follicles or corpus lutea are observed, indicating that ovulation never takes place.[6] The impairment in follicle maturation in Klotho-deficient mice is not due to an intrinsic defect in the ovary but due to a defect in pituitary and/or hypothalamus function, because:

- ◆ Klotho-deficient mice have significantly lower serum gonadotropin levels (LH and FSH) than wild-type mice;
- ◆ gonadotropin treatment of Klotho-deficient mice partially restores maturation of follicles and growth of uteri;
- ◆ ovaries of Klotho-deficient mice function normally when transplanted into wild-type female mice.[19]

Thus, Klotho-deficient mice suffer hypogonadotropic hypogonadism. Since Klotho-deficient mice that lack the 1α-hydroxylase gene (double knockout of Klotho and 1α-hydroxylase) are fertile,[35] hypogonadism in Klotho-deficient mice is due to vitamin D and/or phosphate toxicity. However, the fact that Klotho is expressed in the pituitary gland and hypothalamus suggests that Klotho may be involved in the fine regulation of gonadotropin and/or gonadotropin releasing hormone production/secretion in normal animals.

Premature thymic involution

Thymus develops normally up to 3–4 weeks of age in Klotho-deficient mice. It then undergoes disorganization much more rapidly than that observed in chronologically aged mice and shrinks until it becomes undetectable by 6–9 weeks of age.[6] The thymopoietic insufficiency is not caused by an intrinsic defect in lymphohematopoietic progenitors, because hematopoietic stem cells from Klotho-deficient mice can differentiate into normal lymphoid cells when transplanted into SCID mice.[36] Thus, Klotho-deficiency may lead to a defect in microenvironment that supports thymopoiesis, which shares similarity with the pathophysiology observed in thymic involution associated with chronological aging. Thymic epithelial cells are an important component of the micro-environment that supports thymocyte proliferation and survival. KGF (keratinocyte growth factor, aka FGF7; fibroblast growth factor-7) has been identified as an epithelial cell-specific growth factor that induces proliferation of thymic epithelial cells and increase thymopoietic capacity. Interestingly, injection of KGF rescues thymic degeneration not only in Klotho-deficient mice but also in aged wild-type mice.[36] Since thymic involution is also rescued by ablating vitamin D,[35] toxicity of vitamin D or phosphate may have perturbed thymic epithelial cell function, proliferation, and/or survival.

Ectopic calcification

Ectopic calcification is observed in various soft tissues of Klotho-deficient mice, including gastric mucosa, trachea, and renal tubules. Vascular calcification is observed in small arteries in the kidney as well as larger arteries and aorta. Vascular calcification typically occurs in the media and is not associated with intimal thickening or accumulation of foam cells. Thus, these vascular changes associated with Klotho-deficiency are not atherosclerosis, but arteriosclerosis of Mönckeberg-type, which is often observed in the aged, as well as in patients with diabetes and chronic kidney disease in humans.[6] Vascular calcification in Klotho-deficient was discussed above.

Impaired bone mineralization

Klotho-deficient mice display atypical osteopenia.[6,37] Cortical bone thickness of femur, tibia, and vertebrae is decreased by 20–40% when compared with wild-type mice. Histomorphometric analysis of the bone shows marked decrease in both bone formation and resorption, suggesting a low turnover of the bone metabolism. The net bone loss in cortical bones may be due to the decrease in bone formation that exceeds the decrease in bone resorption. This pathophysiology is similar to that observed in senile osteoporosis in the aged, but distinct from post-menopausal osteoporosis in women. Post-menopausal osteoporosis is primarily triggered by estrogen withdrawal that causes increase in osteoclast number and function and promotes bone resorption, leading to high bone turnover. It is not clear whether the osteopenia in Klotho-deficient mice is due to phosphate and/or vitamin D toxicity, as well as many other aging-like phenotypes because of the lack of precise evaluation of bone phenotype in Klotho-deficient mice rescued by vitamin D ablation.

Although cortical bones are reduced in Klotho-deficient mice, they have paradoxically increased trabecular bones in vertebrae and the metaphysis of tibia and femur.[19] The mechanism by which Klotho deficiency affects cortical and trabecular bones in a different way may involve dysregulation of Wnt signaling pathway. Secreted Klotho protein was reported to bind to multiple Wnt ligands and inhibit their ability to activate Wnt signaling, potentially through preventing Wnt binding to its cognate cell-surface receptor.[32] In general, Wnt signaling activation is essential for stem cells to proliferate and survive. However, continuous activation of Wnt signaling can cause rapid exhaustion and depletion of stem cells. Since stem cell dysfunction limits tissue regeneration and potentially affcts aging processes, the ability of secreted Klotho protein to inhibit Wnt signaling may contribute to some aging-like phenotypes in Klotho-deficient mice. Klotho-deficient mice exhibit reduced cortical bone thickness associated with paradoxically increased trabecular bone at the metaphysis of tibia, where Wnt signaling is selectively enhanced when compared with wild-type mice. Since Wnt signaling promotes proliferation/survival of osteoblasts, the selective enhancement of Wnt signaling may explain why Klotho-deficient mice have increased bone only in the trabecular bone.

Skin atrophy

The skin of Klotho-deficient mice is thin and atrophic. Histological examination shows reduced number of hair follicles and reduced thickness of the dermal and epidermal layers. No subcutaneous fat is observed. These findings are similar to those observed in senile atrophoderma in the aged.[6] These aging-like changes in Klotho-deficient mice are associated with significant reduction in the number of CD34-positive epidermal stem cells in hair follicles.[32] Again, dysregulation of Wnt signaling may be involved in the decrease in the stem cells. In addition, hair follicles of Klotho-deficient mice contain increased number of senescent cells that are positive for senescence-associated endogenous β-galactosidase (SAβ-gal) staining. These senescent cells are also positive for nuclear foci of phosphorylated histone (H2AX) and p53 binding protein-1 (53BP1), indicating activation of the DNA damage response pathway. Thus, Klotho-deficiency is associated with increased DNA damage and depletion of stem cells in the skin. Skin atrophy is also rescued by ablation of vitamin D, indicating that phosphate and/or vitamin D toxicity is primarily responsible for increased DNA damage, dysregulation of Wnt signaling, and depletion of stem cells.

Pulmonary emphysema

Histology of the lung of Klotho-deficient mice is indistinguishable from that of wild-type littermates up to 2 weeks of age, by which time the lung becomes mature. Progressive emphysematous changes become evident around 4 weeks of age characterized by enlargement of air spaces and reduction of lung elastic recoil.[6] An increase in the number of apoptotic cells is observed in airway walls. In addition to these histological changes, the respiratory function of Klotho-deficient mice is compatible with pulmonary emphysema and exhibits increased compliance and expiratory time. Aging and smoking have been identified as the two major risk factors for pulmonary emphysema. A mathematical model suggests that the pattern of alveolar destruction in Klotho-deficient mice is consistent with a random destruction caused by a systemic factor(s), rather than a correlated destruction caused by a local factor(s), such as smoking. Thus, the lung of Klotho-deficient mice may represent aging-related pulmonary emphysema.[38] Again, these changes in lung are rescued by ablation of vitamin D, indicating that phosphate and/or vitamin D toxicity is responsible for the lung phenotypes.

Neurodegeneration

Klotho-deficient mice have impairment in cognitive function measured by novel-object recognition and conditioned-fear tests when compared with wild-type mice.[39] The cognition impairment in Klotho-deficient mice is associated with increased number of apoptotic cells, and increased levels of oxidized lipid and DNA in the hippocampus. Furthermore, treatment of Klotho-deficient mice with an antioxidant α-tocopherol improves cognition impairment and reduces oxidative damage and apoptotic cells in hippocampus, suggesting that Klotho may function as a neuroprotective factor through preventing neurons from oxidative damage. In addition, Klotho-deficient mice exhibited degenerative changes of anterior horn cells (AHCs) in the spinal cord. This is similar to the finding observed in patients with amyotrophic lateral sclerosis (ALS). AHCs of Klotho-deficient mice show significant decrease in cytoplasmic RNA, ribosomes, and rough endoplasmic reticulum and accumulation of neurofilaments as those of ALS patients.[40] Recent studies have indicated that increased oxidative stress may be a common mechanism behind many neurodegenerative disorders including Alzheimer's disease, Parkinson's disease, and ALS. The ability of Klotho protein to alleviate oxidative stress may contribute to the neuroprotective properties of Klotho.[38]

Hearing loss

The *klotho* gene is expressed in the stria vascularis and spiral ligament of the inner ear. Although Klotho-deficient mice have no morphological abnormalities in the inner ear, they have significantly higher threshold for auditory brainstem response than wild-type mice, indicating the existence of hearing disorder.[41] Although function of Klotho in the inner ear is not known, it is possible that Klotho protein may be involved in the electrolyte homeostasis of endolymph in the cochlear duct through its activity that regulates ion channels. Klotho expression in the inner ear decreases with age, suggesting the involvement of Klotho in age-dependent loss of hearing.

Typical aging-like phenotypes not observed in Klotho-deficient mice

There is no report so far indicating that Klotho-deficient mice have an increased incidence of malignant tumors or increased amyloid plaques or neurofibrillary tangles in the brain, which are common features of aging. It is possible that they might die too early (around 2 months of age) to develop these diseases. Although there are differences between pathophysiology observed in Klotho-deficient mice and that in natural aging, Klotho-deficient mice have been used as one of the best characterized mammalian models for premature-aging syndromes that manifests multiple aging-like phenotypes in a single individual.

In contrast to Klotho-deficient mice, Klotho-over expressing transgenic mice have extended life spans.[30] Two independent transgenic mouse lines were established that

over-expressed the membrane form of Klotho protein under the control of a ubiquitous promoter (human elongation factor-1α promoter).[6] One of them (*EFmKL46*)
expressed exogenous Klotho in every tissue so far examined, while the other line
(*EFmKL48*) expressed the transgene only in several tissues including brain and testis,
but not in the kidney, probably due to a position effect of the transgene integration
site. Despite the lack of Klotho transgene expression in the kidney where endogenous
Klotho expression is most abundant, the *EFmKL48* allele was able to rescue the aging-
like phenotypes when introduced into the Klotho-deficient mice, indicating that
expression in the kidney may not be essential for Klotho protein function. This is
consistent with the notion that a humoral factor(s) may mediate Klotho protein function. Both *EFmKL46* and *EFmKL48* transgenic mice appeared normal and lived
20–30% longer on average than wild-type mice.[30] Life span extension observed in
these mice is not as robust as that observed in *dwarf* mice carrying defects in the soma-
totroph axis and remains to be confirmed under different housing conditions.
Nonetheless, the *klotho* gene is considered as one of the aging-suppressor genes
identified in mammals that extends life span when over-expressed and causes a premature-aging syndrome when disrupted. Since food consumption of the transgenic
mice is not decreased, it is unlikely that they lived longer simply because they ate less
and voluntarily restricted calorie intake.[30] As discussed later, the transgenic mice that
over-express Klotho exhibit significant resistance to oxidative stress associated with
moderate resistance to insulin/IGF-1, which may partly explain why these mice live
longer than wild-type mice.

Another set of transgenic mice that over-express Klotho was established using an
inducible promoter (mouse metallothionein-1 promoter) to drive expression of the
transmembrane form of Klotho.[42] Klotho-deficient mice carrying this inducible transgene largely depend on zinc water feeding for Klotho expression. When left untreated,
these mice develop premature-aging symptoms as Klotho-deficient mice do. When
given 25mM $ZnSO_4$ solution as a drinking water, these mice express exogenous Klotho
primarily in the gastrointestinal tract, which rescues all the aging-like phenotypes.
More importantly, many advanced aging-like phenotypes are rescued when Klotho
expression is induced by zinc feeding even after they have already developed multiple
aging-like phenotypes. In addition, reduction of Klotho expression by zinc removal in
these rescued Klotho-deficient mice rapidly induces several aging-like phenotypes
including ectopic calcification and pulmonary emphysema. These observations indicate
that reduction of Klotho expression in adulthood can be a cause of several aging-like
disorders and that Klotho replacement may be useful for the treatment of these disorders. In fact, Klotho was recently identified as one of the genes whose expression was
significantly down-regulated with age in the brain of rodents and primates (rhesus
monkey).[43]

Aging is associated with increased oxidative damages to important biological
macromolecules including DNA, protein, and lipid, which potentially cause dysfunction of these molecules and eventually lead to aging. Oxidative damages are primarily
caused by highly reactive oxygen radicals called reactive oxygen species (ROS) elicited
from electron transport chain in mitochondria upon oxidative phosphorylation.
Enzymes have evolved that detoxify harmful ROS, including catalase, superoxide

dismutase, and glutathione peroxidase. Expression of these enzymes is negatively regulated by insulin/IGF-1 signaling pathway. Activation of insulin/IGF-1 signaling increases activity of a serine-threonine kinase Akt, which in turn phosphorylates Forkhead box O (FOXO) transcription factors, FOXO1, FOXO3a, and FOXO4. Phosphorylated FOXOs are excluded from nucleus and unable to function as transcription factors. FOXOs up-regulate expression of multiple target genes, including ROS-removing enzymes such as catalase and mitochondrial manganese-superoxide dismutase (SOD2). Thus, activation of FOXOs by inhibiting insulin/IGF-1 signaling can increase cellular protection against oxidative stress and may contribute to the suppression of aging.[38]

Consistent with this notion, recent studies have shown that increased insulin resistance does not necessarily mean diabetes and short life span. Rather, it has become increasingly clear that adequate suppression of insulin-like signaling pathway is an evolutionarily conserved mechanism for anti-aging and life span extension.[19,44] Reduction-of-function mutations in the genes encoding orthologs of insulin receptor, insulin receptor substrates (IRS), and PI3-kinase has been known to extend life span in *C. elegans* and *Drosophila*. In mammals, increased longevity is reported in mice lacking insulin receptor in adipose tissues, mice heterozygous for a null allele of the insulin-like growth factor-1 (IGF-1) receptor gene, mice lacking IRS-1, mice lacking IRS-2 in the brain, and *dwarf* mice with impaired growth hormone (GH)-IGF-1 endocrine axis. In humans, some centenarians show resistance to IGF-1, short stature, and high serum IGF-1 associated with loss-of-function mutations in the IGF-1 receptor gene. Importantly, some long-lived animals exhibit insulin resistance, indicating that increased insulin sensitivity is not a prerequisite for long life span and anti-aging. Although many long-lived animals indeed exhibit increased insulin sensitivity, it is always associated with hypoinsulinemia and attenuated insulin/IGF-1 signaling activity in tissues. Thus, attenuated insulin/IGF-1 signaling activity in tissues shows closer association with life span extension than increased insulin sensitivity.

Because secreted Klotho has an activity that inhibits insulin/IGF-1 receptor activity, it may alleviate oxidative stress, protect tissues from oxidative damages, and contribute to suppression of aging. In fact, Klotho-over expressing transgenic mice have higher SOD2 expression in muscles and less phosphorylated FOXOs than wild-type mice, associated with less oxidative stress as evidenced by lower levels of urinary 8-OHdG, a marker of oxidative damages to DNA.[45] In addition, Klotho-over expressing transgenic mice survive a sub-lethal dose of paraquat, a herbicide that generates superoxide, significantly longer than wild-type mice, indicating that Klotho over expression induces resistance to oxidative stress. Furthermore, treatment of cultured cells with the secreted Klotho protein inhibits insulin/IGF-1 signaling, activates FOXOs, induces SOD2 expression, and reduces oxidative damages and apoptosis induced by paraquat or hydrogen peroxide.[38] It remains to be determined whether the ability of Klotho to reduce oxidative stress primarily depends on up-regulation of anti-oxidant enzymes.

Summary

Klotho protein, originally identified as a product of the aging suppressor gene, functions in the kidney as an obligatory co-receptor for FGF23, a bone-derived hormone that suppresses renal phosphate reabsorption and vitamin D synthesis. In addition, the extracellular domain of Klotho protein is clipped on the cell surface and released into systemic circulation. The secreted Klotho functions as a kidney-derived endocrine factor that regulates activity of multiple cell-surface glycoproteins including ion channels and growth factor receptors in various tissues. These diverse activities of membrane and secreted Klotho protein collectively contributes to anti-aging properties of Klotho, including reduction of oxidative stress, prevention of vascular calcification, and preservation of renal function.

References

1. Schiavi SC, Kumar R. The phosphatonin pathway: new insights in phosphate homeostasis. *Kidney Int* 2004;**65**:1–14.
2. Dusso AS, Brown AJ, Slatopolsky E. Vitamin D. *Am J Physiol Renal Physiol* 2005;**289**:F8–28.
3. Berndt T, Kumar R. Phosphatonins and the regulation of phosphate homeostasis. *Ann Rev Physiol* 2007;**69**:341–59.
4. Quarles LD. Endocrine functions of bone in mineral metabolism regulation. *J Clin Invest* 2008;**118**:3820–8.
5. Kuro-o M. Endocrine FGFs and Klothos: emerging concepts. *Trends Endocrinol Metab* 2008;**19**:239–45.
6. Kuro-o M, Matsumura Y, Aizawa H, et al. Mutation of the mouse klotho gene leads to a syndrome resembling ageing. *Nature* 1997;**390**:45–51.
7. Goetz R, Beenken A, Ibrahimi OA, et al. Molecular insights into the Klotho-dependent, endocrine mode of action of FGF19 subfamily members. *Mol Cell Biol* 2007;**27**:3417–28.
8. White KE, Evans WE, O'Riordan JLH, et al. Autosomal dominant hypophosphatemic rickets is associated with mutations in FGF23. *Nat Genet* 2000;**26**:345–8.
9. Kuro-o M. Klotho as a regulator of fibroblast growth factor signaling and phosphate/calcium metabolism. *Curr Opin Nephrol Hypertens* 2006;**15**:437–41.
10. Shimada T, Kakitani M, Yamazaki Y, et al. Targeted ablation of Fgf23 demonstrates an essential physiological role of FGF23 in phosphate and vitamin D metabolism. *J Clin Invest* 2004;**113**:561–8.
11. Kurosu H, Ogawa Y, Miyoshi M, et al. Regulation of fibroblast growth factor-23 signaling by klotho. *J Biol Chem* 2006;**281**:6120–3.
12. Urakawa I, Yamazaki Y, Shimada T, et al. Klotho converts canonical FGF receptor into a specific receptor for FGF23. *Nature* 2006;**444**:770–4.
13. Bastepe M, Juppner H. Inherited hypophosphatemic disorders in children and the evolving mechanisms of phosphate regulation. *Rev Endocr Metab Disord* 2008;**9**:171–80.
14. Segawa H, Kawakami E, Kaneko I, et al. Effect of hydrolysis-resistant FGF23-R179Q on dietary phosphate regulation of the renal type-II Na/Pi transporter. *Pflügers Arch* 2003;**446**:585–92.
15. Segawa H, Yamanaka S, Ohno Y, et al. Correlation between hyperphosphatemia and type II Na-Pi cotransporter activity in klotho mice. *Am J Physiol Renal Physiol* 2007;**292**:F769–79.
16. Perwad F, Zhang MY, Tenenhouse HS, et al. Fibroblast growth factor 23 impairs phosphorus and vitamin D metabolism *in vivo* and suppresses 25-hydroxyvitamin D-1alpha-hydroxylase expression *in vitro*. *Am J Physiol Renal Physiol* 2007;**293**:F1577–83.
17. Liu S, Vierthaler L, Tang W, et al. FGFR3 and FGFR4 do not mediate renal effects of FGF23. *J Am Soc Nephrol* 2008;**19**:2342–50.

18. Ben-Dov IZ, Galitzer H, Lavi-Moshayoff V, et al. The parathyroid is a target organ for FGF23 in rats. *J Clin Invest* 2007;**117**:4003–8.

19. Kuro-o M. Klotho and ageing. *Biochim Biophys Acta* 2009;**1790**:1049–58.

20. Tonelli M, Sacks F, Pfeffer M, et al. Relation between serum phosphate level and cardiovascular event rate in people with coronary disease. *Circulation* 2005;**112**:2627–33.

21. Ganesh SK, Stack AG, Levin NW, et al. Association of elevated serum PO(4), Ca × PO(4) product, and parathyroid hormone with cardiac mortality risk in chronic hemodialysis patients. *J Am Soc Nephrol* 2001;**12**:2131–8.

22. Meyer KB, Levey AS. Controlling the epidemic of cardiovascular disease in chronic renal disease: report from the National Kidney Foundation Task Force on cardiovascular disease. *J Am Soc Nephrol* 1998;**9**:S31–42.

23. Sarnak MJ, Levey AS, Schoolwerth AC, et al. Kidney disease as a risk factor for development of cardiovascular disease: a statement from the American Heart Association Councils on Kidney in Cardiovascular Disease, High Blood Pressure Research, Clinical Cardiology, and Epidemiology and Prevention. *Circulation* 2003;**108**:2154–69.

24. Kuro-o M. Klotho in chronic kidney disease—What's new? *Nephrol Dial Transplant* 2009;**24**:1705–08.

25. Haruna Y, Kashihara N, Satoh M, et al. Amelioration of progressive renal injury by genetic manipulation of Klotho gene. *Proc Natl Acad Sci USA* 2007;**104**:2331–6.

26. Sugiura H, Yoshida T, Tsuchiya K, et al. Klotho reduces apoptosis in experimental ischemic acute renal failure. *Nephrol Dial Transplant* 2005;**20**:2636–45.

27. Gutierrez OM, Mannstadt M, Isakova T, et al. Fibroblast growth factor 23 and mortality among patients undergoing hemodialysis. *N Engl J Med* 2008;**359**:584–92.

28. Gutierrez O, Isakova T, Rhee E, et al. Fibroblast growth factor-23 mitigates hyperphosphatemia but accentuates calcitriol deficiency in chronic kidney disease. *J Am Soc Nephrol* 2005;**16**:2205–15.

29. Chen CD, Podvin S, Gillespie E, et al. Insulin stimulates the cleavage and release of the extracellular domain of Klotho by ADAM10 and ADAM17. *Proc Natl Acad Sci USA* 2007;**104**:19796–801.

30. Kurosu H, Yamamoto M, Clark JD, et al. Suppression of Ageing in Mice by the Hormone Klotho. *Science* 2005;**309**:1829–33.

31. Imura A, Tsuji Y, Murata M, et al. alpha-Klotho as a regulator of calcium homeostasis. *Science* 2007;**316**:1615–18.

32. Liu H, Fergusson MM, Castilho RM, et al. Augmented Wnt signaling in a mammalian model of accelerated ageing. *Science* 2007;**317**:803–6.

33. Chang Q, Hoefs S, van der Kemp AW, et al. The beta-glucuronidase klotho hydrolyzes and activates the TRPV5 channel. *Science* 2005;**310**:490–3.

34. Cha SK, Ortega B, Kurosu H, et al. Removal of sialic acid involving Klotho causes cell-surface retention of TRPV5 channel via binding to galectin-1. *Proc Natl Acad Sci USA* 2008;**105**:9805–10.

35. Ohnishi M, Nakatani T, Lanske B, et al. Reversal of mineral ion homeostasis and soft-tissue calcification of klotho knockout mice by deletion of vitamin D 1alpha-hydroxylase. *Kidney Int* 2009;**75**:1166–72.

36. Min D, Panoskaltsis-Mortari A, Kuro-o M, et al. Sustained thymopoiesis and improvement in functional immunity induced by exogenous KGF administration in murine models of ageing. *Blood* 2007;**109**:2529–37.

37. Kawaguchi H, Manabe N, Miyaura C, et al. Independent impairment of osteoblast and osteoclast differentiation in klotho mouse exhibiting low-turnover osteopenia. *J Clin Invest* 1999;**104**:229–37.

38. Kuro-o M. Klotho as a regulator of oxidative stress and senescence. *Biol Chem* 2008;**389**:233–41.

39. Nagai T, Yamada K, Kim HC, et al. Cognition impairment in the genetic model of ageing klotho gene mutant mice: a role of oxidative stress. *FASEB J* 2003;**17**:50–2.

40. Anamizu Y, Kawaguchi H, Seichi A, et al. Klotho insufficiency causes decrease of ribosomal RNA gene transcription activity, cytoplasmic RNA and rough ER in the spinal anterior horn cells. *Acta Neuropathol (Berl)* 2005;**109**:457–66.

41. Kamemori M, Ohyama Y, Kurabayashi M, et al. Expression of Klotho protein in the inner ear. *Heart Res* 2002;**171**:103–10.

42. Masuda H, Chikuda H, Suga T, et al. Regulation of multiple ageing-like phenotypes by inducible klotho gene expression in klotho mutant mice. *Mech Ageing Dev* 2005;**126**: 1274–83.

43. Duce JA, Podvin S, Hollander W, et al. Gene profile analysis implicates Klotho as an important contributor to ageing changes in brain white matter of the rhesus monkey. *Glia* 2008;**56**:106–17.

44. Kenyon C. The plasticity of ageing: insights from long-lived mutants. *Cell* 2005;**120**: 449–60.

45. Yamamoto M, Clark JD, Pastor JV, et al. Regulation of oxidative stress by the anti-ageing hormone Klotho. *J Biol Chem* 2005;**280**:38029–34.

Chapter 22

Physiology and pathology of calcium and magnesium transport

Yoshiro Suzuki, Marc Bürzle, and
Matthias A. Hediger

Calcium homeostasis

Calcium (Ca^{2+}) is crucial for innumerous biological functions in our body. Therefore, the total body calcium homeostasis is intricately regulated by the co-ordination of intestinal absorption, renal reabsorption, placental transport, and bone formation and resorption. Calcium is distributed in bones (1300g, 99%), intracellular fluids (1%) and extracellular fluids (0.1 %). From a daily calcium intake of 1000mg, 175mg Ca^{2+} is absorbed by the intestine and the same amount is excreted in young normal subjects by the kidney into the urine (Fig. 22.1).

In the intestine, the duodenum is the predominant site for Ca^{2+} absorption.[1] This absorption is regulated by 1,25-dihydroxyvitamin D_3 (1,25-vitamin D). The jejunum, the ileum, and the colon absorb smaller amounts of Ca^{2+} as well. In the kidney, ionized Ca^{2+} is filtered at the glomerulus and the majority (70 %) of filtered Ca^{2+} is reabsorbed in the proximal tubules via the paracellular route. Another 20% is reabsorbed in the thick ascending limbs of Henle's loop also via the paracellular route. Finally, the rest is reabsorbed in the distal convoluted tubules and connecting tubules via the transcellular pathway, which is regulated by parathyroid hormone (PTH) and 1,25-vitamin D. Although small amount of Ca^{2+} (1–3%) also appears to be reabsorbed in the collecting ducts.[2]

To maintain appropriate blood Ca^{2+} levels, PTH, 1,25-vitamin D and calcitonin play a central role. The blood Ca^{2+} level is monitored by the Ca^{2+}-sensing receptor (CaR) in the parathyroid gland. When the blood Ca^{2+} goes down, CaR detects a decreased blood Ca^{2+} level. Then PTH in secreted into the blood to trigger Ca^{2+} release from the bones. PTH also enhances 1,25-vitamin D production, which stimulates the intestinal Ca^{2+} absorption. When the blood Ca^{2+} goes up, calcitonin is secreted to enhance the bone formation. Under these mechanisms the blood Ca^{2+} level is maintained in a normal range (Fig. 22.2).

Magnesium homeostasis

Magnesium (Mg^{2+}) is also essential for many bodily processes. For that reason, the total body magnesium homeostasis should be thoroughly maintained. Magnesium (20–28g

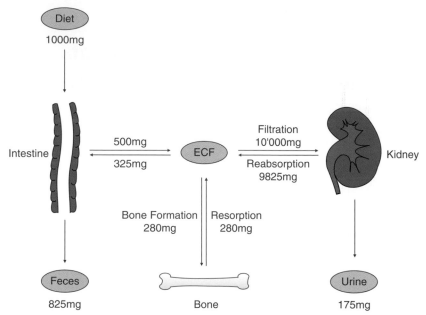

Fig. 22.1 Daily Ca^{2+} balance in human. 175mg Ca^{2+} is absorbed each day in the intestine, and the same amount of Ca^{2+} is excreted into the urine. Total body Ca^{2+} balance is maintained through the co-ordination of intestinal absorption, renal reabsorption, and bone metabolism.

in total) is localized in the bones (60%), muscles (19%), non-muscular soft tissues (19%), and the extracellular space (2%).[3] From a typical daily magnesium intake of 200mg, 30–50% is absorbed by the intestine, mainly by the jejunum and the ileum, and an equal amount of the absorbed Mg^{2+} is excreted by the kidney into the urine. In the kidney, the ionized Mg^{2+} (55% of serum magnesium) is filtered at the glomerulus, then 10–20% of the filtered Mg^{2+} is reabsorbed in the proximal tubules via the paracellular pathway, the majority (50–70%) is reabsorbed in the cortical thick ascending limb of Henle's loop via the paracellular route, and the rest (~10%) is reabsorbed in the distal convoluted tubules via the transcellular pathway. Total Mg^{2+} in plasma is around 0.75–1.05mM. Hypomagnesemia can cause neuromuscular irritabilities (e.g. muscle cramps), hyper-excitability of the central nervous system, cardiac arrhythmias, and seizures in neonates. However, despite the importance of the divalent metal ion, the mechanism of regulation of the magnesium homeostasis is largely unknown.

Transepithelial Ca^{2+} and Mg^{2+} transport

Current findings provide evidence for two different transport pathways for the transepithelial Ca^{2+} and Mg^{2+} transport (Fig. 22.3). One is a paracellular passive pathway that is predominant under high luminal Ca^{2+} or Mg^{2+} concentration. The second is a transcellular active transport pathway. It is the major route under low luminal Ca^{2+} or Mg^{2+} concentration and, therefore, it is regulated by the body's need.

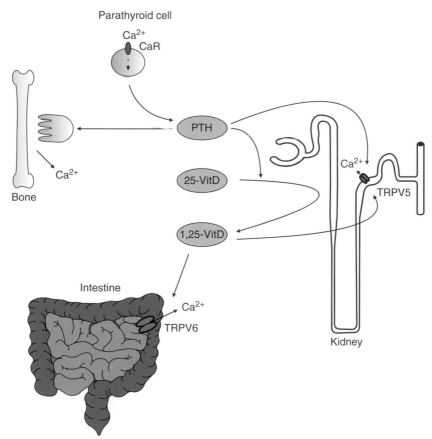

Fig. 22.2 Mechanism of total body Ca^{2+} homeostasis. A decrease in blood Ca^{2+} level triggers the release of the parathyroid hormone (PTH) via the Ca^{2+}-sensing receptor (CaR) in parathyroid cells. This leads to Ca^{2+} release from bone and also enhanced 1,25-dihydroxyvitamin D$_3$ (1,25-vitamin D) production in the renal proximal tubules. 1,25-vitamin D increases the expression of the epithelial Ca^{2+} channel TRPV6 in the intestine, and together with PTH, 1,25-vitamin D increases TRPV5 expression in the kidney. TRPV6 takes Ca^{2+} into the body in the small intestine, whereas TRPV5 enhances Ca^{2+} reabsorption in the distal convoluted tubules in the kidney.

The paracellular pathway is composed only of the tight junctions. This pathway is driven by the transepithelial Ca^{2+} or Mg^{2+} gradient and the electrical potential difference between the lumen and the blood. In the thick ascending limb of Henle's loop in the kidney, it has been shown that mutations in a tight junction protein paracellin-1/claudin-16 cause familial hypomagnesemia with hypercalciuria and nephrocalcinosis (HHN, OMIM #248250), suggesting that this molecule is responsible for the tight junction Mg^{2+} (> Ca^{2+}) permeability in this renal tubule segment.

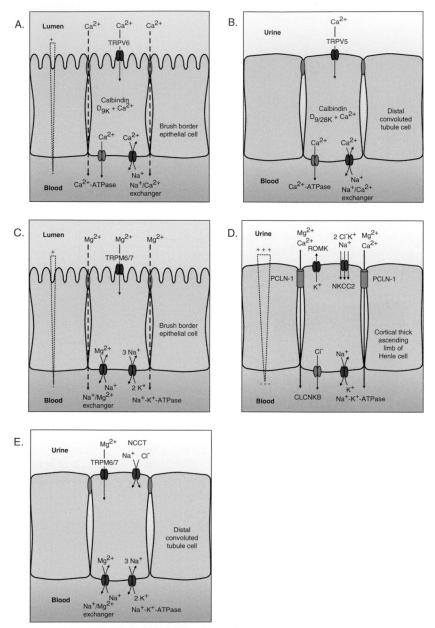

Fig. 22.3 Mechanism of epithelial Ca^{2+} and Mg^{2+} absorption in the intestine and kidney. (A) In the intestine, TRPV6 mediates apical Ca^{2+} uptake into the epithelial cells. Once inside the cells, Ca^{2+} binds to calbindin D_{9K}, which serves as an intracellular Ca^{2+} buffer to diffuse Ca^{2+} to the basolateral side without increasing free intracellular Ca^{2+} concentration. At the basolateral membrane, Ca^{2+} is released through the Ca^{2+}-ATPase PMCA1b or the Na^+/Ca^{2+} exchanger NCX1 (SLC8A1). Under high luminal Ca^{2+} conditions, Ca^{2+} is absorbed via the paracellular pathway. (B) Ca^{2+} reabsorption in the

On the other hand, the transcellular pathway consists of 3 components:

- apical entry via Ca^{2+} or Mg^{2+}-selective channels (TRPV5/6 or TRPM6/7, respectively) driven by the Ca^{2+} or Mg^{2+}-electrochemical gradient from the lumen to the cytosol;

- binding of the absorbed divalent cations to intracellular Ca^{2+} or Mg^{2+}-buffers (calbindin D or ATP, respectively);

- basolateral extrusion via Ca^{2+}-ATPase, Na^+/Ca^{2+} exchanger or the Na^+/Mg^{2+} exchanger.

When the body is in high demand of Ca^{2+}, 1,25-vitamin D increases the expression of intestinal TRPV6 and calbindin D_{9K} to increase the transcellular Ca^{2+} absorption.[4] When the body is in high demand for Mg^{2+}, the expression of the renal and intestinal TRPM6 channels are likely to be increased. However, the molecular mechanism for the regulation of TRPM6 is still poorly understood.[5]

Molecular components of the apical entry for the transcellular pathways

TRPV6

TRPV6 was identified in 1999 by the expression cloning approach using *Xenopus* oocytes.[6] TRPV6 is a Ca^{2+}-selective channel ($Ca^{2+} \gg Ba^{2+}$, Sr^{2+}), which has six membrane-spanning domains and a long C-terminal tail. To avoid intracellular Ca^{2+} overload, there are at least two mechanisms for inactivation by intracellular Ca^{2+} concentration. TRPV6 is predominantly expressed in the apical membrane of duodenum and its expression is high dependent on 1,25-vitamin D.[7] Several vitamin D responsive elements (VDRE) have been identified in the up-stream region of the TRPV6 gene.[8]

---

distal convoluted tubules of the kidney proceeds in a similar fashion, but with TRPV5 as a Ca^{2+} entry channel and both calbindin D_{9K} and calbindin D_{28K} as intracellular Ca^{2+} buffers. (C) Intestinal Mg^{2+} absorption is mediated by TRPM6 as an apical Mg^{2+} entry channel (possibly together with TRPM7). ATP serves as an intracellular Mg^{2+} buffer. A Na^+/Mg^{2+} exchanger facilitates basolateral Mg^{2+} exit. The molecular basis of this Na^+/Mg^{2+} exchange has not yet been determined. Under high luminal Mg^{2+} conditions, Mg^{2+} is absorbed via the paracellular pathway through the tight junctions, down the transepithelial Mg^{2+} gradient. (D) Ca^{2+} and Mg^{2+} reabsorption in the thick ascending limb of Henle's loop (TAL) in the kidney. This transport is mediated by the paracellular pathway through a tight junction protein named paracellin-1 (PCLN-1)/claudin 16 (CLDN16) which is thought to form a divalent cation-specific tight junction channel.[18] The driving force of this transport is likely a lumen-positive potential generated by the transcellular monovalent ion transport (Na^+, K^+ and Cl^-). (E) Mg^{2+} reabsorption in the distal convoluted tubules proceeds in a similar fashion as that in the intestine: TRPM6 serves as Mg^{2+} entry channel and a Na^+/Mg^{2+} exchanger facilitates basolateral exit.

The *trpv6* knockout mice exhibited reduced intestinal Ca^{2+} absorption, resulting in secondary hyperparathyroidism.[9] On the contrary, it has been reported that a gain-of-function haplotype of TRPV6 is associated with absorptive hypercalciuria with renal calcium stone formation, which is likely caused by an increased Ca^{2+} absorption in the intestine.[10] These findings support the view that TRPV6 plays a key role in intestinal Ca^{2+} absorption in order to maintain proper total body calcium homeostasis. However, it seems that the *trpv6* knockout mice can still absorb a significant amount of Ca^{2+} via the transcellular pathway, suggesting that there is an additional apical Ca^{2+} entry channel in the intestine.

In the placenta, TRPV6 is important for the maternal-fetal Ca^{2+} transport in order to sustain the fetal bone mineralization. The blood Ca^{2+} level, bone mineral weight, maternal-fetal Ca^{2+} transport rate were lower in *trpv6* knockout fetuses compared to the wild types.[11]

TRPV5

TRPV5 has also been identified by expression cloning and was found to represent another Ca^{2+}-selective ion channel which shares a moderate sequence homology with TRPV6 (73% identity at the amino acid level).[12] TRPV5 is localized in the apical membrane of the distal convoluted tubules of the kidney where transcellular active Ca^{2+} reabsorption occurs.[13] The TRPV5 expression is also 1,25-vitamin D-dependent, although the range of the induction is much lower compared to TRPV6 in the intestine.[14]

The *trpv5* knockout mice showed reduced Ca^{2+} reabsorption in the distal convoluted tubules. To compensate for this renal Ca^{2+} leak, the intestinal TRPV6 expression was found to be increased in the *trpv5* knockout mice.[15] This compensation is likely due to the effect of a increased 1,25-vitamin D levels because the double-knockout mice of *trpv5* and 1-α-OHase resulted in a disrupted TRPV6 induction, severe hypocalcemia (knockouts: 1.10 ± 0.02 mM, wild types: 2.54 ± 0.01 mM), secondary hyperparathyroidism and rickets.[16] These findings highlight the importance of TRPV5 in the regulation of the final Ca^{2+} reabsorption in order to properly maintain body calcium homeostasis. However, there is no evidence thus far of an association between TRPV5, and renal leak hypercalciuria with nephrolithiasis or other human diseases.

TRPV5 is expressed in osteoclasts as well. Indeed, *trpv5* knockout mice exhibited a reduced bone thickness,[15] resulting from impaired osteoclastic bone resorption.[17] TRPV5 is likely involved in transcellular Ca^{2+} transport during bone resorption, functioning as a Ca^{2+} channel at the ruffled border of resorbing osteoclasts. Future human genetic studies should reveal whether there is a link between TRPV5 mutations and patients with impaired bone mineral density, and/or bone quality such as osteopetrosis or osteoporosis.

TRPM6/TRPM7

TRPM6 and TRPM7 are unique Mg^{2+}-permeable ion channels. They have a typical 6TM channel structure with a kinase domain at the C-terminus. They were initially identified by a homology screening of eukaryotic elongation factor 2 kinase.[18] TRPM7 is a ubiquitously expressed Mg^{2+}-permeable cation channel ($Mg^{2+} > Ca^{2+} \gg Zn^{2+}$,

Co^{2+}, Mn^{2+}), which can be inhibited by intracellular free Mg^{2+} and Mg-ATP. It has been proposed that TRPM7 is critical for cellular magnesium homeostasis.[18] However, *trpm7* knockout mice did not exhibit impaired magnesium homeostasis.[19] TRPM7 is implicated in the thymocyte development at the double-negative stage.[19]

TRPM6 is another Mg^{2+} channel with higher permeability for Mg^{2+}. TRPM6 is localized in the apical membrane of the gastrointestinal tract and the distal convoluted tubules in the kidney. The colonic and renal TRPM6 expression was induced by Mg^{2+}-deficient diet.[5] These results suggest that TRPM6 is involved in intestinal Mg^{2+} absorption and renal Mg^{2+} reabsorption in order to maintain total body magnesium homeostasis.

Hypomagnesemia with secondary hypocalcemia (HSH, OMIM #602014) is an autosomal recessive disease with extremely low blood Mg^{2+} levels (0.2mM). The hypocalcemia in this disease is thought to be caused by the inhibition of the PTH synthesis due to the lower blood Mg^{2+} levels.[18] HSH is likely to be caused by an impaired intestinal Mg^{2+} absorption. Positional cloning revealed that TRPM6 is the responsible gene for HSH.[20,21] These findings support the view that TRPM6 is involved in total body Mg^{2+} homeostasis, functioning as an apical Mg^{2+} entry channel.

Molecular components affecting transcellular Mg^{2+} transport

FXYD2

A mutation (G41R) has been found in FXYD2 gene encoding γ subunit of Na^+, K^+-ATPase in the patients with renal hypomagnesemia with hypocalciuria (OMIM #154020).[22] It suggests that there is a problem in the membrane potential that is generated by Na^+, K^+-ATPase in the basolateral membrane in the distal convoluted tubules. The membrane potential can be used for the effective transcellular Mg^{2+} transport. Therefore, the Mg^{2+} transport can be impaired by the mutation. It was also reported that mutations in the gene for hepatocyte nuclear factor 1B (HNF1B), a transcription factor which could activate the transcription of FXYD2, caused tetany and hypomagnesemia with hypocalciuria.[23] This suggests that HNF1B regulates TRPM6-mediated Mg^{2+} transport by the regulation of transcription of FXYD2.

KCNA1

A voltage-gated K^+ channel Kv1.1 is likely to be important for maintaining the membrane potential across the apical membrane in the distal convoluted tubules in the kidney to support transcellular Mg^{2+} transport. The N255D mutation was reported to be linked to autosomal dominant hypomagnesemia,[24] suggesting a decreased TRPM6-mediated Mg^{2+} reabsorption by a decreased electrochemical driving force in the distal convoluted tubules.

EGF

In patients with recessive hypomagnesemia (OMIM #611718), one mutation was found in the gene for the epidermal growth factor (EGF).[25] The sorting of pro-EGF into the basolateral membrane might be impaired. EGF may regulate TRPM6 channel activity via phosphorylation.

Summary

Calcium (Ca^{2+}) and magnesium (Mg^{2+}) are essential for innumerous functions in the body. Therefore the total body calcium and magnesium levels are finely regulated by the co-ordination of intestinal absorption, renal reabsorption and bone metabolism. In the intestine and kidney (i.e. distal convoluted tubules), the transcellular pathway plays a key role in regulating the absorption of Ca^{2+} and Mg^{2+}, and the apical entry channels (TRPV5/6 for calcium and TRPM6/7 for magnesium) are likely to be rate-limiting steps in this process. Both *trpv5* and *trpv6* knockout mice exhibited calcium deficiency with decreased bone mineral density. Several mutations were found in the gene encoding TRPM6, as well as other genes (*FXYD2, HNF1B, KCNA1, EGF*) concerning the TRPM6-mediated transcellular Mg^{2+} reabsorption in patients with renal hypomagnesemia. These findings strongly suggest that the above mentioned apical entry channels are involved in total body calcium or magnesium homeostasis.

References

1. Bronner F, Pansu D, Stein WD. An analysis of intestinal calcium transport across the rat intestine. *Am J Physiol* 1986;**250**:G561–9.
2. Friedman PA, Gesek FA. Calcium transport in renal epithelial cells. *Am J Physiol* 1993;**264**:F181–98.
3. Satoh J, Romero MF. Mg^{2+} transport in the kidney. *Biometals* 2002;**15**:285–95.
4. Suzuki Y, Landowski CP, Hediger MA. Mechanisms and regulation of epithelial $Ca2+$ absorption in health and disease. *Ann Rev Physiol* 2008;**70**:257–71.
5. Rondon LJ, Groenestege WM, Rayssiguier Y, et al. Relationship between low magnesium status and TRPM6 expression in the kidney and large intestine. *Am J Physiol Regul Integr Comp Physiol* 2008;**294**:R2001–7.
6. Peng JB, Chen XZ, Berger UV, et al. Molecular cloning and characterisation of a channel-like transporter mediating intestinal calcium absorption. *J Biol Chem* 1999;**274**:22739–46.
7. van Cromphaut SJ, Dewerchin M, Hoenderop JG, et al. Duodenal calcium absorption in vitamin D receptor-knockout mice: functional and molecular aspects. *Proc Natl Acad Sci USA* 2001;**98**:13324–9.
8. Meyer MB, Watanuki M, Kim S, et al. The human transient receptor potential vanilloid type 6 distal promoter contains multiple vitamin D receptor binding sites that mediate activation by 1, 25-dihydroxyvitamin D3 in intestinal cells. *Mol Endocrinol* 2006;**20**:1447–61.
9. Bianco SD, Peng JB, Takanaga H, et al. Marked disturbance of calcium homeostasis in mice with targeted disruption of the Trpv6 calcium channel gene. *J Bone Miner Res* 2007;**22**:274–85.
10. Suzuki Y, Pasch A, Bonny O, et al. Gain-of-function haplotype in the epithelial calcium channel TRPV6 is a risk factor for renal calcium stone formation. *Hum Mol Genet* 2008;**17**:1613–18.
11. Suzuki Y, Kovacs CS, Takanaga H, et al. Calcium channel TRPV6 is involved in murine maternal-fetal calcium transport. *J Bone Miner Res* 2008;**23**:1249–56.

12. Hoenderop JG, van der Kemp AW, Hartog A, et al. Molecular identification of the apical Ca^{2+} channel in 1, 25-dihydroxyvitamin D3-responsive epithelia. *J Biol Chem* 1999;**274**:8375–8.

13. Loffing J, Loffing-Cueni D, Valderrabano V, et al. Distribution of transcellular calcium and sodium transport pathways along mouse distal nephron. *Am J Physiol Renal Physiol* 2001;**281**:F1021–7.

14. Hoenderop JG, Mueller D, van der Kemp AW, et al. Calcitriol controls the epithelial calcium channel in kidney. *J Am Soc Nephrol* 2001;**12**:1342–9.

15. Hoenderop JG, van Leeuwen JP, van der Eerden BC, et al. Renal Ca^{2+} wasting, hyperabsorption, and reduced bone thickness in mice lacking TRPV5. *J Clin Invest* 2003;**112**:1906–14.

16. Renkema KY, Nijenhuis T, van der Eerden BC, et al. Hypervitaminosis D mediates compensatory Ca2^{+} hyperabsorption in TRPV5 knockout mice. *J Am Soc Nephrol* 2005;**16**:3188–95.

17. van der Eerden BC, Hoenderop JG, de Vries TJ, et al. The epithelial Ca2^{+} channel TRPV5 is essential for proper osteoclastic bone resorption. *Proc Natl Acad Sci USA* 2005;**102**:17507–12.

18. Schlingmann KP, Waldegger S, Konrad M, et al. TRPM6 and TRPM7 – Gatekeepers of human magnesium metabolism. *Biochim Biophys Acta* 2007;**1772**:813–21.

19. Jin J, Desai BN, Navarro B, et al. Deletion of Trpm7 disrupts embryonic development and thymopoiesis without altering Mg2^{+} homeostasis. *Science* 2008;**322**:756–60.

20. Schlingmann KP, Weber S, Peters M, et al. Hypomagnesemia with secondary hypocalcemia is caused by mutations in TRPM6, a new member of the TRPM gene family. *Nat Genet* 2002;**31**:166–70.

21. Walder RY, Landau D, Meyer P, et al. Mutation of TRPM6 causes familial hypomagnesemia with secondary hypocalcemia. *Nat Genet* 2002;**31**:171–4.

22. Meji IC, Koenderink JB, vanBokhoven H, et al. Dominant isolated renal magnesium loss is caused by misrouting of the Na^{+},K^{+}-ATPase γ subunit. *Nat Genet* 2000;**26**:265–6.

23. Adalat S, Woolf AS, Johnstone KA, et al. HNF1B mutations associate with hypomagnesemia and renal magnesium wasting. *J Am Soc Nephrol* 2009;**20**:1123–31.

24. Glaudemans B, van der Wijst J, Scola RH, et al. A missense mutation in the Kv1.1 voltage-gated potassium channel-encoding gene *KCNA1* is linked to human autosomal dominant hypomagnesemia. *J Clin Invest* 2009;**119**:936–42.

25. Groenestege WMT, Thébault S, van der Wijst J, et al. Impaired basolateral sorting of pro-EGF causes isolated recessive renal hypomagnesemia. *J Clin Invest* 2007;**117**:2260–7.

Chapter 23

Phosphatonins in health and disease

Leslie Thomas, Mukesh Sinha, and Rajiv Kumar

Introduction

In recent years, investigations of rare, inherited bone diseases have greatly contributed to a rapidly evolving model of phosphorus homeostasis. This chapter synthesizes well known and newer concepts of phosphorus adaptation and their abnormalities in various diseases associated with altered phosphate homeostasis. Emphasis is given to the phosphatonins, peptides that reduce serum phosphate concentrations by multiple mechanisms.[1] This group includes fibroblast growth factor-23 (FGF23), secreted frizzled receptor protein-4 (sFRP-4), matrix extracellular phosphoglycoprotein (MEPE), and fibroblast growth factor-7 (FGF7).

Normal phosphorus homeostasis in health

The distribution of phosphorus in *Homo sapiens*

Cadaveric studies performed more than 50 years ago revealed phosphorus to comprise between 0.8 and 1% of total body mass (1.35% of fat-free tissue mass). Eighty-five per cent of total body phosphorus resides in bone, where it crystallizes with calcium as $Ca_{10}(PO_4)_6(OH)_2$ (hydroxyapatite). Soft tissues contain almost all of the remaining phosphorus within the body, while the blood compartment contains only 1% of total body stores. In the blood, freely circulating, inorganic phosphate (Pi) compounds exist in several forms, a substantial portion forming complexes with sodium, magnesium, and calcium with the remaining Pi existing as dihydrophosphate ($H_2PO_4^-$) or monohydrophosphate (HPO_4^{2-}). At physiologic pH, the ratio of $H_2PO_4^-$ to HPO_4^{2-} is approximately 4:1.

Major mechanisms by which Pi homeostasis is regulated

In the healthy adult, body phosphorus content is stable, and dietary intake of phosphorus is balanced by excretion of phosphorus in the feces and urine. Alterations in dietary phosphorus influence the concentrations of extracellular Pi, which stimulate a variety of adaptive processes. Serum Pi levels increase following the ingestion of Pi. Superimposed upon circadian variations, acute increases occur immediately following a meal (Fig. 23.1).[2] Signals and factors originating from the small intestine, parathyroid glands, bone, and kidneys lead to alterations of enteral Pi absorption,

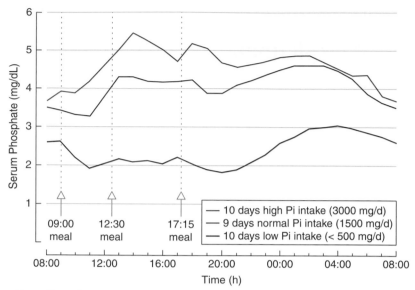

Fig. 23.1 Effect of dietary phosphorus on diurnal serum phosphate concentrations. Healthy men were given meals of varying phosphorus content at 09.00, 12:30, and 17:15 hours. Serum phosphate levels measured after 9 days of normal phosphorus intake (1500mg/day), 10 days of high phosphorus intake (3000mg/day), and 10 days of low phosphorus intake (< 500mg/day) are depicted by black, red, and blue lines, respectively. Meal times are shown by green arrows. Data from Portale AA, et al. *J Clin Invest* 1987;**80**(4):1147–54.[2]

bone mineralization, and renal Pi reabsorption, and result in the maintenance of the extracellular Pi concentrations within narrow limits (Fig. 23.2).[3]

Interactions between the calcium and phosphorus regulatory axes

The primary regulators of extracellular calcium (Ca) concentrations, namely parathyroid hormone (PTH) (via its actions on bone resorption and renal calcium reabsorption) and $1\alpha,25$-dihydroxyvitamin D_3 [$1,25(OH)_2D_3$] (via its effects on intestinal calcium absorption and bone calcium mobilization) also influence phosphorus homeostasis. Fluctuations in the concentration of serum Ca alter the release and production of PTH and the production of $1,25(OH)_2D_3$ (Fig. 23.3). The interested reader is referred to more extensive reviews with appropriate primary citations regarding the interactions between calcium, PTH and the vitamin D endocrine system.[4–9]

Changes in concentrations of serum Pi also alter production of PTH and $1,25(OH)_2D_3$, resulting in correction of Pi concentrations (Fig. 23.4A).[10] Some, but not all reports, have suggested that dietary Pi intake also regulates the concentration of the phosphatonin, FGF23.[10] FGF23 inhibits expression of the 25-hydroxyvitamin D_3 1α-hydroxylase [$25(OH)D$-$1\alpha(OH)ase$] and reduces $1,25(OH)_2D_3$ production. Other growth factors, such as IGF-1 stimulate the $25(OH)D$-$1\alpha(OH)ase$ and increase

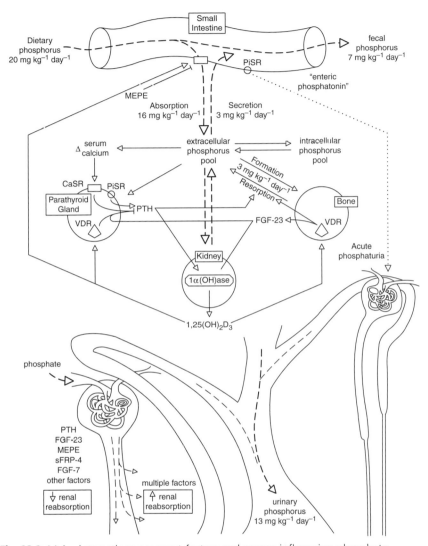

Fig. 23.2 Major interactions amongst factors and organs influencing phosphate homeostasis.

$1,25(OH)_2D_3$ production. $1,25(OH)_2D_3$ stimulates the production of FGF23 thus providing a potential feedback loop (Fig. 23.4B).[11]

Regulation of intestinal Pi absorption

Pi absorption in the intestine occurs by both sodium-independent paracellular and sodium-dependent transcellular mechanisms. At a concentration of 0.1mM Pi, transcellular transport accounts for approximately 80% of total absorption in the rat jejunum.[12] Contributions of transcellular and paracellular pathways likely differ

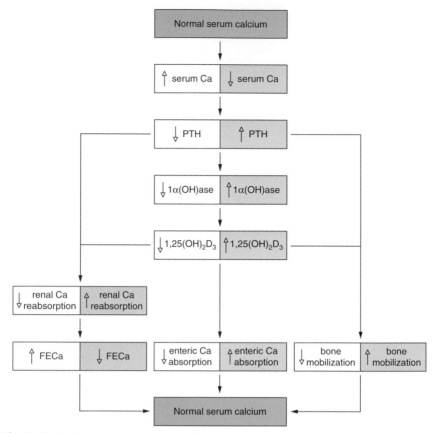

Fig. 23.3 Physiological adaptations to alterations in serum Ca concentrations.

significantly with changing local Pi concentrations and between duodenal, jejunal, and ileal segments of the small intestine.

Sodium-dependent cellular uptake of Pi is mediated by proteins which are encoded by genes of the solute carrier series (SLC). *SLC34A1*, *SLC34A2*, and *SLC34A3* encode NPT2a, NPT2b, and NPT2c, respectively. While NPT2a and NPT2c are found in the renal proximal tubule and facilitate renal reabsorption of phosphate, NPT2b is found in various tissues of the body including the lungs, kidneys, testes, and throughout the small intestine. Regulation of intestinal Pi absorption may be secondary to changes in either *SCL34A2* transcription or localization of NPT2b to or from the enterocyte brush border membrane (BBM). Table 23.1 outlines factors either promoting or inhibiting intestinal Pi absorption. While NTP2b has been conclusively shown in multiple studies to increase Pi transport, the impact of this activity in the maintenance of serum Pi concentrations in humans may not be significant as individuals with mutations of *SCL34A2* gene exhibit no bony abnormalities or alterations in serum Pi (personal observations).[13,14] Other non-sodium dependent mechanisms may also exist for the movement of Pi across the enterocyte.[15]

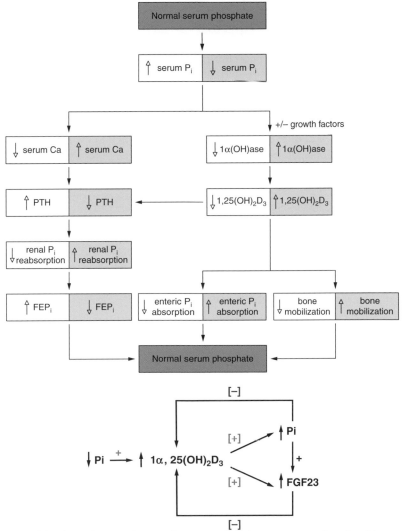

Fig. 23.4 (A) Adaptations to changes in serum phosphate concentrations involving the vitamin D endocrine system, PTH and growth factors such as FGF23 and IGF-1. (B) A feedback loop between 1,25(OH)$_2$D and FGF23.

Table 23.1 Factors affecting intestinal phosphorous absorption

Stimulators of intestinal phosphorus absorption	Inhibitors of intestinal phosphorus absorption
Low dietary phosphorus	MEPE
Vitamin D	Glucocorticoids
Acidosis	EGF
Thyroid hormone	Phosphonoformic acid
Estrogen	

Factors that promote intestinal Pi absorption Various factors have been shown to increase Pi absorption, including dietary phosphorus, vitamin D, acidosis, thyroid hormone, and estrogen.

- *Dietary phosphorus.* Dietary phosphorus content largely determines net phosphorus absorption. While it is well established that $1,25(OH)_2D_3$ increases intestinal Pi absorption and increases the expression of NPT2b, it is also clear that NPT2b expression is regulated directly by dietary Pi.[16,17] VDR-null mice and 25(OH) D-1α(OH)ase-deficient mice fed a low phosphorus diet demonstrate increased *npt2b* mRNA expression and increased npt2b localization to the enterocyte BBM, suggesting an independent role of dietary phosphorus in absorptive efficiency. Furthermore, gut luminal phosphorus concentration may override the effects of $1,25(OH)_2D_3$, even leading to net secretion rather than absorption, suggesting that acute and significant local regulatory effects may be stimulated by the mineral itself.[18] However, an animal model of CKD showed no change in intestinal Pi absorption or *npt2b* mRNA expression compared with rodents with normal renal function either before or after dietary restriction of phosphorus, despite increased expression of renal *npt2a* mRNA, suppression of PTH, and stimulation of $1,25(OH)_2D_3$ production.[19] These data suggest the presence of complex regulatory pathways that are not completely understood.

- *Vitamin D.* $1,25(OH)_2D_3$ increases intestinal Pi absorption.[20] In weanling rats, $1,25(OH)_2D_3$ enhances both *slc34a2* transcription and npt2b BBM localization.[21] In the adult rat, $1,25(OH)_2D_3$ increases localization of npt2b to the enterocyte BBM.[22] Age influences the enterocyte response to $1,25(OH)_2D_3$ in as much as both intestinal and renal npt2 expression, and the effect of $1,25(OH)_2D_3$ are enhanced in young animals.[23] Teleologically, this age-dependent phenomenon may be explained by the increased relative need of the growing organism to maintain a positive balance of Ca and Pi for bone growth and mineralization.

Factors that inhibit intestinal Pi absorption

- *Phosphatonin peptides.* While the roles of the various phosphatonins in the regulation of renal Pi handling have been confirmed over the past several years, recent evidence has also shown that some peptides affect intestinal Pi handling. For instance, FGF23 reduces npt2b expression and activity through its inhibition of $1,25(OH)_2D_3$ synthesis.[24] Short-term MEPE infusion inhibits jejunal Pi absorption in a dose-dependent manner without changes in serum levels of $1,25(OH)_2D_3$, PTH, or FGF23.[25] The actions of sFRP-4 and FGF7 upon intestinal phosphorus absorption have not yet been reported.

- *Other factors.* Glucocorticoids and epidermal growth factor (EGF) inhibit intestinal Pi absorption via their actions on npt2b.

Regulation of normal Pi distribution

In health, multiple regulatory elements govern the distribution of phosphorus within the body compartments, including the intracellular space and mineralized bone. A detailed discussion of the regulation of bone mineralization is beyond the scope of this chapter. However, various factors affecting the distribution of phosphorus have been identified in the context of clinical disease, and specific examples of pathological *redistribution* are outlined below.

Regulation of renal Pi reabsorption

NPT2a and NPT2c   The major site of Pi reabsorption within the nephron is the proximal tubule (PT).[26] NPT2a and NPT2c facilitate reabsorption across the renal PT BBM. The process by which Pi passes across the basolateral membrane into the extracellular space is not clearly delineated. The activity and regulation of NPT2a and NPT2c have been intensively studied and appear to differ in several ways. NPT2a is electrogenic (3 Na^+:1 PO_1^{2-}), is responsible for 70% of PT reabsorption, and is localized throughout the PT. In addition, internalization of the protein from the BBM occurs in a microtubule-independent fashion and leads to lysosomal degradation of the protein. NPT2a localization appears to rely upon interactions with the sodium-hydrogen exchanger regulatory factor 1 (NHERF1), a protein that contains PSD-95, discs-large, and ZO-1 (PDZ) domains. NPT2a interacts with NHERF1 through three carboxyl terminal residues (TRL), which stabilize its position at the BBM.[27] Phosphorylation of NHERF1 promotes internalization of NPT2a.[28] Notably, NPT2a may interact with other proteins containing PDZ domains, although the significance of these interactions is not currently understood. In comparison, NPT2c is found only in the S1 segment of the PT, is electroneutral (2 Na^+:1 PO_4^{2-}), and is estimated to account for 30% of Pi reabsorption, although activity is age-dependent with greater activity being observed in young, weanling animals.[29] Internalization of NPT2c occurs in a microtubule-dependent manner and does not lead to protein degradation. The C terminal residues of NPT2c (QQL) do not comprise a PDZ-binding site, although NPT2c has been shown to interact with both NHERF1 and NHERF3. However, the significance of these interactions is not yet determined.[27]

Major signals regulating the action of these transporters include multiple hormones and other factors. Promoters and inhibitors of renal Pi reabsorption are listed in Table 23.2.

Factors that stimulate renal Pi reabsorption   Low dietary phosphorus content, chronic alkalosis, electrolyte disturbances including hypophosphatemia and hypermagnesemia, and hormones including thyroid hormone, insulin, growth hormone, and insulin-like growth factor-1 each stimulate Pi reabsorption by the kidney.

Factors that inhibit renal Pi reabsorption   Multiple factors have been demonstrated to inhibit renal Pi reabsorption. Among these are high dietary phosphorus content, renal denervation, acidosis, electrolyte disturbances including hyperphosphatemia and hypomagnesemia, and various hormonal factors including atrial natriuretic peptide, dopamine, calcitonin, parathyroid hormone-related peptide, estrogen, glucocorticoids, EGF, and transforming growth factor α. The activities of PTH, the known phosphatonin peptides and the newly described enteric phosphatonin also lead to inhibition of renal Pi reabsorption.

PTH   PTH has a profound effect on renal reabsorption of both Ca and Pi. With regard to Pi handling, PTH signals via the type 1 PTH receptor (PTH1R) in the renal

Table 23.2 Factors affecting renal phosphate reabsorption

Stimulators of renal phosphate reabsorption	Inhibitors of renal phosphate reabsorption
Low dietary phosphate	High dietary phosphate
Alkalosis	Renal denervation
Extracellular magnesium	Acidosis
Thyroid hormone	Extracellular phosphate
Insulin	Hypomagnesemia
Growth hormone	Atrial natriuretic peptide
IGF-1	Dopamine
	Calcitonin
	PTH
	Parathyroid hormone related peptide
	FGF23
	sFRP-4
	MEPE
	FGF7
	Estrogen
	Glucocorticoids
	EGF
	Transforming growth factor-α

PT cell. Similar to NPT2a, this receptor interacts with NHERF1 and is regulated by it.[30] Signaling via PTH1R leads to the activation of both protein kinase A (PKA) and protein kinase C (PKC). PKA and PKC appear to phosphorylate NHERF1, resulting in internalization of NTP2a from the BBM.[30,31]

The three major organs involved in Ca and Pi balance directly communicate with the parathyroid glands to regulate PTH levels. Enteric hormones including secretin and vasoactive intestinal peptide stimulate PTH release. The bone derived peptide, FGF23, decreases PTH mRNA levels and PTH secretion in cultured cells. Furthermore, the local expression of 25(OH)D-1α(OH)ase within parathyroid cell culture *increases* in response to FGF23, which may contribute to the inhibition of PTH.[32] The kidney via its production of $1,25(OH)_2D_3$ decreases PTH synthesis.

Other factors that have been found to influence PTH levels include exercise, which leads to an increase of PTH, and both hyper- and hypomagnesemia, states which are both associated with decreased PTH. In addition, α-Klotho, a protein involved with FGF23 activity, may also regulate PTH secretion (discussed below).[33]

Phosphatonin peptides

- *FGF23.* The osteocyte-derived phosphaturic peptide FGF23 was originally identified from tumors associated with the Pi-wasting disease, tumor-induced osteomalacia (TIO).[1] Mutations of *FGF23* that enhance FGF23 resistance to proteolysis were also identified as the causative factor underlying the development of autosomal dominant hypophosphatemic rickets (ADHR).[34,35] FGF23 reduces serum Pi. Transgenic mice over-expressing FGF23 demonstrate hypophosphatemia, hyperphosphaturia, reduced production of $1,25(OH)_2D_3$, and rickets. FGF23 reduces serum Pi directly, and indirectly through interactions with the kidney and parathyroid gland. In the kidney, FGF23 stimulation leads to phosphaturia via internalization of both NPT2a and NPT2c. Also, FGF23 reduces $1,25(OH)_2D_3$ via the inhibition of 25(OH)D-1α(OH)ase and stimulation of 25(OH)D-24(OH)ase. Through the regulation of $1,25(OH)_2D_3$ production, FGF23 reduces intestinal NPT2b activity and Pi absorption.[24] The significance of the interaction between FGF23 and the vitamin D endocrine system was demonstrated by Hesse et al. who showed a rescue of the FGF23 null mice phenotype in the absence of the VDR.[36] In the parathyroid gland, FGF23 inhibits PTH mRNA transcription and PTH secretion.[37] In addition, FGF23 appears to *increase* 25(OH) D-1α(OH)ase within parathyroid tissue, possibly contributing to the reduction in PTH.[32] The relationship between FGF23 and $1,25(OH)_2D_3$ is reciprocal (Fig. 23.4B). As elevations or reductions in $1,25(OH)_2D_3$ occur, FGF23 expression is increased or decreased, respectively (Fig. 23.4B). Additionally, while dietary phosphorus does not appear to alter the short-term expression of FGF23 in rats or humans, long-term FGF23 regulation appears sensitive to alterations in dietary Pi as demonstrated in mice and humans provided varying levels of dietary Pi.[3] The action of FGF23 is dependent on its interaction with fibroblast growth factor receptors (FGFRs). FGF23 displays limited affinity for the FGFR and requires a cofactor, α-Klotho (α-Kl), for significant interaction and signaling.[38,39] The α-*kl* gene is predominantly expressed in the parathyroid glands, kidneys, and the choroid plexus of the brain.[40] In the kidney, α-Kl is located in the distal convoluted tubule where Ca absorption is actively regulated, and it is co-expressed with Ca permeable transient receptor potential V5 (TRPV5) channels, sodium Ca exchanger 1, and calbindin-D_{28K}. Via interactions with TRPV5, which promotes apical Ca entry, and the sodium/potassium adenosine triphosphatase (Na^+,K^+-ATPase), which indirectly promotes basolateral Ca exit, α-Kl appears to regulate Ca reabsorption in the distal convoluted tubule in response to local concentrations of Ca.[33] In a somewhat analogous fashion, α-Kl:Na^+,K^+-ATPase interactions have been postulated to contribute to the regulation of PTH secretion by the parathyroid glands.[33] The importance of α-Kl to FGF23 action is seen in α-*kl*-null mice, which exhibit many characteristics of *fgf23*-null mice, namely hypercalcemia and hyperphosphatemia, increased $1,25(OH)_2D_3$, ectopic calcification, osteoporosis, and shortened life spans.[38,40] Although FGF23 appears to interact with FGFR1, FGFR3, and FGFR4, recent data suggests the main target of FGF23 may be FGFR1.[41,42] Despite FGF23 actions on the PT, FGFR1 appears to be located mainly in the distal tubule along with α-Kl.[42] The mechanism by which FGF23 signaling to the PT occurs is unclear and may be accomplished indirectly *in vivo*.

◆ *sFRP-4.* sFRP-4, a member of the secreted frizzled-related family of proteins that modulate Wnt signaling, was found to be over-expressed by tumors in patients with TIO.[43] The phosphaturic nature of SFRP-4 is linked to its action to internalise NPT2a, as seen in both OK cells and in the renal PT.[44,45] As with FGF23, sFRP4 inhibits 25(OH)D-1α(OH)ase.[46] In rodents, renal sFRP-4 concentrations increase in response to a diet high in phosphorus in comparison to animals fed a diet containing either low or normal levels of phosphorus.[46] However, the significance of this finding in humans is not known. sFRP-4 levels before and after kidney transplantation in humans were not correlated with either renal clearance or serum Pi level.[47] Interestingly, sFRP-4 is up-regulated in autosomal dominant polycystic kidney disease, suggesting it may play a role in cyst formation.[48]

- ◆ *MEPE.* MEPE, a non-collagenous protein (NCP) found in bone extracellular matrix, belongs to the small integrin binding ligand N-linked glycoprotein (SIBLING) family.[49] The C-terminal residues of MEPE make up an acidic serine-aspartate-rich MEPE-associated (ASARM) motif, which is also found in other SIBLING NCPs[18]. MEPE appears to play a role in bone mineralization. Of note, Martin *et al.* recently showed how addition of ASARM peptide to bone marrow stromal cells resulted in their failure to mineralize properly, suggesting that ASARM peptide may act as an inhibitor of mineralization *in vivo*.[50] MEPE transcription decreases in response to fibroblast growth factor-2, 1,25(OH)$_2$D$_3$, and bone morphogenetic protein-2. MEPE is increased in VDR-null mice.[51] Regulation of MEPE is affected by interactions with PHEX, a protease product of Pi-regulating gene with homologies to endopeptidases on the X chromosome (*PHEX*) that is mutated in X-linked hypophosphatemic rickets. PHEX appears to bind to the ASARM motif of MEPE, thus inhibiting cleavage of MEPE and release of ASARM peptide.[52] MEPE is over-expressed in tumors of individuals with TIO and inhibits renal Pi reabsorption via a reduction in NPT2a protein.[25] In contrast to the known activity of FGF23 and sFRP-4, MEPE does not appear to appreciably inhibit 25(OH)D-1α(OH)ase, but it has been uniquely shown to directly inhibit npt2b and result in decreased Pi absorption in the jejunum in a vitamin D-independent manner.[25] MEPE appears to have a significant physiological role in humans, as levels correlate to serum Pi, PTH, and bone mineral density.[53]

- ◆ *FGF7.* FGF7, previously found to have mitogenic effects on epithelial cells, was also identified in 2005 as a phosphatonin by Carpenter et al.[54] FGF7 was found to inhibit sodium-dependent Pi uptake in opossum kidney cells, and *in vivo* studies demonstrated inhibition of renal Pi reabsorption (personal observations). FGF7 levels are correlated with renal clearance in individuals with chronic kidney disease (CKD) and ESRD (personal observations).

Dietary phosphorus and the phosphaturic enteral axis.   Significant progress has been made in our understanding of the regulation of enteric absorption of Pi. Initial studies determined that absorption is dependent on the presence of sodium and that transmembrane conductance is actively increased by the vitamin D endocrine system, although recent data have challenged the central role of sodium in Pi absorption.[15] Inded, it is clear that the semi-regulated diffusion of Pi along the length of the small intestine is not a complete model of post-cibal adaptation. Steele et al. demonstrated that the renal response to alterations in dietary phosphorus occurred efficiently in the absence of PTH.[55] Calvo et al. showed marked changes in fractional excretion of Pi (FEPi) following ingestion of high Pi diets were associated with only modest changes in PTH, nephrogenous cyclic adenosine 3',5'-monophosphate (cAMP) and 1,25(OH)$_2$D$_3$.[56,57] More recent data suggest the administration of Pi within the lumen of the small intestine stimulates rapid changes in both serum PTH secretion and renal Pi reabsorption. Rapid increases in PTH occur after enteric administration of both sodium Pi and phosphonoformate, a poorly absorbed Pi analog.[58] In individuals with end-stage renal disease (ESRD) and secondary hyperparathyroidism an acute *decrease* in PTH occurs shortly after a meal.[59] These findings suggest the presence of a rapid signaling mechanism between the enteric system and parathyroid glands.

An acute enteric-renal signaling mechanism also appears to exist. Nishida et al. showed that healthy men who received increasing levels of dietary Pi were found to have rapid increases in FEPi associated with only modest changes in PTH and FGF23.[60] More recently, data from our laboratory reveal an acute elevation in the fractional excretion of Pi (FEPi) in rats following duodenal infusion of Pi (Fig. 23.5). The increase in FEPi occurs without changes in serum Pi, PTH, FGF23, and sFRP-4 and is not affected by thyroparathyroidectomy or ablation of renal innervation. Furthermore, infusion of saline extracts of duodenal mucosa results in rapid phosphaturia.[61] Together, these data indicate the presence of a novel, rapidly-acting stimulus originating in the small intestine that may act independently of previously described regulatory elements. This 'enteric phosphatonin' may be analogous to previously described signals that also potentially originate in the gastrointestinal tract that act to mediate natriuretic and kaliuretic responses.[62]

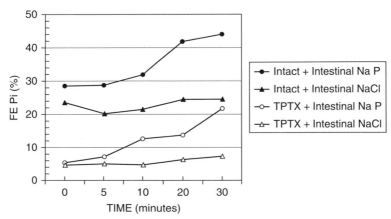

Fig. 23.5 Mean FEPi in intact or thyro-parathyroidectomized rats after the intestinal administration of sodium phosphate or sodium chloride. Reproduced from Berndt T, et al. *Proc Natl Acad Sci USA* 2007;**104:**11085–90.[61]

Abnormal phosphorus homeostasis in disease

Maintenance of serum Pi within a narrow range is critically important to the health and survival of *Homo sapiens*. A number of physiologic elements are promoted by or dependent upon phosphorus and include cellular membrane integrity, cellular signaling, enzyme activity, energy metabolism, nucleic acid, lipid and muscle function, and bone mineralization. Considering its ubiquitous nature in an array of biophysical and biochemical processes, it is not unusual that minor alterations in the homeostasis of phosphorus lead to significant and even devastating consequences in the affected individual. Derangements in phosphorus homeostasis leading to either hypophosphatemia or hyperphosphatemia are encountered in many disease states as outlined in Table 23.3.

Consequences of hypophosphatemia

Moderate hypophosphatemia is defined as a serum Pi concentration between the lower limit of normal and 1mg/dL (0.33 mmol/L). Symptoms associated with the acute development of moderate hypophosphatemia are uncommon. Severe hypophosphatemia may be defined as a Pi concentration less than 1mg/dL. Findings associated with severe hypophosphatemia include confusion, paresthesias, weakness, seizures, and coma. Rhabdomyolysis, hemolysis, left ventricular dysfunction, and respiratory failure are also conditions that have been attributed to severe hypophosphatemia.[63] Hypophosphatemia may be found in up to two percent of hospitalized patients, but a retrospective analysis of 10,197 patients revealed that severe hypophosphatemia occurred with an incidence of 0.4% and in some patients more than others.[64] Severe hypophosphatemia occurred with an incidence of 0.9% in alcoholics, 2.4% in septic patients, 10.4% in the malnourished, and 14.6% in individuals with diabetic ketoacidosis, and severe hypophosphatemia was associated with a four-fold increased risk of death.[64]

Hypophosphatemic disease

Hypophosphatemia may result from a decreased intake of phosphorus, decreased intestinal absorption of phosphorus, pathological redistribution of phosphorus to the intracellular compartment or increased renal Pi excretion.

Decreased phosphorus intake

Decreased phosphorus intake may be secondary to inadequate dietary phosphorus intake or use of total parenteral nutrition with solutions containing inadequate phosphorus content. An associated condition may be chronic alcohol abuse. Chronic negative phosphorus balance from this or other causes may lead to defective bone mineralization, rickets, or osteomalacia.

Decreased intestinal phosphorus absorption

Decreased intestinal absorption of dietary Pi may be caused by the use or overuse of Pi binding agents or with acquired or inherited deficiency of vitamin D. Inherited forms of vitamin D deficiency include pseudovitamin D deficiency rickets (PDDR) and

Table 23.3 Disorders resulting in abnormal serum Pi concentrations

Hypophosphatemic disease	Hyperphosphatemic disease
Decreased phosphorus intake	Increased phosphorus intake

Decreased enteric phosphorus absorption
  Use of phosphate binders
  Vitamin D deficiency
  PDDR
  HVDRR	

Pathological redistribution
  Acute alkalosis
  Hypokalemic periodic paralysis
  Refeeding syndrome
  Acute leukemia
  Stem cell transplantation
	Pathologic redistribution
	  Crush injuries
	  Rhabdomyolysis
	  Tumor lysis syndrome

Increased renal phosphate excretion
  Hypothermia
  Hypokalemia
  Hypomagnesemia
  Hyperparathyroidism
  Generalized renal tubulopathies
    Ethanol use
    Fanconi syndrome
  Specific renal tubulopathies
    NPT2a mutation
    NPT2c mutation
    NHERF1 mutation
    ClC-5 mutation
  Tumor-induced osteomalacia
  ADHR
  ARHR
  XLH
  Hypophosphatemia after renal transplantation
  Nephrolithiasis with "renal phosphate leak"
  Fibrous dysplasia and McCune Albright syndrome
  Epidermal nevus syndromes
  Osteoglophonic dysplasia
  Jansen's metaphyseal chrondrodysplasia
	Decreased renal phosphate excretion
	  Chronic alkalosis
	  Hypoparathyroidism
	  Pseudohypoparathyroidism
	  Tumoral calcinosis
	  CKD and ESRD

hereditary vitamin D-resistant rickets (HVDRR). PDDR, previously referred to as type I vitamin D-resistant rickets (VDDR), is a recessively inherited disorder associated with normal plasma levels of $25(OH)D_3$ and low or undetectable levels of $1,25(OH)_2D_3$. Defective $25[OH]D\text{-}1\alpha(OH)ase]$ activity is the underlying trait responsible for this disorder.[65] HVDRR, previously referred to as type II VDDR, is also inherited recessively and is secondary to a defective VDR. HVDRR is associated with normal levels of $25(OH)D_3$ and elevated levels of $1,25(OH)_2D_3$.[66]

Pathological redistribution

Redistribution of Pi to the intracellular compartment may be secondary to a variety of etiologies, including acute alkalosis, hypokalemic periodic paralysis, refeeding syndrome, acute leukemia, and following stem cell transplantation.

Increased renal Pi excretion

Disorders without known phosphatonin dysregulation   Increased renal Pi excretion may also be caused by a variety of conditions. Hypothermia, hypokalemia, hypomagnesemia, and hyperparathyroidism may each lead to excessive Pi excretion and the development of hypophosphatemia. Generalized renal PT disease, such as may occur with chronic ethanol abuse or Fanconi syndrome, is associated with hyperphosphaturia. Specific tubulopathies may also lead to excessive renal Pi wasting. For instance, mutation of NPT2a has been associated with some cases of nephrolithiasis and osteoporosis.[67] Mutation of NPT2c has been identified as the underlying abnormality leading to hereditary hypophosphatemic rickets with hypercalciuria (HHRH), an autosomal recessive disorder characterized by hypophosphatemia and phosphaturia, muscle weakness, significant bone disease that may manifest as rickets or bone pain, and nephrolithiasis.[68] Karim *et al.* have shown that mutations of NHERF1 may contribute to the development of nephrolithiasis and osteopenia.[69] Mutation of the Cl^-/H^+ exchanger, ClC-5, which plays a crucial role in PT endocytosis, is the underlying genetic defect leading to Dent's disease, which is characterized by kidney stones, nephrocalcinosis, low molecular weight proteinuria, hypophosphatemia, and hyperphosphaturia.[70] Abnormally high serum concentrations of the phosphatonin peptides have not been described in the above conditions, although the relative contributions of the phosphatonins in these conditions of abnormal phosphaturia are largely unreported.

Disorders associated with phosphatonin dysregulation and/or abnormal phosphatonin concentration

◆ *Tumor-induced osteomalacia.* Excessive phosphaturia stemming from excessive generation of tumor-derived phosphatonins may eventually lead to hypophosphatemia and clinically evident bone disease, a syndrome referred to as tumor-induced osteomalacia (TIO). Patients with these tumors exhibit hypophosphatemia with hyperphosphaturia and a relative deficiency of $1,25(OH)_2D_3$. With removal of the tumor, phosphatonin excess is abolished, and hypophosphatemia and osteomalacia generally resolve. Phosphatonins identified from tumors include the aforementioned FGF23, sFRP-4, MEPE, and FGF7.

◆ *Autosomal dominant hypophosphatemic rickets.* In 2000, mutations in the gene encoding *FGF23* were found to be associated with the development of autosomal dominant hypophosphatemic rickets (ADHR).[34] Mis-sense mutations in the *FGF23* gene lead to replacement of arginine (R) residues within a subtilisin-like proprotein convertase cleavage site (176RHTR179) within the encoded protein with other amino-acid residues. The mutant FGF23 protein is resistant to proteolysis and has an abnormally long half-life.[35] ADHR is characterized by renal Pi wasting and inappropriately normal $1,25(OH)_2D_3$ concentrations. Clinical manifestations of ADHR are variable, with some affected individuals presenting in childhood with rickets or lower extremity deformity, and others presenting in adulthood with weakness, bone pain, and insufficiency fractures.

♦ *Autosomal recessive hypophosphatemic rickets.* Individuals with autosomal recessive hypophosphatemic rickets (ARHR) have biochemical derangements similar to individuals with TIO and ADHR and manifest hypophosphatemia, hyperphosphaturia, and low or inappropriately normal serum $1,25(OH)_2D_3$ concentrations. However, the underlying pathogenesis of ARHR is related to inactivating mutations of *DMP1*, the gene encoding dentin matrix acidic phosphoprotein 1 (DMP1).[71] Similar to MEPE, DMP1 is a SIBLING family NCP and contains an ASARM motif.[72] Furthermore, mutation of DMP1 leads to increases in FGF23 expression, although the pathway by which this occurs is presently unclear.

♦ *X-linked hypophosphatemia.* X-linked hypophosphatemia (XLH) may present in a similar fashion to ADHR and ARHR and is also associated with elevated levels of FGF23. However, the underlying defect in this disorder is a mutation in *PHEX* that encodes a membrane-bound Zn-metalloprotease expressed mainly by osteoblasts and odontoblasts, PHEX.[73] Patients with XLH demonstrate increased circulating levels of FGF23, as well as MEPE in some. The Hyp mouse, a rodent model of unstable PHEX transcription in which the XLH phenotype is recapitulated, also demonstrates increased circulating levels of the intact form of FGF23. Global deletion of the *Phex* gene in mice results in an increase in circulating FGF23, sFRP-4 and MEPE, whereas an osteoblast specific deletion of *Phex* results in an increase in FGF23 alone.74]. Both the knock out models have hypophosphatemia, increased urinary phosphate losses and a mineralization defect. Evidence demonstrating the relationship between PHEX and FGF23 has been conflicting. Bowe *et al.* showed that FGF23 is a PHEX substrate and that mutant PHEX may lead to increased intact FGF23 concentrations.[75] Others have not shown that FGF23 is a PHEX substrate.[76,77] Furthermore, reduction in PHEX activity may also lead to decreased PHEX:ASARM motif interactions with subsequent increase in degradation of MEPE and DMP1 along with other changes.[50] Accumulation of ASARM peptide likely accounts for defective mineralization seen in XLH and may also contribute to phosphaturia.

♦ *Hypophosphatemia after renal transplantation.* While hyperphosphatemia occurs commonly in patients with CKD and ESRD, individuals who receive renal allografts typically demonstrate hypophosphatemia with hyperphosphaturia. This phosphaturic state may persist for months following transplantation. Persistent elevations of PTH are often present and account for most of the hypophosphatemia but some data has shown that the etiology is related to chronic elevation of FGF23.

♦ *Nephrolithiasis with 'renal Pi leak'.* As described above, altered PT handling of Pi secondary to changes in the normal function of NPT2a, NPT2c, NHERF1, and ClC-5, may lead to the development of kidney stones. The relationship of nephrolithiasis and FGF23 was explored in a prospective study examining nephrolithiasis patients who had hypophosphatemia and renal Pi leak (renal Pi threshold < 2.2mg/L), with nephrolithiasis patients without hypophosphatemia and renal Pi leak, and normal subjects. FGF23 concentrations were significantly different in the three groups (83 RU/mL versus 32.1 and 24.5, respectively), suggesting that aberrant FGF23 may contribute to hypophosphatemia in some patients with nephrolithiasis. The presence of elevated $1,25(OH)_2D_3$ concentrations is not satisfactorily explained in such patients in the presence of elevated FGF23 concentrations.

- *Fibrous dysplasia and McCune-Albright syndrome.* A post-zygotic point mutation of *GNAS1* is the underlying etiology of both isolated fibrous dysplasia (FD) and McCune-Albright syndrome (MAS), a disease characterized by FD in association with café-au-lait spots and multiple endocrinopathies. The particular *GNAS1* mutation responsible for FD and MAS results in constitutive activation of the alpha subunit of stimulatory G protein (Gsα), which, in turn, leads to an increased intracellular concentration of cAMP. The subsequent increase in cAMP signaling enhances the cellular response to hormones that utilize Gsα protein. In MAS, augmented effects of luteinizing hormone (LH), thyroid-stimulating hormone (TSH), adrenocorticotropin hormone (ACTH), and growth hormone-releasing hormone (GHRH) may be encountered. In addition, a bleeding diathesis secondary to platelet dysfunction and severe hypertension have been described in some cases. Abnormal bone findings include FD lesions, which consist of immature osteogenic cells and abnormal trabeculae associated with abnormal osteoblasts and osteocytes. In some cases, rickets or osteomalacia has been described. The proximate etiology of these bony abnormalities appears to, in part, be related to an increase in interleukin-6 (IL-6) expression, which may itself be stimulated by cAMP, with resultant enhancement of osteoclastogenesis. Increased serum levels of FGF23 may be secondary to either abnormal production, as a result of maturation defects related to IL-6 expression, or normal production by abnormally high numbers of FGF23-producing cells within the fibrous lesions. Hypophosphatemia and decreased $1,25(OH)_2D_3$ seen in patients with FD or MAS appear to result from elevation of FGF23. These conditions may lead to the development of rickets or osteomalacia, as has been described in some cases, and they may contribute to the formation of FD lesions.

- *The epidermal nevus syndromes.* The epidermal nevus syndromes (ENS) encompasses a variety of rare, sporadic disorders characterized by congenital hamartomas of ectodermal origin (epidermal nevi) with associated isolated or combined ectodermal defects of the skin, brain, eyes, and skeleton. Skeletal lesions may be focal and similar to fibrous dysplasia lesions by some accounts. The underlying pathogenesis of ENS appears to stem from post-zygotic mutations, similar to the pathogenesis of fibrous dysplasia and MAS. Interestingly, cases of MAS and ENS may present with hypophosphatemic rickets. Recent case reports of individuals who had ENS and associated hypophosphatemic rickets also had elevations in FGF23. The underlying cause of increased FGF23 concentrations seen in these specific cases of ENS is presently unknown.

- *Osteoglophonic dysplasia.* Mis-sense mutations of FGFR1 lead to osteoglophonic dysplasia (OD), a disorder characterized by multiple abnormalities including abnormal bone mineralization at the metaphyses of long bones that may be similar to FD lesions, rhizomelic dwarfism, and craniosynostosis. One report showed that three of four individuals with OD demonstrated renal Pi wasting and low $1,25(OH)_2D_3$ concentrations. FGF23 was found to be elevated in one individual with OD.[78]

♦ *Jansen's metaphyseal chondrodysplasia.* Jansen's metaphyseal chondrodysplasia is a rare, autosomal dominant disorder caused by activating mutations of PTH1R. Hypercalcemia, hypophosphatemia, low or undetectable PTH and PTHrP, and short-limbed dwarfism along with other skeletal abnormalities characterize the disorder. FGF23 levels were found to be elevated in one reported case.[79]

Potential mechanisms by which hypophosphatemia occurs in some of the acquired and inherited rickets are shown in Fig. 23.6.

Consequences of hyperphosphatemia

Increased serum phosphate concentrations are associated with increased mortality and coronary artery disease (CAD). Hyperphosphatemia in ESRD has long been shown to independently associate with mortality and cardiovascular events.[80–82] A reduction in serum Pi by use of Pi binders is associated with lower mortality.[83] The possible mechanisms by which an increased serum Pi may influence mortality and CAD in ESRD include alterations in PTH, a reduction in $1,25(OH)_2D_3$ formation, an elevation of FGF23 concentrations, the development of cardiac fibrosis and micro-vascular and macrovascular calcification. Although the pathogenesis of this abnormal vascular calcification is not completely understood, the role of extracellular Pi is crucial as it promotes the expression of an osteogenic phenotype in vascular myocytes.[84,85] The development of vascular calcification is not limited to individuals afflicted with severe kidney dysfunction or others who may have extremes of serum Pi concentration.

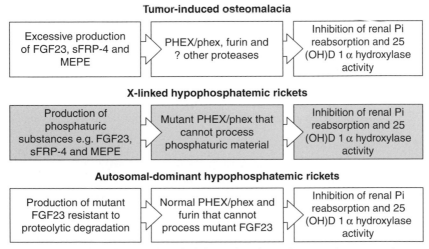

Fig. 23.6 Potential mechanisms by which hypophosphatemia occurs in some patients with acquired and inherited rickets.

The relationship of serum Pi to the development of vascular calcification is maintained in lower risk populations. In individuals with chronic kidney disease (CKD) of moderate severity (estimated glomerular filtration rate < 60mL/min/1.73m^2) higher Pi levels are associated with the prevalence of vascular calcification, calcification of cardiac valves, and death.[86,87] Even in individuals with normal kidney function, serum Pi levels are associated with the long-term development of vascular calcification.[88] A *post hoc* analysis of over 4000 patients with hyperlipidemia and previous myocardial infarction who were followed on average for 5 years revealed a graded, independent relationship between higher serum Pi levels and the risk of all-cause death. This study also showed that a higher Pi level in individuals from this select, high risk population is associated with increased risk of new onset symptomatic heart failure, fatal or non-fatal myocardial infarction, and fatal coronary disease or non-fatal myocardial infarction.[89] Data taken from the Framingham cohort were consistent with these findings and revealed a significant graded association of higher serum Pi levels with incident cardiovascular disease.[90]

Hyperphosphatemic disease

Hyperphosphatemia is defined by a serum Pi concentration greater than the upper range of normal, usually defined as greater than 4.5mg/dL (1.50 mmol/L). Findings associated with hyperphosphatemia may be acute or chronic. Acute symptoms are related to hypocalcemia which may occur as a result of reduced intestinal absorption of calcium secondary to inhibition of $1,25(OH)_2D_3$ production by elevated Pi levels and from the formation of calcium Pi complexes and extraskeletal calcification. Chronic changes are seen commonly in individuals afflicted with CKD or ESRD, and include vascular calcification, secondary hyperparathyroidism, and metabolic bone disease. Analogous to the disease states associated with hypophosphatemia, hyperphosphatemic diseases may be grouped by the mechanism by which high Pi levels develop.

Increased phosphorus intake

Whether via the use of Pi salts commonly prescribed for their laxative effects or via total parenteral nutrition, phosphorus intake exceeding the ability of the kidneys to clear it from the body will inexorably lead to hyperphosphatemia. Notably, the use of Pi salts for bowel preparation prior to colonoscopy or other procedures has fallen out of favor secondary to the association with acute nephrocalcinosis (acute Pi nephropathy).

Pathologic redistribution

Phosphorus is the major intracellular anion. While normal serum Pi concentration ranges from 3 to 5mg/dL, intracellular concentrations are approximately 150mg/dL. Processes that destroy cellular membranes expose the extracellular environment to intracellular components, including high relative concentrations of Pi. Cellular lysis may occur in a variety of settings including after crush injuries or during rhabdomyolysis. Chemotherapy, especially when employed in cases of massive tumor burden, may lead to tumor lysis syndrome which includes the development of hyperphosphatemia.

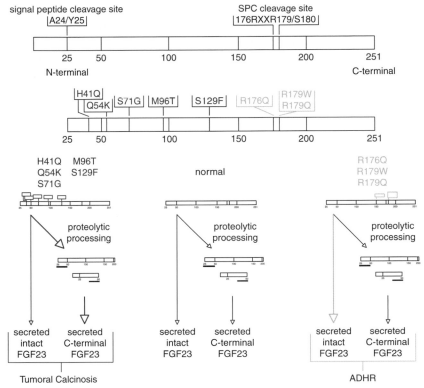

Fig. 23.7 Processing of FGF23 in TC and ADHR. TC results from decreased FGF23 activity, which may occur secondary to mutation in *FGF23*, α-*kl*, or *GALNT3* (see text). *FGF23* mutations (S71G or S129F) in TC lead to altered peptide folding, decreased secretion, and increased proteolytic cleavage and result in increased C-terminal peptide secretion and decreased overall FGF23 activity. ADHR results from mutations at the proteolytic cleavage site, leading to reduced intact mutant FGF23 enzymatic processing and subsequent secretion of mutant FGF23 with prolonged bioactivity.

Decreased renal phosphorus excretion

Chronic respiratory alkalosis, hypoparathyroidism, pseudohypoparathyroidism, tumoral calcinosis (TC), CKD, and ESRD may each lead to hyperphosphatemia. Of these disorders, altered FGF23 concentrations or regulation has been demonstrated in some cases of hypoparathyroidism, TC, CKD, and ESRD. It is not presently known whether increased concentrations of FGF23 seen in some cases of hypoparathyroidism may contribute to the pathogenesis of the disorder or are simply a result of the disorder. TC and CKD and ESRD are discussed in detail below.

◆ *Tumoral calcinosis.* TC is a disorder of deranged phosphorus metabolism characterized by severe ectopic calcifications. Individuals with TC have hyperphosphatemia, elevated or inappropriately normal serum $1,25(OH)_2D_3$ concentrations, and normal serum calcium and PTH concentrations. Inactivating mutations of *FGF23*, α-*kl*, and UDP-N-acetyl-alpha-D-galactosamine:polypeptide N-acetylgalactosaminyltransferase 3 (*GALNT3*) have been associated with the development of TC. As shown in Fig. 23.7, mutations of *FGF23* have been shown to decrease secretion of intact (active) FGF23 and increase secretion of C-terminal (inactive) FGF23.[91-93] Mutation of α-*kl* is thought to decrease the affinity of FGF23 to its co-receptor while mutation of *GALNT3* also leads to decreased secretion of intact peptide via alterations of normal peptide glycosylation.[94]

◆ *Renal failure.* With a moderate reduction in renal function, the ability of the kidneys to excrete ingested phosphorus declines. At first, this situation results in a relative, if not an absolute, hyperphosphatemia which stimulates multiple changes described above, including a decrease in serum calcium concentrations, an increase in PTH and FGF23, and a reduction in $1,25(OH)_2D_3$. For example, we demonstrated that plasma FGF23 correlated with creatinine clearance ($r^2 = -0.584$, $p < 0.0001$) and plasma phosphorus ($r^2 = 0.347$, $p < 0.001$) in CKD patients and with plasma phosphorus ($r^2 = 0.448$, $p < 0.001$) in end-stage renal disease patients.[47] Phosphate binder withdrawal increased FGF23 levels. sFRP-4 levels did not change with creatinine clearance or hyperphosphatemia in CKD or end-stage renal disease patients, and no relationship was noted between post-transplant sFRP-4 levels and hypophosphatemia. While several investigators have noted increased FGF23 concentrations in CKD and ESRD, and increased FGF23 concentrations increase renal Pi excretion in normal subjects, it is uncertain to what extent the elevated FGF23 concentrations are effective because a significant proportion of FGF23 in the circulation is in the form of inactive fragments and because the nephron may fail to respond to the intact form of FGF23. The effect of FGF23 on the pathogenesis of bone disease in renal failure is not completely understood. In peritoneal dialysis patients, higher FGF23 concentrations were associated with decreased osteoid thickness and shorter osteoid maturation time, that is, improved mineralization.[95]

Summary

The model of phosphorus homeostasis has evolved significantly in the past few years and will improve further as new insights are made. The discovery of phosphatonin peptides marks an important milestone in our understanding of the greater scheme of Pi metabolism. Further elucidation of the complex regulatory elements of phosphorus balance may lead to novel therapies for those afflicted with derangements of phosphorus handling, including those with advanced CKD and ESRD.

References

1. Cai Q, Hodgson SF, Kao PC, et al. Brief report: inhibition of renal phosphate transport by a tumor product in a patient with oncogenic osteomalacia. *N Engl J Med* 1994;**330**(23):1645–9.
2. Portale AA, Halloran BP, Morris RC, Jr. Dietary intake of phosphorus modulates the circadian rhythm in serum concentration of phosphorus. Implications for the renal production of 1,25-dihydroxyvitamin D. *J Clin Invest* 1987;**80**:1147–54.

3. Berndt, T, Kumar R. Phosphatonins and the regulation of phosphate homeostasis. *Ann Rev Physiol* 2007;**69:**341–59.

4. Kumar R. Metabolism of 1,25-dihydroxyvitamin D3. *Physiol Rev* 1984;**64:**478–504.

5. Tebben PJ, Kumar R. The hormonal regulation of calcium metabolism. In: R. J. Alpern & S. C. Hebert (eds), *The Kidney: Physiology and Pathophysiology*. Amsterdam: Elsevier Academic Press, 2008;1891–910.

6. Kumar R. Calcium disorders. In: J. P. Kokko & R. L. Tannen (eds) *Fluids and Electrolytes*. Philadelphia: W.B. Saunders Co, 1996;391–419.

7. Kumar, R. Vitamin D and the kidney. In: D. Feldman, F. H. Glorieux, and J. W. Pike (eds). *Vitamin D*. San Diego: Academic Press, 1997;275–92.

8. Kumar R, Craig T. Vitamin D metabolism. In: R. L. Jamison & R. Wilkinson (eds), *Nephrology*. London: Chapman & Hall, 1997;205–14.

9. Popovtzer MM, Knochel JP, Kumar R. Disorders of calcium phosphorus, vitamin D, and parathyroid hormone activity. In: R. W. Schrier (ed.), *Renal and Electrolyte Disorders*. Little: Lippincott-Raven, 1997;241–319.

10. Berndt T, Kumar R. Novel mechanisms in the regulation of phosphorus homeostasis. *Physiol (Bethesda)* 2009;**24:**17–25.

11. Kolek OI, Hines ER, Jones MD, et al. 1 α,25-dihydroxyvitamin D3 upregulates *FGF23* gene expression in bone: the final link in a renal-gastrointestinal-skeletal axis that controls phosphate transport. *Am J Physiol Gastrointest Liver Physiol* 2005;**289:**G1036–42.

12. Eto N, Tomita M, Hayashi M. NaPi-mediated transcellular permeation is the dominant route in intestinal inorganic phosphate absorption in rats. *Drug Metab Pharmacokinet* 2006;**21**(3):217–21.

13. Corut A, Senyigit A, Ugur SA, et al. Mutations in SLC34A2 cause pulmonary alveolar microlithiasis and are possibly associated with testicular microlithiasis. *Am J Hum Genet* 2006;**79**(4):650–6.

14. Huqun, Izumi S, Miyazawa H, et al. Mutations in the SLC34A2 gene are associated with pulmonary alveolar microlithiasis. *Am J Respir Crit Care Med* 2007;**175**(3):263–8.

15. Williams KB, DeLuca HF. Characterisation of intestinal phosphate absorption using a novel *in vivo* method. *Am J Physiol Endocrinol Metab* 2007;**292:**E1917–21.

16. Segawa H, Kaneko I, Yamanaka S, et al. Intestinal Na-P(i) cotransporter adaptation to dietary P(i) content in vitamin D receptor null mice. *Am J Physiol Renal Physiol* 2004;**287:**F39–47.

17. Capuano P, Radanovic T, Wagner CA, et al. Intestinal and renal adaptation to a low-Pi diet of type II NaPi cotransporters in vitamin D receptor- and 1alphaOHase-deficient mice. *Am J Physiol Cell Physiol* 2005;**288:**C429–34.

18. Lee DB, Hardwick LL, Hu MS, Jamgotchian N. Vitamin D-independent regulation of calcium and phosphate absorption. *Miner Electrolyte Metab* 1990;**16**(2–3):167–73.

19. Marks J, Churchill LJ, Srai SK, et al. Intestinal phosphate absorption in a model of chronic renal failure. *Kidney Int* 2007;**72**(2):166–73.

20. Tanaka Y, Frank H, DeLuca HF. Biological activity of 1,25-dihydroxyvitamin D3 in the rat. *Endocrinology* 1973;**92**(2):417–22.

21. Xu H, Bai L, Collins JF, Ghishan FK. Age-dependent regulation of rat intestinal type IIb sodium-phosphate cotransporter by 1,25-(OH)(2) vitamin D(3). *Am J Physiol Cell Physiol* 2002;**282**(3):C487–93.

22. Hattenhauer O, Traebert M, Murer H, Biber J. Regulation of small intestinal Na-P(i) type IIb cotransporter by dietary phosphate intake. *Am J Physiol* 1999;**277**(4 Pt 1):G756–62.

23. Segawa H, Kaneko I, Takahashi A, et al. Growth-related renal type II Na/Pi cotransporter. *J Biol Chem* 2002;**277**(22):19665–72.

24. Miyamoto K, Ito M, Kuwahata M, Kato S, Segawa H. Inhibition of intestinal sodium-dependent inorganic phosphate transport by fibroblast growth factor 23. *Ther Apher Dial* 2005;**9**(4):331–5.

25. Marks J, Churchill LJ, Debnam ES, Unwin RJ. Matrix extracellular phosphoglycoprotein inhibits phosphate transport. *J Am Soc Nephrol* 2008;**19**(12):2313–20.

26. Knox FG, Haas J, Berndt T. An evaluation of possible sites of phosphate secretion in the rat nephron. *Adv Exp Med Biol* 1978;**103**:65–9.

27. Villa-Bellosta R, Barac-Nieto M, Breusegem SY, Barry NP, Levi M, Sorribas V. Interactions of the growth-related, type IIc renal sodium/phosphate cotransporter with PDZ proteins. *Kidney Int* 2008;**73**(4):456–64.

28. Weinman EJ, Biswas RS, Peng G, et al. Parathyroid hormone inhibits renal phosphate transport by phosphorylation of serine 77 of sodium-hydrogen exchanger regulatory factor-1. *J Clin Invest* 2007;**117**(11):3412–20.

29. Biber J, Hernando N, Forster I, Murer H. Regulation of phosphate transport in proximal tubules. *Pflugers Arch* 2009;**458**(1):39–52.

30. Wang B, Yang Y, Abou-Samra AB, Friedman PA. NHERF1 regulates parathyroid hormone receptor desensitisation; interference with beta-arresting binding. *Mol Pharmacol* 2009;**75**(5):1189–97.

31. Cunningham R, Biswas R, Brazie M, Steplock D, Shenolikar S, Weinman EJ. Signaling pathways utilized by PTH and dopamine to inhibit phosphate transport in mouse renal proximal tubule cells. *Am J Physiol Renal Physiol* 2009;**296**(2):F355–61.

32. Krajisnik T, Bjorklund P, Marsell R, et al. Fibroblast growth factor-23 regulates parathyroid hormone and 1alpha-hydroxylase expression in cultured bovine parathyroid cells. *J Endocrinol* 2007;**195**:125–31.

33. Nabeshima Y, Imura H. Alpha-Klotho: a regulator that integrates calcium homeostasis. *Am J Nephrol* 2008;**28**(3):455–64.

34. The ADHR Consortium. Autosomal dominant hypophosphatemic rickets is associated with mutations in FGF23. *Nat Genet* 2000;**26**(3):345–8.

35. White KE, Jonsson KB, Carn G, et al. The autosomal dominant hypophosphatemic rickets (ADHR) gene is a secreted polypeptide overexpressed by tumors that cause phosphate wasting. *J Clin Endocrinol Metab* 2001;**86**(2):497–500.

36. Hesse M, Frohlich LF, Zeitz U, Lanske B, Erben RG. Ablation of vitamin D signaling rescues bone, mineral, and glucose homeostasis in Fgf23 deficient mice. *Matrix Biol* 2007;**26**(2):75–84.

37. Ben-Dov IZ, Galitzer H, Lavi-Moshayoff V, et al. The parathyroid is a target organ for FGF23 in rats. *J Clin Invest* 2007;**117**(12):4003–8.

38. Kurosu H, Ogawa Y, Miyoshi M, et al. Regulation of fibroblast growth factor-23 signaling by klotho. *J Biol Chem* 2006;**281**(10):6120–3.

39. Nakatani T, Sarraj B, Ohnishi M, et al. In vivo genetic evidence for klotho-dependent, fibroblast growth factor 23 (Fgf23)-mediated regulation of systemic phosphate homeostasis. *FASEB J* 2009;**23**(2):433–41.

40. Kuro-o M. Klotho as a regulator of fibroblast growth factor signaling and phosphate/calcium metabolism. *Curr Opin Nephrol Hypertens* 2006;**15**(4):437–41.

41. Urakawa I, Yamazaki Y, Shimada T, et al. Klotho converts canonical FGF receptor into a specific receptor for FGF23. *Nature*, 2006;**444**(7120):770–4.

42. Liu S, Vierthaler L, Tang W, Zhou J, Quarles LD. FGFR3 and FGFR4 do not mediate renal effects of FGF23. *J Am Soc Nephrol* 2008;**19**(2):2342–50.

43. De Beur SM, Finnegan RB, Vassiliadis J, et al. Tumors associated with oncogenic osteomalacia express genes important in bone and mineral metabolism. *J Bone Miner Res* 2002;**17**(6):1102–10.

44. Berndt T, Craig TA, Bowe AE, et al. Secreted frizzled-related protein 4 is a potent tumor-derived phosphaturic agent. *J Clin Invest* 2003;**112**(5):785–94.

45. Berndt TJ, Bielesz B, Craig TA, et al. Secreted frizzled-related protein-4 reduces sodium-phosphate co-transporter abundance and activity in proximal tubule cells. *Pflugers Arch* 2006;**451**(4):579–87.

46. Sommer S, Berndt T, Craig T, Kumar R. The phosphatonins and the regulation of phosphate transport and vitamin D metabolism. *J Steroid Biochem Mol Biol* 2007;**103**(3–5):497–503.

47. Pande S, Ritter CS, Rothstein M, et al. FGF23 and sFRP-4 in chronic kidney disease and post-renal transplantation. *Nephron Physiol* 2006;**104**(1):23–32.

48. Romaker D, Puetz M, Teschner S, et al. Increased expression of secreted frizzled-related protein 4 in polycystic kidneys. *J Am Soc Nephrol* 2009;**20**(1):48–56.

49. Fisher LW, Fedarko NS. Six genes expressed in bones and teeth encode the current members of the SIBLING family of proteins. *Connect Tissue Res* 2003;**44**(Suppl 1): 33–40.

50. Martin A, David V, Laurence JS, et al. Degradation of MEPE, DMP1, and release of SIBLING ASARM-peptides (minhibins): ASARM-peptide(s) are directly responsible for defective mineralization in HYP. *Endocrinology*, 2008;**149**(4):1757–72.

51. Liu S, Brown TA, Zhou J, et al. Role of matrix extracellular phosphoglycoprotein in the pathogenesis of X-linked hypophosphatemia. *J Am Soc Nephrol* 2005;**16**(6): 1645–53.

52. Rowe PS, Garrett IR, Schwartz PM, et al. Surface plasmon resonance (SPR) confirms that MEPE binds to PHEX via the MEPE-ASARM motif: a model for impaired mineralization in X-linked rickets (HYP). *Bone* 2005;**36**(1):33–46.

53. Jain A, Fedarko NS, Collins MT, et al. Serum levels of matrix extracellular phosphoglyco-protein (MEPE) in normal humans correlate with serum phosphorus, parathyroid hormone and bone mineral density. *J Clin Endocrinol Metab* 2004;**89**(8):415–61.

54. Carpenter TO, Ellis BK, Insogna KL, Philbrick WM, Sterpka J, Shimkets R. Fibroblast growth factor 7: an inhibitor of phosphate transport derived from oncogenic osteomalacia-causing tumors. *J Clin Endocrinol Metab* 2005;**90**(2):1012–20.

55. Steele TH, DeLuca HF. Influence of dietary phosphorus on renal phosphate reabsorption in the parathyroidectomised rat. *J Clin Invest* 1976;**57**(4):867–74.

56. Calvo MS, Kumar R, Heath H, 3rd, Elevated secretion and action of serum parathyroid hormone in young adults consuming high phosphorus, low calcium diets assembled from common foods. *J Clin Endocrinol Metab* 1988;**66**(4):823–9.

57. Calvo MS, Kumar R, Heath H. Persistently elevated parathyroid hormone secretion and action in young women after four weeks of ingesting high phosphorus, low calcium diets. *J Clin Endocrinol Metab* 1990;**70**(5):1334–40.

58. Martin DR, Ritter CS, Slatopolsky E, Brown AJ. Acute regulation of parathyroid hormone by dietary phosphate. *Am J Physiol Endocrinol Metab* 2005;**289**(4):E729–34.

59. Brown AJ, Koch MJ, Coyne DW. Oral feeding acutely down-regulates serum PTH in hemodialysis patients. *Nephron Clin Pract* 2006;**103**(3):c106–13.

60. Nishida Y, Taketani Y, Yamanaka-Okumura H, et al. Acute effect of oral phosphate loading on serum fibroblast growth factor 23 levels in healthy men. *Kidney Int* 2006;**70**(12):2141–7.

61. Berndt T, Thomas LF, Craig TA, et al. Evidence for a signaling axis by which intestinal phosphate rapidly modulates renal phosphate reabsorption. *Proc Natl Acad Sci USA* 2007;**104**(26):11085–90.

62. Thomas L, Kumar R. Control of renal solute excretion by enteric signals and mediators. *J Am Soc Nephrol* 2008;**19**(2):207–12.

63. Amanzadeh J, Reilly RF, Jr. Hypophosphatemia: an evidence-based approach to its clinical consequences and management. *Nat Clin Pract Nephrol* 2006;**2**(3):136–48.

64. Camp MA, Allon M. Severe hypophosphatemia in hospitalised patients. *Miner Electrolyte Metab* 1990;**16**(6):365–8.

65. Fu GK, Lin D, Zhang MY, et al. Cloning of human 25-hydroxyvitamin D-1 alpha-hydroxylase and mutations causing vitamin D-dependent rickets type 1. *Mol Endocrinol* 1997;**11**(13):1961–70.

66. Hochberg Z, Weisman Y. Calcitriol-resistant rickets due to vitamin D receptor defects. *Trends Endocrinol Metab* 1995;**6**(6):216–20.

67. Prie D, Huart V, Bakouh N, et al. Nephrolithiasis and osteoporosis associated with hypophosphatemia caused by mutations in the type 2a sodium-phosphate cotransporter. *N Engl J Med* 2002;**347**(13):983–91.

68. Bergwitz C, Roslin NM, Tieder M, et al. SLC34A3 mutations in patients with hereditary hypophosphatemic rickets with hypercalciuria predict a key role for the sodium-phosphate cotransporter NaPi-IIc in maintaining phosphate homeostasis. *Am J Hum Genet* 2006;**78**(2):179–92.

69. Karim Z, Gerard B, Bakouh N, et al. NHERF1 mutations and responsiveness of renal parathyroid hormone. *N Engl J Med* 2008;**359**(11):1128–35.

70. Plans V, Rickheit G, Jentsch TJ. Physiological roles of CLC Cl(−)/H (+) exchangers in renal proximal tubules. *Pflugers Arch* 2009;**458**(1):23–37.

71. Feng JQ, Ward LM, Liu S, et al. Loss of DMP1 causes rickets and osteomalacia and identifies a role for osteocytes in mineral metabolism. *Nat Genet* 2006;**38**(11):1310–5.

72. Farrow EG, Davis SI, Ward LM, et al. Molecular analysis of DMP1 mutants causing autosomal recessive hypophosphatemic rickets. *Bone* 2009;**44**(2):287–94.

73. A gene (PEX) with homologies to endopeptidases is mutated in patients with X-linked hypophosphatemic rickets. The HYP Consortium. *Nat Genet* 1995;**11**(2):130–6.

74. Yuan B, Takaiwa M, Clemens TL, et al. Aberrant Phex function in osteoblasts and osteocytes alone underlies murine X-linked hypophosphatemia. *J Clin Invest* 2008;**118**(2):722–34.

75. Bowe AE, Finnegan R, Jan de Beur SM, et al. FGF23 inhibits renal tubular phosphate transport and is a PHEX substrate. *Biochem Biophys Res Commun* 2001;**284**(4):977–81.

76. Liu S, Guo R, Simpson LG, Xiao ZS, Burnham CE, Quarles LD. Regulation of fibroblastic growth factor 23 expression but not degradation by PHEX. *J Biol Chem* 2003;**278**(39):37419–26.

77. Benet-Pages A, Lorenz-Depiereux B, Zischka H, White KE, Econs MJ, Strom TM. FGF23 is processed by proprotein convertases but not by PHEX. *Bone* 2004;**35**(2):455–62.

78. White KE, Cabral JM, Davis SI, et al. Mutations that cause osteoglophonic dysplasia define novel roles for FGFR1 in bone elongation. *Am J Hum Genet* 2005;**76**(2):361–7.

79. Brown WW, Juppner H, Langman CB, et al., Hypophosphatemia with elevations in serum fibroblast growth factor 23 in a child with Jansen's metaphyseal chondrodysplasia. *J Clin Endocrinol Metab* 2009;**94**(1):17–20.

80. Stevens LA, Djurdjev O, Cardew S, Cameron EC, Levin A. Calcium, phosphate, and parathyroid hormone levels in combination and as a function of dialysis duration predict mortality: evidence for the complexity of the association between mineral metabolism and outcomes. *J Am Soc Nephrol* 2004;**15**(3):770–9.

81. Slinin Y, Foley RN, Collins AJ. Calcium, phosphorus, parathyroid hormone, and cardiovascular disease in hemodialysis patients: the USRDS waves 1, 3, and 4 study. *J Am Soc Nephrol* 2005;**16**(6):1788–93.

82. Ganesh SK, Stack AG, Levin NW, Hulbert-Shearon T, Port FK. Association of elevated serum PO(4), Ca × PO(4) product, and parathyroid hormone with cardiac mortality risk in chronic hemodialysis patients. *J Am Soc Nephrol* 2001;**12**(10):2131–8.

83. Isakova T, Gutierrez OM, Chang Y, et al. Phosphorus Binders and Survival on Hemodialysis. *J Am Soc Nephrol* 2009;**20**(2):388–96.

84. Jono S, McKee MD, Murry CE, et al. Phosphate regulation of vascular smooth muscle cell calcification. *Circ Res* 2000;**87**(7):E10–7.

85. Chen NX, O'Neill KD, Duan D, Moe SM. Phosphorus and uremic serum up-regulate osteopontin expression in vascular smooth muscle cells. *Kidney Int* 2002;**62**(5):1724–31.

86. Adeney KL, Siscovick DS, Ix JH, et al. Association of serum phosphate with vascular and valvular calcification in moderate CKD. *J Am Soc Nephrol* 2009;**20**(2):381–7.

87. Kestenbaum B, Sampson JN, Rudser KD, et al. Serum phosphate levels and mortality risk among people with chronic kidney disease. *J Am Soc Nephrol* 2005;**16**(2):520–8.

88. Foley RN, Collins AJ, Herzog CA, Ishani A, Kalra PA. Serum phosphorus levels associate with coronary atherosclerosis in young adults. *J Am Soc Nephrol* 2009;**20**(2):397–404.

89. Tonelli M, Sacks F, Pfeffer M, Gao Z, Curhan G. Relation between serum phosphate level and cardiovascular event rate in people with coronary disease. *Circulation* 2005;**112**(17):2627–33.

90. Dhingra R, Sullivan LM, Fox CS, et al. Relations of serum phosphorus and calcium levels to the incidence of cardiovascular disease in the community. *Arch Intern Med* 2007;**167**(9):879–85.

91. Araya K, Fukumoto S, Backenroth R, et al. A novel mutation in fibroblast growth factor 23 gene as a cause of tumoral calcinosis. *J Clin Endocrinol Metab* 2005;**90**(10):5523–7.

92. Benet-Pages A, Orlik P, Strom TM, Lorenz-Depiereux B. An FGF23 missense mutation causes familial tumoral calcinosis with hyperphosphatemia. *Hum Mol Genet* 2005;**14**(3):385–90.

93. Larsson T, Davis SI, Garringer HJ, et al. Fibroblast growth factor-23 mutants causing familial tumoral calcinosis are differentially processed. *Endocrinology* 2005;**146**(9):3883–91.

94. Kato K, Jeanneau C, Tarp MA, et al. Polypeptide GalNAc-transferase T3 and familial tumoral calcinosis. Secretion of fibroblast growth factor 23 requires O-glycosylation. *J Biol Chem* 2006;**281**(27):18370–7.

95. Wesseling-Perry K, Pereira RC, Wang H, et al. Relationship between plasma fibroblast growth factor-23 concentration and bone mineralization in children with renal failure on peritoneal dialysis. *J Clin Endocrinol Metab* 2009;**94**(2):511–17.

Chapter 24

FGF23 in renal failure

Katherine Wesseling-Perry and Myles Wolf

Introduction

Fibroblast growth factor 23 (FGF23) is a key regulator of phosphorus metabolism whose effects in patients with chronic kidney disease (CKD) have only recently begun to be appreciated. Recent study of this phosphaturic hormone has revealed new pathways of mineral regulation in both individuals with normal kidney function and in patients with CKD. While the effects of FGF23 on mineral metabolism in CKD appears to be similar to its effects in individuals with normal kidney function, elevated levels of the protein in the CKD population have also been linked to kidney disease progression, altered skeletal histology, and increased mortality rates, relationships that have not been examined in the general population.[1–3] Thus, potential differences in FGF23 metabolism accompany the elevated levels found in CKD patients and, although the exact pathophysiological consequences remain mostly unknown, elevated FGF23 levels appear to contribute to major complications of CKD that plague both adults and children.

FGF23 physiology

The fibroblast growth factor (FGF) family is comprised of 22 structurally-related mammalian proteins with a variety of functions in angiogenesis, tissue remodeling, and nervous system control;[4–7] the FGF19 subfamily, including FGF19, FGF21, and FGF23, consists of metabolic regulators.[8] FGF23 is expressed in a variety of tissues, although the majority of circulating FGF23 is derived from osteocytes and osteoblasts in bone.[9] Degradation of the FGF23 molecule relies on proteolytic cleavage between arginine 179 and serine 180, generating two inactive fragments.[10,11] The intact FGF23 protein binds to various FGF receptors, including FGFR1, FGFR3, and FGFR4;[12;13] however, only FGFR1 mediates the effects of FGF23 on mineral metabolism.[14] Indeed, a co-receptor, Klotho, which is expressed in distal tubular cells of the kidney, in the parathyroid glands, and in epithelial cells of the choroid plexus,[15–17] transforms the FGFR1c into a receptor specific for FGF23[18,19] and is necessary for FGF23 site-specific effects. Klotho deficient and FGF23 deficient mice display similar phenotypes[15,20,21] and inhibition of Klotho removes the effect of FGF23 on target tissues.[19]

The physiological importance of the FGF23 was first identified in human genetic and acquired rachitic diseases,[22–25] where increased levels of the protein are accompanied by impaired tubular phosphate reabsorption, hypophosphatemia, low (or inappropriately

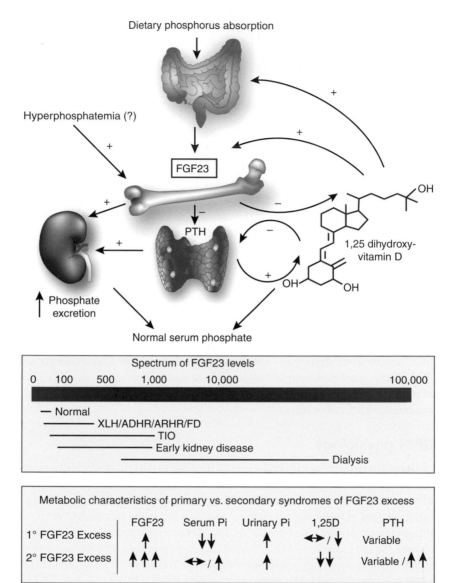

Dietary phosphorus absorption

Hyperphosphatemia (?)

FGF23

PTH

OH

1,25 dihydroxy-
vitamin D

OH   OH

Phosphate
excretion

Normal serum phosphate

Spectrum of FGF23 levels						
0	100	500	1,000	10,000		100,000

— Normal
———— XLH/ADHR/ARHR/FD
——————— TIO
—————— Early kidney disease
————————————— Dialysis

Metabolic characteristics of primary vs. secondary syndromes of FGF23 excess

	FGF23	Serum Pi	Urinary Pi	1,25D	PTH
1° FGF23 Excess	↑	↓↓	↑	↔ / ↓	Variable
2° FGF23 Excess	↑↑↑	↔ / ↑	↑	↓↓	Variable / ↑↑

Fig. 24.1 Fibroblast growth factor 23 (FGF23) regulates serum phosphate levels within a narrow range despite wide fluctuation in dietary intake via a series of classic negative endocrine feedback loops involving 1,25-dihydroxyvitamin D (1,25D), PTH, urinary phosphate excretion, and dietary phosphorus absorption. FGF23 secretion by osteocytes is primarily stimulated (+) by increased dietary phosphorus intake, exposure to 1,25D, and possibly, by increased serum phosphate levels; FGF23 is inhibited (–) by low dietary phosphorus intake, hypophosphatemia, and low 1,25D levels. FGF23 binds FGF receptor with highest affinity in the presence of the co-receptor Klotho. In the renal proximal tubule, FGF23 binding increases urinary phosphate excretion by down-regulating expression of luminal sodium-phosphate co-transporters, NaPi-2a and NaPi-2c. In addition, FGF23 inhibits secretion of PTH and inhibits 25-hydroxyvitamin

normal) levels of 1,25 (OH)$_2$vitamin D, and impaired skeletal mineralization (rickets or osteomalacia).[21,26-29] Increased circulating levels of FGF23 are necessary and sufficient to account for these abnormalities since infusion of FGF23 into rats with normal renal function results in renal phosphate wasting and direct suppression of 1α hydroxylase activity,[28] while the complete lack of functional FGF23 results in the inverse phenotype. Indeed, patients with genetic forms of tumoral calcinosis, caused either by defects in GALNT3, a protein involved in post-translational O-glycosylation FGF23, or by destabilizing mutations in the FGF23 molecule itself,[30-33] have increased circulating values of calcitriol, despite hyperphosphatemia and hypercalcemia.[21,29] More recently, FGF23 has also been shown to regulate PTH metabolism, FGF23 suppressing PTH secretion both *in vitro* and *in vivo*.[34,35]

Under conditions of normal renal function, FGF23 is regulated by both phosphorus and vitamin D.[36,37] Sustained increases in dietary phosphorus are associated with an increase in FGF23 and a decline in 1,25(OH)$_2$ vitamin D,[38,39] while dietary phosphorus restriction reverses these trends.[38,39] The rise in FGF23 in response typically occurs over the course of days. The earliest changes in FGF23 have been observed 8h after ingestion of a supraphysiological oral phosphate load, administered to stimulate a rapid increase in FGF23 levels.[38,40] In both animals and humans, the administration of 1,25(OH)$_2$vitamin D also increases circulating FGF23 levels,[37] mediated by a vitamin D response element located upstream of the FGF23 gene (Fig. 24.1).[36] Parathyroid hormone levels may also stimulate FGF23 expression,[41] although whether this is a direct effect or mediated through 1,25(OH)$_2$vitamin D remains to be established.

D-1-α-hydroxylase leading to decreased circulating levels of 1,25D. Decreased 1,25D levels, in turn, lower gut phosphorus absorption and release the parathyroid glands from feedback inhibition, thereby increasing circulating PTH levels, which further augment urinary phosphate excretion. The direct effects of FGF23 on bone mineralization and other organs are less clear. The upper insert illustrates the spectrum of FGF23 levels that can be observed under normal conditions and in a variety of syndromes of FGF23 excess. Circulating FGF23 levels are 10- to 20-fold above normal (~30–60RU/mL using a C-terminal FGF23 assay) in patients with hereditary hypophosphatemic rickets syndromes, including X-linked hypophosphatemia (XLH), autosomal dominant hypophosphatemic rickets (ADHR), autosomal recessive hypophosphatemic rickets (ARHR), and fibrous dysplasia (FD). While FGF23 levels are often even higher in patients with tumor-induced osteomalacia (TIO), the highest levels are encountered in patients with kidney disease and especially those on dialysis, in whom levels can reach concentrations more than 1000-fold above the normal range. The lower insert illustrates the differences in the metabolic characteristics of 'primary' syndromes of FGF23 excess, such as the hereditary diseases and TIO, versus 'secondary' syndromes of FGF23 excess, such as kidney disease. In addition to the severity of the FGF23 increase, the primary difference is normal to high serum phosphate (Pi) levels in patients with kidney disease compared with hypophosphatemia, which is the sine qua non of the hereditary syndromes. Although variable, 1,25D levels tend to be lower and PTH levels higher in patients with kidney disease compared with the hereditary syndromes. Urinary fractional excretion of phosphate is high in both pre-dialysis kidney disease and genetic hypophosphatemic disorders.

FGF23 and mineral metabolism in patients with chronic kidney disease

Circulating levels of FGF23 rise progressively as renal function declines.[42,43] Several potential mechanisms have been proposed, including a decreased capacity for renal phosphate excretion and decreased renal clearance of FGF23. Vitamin D sterol therapy, which is commonly used to treat elevated PTH levels in CKD patients, would also be expected to increase FGF23 levels, but FGF23 levels are elevated in CKD even in the absence of treatment. Recent evidence suggest that the rise in circulating FGF23 is linked to declining 1,25(OH)$_2$vitamin D values and, thus, may play a critical role in the initial development of secondary hyperparathyroidism. In a cross-sectional analysis of 80 adult patients with CKD stages 1–4, FGF23 levels were independently associated with decreasing kidney function, and levels of the protein rose before any abnormalities in serum calcium, phosphorus or PTH were apparent.[43] In this cohort of patients, increased FGF23 values were associated with low 1,25(OH)$_2$vitamin D levels, independent of glomerular filtration rate and serum phosphate concentration. Moreover, increases in FGF23 and decreases in circulating calcitriol were observed long before the need for erythropoietin therapy, suggesting that the decline in 1,25(OH)$_2$vitamin D was due to an increasing burden of circulating FGF23 and not solely to loss of functional renal mass.[43] Since normal serum phosphate levels are typically maintained until late in the course of CKD,[43] increasing concentrations of FGF23 appear to represent a compensatory response to maintain normal serum phosphate levels in the face of declining nephron mass; the decline in calcitriol levels associated with this response subsequently leads to the development of secondary hyperparathyroidism. These hypotheses are supported by similar results from other studies in pre-dialysis CKD populations.[1,44]

After successful renal transplantation, serum phosphorus levels decrease to below the normal range in many adult and pediatric patients. Although values gradually increase over time in most patients, hypophosphatemia may persist in some individuals for months to years after the transplant, despite the resolution of secondary hyperparathyroidism.[45] Persistent elevation of circulating levels of FGF23 may contribute to post-transplant hypophosphatemia and the relationship between FGF23, phosphorus, and calcitriol levels during the first year post-transplantation has been investigated by several groups. FGF23 values decline rapidly within days and values are similar to those observed in patients with CKD by 3 months post-transplantation.[46,47] In the early post-transplant period, increased serum FGF23 levels predict hypophosphatemia and low calcitriol levels,[46,48] and thus, at least early on, a residual excess of FGF23 may contribute to post-transplantation alterations in mineral metabolism. The clinical consequences of these findings are uncertain. Indeed, although bone loss and cardiovascular disease are significant complications in the post-transplant period, little information exists as to the role, if any, that FGF23 and its effect on mineral metabolism play in these processes. Nevertheless, these studies support a central role for increased FGF23 levels in the pathogenesis of calcitriol deficiency in CKD in general. Indeed, in recipients of functioning allografts, hypophosphatemia and elevated PTH levels should be associated with maximal stimulation of 1α hydroxylase activity.

However, serum calcitriol levels increase to the normal range only after FGF23 levels decline.[45,46–48]

Systemic implications of increased levels of FGF23

While increased circulating FGF23 levels appear to modulate mineral metabolism similarly in patients with CKD as compared with those in individuals with normal kidney function,[43] systemic consequences of elevated FGF23 have been reported only in patients with CKD. Differences in FGF23 physiology in the context of renal failure are not entirely surprising; indeed, circulating levels may be hundreds- to thousands-fold higher in patients with renal failure as compared with those detected in individuals with normal kidney function.[42] In the CKD population, increased FGF23 levels have been associated with progression of renal disease, changes in parathyroid gland responsiveness, alterations in skeletal mineralization, and increased mortality rates.[1–3] Whether these associations reflect direct FGF23 toxicity or whether increased FGF23 serves as a sensitive biomarker of disordered phosphorus metabolism is unknown. Importantly, high FGF23 has been associated with toxicity in some tissues that do not express Klotho; thus, potential mechanisms through which FGF23 might mediate these changes in CKD require further study.

Progression of renal disease

In the early 1980s, a link between dietary phosphate intake in CKD patients and the rate of progression to renal failure was established[49] and more recent evidence suggests increased levels of FGF23—potentially reflecting chronically increased dietary phosphate loads—may also predict a more rapid deterioration of renal function. Consistent with prior reports,[43,44] in a cross-sectional evaluation of 227 non-diabetic adult patients with CKD stages 1–4, higher serum values for the Ca × P ion product, PTH, and FGF23 were observed with progressive CKD stages. In a subsequent 53-month longitudinal analysis of 177 patients from this cohort, older age, higher protein excretion rates, lower glomerular filtration rates, along with higher serum phosphorus, PTH, and FGF23 levels, were all associated with an increased rate of CKD progression—as defined by a doubling of serum creatinine or the need for renal replacement therapy during the follow-up period. However, in multivariable analysis, only baseline GFR and FGF23 were independent predictors of progression.[1] The etiology of the association between increased FGF23 and renal failure progression is incompletely understood, but may reflect some deleterious effect of phosphate itself, such as progressive tissue calcification or some, as yet uncharacterized, toxic effects of FGF23 on the renal parenchyma.

Parathyroid gland

The ability of serum FGF23 levels to suppress PTH secretion in animals with intact renal function[34,35] suggests a cross-talk between bone and parathyroids. The presence of CKD complicates this relationship; levels of PTH and FGF23 both become markedly elevated and end-organ 'resistance' to the actions of both hormones likely develops as renal function declines. In 2005, two studies reported an association between serum

FGF23 levels and the response of the parathyroid gland to vitamin D sterol and phosphate binder therapy, suggesting a continued, although altered, interaction between the parathyroid gland and skeleton in uremic patients. In two longitudinal studies of non-diabetic hemodialysis patients—one group of 103 subjects with base-line serum PTH levels <300pg/ml receiving 2 years of treatment and one group of 62 patients with PTH values >300pg/ml who received 24 weeks of medication—pre-treatment FGF23 levels predicted parathyroid response to therapy. Significantly higher baseline FGF23 values were present in patients with subsequent refractory secondary hyperparathyroidism—defined as final serum PTH levels greater than 300pg/ml or those needing a parathyroidectomy.[50,51] Whether FGF23 levels counter-act the suppressive effects of vitamin D therapy on the parathyroid gland or whether higher PTH values despite increased FGF23 levels identifies patients with refractory secondary hyperparathyroidism remains unknown.

Bone

The poor skeletal mineralization (rickets or osteomalacia) associated with primary increases in circulating FGF23 is mediated by low circulating levels of phosphate and vitamin D, which limit substrate for skeletal mineralization.[22] Defective skeletal min-eralization is also common in patients with end-stage renal disease, in whom increased circulating levels of FGF23 occur in the presence of normal or elevated serum phos-phorus values. However, the association between FGF23 and bone in this population differs greatly from that in the general population. A cross-sectional analysis of 49 pediatric dialysis patients with secondary hyperparathyroidism suggested that high circulating levels of FGF23 in these patients were associated with improved indices of skeletal mineralization.[3] Although these results contrast with findings in patients with normal kidney function, they are not unprecedented. Indeed, rodents who completely lack FGF23 display defects in skeletal mineralization, despite increased serum phos-phate, low PTH, and high $1,25(OH)_2$ vitamin D levels,[21,29] suggesting that some FGF23 expression may be necessary for proper skeletal mineralization. Mineralized bone is the primary source of FGF23[9] and FGF23 secretion appears to be locally regulated by some members of the small integrin-binding ligand N-linked glycopro-tein (SIBLING) family of proteins. Several of these proteins, including MEPE and dentrin matrix protein 1 (DMP1) are exclusively expressed in osteoblasts, osteocytes, and odontoblasts.[52] MEPE inhibits mineralization *in vitro*[53] and is associated with changes in FGF23 expression.[54,55] Loss of DMP1 expression or activity results in hypophosphatemia and osteomalacia due to increased FGF23 expression.[56] Other proteins, including PHEX[57,58] and NHERF1[59] have also been implicated in phosphate and FGF23 metabolism. How these and other proteins are expressed in bone, how their expression is altered by FGF23, and how this system is modified by the presence of CKD remains to be determined.

Mortality

The association between phosphate metabolism and mortality rates in both the gen-eral and CKD populations has been observed repeatedly during the past decade.[60–66]

Hyperphosphatemia is associated with soft-tissue and vascular calcifications,[64] and, at the molecular level, phosphate plays a major role in the genesis of these lesions.[65] Recently, FGF23 has also been associated with increased mortality. In a prospective, nested, case-control study of 400 adult patients new to dialysis, the greatest increases in baseline serum phosphate levels were modestly associated with an increased mortality rate during the first year of dialysis. However, concomitant levels of FGF23 were independently associated with future risk of death in a dose-dependent fashion. Furthermore, increased FGF23 was associated with increased risk of mortality in every quartile of serum phosphorus value except the highest and this included phosphate levels in the 'normal' range for dialysis patients.[2] This association between FGF23 and mortality was independent of serum phosphate levels, prior phosphate binder use, and follow-up treatment with active vitamin D, all of which have themselves been associated with improved survival in other studies.[67–70] While further studies are needed, these findings suggest that FGF23 may have physiological importance, independent of its traditional role in mineral metabolism, in affecting survival. Alternatively, FGF23 may be a superior biomarker of net phosphorus exposure than even serum phosphate itself.

Summary

FGF23 plays a central role in phosphorus metabolism. This role was initially delineated by the study of genetic and acquired conditions of hypophosphatemic rickets but the greatest clinical impact of the discovery of FGF23 may be in the management of CKD patients. In patients with CKD, FGF23 levels rise as renal function declines, likely due to decreasing capacity of the damaged kidney to excrete dietary phosphorus loads. Rising FGF23 levels appear to contribute to the initiation of secondary hyperparathyroidism in CKD patients; however, increased levels of FGF23 also appear to contribute to or serve as markers of accelerated progression to renal failure, increased rates of mortality, and alterations in skeletal mineralization. Collectively, these results suggest that the effects of FGF23 on end-organ function in the context of chronic kidney disease differ markedly from the physiology observed in individuals with normal renal function.

References

1. Fliser D, Kollerits B, Neyer U, et al. Fibroblast growth factor 23 (FGF23) predicts progression of chronic kidney disease: the Mild to Moderate Kidney Disease (MMKD) Study. *J Am Soc Nephrol* 2007;**18**:2600–8.
2. Gutierrez O, Mannstadt M, Isakova T, et al. Fibroblast growth factor 23 and mortality among patients undergoing hemodialysis. *N Engl J Med* 2008;**359**:584–92.
3. Wesseling-Perry K, Pereira RC, Wang H, et al. Relationship between plasma FGF23 concentration and bone mineralization in children with renal failure on peritoneal dialysis. *J Clin Endocrinol Metab* 2009;**94**:511–17.
4. Genbank. *Ref Type: Catalog*, 2009. http://www.ncbi.nlm.nih.gov/genbank/index.html
5. Online Mendelian Inheritance in Man. *Ref Type: Catalog*, 2009. http://www.ncbi.nlm.nih.gov/sites/entrez?ub=omim

6. Itoh N, Ornitz DM. Evolution of the FGF and FGFR gene families. *Trends Genet* 2004;**20**:563–9.

7. Ornitz DM, Itoh N. Fibroblast growth factors. *Genome Biol* 2001;**2**:REVIEWS3005.

8. Inagaki T, Choi M, Moschetta A, et al. Fibroblast growth factor 15 functions as an enterohepatic signal to regulate bile acid homeostasis. *Cell Metab* 2005;**2**:217–25.

9. Yoshiko Y, Wang H, Minamizaki T, et al. Mineralized tissue cells are a principal source of FGF23. *Bone* 2007;**40**:1565–73.

10. White KE, Carn G, Lorenz-Depiereux B, et-Pages A, Strom TM, Econs MJ. Autosomal-dominant hypophosphatemic rickets (ADHR) mutations stabilise FGF23. *Kidney Int* 2001;**60**:2079–86.

11. Shimada T, Muto T, Urakawa I, et al. Mutant FGF23 responsible for autosomal dominant hypophosphatemic rickets is resistant to proteolytic cleavage and causes hypophosphatemia *in vivo*. *Endocrinology* 2002;**143**:3179–82.

12. Yamashita T, Konishi M, Miyake A, Inui K, Itoh N. Fibroblast growth factor (FGF)-23 inhibits renal phosphate reabsorption by activation of the mitogen-activated protein kinase pathway. *J Biol Chem* 2002;**277**:28265–70.

13. Yu X, Ibrahimi OA, Goetz R, et al. Analysis of the biochemical mechanisms for the endocrine actions of fibroblast growth factor-23. *Endocrinology* 2005;**146**:4647–56.

14. Liu S, Vierthaler L, Tang W, Zhou J, Quarles LD. FGFR3 and FGFR4 do not mediate renal effects of FGF23. *J Am Soc Nephrol* 2008;**19**:2342–50.

15. Kuro-o M, Matsumura Y, Aizawa H, et al. Mutation of the mouse klotho gene leads to a syndrome resembling ageing. *Nature* 1997;**390**:45–51.

16. Kurosu H, Yamamoto M, Clark JD, et al. Suppression of aging in mice by the hormone Klotho. *Science* 2005;**309**:1829–33.

17. Imura A, Tsuji Y, Murata M, et al. alpha-Klotho as a regulator of calcium homeostasis. *Science* 2007;**316**:1615–18.

18. Kurosu H, Ogawa Y, Miyoshi M, et al. Regulation of fibroblast growth factor-23 signaling by klotho. *J Biol Chem* 2006;**281**:6120–3.

19. Urakawa I, Yamazaki Y, Shimada T, et al. Klotho converts canonical FGF receptor into a specific receptor for FGF23. *Nature* 2006;**444**:770–4.

20. Yoshida T, Fujimori T, Nabeshima Y. Mediation of unusually high concentrations of 1,25-dihydroxyvitamin D in homozygous klotho mutant mice by increased expression of renal 1alpha-hydroxylase gene. *Endocrinology* 2002;**143**:683–9.

21. Shimada T, Kakitani M, Yamazaki Y, et al. Targeted ablation of Fgf23 demonstrates an essential physiological role of FGF23 in phosphate and vitamin D metabolism. *J Clin Invest* 2004;**113**:561–8.

22. ADHR Consortium. Autosomal dominant hypophosphatemic rickets is associated with mutations in FGF23. *Nat Genet* 2000; **26**: 345-348

23. Shimada T, Mizutani S, Muto T, et al. Cloning and characterisation of FGF23 as a causative factor of tumor-induced osteomalacia. *Proc Natl Acad Sci USA* 2001;**98**: 6500–5.

24. Jonsson KB, Zahradnik R, Larsson T, et al. Fibroblast growth factor 23 in oncogenic osteomalacia and X-linked hypophosphatemia. *N Engl J Med* 2003;**348**:1656–63.

25. Yamazaki Y, Okazaki R, Shibata M, et al. Increased circulatory level of biologically active full-length FGF23 in patients with hypophosphatemic rickets/osteomalacia. *J Clin Endocrinol Metab* 2002;**87**:4957–60.

26. White KE, Jonsson KB, Carn G, et al. The autosomal dominant hypophosphatemic rickets (ADHR) gene is a secreted polypeptide overexpressed by tumors that cause phosphate wasting. *J Clin Endocrinol Metab* 2001;**86:**497–500

27. De Beur SM, Finnegan RB, Vassiliadis J, et al. Tumors associated with oncogenic osteomalacia express genes important in bone and mineral metabolism. *J Bone Miner Res* 2002;**17:**1102–10

28. Shimada T, Hasegawa H, Yamazaki Y, et al. FGF23 is a potent regulator of vitamin D metabolism and phosphate homeostasis. *J Bone Miner Res* 2004;**19:**429–35.

29. Sitara D, Razzaque MS, Hesse M, et al. Homozygous ablation of fibroblast growth factor-23 results in hyperphosphatemia and impaired skeletogenesis, and reverses hypophosphatemia in Phex-deficient mice. *Matrix Biol* 2004;**23:**421–32.

30. Kato K, Jeanneau C, Tarp MA, et al. Polypeptide GalNAc-transferase T3 and familial tumoral calcinosis. Secretion of fibroblast growth factor 23 requires O-glycosylation. *J Biol Chem* 2006;**281:**18370–7.

31. Araya K, Fukumoto S, Backenroth R, et al. A novel mutation in fibroblast growth factor 23 gene as a cause of tumoral calcinosis. *J Clin Endocrinol Metab* 2005;**90:**5523–7.

32. Benet-Pages A, Orlik P, Strom TM, Lorenz-Depiereux B. An FGF23 missense mutation causes familial tumoral calcinosis with hyperphosphatemia. *Hum Mol Genet* 2005;**14:** 385–90.

33. Larsson T, Yu X, Davis SI, et al. A novel recessive mutation in fibroblast growth factor-23 causes familial tumoral calcinosis. *J Clin Endocrinol Metab* 2005;**90:**2424–7.

34. Krajisnik T, Bjorklund P, Marsell R, et al. Fibroblast growth factor-23 regulates parathyroid hormone and 1alpha-hydroxylase expression in cultured bovine parathyroid cells. *J Endocrinol* 2007;**195:**125–31.

35. Ben-Dov IZ, Galitzer H, Lavi-Moshayoff V, et al. The parathyroid is a target organ for FGF23 in rats. *J Clin Invest* 2007;**117:**4003–8.

36. Barthel TK, Mathern DR, Whitfield GK, et al. 1,25-Dihydroxyvitamin D3/VDR-mediated induction of FGF23 as well as transcriptional control of other bone anabolic and catabolic genes that orchestrate the regulation of phosphate and calcium mineral metabolism. *J Steroid Biochem Mol Biol* 2007;**103:**381–8.

37. Yu X, Sabbagh Y, Davis SI, Demay MB, White KE. Genetic dissection of phosphate- and vitamin D-mediated regulation of circulating FGF23 concentrations. *Bone* 2005;**36:**971–7.

38. Antoniucci DM, Yamashita T, Portale AA. Dietary phosphorus regulates serum fibroblast growth factor-23 concentrations in healthy men. *J Clin Endocrinol Metab* 2006;**91:**3144–9.

39. Burnett SA, Gunawardene SC, Bringhurst FR, Juppner H, Lee H, Finkelstein JS. Regulation of C-terminal and intact FGF23 by dietary phosphate in men and women. *J Bone Miner Res* 2006;**21:**1187–96.

40. Isakova T, Gutierrez O, Shah A, et al. Postprandial mineral metabolism and secondary hyperparathyroidism in early CKD. *J Am Soc Nephrol* 2008;**19:**615–23.

41. Kawata T, Imanishi Y, Kobayashi K, et al. Parathyroid hormone regulates fibroblast growth factor-23 in a mouse model of primary hyperparathyroidism. *J Am Soc Nephrol* 2007;**18:**2683–8.

42. Larsson T, Nisbeth U, Ljunggren O, Juppner H, Jonsson KB. Circulating concentration of FGF23 increases as renal function declines in patients with chronic kidney disease, but does not change in response to variation in phosphate intake in healthy volunteers. *Kidney Int* 2003;**64:**2272–9.

43. Gutierrez O, Isakova T, Rhee E, et al. Fibroblast growth factor-23 mitigates hyperphosphatemia but accentuates calcitriol deficiency in chronic kidney disease. *J Am Soc Nephrol* 2005;**16**:2205–15.

44. Shigematsu T, Kazama JJ, Yamashita T, et al. Possible involvement of circulating fibroblast growth factor 23 in the development of secondary hyperparathyroidism associated with renal insufficiency. *Am J Kidney Dis* 2004;**44**:250–6.

45. Rosenbaum RW, Hruska KA, Korkor A, Anderson C, Slatopolsky E. Decreased phosphate reabsorption after renal transplantation: Evidence for a mechanism independent of calcium and parathyroid hormone. *Kidney Int* 1981;**19**:568–78.

46. Bhan I, Shah A, Holmes J, et al. Post-transplant hypophosphatemia: tertiary 'hyper-phosphatoninism'? *Kidney Int* 2006;**70**:1486–94.

47. Evenepoel P, Meijers BK, de JH, et al. Recovery of hyperphosphatoninism and renal phosphorus wasting one year after successful renal transplantation. *Clin J Am Soc Nephrol* 2008;**3**:1829–36.

48. Evenepoel P, Naesens M, Claes K, Kuypers D, Vanrenterghem Y. Tertiary 'hyperphosphatoninism' accentuates hypophosphatemia and suppresses calcitriol levels in renal transplant recipients. *Am J Transplant* 2007;**7**:1193–200.

49. Haut LL, Alfrey AC, Guggenheim S, Buddington B, Schrier N. Renal toxicity of phosphate in rats. *Kidney Int* 1980;**17**:722–31.

50. Kazama JJ, Sato F, Omori K, et al. Pretreatment serum FGF23 levels predict the efficacy of calcitriol therapy in dialysis patients. *Kidney Int* 2005;**67**:1120–5.

51. Nakanishi S, Kazama JJ, Nii-Kono T et al. Serum fibroblast growth factor-23 levels predict the future refractory hyperparathyroidism in dialysis patients. *Kidney Int* 2005;**67**:1171–8.

52. Petersen DN, Tkalcevic GT, Mansolf AL, Rivera-Gonzalez R, Brown TA. Identification of osteoblast/osteocyte factor 45 (OF45), a bone-specific cDNA encoding an RGD-containing protein that is highly expressed in osteoblasts and osteocytes. *J Biol Chem* 2000;**275**: 36172–80.

53. Rowe PS, Kumagai Y, Gutierrez G, et al. MEPE has the properties of an osteoblastic phosphatonin and minhibin. *Bone* 2004;**34**:303–19.

54. Liu S, Rowe PS, Vierthaler L, Zhou J, Quarles LD. Phosphorylated acidic serine-aspartate-rich MEPE-associated motif peptide from matrix extracellular phosphoglycoprotein inhibits phosphate regulating gene with homologies to endopeptidases on the X-chromosome enzyme activity. *J Endocrinol* 2007;**192**:261–7.

55. Rowe PS, Matsumoto N, Jo OD, et al. Correction of the mineralization defect in hyp mice treated with protease inhibitors CA074 and pepstatin. *Bone* 2006;**39**:773–86.

56. Feng JQ, Ward LM, Liu S, et al. Loss of DMP1 causes rickets and osteomalacia and identifies a role for osteocytes in mineral metabolism. *Nat Genet* 2006;**38**:1310–15.

57. Ichikawa S, Traxler EA, Estwick SA, et al. Mutational survey of the PHEX gene in patients with X-linked hypophosphatemic rickets. *Bone* 2008;**43**:663–6.

58. Addison WN, Nakano Y, Loisel T, Crine P, McKee MD. MEPE-ASARM peptides control extracellular matrix mineralization by binding to hydroxyapatite: an inhibition regulated by PHEX cleavage of ASARM. *J Bone Miner Res* 2008;**23**:1638–49.

59. Karim Z, Gerard B, Bakouh N, et al. NHERF1 mutations and responsiveness of renal parathyroid hormone. *N Engl J Med* 2008;**359**:1128–35.

60. Goodman WG, Goldin J, Kuizon BD, et al. Coronary-artery calcification in young adults with end-stage renal disease who are undergoing dialysis. *N Engl J Med* 2000;**342**:1478–83.

61. K/DOQI clinical practice guidelines for bone metabolism and disease in children with chronic kidney disease. *Am J Kidney Dis* 2005;**46:**S1–121.

62. Block GA, Spiegel DM, Ehrlich J, et al. Effects of sevelamer and calcium on coronary artery calcification in patients new to hemodialysis. *Kidney Int* 2005;**68:**1815–24

63. Block GA, Raggi P, Bellasi A, Kooienga L, Spiegel DM. Mortality effect of coronary calcification and phosphate binder choice in incident hemodialysis patients. *Kidney Int* 2007;**71:**438–41.

64. Ibels LS, Alfrey AC, Huffer WE, Craswell PW, Anderson JT, Weil R, III. Arterial calcification and pathology in uremic patients undergoing dialysis. *Am J Med* 1979;**66:** 790–6.

65. Giachelli CM, Jono S, Shioi A, Nishizawa Y, Mori K, Morii H. Vascular calcification and inorganic phosphate. *Am J Kidney Dis* 2001;**38:**S34–7.

66. Block GA, Hulbert-Shearon TE, Levin NW, Port FK. Association of serum phosphorus and calcium x phosphate product with mortality risk in chronic hemodialysis patients: a national study. *Am J Kidney Dis* 1998;**31:**607–17.

67. Teng M, Wolf M, Ofsthun MN, et al. Activated injectable vitamin D and hemodialysis survival: a historical cohort study. *J Am Soc Nephrol* 2005;**16:**1115–25.

68. Teng M, Wolf M, Lowrie E, Ofsthun N, Lazarus JM, Thadhani R. Survival of patients undergoing hemodialysis with paricalcitol or calcitriol therapy. *N Engl J Med* 2003;**349:**446–56.

69. Tentori F, Hunt WC, Stidley CA, et al. Mortality risk among hemodialysis patients receiving different vitamin D analogs. *Kidney Int* 2006;**70:**1858–65.

70. Isakova T, Gutierrez OM, Chang Y, et al. Phosphorus binders and survival on hemodialysis. *J Am Soc Nephrol* 2009;**20:**388–96.

Chapter 25

New vitamin D analogs for chronic kidney disease patients

Adriana Dusso, Masanori Tokumoto, Alex J. Brown, and Eduardo Slatopolsky

Introduction

Secondary hyperparathyroidism (2HPT) is a common and serious complication of chronic kidney disease (CKD). Calcitriol (1,25-dihydroxyvitamin D, the hormonal form of vitamin D) deficiency, phosphate retention, and hypocalcemia, all resulting from the progressive decrease in kidney function, are the main contributors to enhanced parathyroid cell growth and elevations in serum parathyroid hormone (PTH). Calcitriol replacement therapy has proven effective in treating 2HPT, but is often limited by hypercalcemia and hyperphosphatemia, which spurred the development and implementation of analogs with wider therapeutic windows. Subsequent observational studies in hemodialysis patients revealed that the analogs conferred a greater survival benefit than calcitriol, and that mortality was highest in patient not receiving any vitamin D therapy. The survival benefits of calcitriol and its less calcemic analogs can be only partially accounted for by their efficacy in suppressing 2HPT; they appear to involve active vitamin D protection from renal and cardiovascular damage. This chapter presents the evidence, gained from animal models of kidney disease and from clinical trials, for the efficacy of the analogs available to treat 2HPT in protecting parathyroid, renal, and cardiovascular function, as well as the current limited understanding of the mechanisms for their selective properties, with the goal of providing solid bases to expedite the design of the pre-clinical studies and prospective trials required to improve outcomes from vitamin D (analog) interventions in early and advanced CKD.

In patients with CKD, the development of 2HPT can be attributed to phosphate retention, progressive reduction in the synthesis of calcitriol and the resulting hypocalcemia. This common and serious disorder is characterized by parathroid hyperplasia and elevations in serum levels of PTH. High serum PTH causes disturbances in mineral and bone metabolism, which are responsible for the decreased quality of life, extra-skeletal calcifications, and markedly increased cardiovascular mortality (reviewed in ref. 1 and summarized in Fig. 25.1). The low serum calcitriol levels increase PTH indirectly via a reduction in intestinal calcium absorption and also directly through the loss of a direct transcriptional repression of the PTH gene.[2] Phosphate retention aggravates both 2HPT and calcitriol deficiency in CKD.

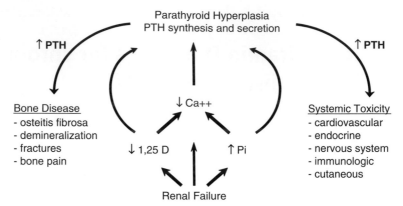

Fig. 25.1 The pathogenesis of secondary hyperparathyroidism in chronic kidney disease and the role of vitamin D therapy. Loss of renal function leads to phosphate (Pi) retention and a decrease in serum 1,25(OH)$_2$D$_3$ (1,25D), both of which reduce serum calcium levels. Hypocalcemia stimulates the PTH synthesis and secretion and, eventually, parathyroid gland hyperplasia. The effects of hyperparathyroidism on bone and other tissues are listed.

Hyperphosphatemia can stimulate parathyroid hyperplasia and PTH secretion directly,[3] and also indirectly by either reducing ionized calcium or by inducing serum levels of the phosphatonin, fibroblast growth factor 23 (FGF23).[4] FGF23 further reduces serum calcitriol through dual mechanisms, inhibition of the already defective renal calcitriol synthesis[5] and enhancement of serum calcitriol degradation through the induction of 24-hydroxylase,[6] the enzyme responsible for calcitriol inactivation.

The efficacy of calcitriol to induce intestinal calcium absorption and to suppress parathyroid cell growth and PTH gene transcription led to its successful use for the treatment of 2HPT for more than two decades in the United States.[2] However, in advanced kidney disease, the severity of parathyroid hyperplasia markedly reduces the efficacy of calcitriol therapy in suppressing parathyroid cell growth and serum PTH through a reduction in parathyroid levels of the vitamin D receptor (VDR) and the calcium sensing receptor. The calcitriol dose escalation required to effectively suppress serum PTH is limited by the development of hypercalcemia and hyperphosphatemia, secondary to increases in intestinal absorption and bone mobilization of calcium and phosphate.[2] The hypercalcemic toxicity of calcitriol is further aggravated by the concomitant use of large doses of calcium-containing phosphate-binders. Hypercalcemia predisposes to extra-osseous calcifications per se, and also through PTH over-suppression causing adynamic bone disease.[7] To minimize the toxicities of calcitriol therapy, structural modifications in the calcitriol molecule led to the development of pro-hormone and calcitriol analogs that retain the capacity to suppress parathyroid function, both PTH synthesis and parathyroid cell growth, with lesser effects on kidney and bone.[8] Section 2 of this chapter presents the relative potencies of a pro-hormone and three calcitriol analogs in the control of 2HPT and in mitigating the abnormalities in mineral and bone disease. Section 3 summarizes the current understanding and the unknowns on the biological and physiological bases for the selective actions of vitamin D analogs for 2HPT.

The improvements in biochemical markers of mineral and bone disease achieved with analog therapy were strongly supported by several retrospective studies in dialysis patients demonstrating that analog usage was associated with a reduced mortality.[9,10] However, the results from a large historical cohort[11] demonstrated not only that calcitriol dosage also conferred a survival advantage compared with non-users of any active vitamin D therapy, but more intriguingly, that the favorable outcome in these patients could only partly be attributed to improvements in the control of 2HPT. The identification of important renal and cardiovascular protective actions of active vitamin D therapy as the main contributors to the favorable outcomes have suggested the potential benefits of either intervening earlier in the course of kidney disease, or of extending vitamin D therapy regardless of serum PTH, calcium, and phosphate levels in advanced kidney disease. However, recent meta-analysis on the survival advantage of active vitamin D therapy has both questioned[12] and confirmed[13] the results from these trials, raising valid concerns as to whether the available level of evidence is sufficient to change current clinical practice. The last section of this chapter analyses the available evidence on the safety and efficacy of the renal and cardioprotective actions of vitamin D therapy obtained exclusively from *in vivo* studies in experimental models of kidney disease and clinical trials, which can help expedite the implementation of safe vitamin D interventions that maximize favorable outcomes in attenuating the progression of renal and cardiovascular damage in the course of kidney disease.

Pro-hormone and vitamin D analogs for secondary hyperparathyroidism

This section presents an update on the structure-function properties for two pro-hormones and three analogs currently in use for the treatment of 2HPT in CKD patients. These compounds were initially selected for their high VDR affinity, their lower calcemic activity in normal rats, and their efficacy in suppressing PTH *in vitro* in cultured parathyroid cells. Fig. 25.2 shows the structures of vitamin D_2 and vitamin D_3, along with the numbering of the carbon atoms, in order to provide a reference for the structural modifications in the analogs that will be described below (see Fig. 25.3). Special focus is directed to the contribution of these structural changes to the differences in potency and selectivity reported in preclinical (the rat model of kidney disease) studies and clinical trials. Please see the comprehensive reviews by Brown et al.[8,14]

1α-hydroxyvitamin D_3 and 1α-hydroxyvitamin D_2

1α-hydroxyvitamin D_3 (1α-D_3) and 1α-hydroxyvitamin D_2 (1α-D_2, doxercalciferol) are pro-hormones that require the hydroxylation of the carbon 25 in the liver to become active 1,25-dihydroxyvitamin $D_{2/3}$.

1α-D_3 was produced by Leo Pharma in 1973, and become available in Europe for oral and intravenous formulations in the middle 1980s. A comprehensive recent review by Brandi[15] provides an update on relative efficacy of different 1α-D_3 regimens

Vitamin D_2 Vitamin D_3

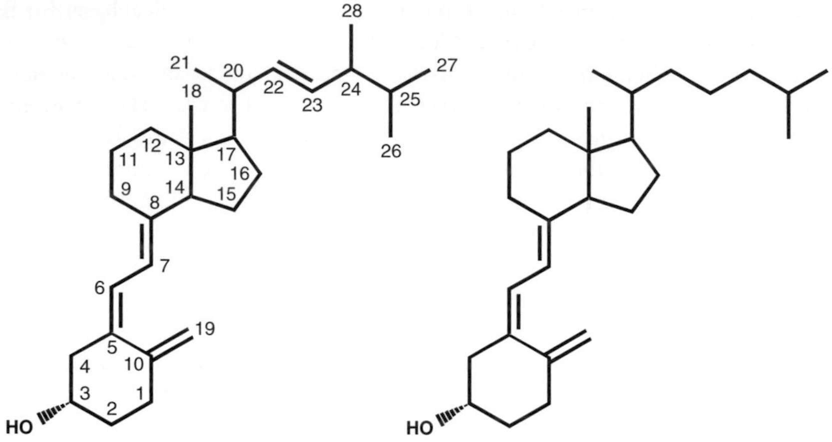

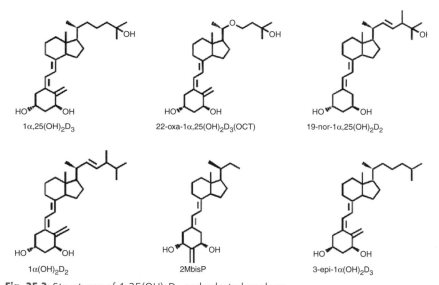

Fig. 25.2 Structures of vitamin D_2 and vitamin D_3. The structures of vitamins D_2 and D_3 are shown with the carbon atoms numbered to provide a reference for the vitamin D analogs presented in this review.

Fig. 25.3 Structures of 1,25$(OH)_2D_3$ and selected analogs.

compared with calcitriol that could improve the prophylaxis and treatment of 2HPT. Briefly, intermittent intravenous 1α-D_3 combined with low calcium in the hemodialysis fluid effectively prevented the development of 2HPT in patients with normal parathyroid function, moderated its progression in those with established 2HPT, and also reduced the loss of bone mineral content. Single doses of 10μg of 1α-D_3 effectively

suppressed serum PTH. Its efficacy, however, was 3 times lower than that of the same dose of calcitriol, a difference attributable to the differential increase in serum calcium. Upon PTH reduction, intermittent dosage with 1α-D3 is sufficient to maintain serum PTH levels. The potential of the oral formulation to mimic intermittent intravenous dosage has not been explored.

In experimental animals, 1α-D_2 is less toxic than 1α-D_3 counterpart in spite of causing a similar stimulation of calcium and phosphate transport. The mechanisms for the selective actions of 1α-D_2 over calcitriol are unclear, but could involve the conversion of high levels of 1α-D_2 to 1,24-dihydroxyvitaminD$_2$, a compound with lower calcemic activity than calcitriol.

Oral and intravenous 1α-D_2 formulations have been effectively used to treat 2HPT.[16,17] In an initial 12-week trial, Tan and collaborators[18] showed that 21 of 24 hemodialysis patients with moderate to severe 2HPT receiving oral $1\alpha(OH)D_2$, daily or thrice weekly, reached the target range for PTH of 130–250pg/mL. However, although serum calcium rose within the normal range (from 8.8 to 9.5mg/dL), and serum phosphate levels remained unchanged, $1\alpha D_2$ treatment caused 13 episodes of hypercalcemia (Ca > 10.5mg/dL) and 30 episodes of hyperphosphatemia (p > 6.9mg/dL). Importantly, the comparison of the number of hyperphosphatemic episodes in 100 weeks between treatment (10.1) and washout (6.9) periods rendered no statistical difference. In a larger open-label study of 99 patients, 82 attained the 150–300pg/mL target goal for PTH,[19] with modest increases in serum calcium (0.7mg/dL) and phosphorus (0.8mg/dL). In the US, oral $1\alpha(OH)D_2$ was approved in 1999 under the brand name Hectorol® (Genzyme, Cambridge, MA). This formulation was effective in reducing PTH levels by 45% in predialysis patients with mild increments in serum calcium (0.44mg/dL), phosphorus (0.25mg/dL), Ca × P product (4.1mg^2/dL^2) and urinary calcium (11.0mg/24h).[20] Intravenous $1\alpha(OH)D_2$ was approved following a trial demonstrating a similar efficacy in the rate and degree of PTH suppression to that of the oral formulation, but causing milder increases in serum calcium and phosphate levels, and fewer hypercalcemic and hyperphosphatemic episodes.[16]

Falecalcitriol

Falecalcitriol [1,25(OH)$_2$-26,27-F$_6$-D$_3$] results from the substitution of fluorine atoms for the hydrogen atoms on carbons 26 and 27, which causes a slower metabolic inactivation. Its 23-hydroxylated metabolite is resistant to further metabolism and also retains high activity. In rats, active 23-hydroxylated falecalcitriol accumulates in the parathyroid glands, but also in the intestine and the kidney, which raised concerns as to whether falecalcitriol would have the wider therapeutic window required to treat advanced human 2HPT. However, two relatively small clinical trials in dialysis patients reported the efficacy of oral falecalcitriol. In 43 dialysis patients for 12 weeks, with dose-adjustments to avoid hypercalcemia, falecalcitriol reduced PTH by 25% with minimal changes in serum calcium (0.30mg/dL).[21] Also, falecalcitriol elicited greater activity compared with alphacalcidol (1α-D_3) in suppressing PTH in patients with moderate to severe 2HPT.[22] Importantly, although serum calcium was similar in patients treated with either compound, the control of serum phosphorus was better with falecalcitriol treatment.[22] Oral falecalcitriol is available in Japan under the brand names Hornel® (Taisho Pharmaceutical Co.) and Fulstan® (Kissei Pharmaceutical Co.).

22-oxacalcitriol

22-oxacalcitriol (OCT), differs from calcitriol in the substitution of an oxygen atom for carbon 22. This structural modification reduces OCT's affinity for two key proteins of the vitamin D endocrine system: the vitamin D receptor (VDR), essential for analog/calcitriol actions, and for the vitamin D binding protein (VDBP), the serum carrier of vitamin D metabolites. The reduced affinity of OCT for VDBP results in a faster clearance of the analog from the circulation compared with calcitriol. Cell-specific degradation rates of intracellular OCT contribute to the prolonged suppression of PTH secretion, but short-lived calcemic effects on intestine and bone that occur upon OCT administration to experimental animals. OCT selectivity in regulating the rate of transcription of vitamin D responsive genes could also be accounted for by a differential recruitment of co-activator molecules to the transcription initiation complex by the VDR bound to OCT compared with the calcitriol/VDR complex, as shown *in vitro* for OCT suppression of the expression of the PTH gene. Indeed, in animal models of kidney disease, OCT is slightly less active than calcitriol in suppressing PTH, but its much lower calcemic activity creates a wider therapeutic window to effectively reverse abnormalities in bone turnover without impairment of bone formation.

Clinical trials in hemodialysis patients confirmed that OCT effectively reduces serum PTH levels.[23–27] The targeted 30% reduction in serum PTH was attained in 51% of the patients in a 1-year protocol,[24] as well as in 44%[25] and 77%[26] of the patients treated for 12 weeks. As expected, a higher frequency of hypercalcemia was reported for the higher doses of OCT that were more effective in suppressing serum PTH.[26] However, comparison of the efficacy of intravenous OCT (thrice weekly) and oral calcitriol (twice weekly) to treat 2HPT over 24 weeks, using dose adjustments to minimize hypercalcemia, yielded similar results not only in the decreases in serum PTH levels (35%), but also in the increases in serum calcium levels (0.7–0.8mg/dL) and in the number of episodes of elevated Ca × P product.[23] A larger 1-year study comparing intravenous (IV) OCT to IV calcitriol also found equivalent reductions in PTH (40%) and similar increases in calcium, phosphate and Ca × P product within their normal ranges.[27] Importantly, a more recent study reporting similar findings in the control of serum PTH, calcium and phosphate, also demonstrated a higher efficacy of OCT compared with calcitriol in reducing markers of bone turnover.[28] OCT (maxacalcitol) is now available in Japan for CKD patients with 2HPT under the brand name Oxarol® (Chugai Pharmvaceuticals).

Paricalcitol

Paricalcitol (19-nor 1,25-dihydroxyvitamin D2) differs from calcitriol in that it has a vitamin D2 side chain and lacks the exocyclic carbon 19. In the rat model of kidney disease, paricalcitol is 10 times less active than calcitriol in mobilizing calcium from bone and in absorbing calcium and phosphate from the gastrointestinal tract while 3 or 4 times less effective in suppressing serum PTH and parathyroid hyperplasia. Paricalcitol inhibits parathyroid hyperplasia in the absence of hypercalcemia through mechanisms that include the induction of the cell cycle inhibitor p21 and the suppression of transforming growth factor α and its receptor, the epidermal growth factor receptor, in parathyroid cells. In uremic rats, the effective control of serum PTH by paricalcitol can prevent and/or reverse the high turnover bone disease without compromising bone formation.[29] Furthermore, although high doses of paricalcitol can increase Ca × P product, leading to vascular calcification, several studies found dramatically less calcification with paricalcitol than with calcitriol or $1\alpha D_2$. The mechanisms for the differential effects on vascular calcification require further investigation, as *in vitro* studies in smooth muscle cell culture have suggested both direct and indirect similar actions of the analogs.

Paricalcitol is also approximately 10 times less calcemic and phosphatemic than $1\alpha D_2$ in normal and uremic rats, as determined by Slatopolsky and collaborators. The mechanisms responsible for paricalcitol selectivity are unknown at present.

Paricalcitol was approved to treat 2HPT in 1998, and is marketed by Abbott Laboratories (Chicago, IL) under the brand name Zemplar. Clinical studies found that paricalcitol effectively reduced PTH with very few hypercalcemic events (2 versus 1% in placebo controls).[30,31] Dose equivalency indicated that paricalcitol was approximately 3 times less potent than calcitriol,[31] and although paricalcitol has less calcemic activity than calcitriol, mild hypercalcemia can occur during therapy. Hypercalcemic episodes were associated with over-treating as suggested by PTH suppression below the desired target range.[32] The widespread use of intravenous paricalcitol in the US has allowed the comparison of the efficacy of therapy with this analog and calcitriol. Studies in hemodialysis patients with end-stage renal disease and in a low calcium diet demonstrated that 8 times more paricalcitol than calcitriol was required to achieve a similar increment in serum calcium, possibly mobilized from bone.[33] Less severe hyperphosphatemia occurred in patients treated with paricalcitol compared with those receiving calcitriol.[34] A double-blind study with 263 dialysis patients randomly chosen to receive paricalcitol or calcitriol in a dose-escalating fashion found that patients receiving paricalcitol reached the target reduction in PTH (–50%) more rapidly, had a lower mean PTH at the end of the 32-week study, and had fewer sustained episodes of hypercalcemia (serum calcium level > 11.5mg/dL) or elevated Ca × P product ($>70mg^2/dL^2$).[35] In CKD patients, paricalcitol was estimated to have 57% of the potency of $1\alpha-D_2$ in suppressing PTH,[36] but to be 10 times less potent in mobilizing bone calcium in patients fed a very low-calcium diet.[37] Their relative potencies for the stimulation of intestinal calcium transport in humans have not been reported. Taken together, these clinical data would predict a wider therapeutic window for paricalcitol, but direct comparison in a controlled trial is clearly warranted.

In 2005, an oral paricalcitol formulation was approved for predialysis patients, following the demonstration of its efficacy in reducing PTH by 45%, with very mild average increases in serum calcium (0.14mg/dL), serum phosphorus (0.18mg/dL), and urinary calcium (2.4mg/24h).[38]

Other potential new analogs for 2HPT

The efforts to generate vitamin D analogs with wider therapeutic windows for 2HPT continue, and several of these new molecules were proven effective in the rat model of kidney disease. $1,25(OH)_2$-dihydrotachysterol elicits the same potency of OCT in suppressing PTH levels, with no increase in serum calcium. Similarly, the 20-epi analogs synthesized by Leo Pharmaceuticals (CB1093, EB1213 and GS1725) effectively suppress serum PTH by 60–80% in uremic rats with minimal calcemic activity. Also, $1,25(OH)_2$-16-ene,23-yne-D_3, which is as effective as calcitriol in suppressing PTH levels in uremic rats, is much less calcemic resulting in a lower Ca × P product, thereby providing a wider therapeutic window compared with calcitriol to treat 2HPT. $1\alpha(OH)$-3-epi-D_3, an analog of alfacalcidol with inverted stereochemistry at carbon 3, is a potent suppressor of PTH levels in uremic rats but with much less calcemic activity than calcitriol or alfacalcidol. Most recently, (20S)-1α-hydroxy-2-methylene-19-nor-bishomopregnacalciferol (2MbisP) was found to be very selective, with potent suppression of PTH levels and no calcemic activity in normal rats or in uremic rats with 2HPT.

In summary, vitamin D analogs elicit a similar or higher potency compared with calcitriol in suppressing serum PTH, while having a better side effect profile of fewer episodes of sustained elevations in calcium and phosphate, which contributes in part to the association between analog usage and reduced mortality in hemodialysis patients. The section below summarizes the current understanding of the mechanisms underlying the selective actions of vitamin D analogs for 2HPT (see Summary in Fig. 25.4).

Analog selectivity: implications for therapy in CKD

The relative potency of vitamin D analogs to exert their biological actions is the net result of the interactions of these compounds with three critical proteins of the vitamin D endocrine system: the VDR, the serum vitamin D binding protein (VDBP), and the vitamin D-24-hydroxylase (and perhaps other metabolizing enzymes). In *in vitro* and *ex-vivo* assays, analog function is also modified by interactions with the membrane receptor(s) that mediate the rapid actions of vitamin D compounds, and with intracellular binding proteins that can facilitate both analog metabolism and VDR activation. The physiological relevance of analog interactions with either the membrane receptor(s) or with intracellular vitamin D binding proteins remains incompletely characterized. This section presents the current understanding on how specific structural modifications affect the interaction of the vitamin D analog with each of these proteins, ultimately determining its biological activity in a cell and gene specific manner (please see the comprehensive reviews by Brown et al[8,14]).

Vitamin D receptor binding and activation

Most biological actions of vitamin D compounds are mediated by the VDR, a member of the nuclear receptor superfamily of transcriptional regulators. Upon calcitriol/analog binding, the VDR undergoes a conformational change that allows interactions with several other macromolecules within the cell, ultimately altering the rate of transcription of target genes.[2] Thus, a fundamental requirement of therapeutically useful vitamin D analogs is that they retain a significant VDR affinity. The key structural

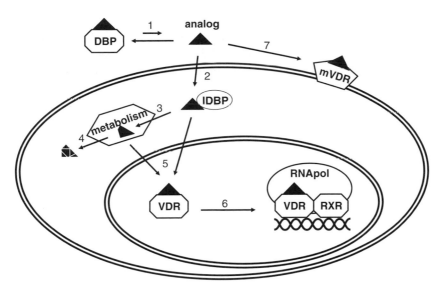

Fig. 25.4 Potential sites of differential actions of 1,25(OH)$_2$D$_3$ and its analogs. The possible steps in the vitamin D activation pathways at which differences in vitamin D analog action could lead to selective activities *in vivo* are shown. The steps diagrammed include: (1) binding to the serum vitamin D binding protein (VDBP); (2) cellular uptake; (3) interaction with intracellular vitamin D binding proteins (IDBPs); (4) mitochondrial conversion to active metabolites or catabolic inactivation; (5) interaction with the nuclear vitamin D receptor (VDR); (6) inducing a conformational change that promotes interaction with the retinoid × receptor (RXR), DNA and co-modulators that regulate gene transcription; and (7) activation of the non-genomic pathway through a putative membrane vitamin D receptor (mVDR).

portion of the vitamin D compound for VDR binding is the A-ring containing the 1α-hydroxyl group, although other groups can be substituted at this position with retention of activity. Other portions of the molecule, such as the side chain, can be greatly modified with minimal effect on VDR binding affinity. However, while high VDR affinity is important, the selective actions of a vitamin D compound at the cell or gene level may also result from the induction of unique conformational changes in the VDR molecule that largely affects VDR function, as demonstrated by the higher activity of the 20-epi analogs compared with calcitriol in spite of their lower VDR affinities. Not only does the VDR bound to 20-epi analogs undergo an *in vitro* proteolytic fragmentation that is different from that of calcitriol-bound VDR,[39] suggesting a differential binding or VDR conformation, but, more significant physiologically, VDR activated with 20-epi analogs forms tighter complexes with retinoid X receptor (RXR), the heterodimer partner of the VDR required for transcriptional regulation. Furthermore, crystal structure analysis of the ligand binding domain of the VDR and in silico modeling of the VDR have confirmed that both the VDR ligand binding pocket and the analogs can adapt to each other, leading to slight differences in the three dimensional VDR conformation, which in turn influence analog-VDR interactions with co-activators and co-repressors required for VDR regulation of the transcription of target genes. In fact, the differential recruitment of co-regulators (activators/repressors) by analog-bound versus $1,25(OH)_2D_3$-bound VDR already described for OCT also occurs with 20-epi analogs. Cell-specific differences in the content of VDR co-activator and co-repressor molecules could contribute to analog selectivity. Furthermore, the ratio of co-activators to co-repressors in a cell can trigger a cell-specific switch of the analog function from VDR agonist to VDR antagonist.

This brief sampling of the varied interactions of vitamin D analogs with the VDR suggest the tremendous potential of further modifications to achieve selectivity at the cellular and perhaps target gene level.

Interaction with the serum vitamin D binding protein

VDBP is the major carrier of natural vitamin D compounds in the circulation. Other proteins such as albumin and lipoproteins can also bind vitamin D compounds, but with lower affinity. In the case of calcitriol, over 99% is protein bound in plasma, mostly to VDBP. The structural elements of vitamin D compounds that affect VDBP binding are different from those determining VDR affinity. Whereas the 1α-hydroxyl group is not required for VDBP binding, side chain modifications tend to greatly alter the association of the analog with VDBP. Higher VDBP binding enhances calcitriol (analog) circulating half-life and decreases its accessibility to target tissues. Therefore, VDBP acts as a reservoir for vitamin D metabolites and guards against vitamin D intoxication. Most analogs are modified in the side chain, which typically reduces their interaction with serum VDBP, causing the analog to be either poorly absorbed into the circulation or rapidly cleared, which greatly influences the activity of vitamin D analogs. OCT is the most studied example of an analog that exerts its selectivity primarily through VDBP-modulated pharmacokinetics. The affinity of OCT for VDBP is about 500 times lower than that of calcitriol. Consequently, upon OCT or calcitriol injection, OCT is cleared more rapidly from the circulation rendering lower serum peak levels compared with calcitriol. In spite of lower peak levels of OCT than calcitriol in the blood, the peak levels of the analog in target tissues, including intestine and the parathyroid glands, are greater than those of calcitriol, but fall quickly after OCT clearance from the circulation. This 'pulse' of OCT in the intestine causes only a transient increase in calcium transport which falls to basal levels soon after OCT disappears from the circulation. In contrast, calcitriol, which is cleared more slowly, produces a prolonged increase in calcium transport. The effects of OCT on bone calcium mobilization were also short-lived compared with those of calcitriol. In contrast to its transient calcemic actions, OCT treatment caused a more prolonged effect on serum PTH levels and PTH mRNA in animal models of hyperparathyroidism. The molecular basis for the short duration of the calcemic responses to OCT in intestine and bone is unclear, but could involve the induction of short-lived proteins. Alternatively, these transient responses could result from the cessation of stimulation of non-genomic pathways as will be discussed below.

Low VDBP binding and rapid clearance from circulation may contribute to the selectivity of 2MbisP in controlling 2HPT. The low calcemic activity of paricalcitol cannot be attributed to its VDBP affinity and pharmacokinetics, as they are similar to those of calcitriol.

Differential metabolism

The metabolic activation or inactivation of vitamin D compounds by target cells plays an important role in analog selectivity. As discussed above, the prodrugs $1\alpha(OH)D_3$ and $1\alpha(OH)D_2$ require hydroxylation of carbon 25 (or carbon 24) in order to bind the VDR with high affinity. These prodrugs are efficiently 25-hydroxylated by the liver yielding the activated compounds 1,25-dihydroxyvitamin D_2 and 1,25-dihydroxy vitamin D_3 in the circulation. However, because the prodrugs do not bind well, if at all to VDBP, they can also be rapidly taken up by peripheral tissues other than the liver. Therefore, cell specific differences in pro-drug activation by 25-hydroxylation in vitamin D responsive targets may also contribute to analog selectivity.

Conversely, cell specific induction of catabolic pathways attenuates the activity of vitamin D compounds. The most important inactivation pathway is the side chain oxidation and cleavage catalyzed by the 24-hydroxylase, an enzyme highly induced by calcitriol (and its analogs) through direct VDR-mediated enhancement of 24-hydroxylase gene transcription. In fact, the biological efficacy of calcitriol or its less calcemic analogs can be easily enhanced if 24-hydroxylase is chemically inhibited or epigenetically silenced. Because the side chain is the most common site of modification of the existing vitamin D analogs, differences in the rates of metabolism, and in the activity of end-products can contribute to analog selectivity. Analogs that are more rapidly catabolized will have lower intracellular levels to activate the VDR compared with more slowly catabolized compounds, as clearly demonstrated for the distinct antiproliferative properties of calcitriol analogs using ketoconazole, a cytochrome P450 inhibitor that blocks 24-hydroxylase activity. The explanation for this cell-specific induction of 24-hydroxylase and analog (calcitriol) degradation is unclear, and certainly deserves further study since exploitation of the catabolic differences between vitamin D compounds could produce highly selective therapeutic agents. In addition, target cell catabolism can also convert some analogs into active metabolites that accumulate in the cell, as shown for $1,25(OH)_2$-16-ene-D_3, and 20-epi-$1,25(OH)_2D_3$.

In view of the importance of 'autocrine/paracrine' actions by locally produced calcitriol, rather than its serum levels in the protection of parathyroid, renal and cardiovascular function,[40,41] the differential cell-specific induction of 24-hydroxylase by calcitriol analogs has important implications for therapy. Increases in 24-hydroxylase activity will not only impact the half-life of the analog in a cell-specific manner, but also the degradation of 25-hydroxyvitamin D, thereby compromising local calcitriol synthesis for autocrine/paracrine actions. This is not mere speculation as OCT administration causes a rapid disappearance of calcitriol from the circulation.[42]

Rapid actions mediated by a cell-surface receptor

In addition to VDR activation to control gene transcription, calcitriol can act at the cell membrane to elicit rapid, apparently non-genomic, responses in target cells (reviewed in reference 2). These rapid actions include vesicular calcium absorption in the intestine, activation of mitogen-activated protein kinases (MAPK) pathways, phosphoinositide signaling and changes in cytosolic calcium, as well as many others. It has also been suggested that the rapid actions of calcitriol could affect genomic actions through the activation of kinase pathways that alter the phosphorylation state and transcriptional activity of either the VDR or of co-regulators of VDR gene transcription. The identity of receptors that mediate the rapid actions is still debated. Current evidence indicates roles for membrane-localized VDR[43] and for a distinct protein designated the MARRS (Membrane-Associated Rapid Response Steroid binding) receptor.[44] The ligand specificity for the rapid actions is distinct from that for regulation of gene transcription. In silico modeling data for the VDR suggests the existence of a second ligand binding pocket on the VDR that may accommodate the 'rapid action' ligands.[43] The predicted transient nature of the ligand interaction with this site prevents typical binding studies.

The relevance of the non-genomic actions of calcitriol in most cell types is still not fully understood. In the intestine, it is well established that exposure of the basolateral membrane to calcitriol stimulates calcium movement from the lumen to the bloodstream, a process called transcaltachia, and rapidly stimulates phosphate uptake into isolated enterocytes. In adult rat cardiomyocytes non-genomic calcitriol actions regulate contractile function,[45] and in endothelial cells, where a reduction in calcium influx regulates vascular tone, they cause a decrease in the synthesis of endothelium-derived contracting factors.[46] Although the role of these rapid response pathways remains controversial, it may explain some of the differential effects of vitamin D analogs. Considering the unique ligand specificity for the rapid responses, this pathway is a potential target for analog design.

Intracellular vitamin D binding proteins

Intracellular binding proteins such as Hsc-70 and Bag-1 can bind vitamin D compounds with high affinity and influence their metabolism and activity. These intracellular vitamin D binding proteins (IDBPs) are relatively ubiquitous and likely play a role in modulating the endocrine and autocrine/paracrine actions of vitamin D compounds. The natural vitamin D metabolites have high affinity for HSC-70, which prefers 25-hydroxyvitamin D_3 over calcitriol. However, several analogs with modified side chains (calcipotriol, EB1089 and KH1060) have no detectable IDBP affinity. The contribution of IDBP affinity to the selectivity of other vitamin D analogs remains unknown.

Additional important consideration for analog actions

Renal calcitriol production is also central to maintain the normal phosphate/calcitriol/FGF23-klotho axis (See summary in Fig. 25.5) required to preventing the excesses in serum P predisposing to ectopic calcification.[47] FGF23 appears to exert an anabolic effect on bone that is independent of serum phosphate.[48] A similar osteomalacic phenotype (i.e. less bone mineralization) occurs in FGF23 (–/–) mice and in the double FGF23(–/–)/NaPi2a (–/–) mice in spite of opposing serum P levels. The contribution of calcitriol (analog) induction of FGF23 to bone anabolism is unknown at present.

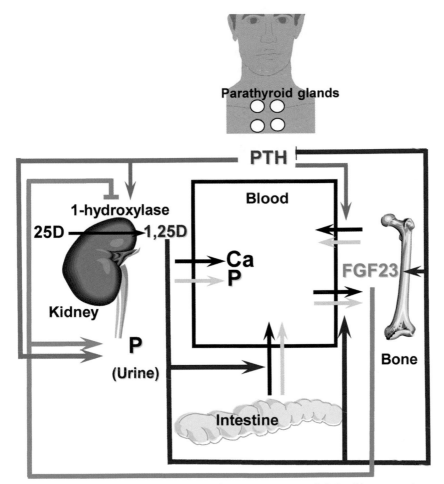

Fig. 25.5 Central role of renal calcitriol production in Ca, P, and skeletal homeostasis. Renal calcitriol (1,25D) production is a central integrator of hormonal feedback loops between PTH and FGF23, as well as Ca (black arrows) and P (gray arrows) fluxes between the intestine, bone, and the kidney that ensure normal mineral metabolism and skeletal integrity, while preventing the excess of both ions predisposing to ectopic calcifications. Hypocalcemia stimulates PTH secretion by the parathyroid glands, which induces Ca and P resorption from bone and stimulates renal 1-hydroxylase to induce calcitriol production thus promoting intestinal and renal Ca and P absorption/ reabsorption. Upon Ca normalization, both Ca and calcitriol close the loop through simultaneous suppression of PTH synthesis and renal 1-hydroxylase. Calcitriol induction of the synthesis of FGF23 in bone helps prevent hyperphosphatemia through FGF23-mediated increases in renal P excretion and suppression of 1-hydroxylase.

Although FGF23 was also shown to suppress PTH secretion,[49,50] it is unclear whether the increase in FGF23 that occur in CKD, induced by hyperphosphatemia, or by a decrease in FGF23 clearance by the damaged kidney, is a protective or a harmful response.[51,52] In fact, in experimental and human kidney disease, elevations in serum FGF23 correlate directly with increases in serum PTH.[52] Therefore, it is unclear at present whether a distinct induction of bone synthesis of FGF23 by vitamin D analogs would have a beneficial or a deleterious impact on bone remodeling, and extra-osseous calcium and phosphate deposition, through mechanisms that are independent of the abnormalities in P homeostasis driven by renal lesions.

Vitamin D analogs and increased survival in dialysis patients

Observational studies

Retrospective analyses of data from dialysis patients revealed increased survival with treatment with vitamin D analogs in the order 19-norD_2 = 1α(OH)D_2 > 1,25(OH)$_2D_3$ > no analog therapy.[10,11,53,54] In the historical cohort study performed by investigators at Massachusetts General Hospital and Fresenius Medical Care (North America), over 60,000 chronic hemodialysis patients throughout the US, naïve to injectable vitamin D, were followed for 36 months after they were started on calcitriol or paricalcitol. Patients were censored when they switched formulations or received a renal transplant. A 16% survival advantage was found among patients treated with paricalcitol compared with those treated with calcitriol.[9] This survival advantage accounted for baseline differences, including mortality rates of the different dialysis centers involved, duration on dialysis before starting injectable active vitamin D therapy, and baseline mineral levels. Furthermore, patients who switched formulations were also studied. Those who switched from paricalcitol to calcitriol had a worse survival over the remaining follow-up period compared with those who switched from calcitriol to paricalcitol. Paricalcitol was found to produce smaller increases in serum calcium and phosphate and a greater decrease in PTH. Similarly, 1α-hydroxyvitamin D_2 therapy has also been associated with an apparent survival advantage when compared with calcitriol.[10] Consistent with these 'observational' survival data, patients treated with paricalcitol or 1α-hydroxyvitamin D_2 had fewer hospitalizations and hospital days per year than those treated with calcitriol.[55,56]

A major shift in the focus on the use and development of vitamin D analogs for CKD came with the observation that treatment with 1,25(OH)$_2D_3$ or its analogs can reduce morbidity and mortality in CKD patients through mechanisms independent of PTH and mineral metabolism. Two very large retrospective studies in Japanese and US end-stage renal disease (ESRD) patients have shown that active vitamin D therapy provide a 20 and 24% survival advantage, respectively, over no active vitamin D interventions.[11,57] All cause mortality, as well as cardiovascular mortality, was lower in the group receiving active vitamin D treatment. In a small cohort of Japanese ESRD patients, the use of 1α-hydroxyvitamin D_3 was associated with a 70% lower risk of death from cardiovascular disease when compared with a group of 1α-hydroxyvitamin D_3 non-users.[58]

In spite of the strong debate regarding the accuracy of these reports on survival, which were both contradicted[12] and confirmed[13] by other investigators (including Young *et al.*,[59] using the Dialysis Outcomes and Practice Patterns Study (DOPPS) database, and Kalantar-Zadeh *et al.*,[60,61] the great interest raised in the field for the identification of the mechanisms underlying the 'apparent' survival benefits associated with vitamin D therapy revealed critical renal and cardiovascular protective properties of the vitamin D endocrine system. The section below presents the current evidence from pre-clinical and clinical trials of the renoprotective and cardioprotective properties of vitamin D analogs that can help expedite the implementation of safe active vitamin D interventions to maximize favorable outcomes in CKD patients.

Renoprotective properties of active vitamin D therapy

Several animal models of kidney disease have demonstrated renoprotective properties of active vitamin D therapy[62–65] that are independent of PTH suppression, as they also occur in parathyroidectomized rats.[63] The renoprotective actions of active vitamin D therapy include:

- suppression of the renin-angiotensin system (RAS);
- prevention/amelioration of chronic renal inflammation;
- attenuation of glomerular injury, tubule-interstitial fibrosis, and proteinuria through direct regulation of specific functions of mesangial cells, podocytes, tubular cells, fibroblasts, resident or infiltrating macrophages, and immune cells, all of which are essential in maintaining a normal kidney.

Active vitamin D metabolites directly suppress the RAS through a VDR-mediated repression of the expression of the renin gene.[66,67] Prolonged RAS activation has been implicated in the development of the glomerular hemodynamic adaptation leading to fibrogenic responses, glomerulosclerosis, tubular hyperplasia, fibrosis, mononuclear cell infiltration, interstitial inflammation, and severe proteinuria.[68] In the rat model of remnant kidney after subtotal nephrectomy (SNX), a classic experimental model of CKD characterized by primary glomerular lesions, administration of active vitamin D not only effectively decreases albuminuria, glomerulosclerosis, glomerular cell proliferation,[62,63,69] but also serum creatinine, suggesting a role for calcitriol (analog) in the preservation of renal function.[69]

Calcitriol renoprotective properties also involve the prevention/amelioration of chronic inflammation, a disorder characterized by infiltration of inflammatory cells into the glomeruli and tubulointerstitium, and a key pathogenic mechanism in the development and progression of CKD, as the decline in renal function correlates closely with the extent of inflammation. Inflammatory cells produce reactive oxygen species and pro-inflammatory cytokines that modulate the response of renal resident cells to injurious stimuli, and pro-fibrotic cytokines such as transforming growth factor-β (TGF-β), all of which induce matrix-producing myofibroblast activation, and tubular cell epithelial-to-mesenchymal transition (EMT), thereby enhancing the propensity for the fibrogenic process. Calcitriol elicits potent anti-inflammatory properties,[70] and the VDR is present in most cells of the immune system including macrophages, dendritic cells, and both CD4+ and CD8+ T-cells.[71,72] In fact, in the rat anti-thy-1 model of mesangial proliferative glomerulonephritis, administration of either calcitriol or 22-oxa-calcitriol reduced mesangial cell proliferation and prevented albuminuria, inflammatory cell infiltration, and the extracellular matrix (ECM) accumulation that accompanies myofibroblast activation.[73,74] Also, calcitriol almost completely abrogates the glomerular infiltration of neutrophils.[73]

In the SNX rat model, paricalcitol inhibits macrophage infiltration via suppression of macrophage chemoattractant protein 1 (MCP-1).[75]

In immune and non-immune rat models of mesangial proliferative glomerulonephritis, calcitriol reduces podocyte injury.[62,76] In the SNX rat model, calcitriol administration effectively reduces podocyte loss and hypertrophy, improves podocyte ultrastructure, and suppresses the expression of desmin, a marker of podocyte injury. Accordingly, a diabetic VDR-null mouse model develops a more severe form of albuminuria and glomerulosclerosis, with reduced nephrin expression in podocytes, and enhanced fibronectin content in mesangial cells.[64] Active vitamin D therapy may also attenuate protein-dependent interstitial inflammation either by decreasing proteinuria, or by inducing tolerance in the renal tubule-associated dendritic cells,[77] which in turn will reduce the active immune responses triggered by filtered albumin in the damaged kidney.[78]

Active vitamin D therapy also prevents tubule-interstitial lesions. Calcitriol (analog) inhibition of the expression of TGF-β1, a well-known mediator of the onset and progression of various forms of renal fibrotic lesions, contributes to calcitriol renoprotection.[76] Myofibroblast activation is a critical event in the diseased kidney, involving the generation of α-smooth muscle actin (α SMA)-positive, matrix-producing effector cells from interstitial fibroblasts. Calcitriol inhibition of myofibroblast activation attenuates/suppresses interstitial fibrosis, a final common pathway for diverse types of causes of CKD. In fact, in the obstructed kidney, paricalcitol elicits a dose-dependent reduction in interstitial volume and the deposition of interstitial matrix components, through inhibition of renal mRNA expression of fibronectin, type I and III collagen, and fibrogenic TGF-β1.[65] Also, paricalcitol directly blocks the epithelial mesenchymal transition of tubular epithelial cells to become myofibroblasts, a process induced by TGF-β1 and common in the fibrotic kidney that follows sustained injury. In in vivo models of obstructive nephropathy, paricalcitol preserves the integrity of the tubular epithelium by restoring E-cadherin and VDR expression, and also by attenuating interstitial fibrosis through the suppression of α-SMA and fibronectin expression.[65] Intriguingly, paricalcitol was shown to increase renal perivascular fibrosis in the rat model of renal insufficiency, an effect attributed to suppression of local calcitriol synthesis,[79] thus indicating caution to avoid excessive dosage of vitamin D analogs that could compromise VDR activation by locally produced calcitriol.

In spite of the multiple renoprotective properties of calcitriol demonstrated in animal models of kidney disease, the use of active vitamin D or its analogs in early stages of KD has been limited by reports on the nephrotoxicity of vitamin D therapy,[80,81] and by the fear of accelerating the decline in renal function with the hypercalcemic and hyperphosphatemic effects of high doses of active vitamin D. Recent studies, including prospective randomized trials in patients with mild to moderate CKD, have demonstrated the benefits of moderate doses of active vitamin D in reducing serum PTH levels and in bone health, with no adverse impact on renal function.[20,82,83]

Furthermore, a randomized, double-blinded and placebo-controlled clinical trial in CKD stages 3 and 4 has shown an anti-proteinuric effect of oral paricalcitol administration.[84] In addition, a retrospective study in renal transplant patients with chronic allograft nephropathy has also demonstrated that calcitriol prolonged the duration of graft survival and lowered the rate of loss of renal function.[85] The very recent demonstration that, in kidney transplant patients, the appropriate correction of vitamin D deficiency (serum 25-hydroxyvitamin D levels above 35ng/mL) is sufficient to prevent elevations in serum PTH and abnormalities in mineral homeostasis, suggests a contribution of 'local' calcitriol production and autocrine/paracrine calcitriol actions to the favorable outcome in kidney transplantation. Consequently, appropriate monitoring of serum 25-hydroxyvitamin D levels to avoid an excess of analog dosage that could compromise autocrine/paracrine calcitriol actions should further improve the impact of active vitamin D therapy on graft survival.

Cardioprotective properties of active vitamin D therapy

At least half of the deaths among dialysis patients are attributed to cardiovascular disease. Thus, it is not surprising that the reported survival benefits of active vitamin D treatment are associated to down regulation of vascular calcification, the RAS, systemic inflammation, atherosclerosis, and cardiac dysfunction, all of which are important contributors to the development and progression of cardiovascular damage. Indeed, not only serum vitamin D and calcitriol levels are inversely correlated with coronary calcification,[86] symptoms of heart failure,[87] and left ventricular hypertrophy (LVH),[88] but more importantly, active vitamin D treatment down-regulates plasma renin activity,[66] left ventricular hypertrophy,[89] and systemic inflammation.[90] Clearly, early interventions with active vitamin D therapy may either prevent the development of clinically adverse cardiovascular signs and symptoms or reverse them.

Preclinical studies using the rat model of kidney disease have reproduced the findings from retrospective studies in kidney disease patients, thereby providing important mechanistic insights into the cardiovascular protection and safety of active vitamin D therapy. As stated earlier, calcitriol and its analogs attenuate vascular calcification, one of the main determinants of cardiovascular damage in CKD, through mechanisms unrelated to their efficacy in suppressing 2HPT, or in preventing increases in serum P, Ca, or Ca × P product. In uremic rats, administration of the analog 22-oxa calcitriol, at doses 50-fold higher than those of calcitriol, conferred a protection from vascular calcification superior to that achieved with calcitriol, in spite of similar increases in serum Ca and P.[69] Mizobuchi and co-workers[91] demonstrated that calcitriol and doxercalciferol increased aortic calcification compared with paricalcitol through mechanisms unrelated to a distinct regulation of serum P, Ca, or Ca × P product, and involved the prevention of increases in Runx2 and osteocalcin mRNA levels in the vasculature. The expression of both genes reflects the acquisition of an osteoblastic phenotype by vascular smooth muscle cells that induces calcification. Abnormalities in the vitamin D endocrine system impair cardiovascular health in spite of normal renal function. In mice with intact kidneys, the absence of either the VDR or the 1-hydroxylase (cyp27b1, the enzyme responsible for calcitriol synthesis) results in up-regulation of the renin-angiotensin system, cardiac hypertrophy, and impaired cardiac function.[66,92] All of these defects can be corrected by calcitriol in the 1-hydroxylase null mice. The suppression of the RAS, with an essential role in cardiovascular pathophysiology, by calcitriol and its less calcemic analogs contributes to cardiovascular protection. In spontaneously hypertensive heart failure rats that carry two copies of a mutant form of the leptin gene, increased dietary salt intake induces LVH and fibrosis with severe hypertension.[93] Treatment of these rats with calcitriol reduces heart weight, myocardial collagen levels, ventricular diameter, and improves cardiac output. In the Dahl-salt sensitive rat model,[94] in which high salt diet induces hypertension, paricalcitol therapy also prevents cardiac hypertrophy and cardiac dysfunction independently of blood pressure control. This cardiovascular protection associated with reduced plasma levels of brain natriuretic peptide, as well as cardiac mRNA expression of brain natriuretic peptide, atrial natriuretic factor, and renin. Direct inhibition of oxidative stress and inflammation by active vitamin D therapy may also provide cardiovascular protection regardless of the efficacy in the control of blood pressure. Activation of the RAS induces oxidative stress in the cardiovascular system, which in turn initiates membrane lipid peroxidation leading to inflammation responsible for cardiovascular dysfunction. In 5/6 nephrectomized rats, paricalcitol was as effective as the angiotensin II converting enzyme (ACE) inhibitor enalapril affording protection against cardiac oxidative stress.[95] Also, the synergy demonstrated by combined therapy with angiotensin II converting enzyme inhibitors and paricalcitol in attenuating the progression of monocyte infiltration and interstitial inflammation of the renal parenchyma, in spite of a defective control of blood pressure,[75] could certainly operate in the cardiovascular system, in which increased TNFα is a key contributor to atherosclerosis and vascular calcification.[96] In fact, while renal ablation in the LDL receptor null mice markedly aggravates the calcification of the atherosclerotic plaques,[97] neointimal vascular calcium content was reduced by calcitriol and paricalcitol treatment. However, high paricalcitol dosage resulted in enhanced calcification. Vascular inflammation enhances the production of matrix metalloproteinases that remodel the vascular wall and the myocardium, destabilizing atherosclerotic plaques and causing thrombosis. The prevention of thromboses is another mechanism by which active vitamin D therapy can reduce mortality, as demonstrated by the development of arterial thrombosis in the VDR null mice in association with the down regulation of antithrombin and thrombomodulin.[98]

Active vitamin D attenuation of proteinuria may also protect the cardiovascular system through a reduction in filtered protein-induced inflammation.[78]

In humans, studies in two CKD patient populations demonstrated an inverse correlation between serum calcitriol levels and coronary artery calcification and moderate risk for coronary heart disease.[86,99] Also, in a small trial in 24 patients (22 CKD stage 3, and 2 CKD 2), oral paricalcitol administration, at doses of 1 and 2μg, reduced albuminuria and systemic inflammation, as demonstrated by serum levels of C reactive protein, through mechanisms unrelated to the control of blood pressure or serum PTH.[90] Importantly, not only serum calcitriol but also serum 25-hydroxyvitamin D levels were correlated negatively with pulse wave velocity and positively correlated with brachial artery distensibility and flow mediated dilation.[100] This suggests that autocrine/paracrine activation of the VDR by locally produced calcitriol may effectively regulate cardiovascular function. In fact, the recent studies by Wolf et al. in hemodialysis patients found a stronger association of increased risk of all cause early mortality with severe vitamin D deficiency than with calcitriol deficiency.[101] More significantly, a very recent report demonstrates that low vitamin D levels affect mortality rates in CKD patients independently of vascular calcification and stiffness[102] supporting the contribution of local calcitriol production to the cardiovascular protection conferred to these patients by a normal vitamin D status.

Future perspectives

Vitamin D analog therapy is widely employed for the treatment of 2HPT, and the additional survival benefits are now appreciated. Several major challenges remain that require both basic and clinical studies to optimize the use of current and future vitamin D analogs. While the analogs currently in use were selected for their efficacy and safety for the treatment of 2HPT, the next generation of analogs will be optimized for promoting survival. A major challenge will be to identify the cellular and molecular targets through which vitamin D compounds exert these beneficial effects. The recent recognition that vitamin D compounds can induce FGF23, a potent phosphaturic hormone that can also modulate parathyroid gland function bears further study. Increases in FGF23 should help ameliorate the hyperphosphatemia in CKD patients, but yet high FGF23 levels are associated with increased mortality. In addition, acute treatment with FGF23, *in vivo* and *in vitro*, reduces PTH, but transgenic mice over-expressing FGF23 develop hyperparathyroidism; this disparity needs to be resolved. Finally, the correction of vitamin D deficiency and insufficiency in CKD patients is becoming a higher priority. The impact of normalizing vitamin D status alone on 2HPT and survival needs to be established as well as the influence it may have on dosing with active vitamin D compounds. Extra-renal production of calcitriol may play a critical role in many of key processes that promote survival, and adequate 25-hydroxyvitamin D is essential. Exogenous vitamin D analog treatment may not fully compensate for these autocrine effects, and could even impair the actions of locally-produced calcitriol by impairing its synthesis or by inducing its catabolism. Thus, optimal dosing with analogs must be established in the context of a normalized vitamin D status. These challenges, though daunting, need to be addressed in order to maximize the efficacy of vitamin D analog therapy in CKD.

References

1. Slatopolsky E, Brown A, Dusso A. Role of phosphorus in the pathogenesis of secondary hyperparathyroidism. *Am J Kidney Dis* 2001;**37**:S54–7.
2. Dusso AS, Brown AJ, Slatopolsky E. Vitamin D. *Am J Physiol Renal Physiol* 2005;**289**:F8–28.
3. Slatopolsky E, Finch J, Denda M, et al. Phosphorus restriction prevents parathyroid gland growth. High phosphorus directly stimulates PTH secretion *in vitro. J Clin Invest* 1996;**97**:2534–40.
4. Perwad F, Azam N, Zhang MY, et al. Dietary and serum phosphorus regulate fibroblast growth factor 23 expression and 1,25-dihydroxyvitamin D metabolism in mice. *Endocrinology* 2005;**146**:5358–64.

5. Schiavi SC. Fibroblast growth factor 23: the making of a hormone. *Kidney Int* 2006;**69**:425–7.

6. Shimada T, Hasegawa H, Yamazaki Y, et al. FGF23 is a potent regulator of vitamin D metabolism and phosphate homeostasis. *J Bone Miner Res* 2004;**19**:429–35.

7. Hruska KA, Saab G, Mathew S, et al. Renal osteodystrophy, phosphate homeostasis, and vascular calcification. *Semin Dial* 2007;**20**:309–15.

8. Brown AJ. Vitamin D analogs for secondary hyperparathyroidism: what does the future hold? *J Steroid Biochem Mol Biol* 2007;**103**:578–83.

9. Teng M, Wolf M, Lowrie E, et al. Survival of patients undergoing hemodialysis with paricalcitol or calcitriol therapy. *N Engl J Med* 2003;**349**:446–56.

10. Tentori F, Hunt WC, Stidley CA, et al. Mortality risk among hemodialysis patients receiving different vitamin D analogs. *Kidney Int* 2006;**70**:1858–65.

11. Teng M, Wolf M, Ofsthun MN, et al. Activated injectable vitamin D and hemodialysis survival: a historical cohort study. *J Am Soc Nephrol* 2005;**16**:1115–25.

12. Palmer SC, McGregor DO, Macaskill P, et al. Meta-analysis: vitamin D compounds in chronic kidney disease. *Ann Intern Med* 2007;**147**:840–53.

13. Autier P, Gandini S. Vitamin D supplementation and total mortality: a meta-analysis of randomised controlled trials. *Arch Intern Med* 2007;**167**:1730–7.

14. Brown AJ, Slatopolsky E. Vitamin D analogs: therapeutic applications and mechanisms for selectivity. *Mol Aspects Med* 2008;**29**:433–52.

15. Brandi L. 1alpha(OH)D3 One-alpha-hydroxy-cholecalciferol—an active vitamin D analog. Clinical studies on prophylaxis and treatment of secondary hyperparathyroidism in uremic patients on chronic dialysis. *Dan Med Bull* 2008;**55**:186–210.

16. Maung HM, Elangovan L, Frazao JM, et al. Efficacy and side effects of intermittent intravenous and oral doxercalciferol (1alpha-hydroxyvitamin D(2)) in dialysis patients with secondary hyperparathyroidism: a sequential comparison. *Am J Kidney Dis* 2001;**37**:532–43.

17. Frazao JM, Elangovan L, Maung HM, et al. Intermittent doxercalciferol (1alpha-hydroxyvitamin D(2)) therapy for secondary hyperparathyroidism. *Am J Kidney Dis* 2000;**36**:550–61.

18. Tan AU, Levine BS, Mazess RB, et al. Effective suppression of parathyroid hormone by 1α-hydroxy-vitamin D2 in hemodialysis patients with moderate to severe secondary hyperparathyroidism. *Kidney Int* 1997;**51**:317–23.

19. Frazao JM, Chesney RW, Coburn JW. Intermittent oral 1αhydroxyvitamin D2 is effective and safe for the suppression of secondary hyperparathyroidism in hemodialysis patients. *Nephrol Dial Transplant* 1998;**3**:68–72.

20. Coburn JW, Maung HM, Elangovan L, et al. Doxercalciferol safely suppresses PTH levels in patients with secondary hyperparathyroidism associated with chronic kidney disease stages 3 and 4. *Am J Kidney Dis* 2004;**43**:877–90.

21. Nishizawa Y, Morii H, Ogura Y, et al. Clinical trial of 26,26,26,27,27,27-hexafluoro-1, 25-dihydroxyvitamin D3 in uremic patients on hemodialysis: preliminary report. *Contrib Nephrol* 1991;**90**:196–203.

22. Akiba T, Marumo F, Owada A, et al. Controlled trial of falecalcitriol versus alfacalcidol in suppression of parathyroid hormone in hemodialysis patients with secondary hyperparathyroidism. *Am J Kidney Dis* 1998;**32**:238–46.

23. Tamura S, Ueki K, Mashimo K, et al. Comparison of the efficacy of an oral calcitriol pulse or intravenous 22-oxacalcitriol therapies in chronic hemodialysis patients. *Clin Exp Nephrol* 2005;**9**:238–43.

24. Akizawa T, Suzuki M, Akiba T, et al. Long-term effect of 1,25-dihydroxy-22-oxavitamin D(3) on secondary hyperparathyroidism in hemodialysis patients. One-year administration study. *Nephrol Dial Transplant* 2002;**17**(Suppl. 10):28–36.

25. Yasuda M, Akiba T, Nihei H. Multicenter clinical trial of 22-oxa-1,25-dihydroxyvitamin D3 for chronic dialysis patients. *Am J Kidney Dis* 2003;**41**:S108–11.

26. Akizawa T, Ohashi Y, Akiba T, et al. Dose-response study of 22-oxacalcitriol in patients with secondary hyperparathyroidism. *Ther Apher Dial* 2004;**8**:480–91.

27. Hayashi M, Tsuchiya Y, Itaya Y, et al. Comparison of the effects of calcitriol and maxacalcitol on secondary hyperparathyroidism in patients on chronic hemodialysis: a randomised prospective multicentre trial. *Nephrol Dial Transplant* 2004;**19**:2067–73.

28. Ogata H, Koiwa F, Shishido K, et al. Effects of 22-oxacalcitriol and calcitriol on PTH secretion and bone mineral metabolism in a crossover trial in hemodialysis patients with secondary hyperparathyroidism. *Ther Apher Dial* 2007;**11**:202–9.

29. Slatopolsky E, Cozzolino M, Lu Y, et al. Efficacy of 19-Nor-1,25-(OH)2D2 in the prevention and treatment of hyperparathyroid bone disease in experimental uremia. *Kidney Int* 2003;**63**:2020–7.

30. Martin KJ, Gonzales EA, Gellens M, et al. 19-Nor-1α,25-dihydroxyvitamin D2 (Paricalcitol) safely and effectively reduces the levels of intact parathyroid hormone in patients on hemodialysis. *J Am Soc Nephrol* 1998;**9**:1427–32.

31. Martin KJ, Gonzalez EA, Gellens ME, et al. Therapy of secondary hyperparathyroidism with 19-nor-1α,25-dihydroxyvitamin D2. *Am J Kidney Dis* 1998;**32**:S 61–6.

32. Martin KJ, Gonzalez E, Lindberg JS, et al. Paricalcitol dosing according to body weight or seventy of hyperparathyroidism: a double-blind, multicenter, randomized study. *Am J Kidney Dis* 2001;**38**:S57–63.

33. Coyne DW, Grieff M, Ahya SN, et al. Differential effects of acute administration of 19-Nor-1,25-dihydroxy-vitamin D2 and 1,25-dihydroxy-vitamin D3 on serum calcium and phosphorus in hemodialysis patients. *Am J Kidney Dis* 2002;**40**:1283–8.

34. Sprague SM, Lerma E, McCormmick D, et al. Suppression of parathyroid hormone secretion in hemodialysis patients: comparison of paricalcitol with calcitriol. *Am J Kidney Dis* 2001;**38**:S51–6.

35. Sprague SM, Llach F, Amdahl M, et al. Paricalcitol versus calcitriol in the treatment of secondary hyperparathyroidism. *Kidney Int* 2003;**63**:1483–90.

36. Zisman AL, Ghantous W, Schinleber P, et al. Inhibition of parathyroid hormone: a dose equivalency study of paricalcitol and doxercalciferol. *Am J Nephrol* 2005;**25**:591–5.

37. Joist HE, Ahya SN, Giles K, et al. Differential effects of very high doses of doxercalciferol and paricalcitol on serum phosphorus in hemodialysis patients. *Clin Nephrol* 2006;**65**:335–41.

38. Coyne D, Acharya M, Qui P, et al. Paricalcitol capsule for treatment of secondary hyperparathyroidism in stages 3 and 4 CKD. *Am J Kidney Dis* 2006;**47**:263–76.

39. Peleg S, Sastry M, Collins ED, et al. Distinct conformational changes induced by 20-epi analogues of 1 alpha,25-dihydroxyvitamin D3 are associated with enhanced activation of the vitamin D receptor. *J Biol Chem* 1995;**270**:10551–8.

40. Heaney RP. Vitamin D in health and disease. *Clin J Am Soc Nephrol* 2008;**3**:1535–41.

41. Jones G. Expanding role for vitamin D in chronic kidney disease: importance of blood 25-OH-D levels and extra-renal 1alpha-hydroxylase in the classical and nonclassical actions of 1alpha,25-dihydroxyvitamin D(3). *Semin Dial* 2007;**20**:316–24.

42. Dusso AS, Negrea L, Finch J, et al. The effect of 22-oxacalcitriol on serum calcitriol. *Endocrinology* 1992;**130:**3129–34.

43. Mizwicki MT, Bula CM, Bishop JE, et al. A perspective on how the Vitamin D sterol/ Vitamin D receptor (VDR) conformational ensemble model can potentially be used to understand the structure-function results of A-ring modified Vitamin D sterols. *J Steroid Biochem Mol Biol* 2005;**97:**69–82.

44. Khanal RC, Nemere I. The ERp57/GRp58/1,25D3-MARRS receptor: multiple functional roles in diverse cell systems. *Curr Med Chem* 2007;**14:**1087–93.

45. Green JJ, Robinson DA, Wilson GE, et al. Calcitriol modulation of cardiac contractile performance via protein kinase C. *J Mol Cell Cardiol* 2006;**41:**350–9.

46. Wong MS, Delansorne R, Man RY, et al. Vitamin D derivatives acutely reduce endothelium-dependent contractions in the aorta of the spontaneously hypertensive rat. *Am J Physiol Heart Circ Physiol* 2008;**295:**H289–96.

47. Barthel TK, Mathern DR, Whitfield GK, et al. 1,25-Dihydroxyvitamin D3/VDR-mediated induction of FGF23 as well as transcriptional control of other bone anabolic and catabolic genes that orchestrate the regulation of phosphate and calcium mineral metabolism. *J Steroid Biochem Mol Biol* 2007;**103:**381–8.

48. Sitara D, Kim S, Razzaque MS, et al. Genetic evidence of serum phosphate-independent functions of FGF23 on bone. *PLoS Genet* 2008;**4:**e1000154.

49. Ben-Dov IZ, Galitzer H, Lavi-Moshayoff V, et al. The parathyroid is a target organ for FGF23 in rats. *J Clin Invest* 2007;**117:**4003–8.

50. Krajisnik T, Bjorklund P, Marsell R, et al. Fibroblast growth factor-23 regulates parathyroid hormone and 1alpha-hydroxylase expression in cultured bovine parathyroid cells. *J Endocrinol* 2007;**195:**125–31.

51. Nagano N, Miyata S, Abe M, et al. Effect of manipulating serum phosphorus with phosphate binder on circulating PTH and FGF23 in renal failure rats. *Kidney Int* 2006;**69:**531–7.

52. Westerberg PA, Linde T, Wikstrom B, et al. Regulation of fibroblast growth factor-23 in chronic kidney disease. *Nephrol Dial Transplant* 2007;**22:**3202–7.

53. Teng M, Wolf M, Lowrie E, et al. Survival of patients undergoing hemodialysis with paricalcitol or calcitriol therapy. *N Engl J Med* 2003;**349:**446–56.

54. Naves-Diaz M, Alvarez-Hernandez D, Passlick-Deetjen J, et al. Oral active vitamin D is associated with improved survival in hemodialysis patients. *Kidney Int* 2008;**74:**1070–8.

55. Tentori F, Hunt WC, Rohrsceib MR, et al. Decreased odds of hospitalisation among hemodialysis patients receiving doxercalciferol and paricalcitol versus calcitriol. *J Am Soc Nephrol* 2005;**16:**279A.

56. Dobrez DG, Mathes A, Amdahl M, et al. Paricalcitol-treated patients experience improved hospitalisation outcomes compared with calcitriol-treated patients in real-world clinical settings. *Nephrol Dial Transplant* 2004;**19:**1174–81.

57. Nakai S, Shinzato T, Nagura Y, et al. An overview of regular dialysis treatment in Japan (as of 31 December (2001)). *Ther Apher Dial* 2004;**8:**3–32.

58. Shoji T, Shinohara K, Kimoto E, et al. Lower risk for cardiovascular mortality in oral 1alpha-hydroxy vitamin D3 users in a hemodialysis population. *Nephrol Dial Transplant* 2004;**19:**179–84.

59. Young EW, Albert JM, Satayathum S, et al. Predictors and consequences of altered mineral metabolism: the Dialysis Outcomes and Practice Patterns Study. *Kidney Int* 2005;**67:**1179–87.

60. Kalantar-Zadeh K, Kuwae N, Regidor DL, et al. Survival predictability of time-varying indicators of bone disease in maintenance hemodialysis patients. *Kidney Int* 2006;**70**:771–80.

61. Tentori F, Albert JM, Young EW, et al. The survival advantage for hemodialysis patients taking vitamin D is questioned: findings from the Dialysis Outcomes and Practice Patterns Study. *Nephrol Dial Transplant* 2009;**24**:963–72.

62. Kuhlmann A, Haas CS, Gross ML, et al. 1,25-Dihydroxyvitamin D3 decreases podocyte loss and podocyte hypertrophy in the subtotally nephrectomised rat. *Am J Physiol Renal Physiol* 2004;**286**:F526–33.

63. Schwarz U, Amann K, Orth SR, et al. Effect of 1,25 (OH)2 vitamin D3 on glomerulosclerosis in subtotally nephrectomised rats. *Kidney Int* 1998;**53**:1696–705.

64. Zhang Z, Sun L, Wang Y, et al. Renoprotective role of the vitamin D receptor in diabetic nephropathy. *Kidney Int* 2008;**73**:163–71.

65. Tan X, Li Y, Liu Y. Paricalcitol attenuates renal interstitial fibrosis in obstructive nephropathy. *J Am Soc Nephrol* 2006;**17**:3382–93.

66. Li YC, Kong J, Wei M, et al. 1,25-Dihydroxyvitamin D(3) is a negative endocrine regulator of the renin-angiotensin system. *J Clin Invest* 2002;**110**:229–38.

67. Li YC, Qiao G, Uskokovic M, et al. Vitamin D: a negative endocrine regulator of the renin-angiotensin system and blood pressure. *J Steroid Biochem Mol Biol* 2004;**89–90**:387–92.

68. Lautrette A, Li S, Alili R, et al. Angiotensin II and EGF receptor cross-talk in chronic kidney diseases: a new therapeutic approach. *Nat Med* 2005;**11**:867–74.

69. Hirata M, Makibayashi K, Katsumata K, et al. 22-Oxacalcitriol prevents progressive glomerulosclerosis without adversely affecting calcium and phosphorus metabolism in subtotally nephrectomised rats. *Nephrol Dial Transplant* 2002;**17**:2132–7.

70. Mathieu C, Adorini L. The coming of age of 1,25-dihydroxyvitamin D(3) analogs as immunomodulatory agents. *Trends Mol Med* 2002;**8**:174–9.

71. Provvedini DM, Tsoukas CD, Deftos LJ, et al. 1,25-dihydroxyvitamin D3 receptors in human leukocytes. *Science* 1983;**221**:1181–3.

72. Veldman CM, Cantorna MT, DeLuca HF. Expression of 1,25-dihydroxyvitamin D(3) receptor in the immune system. *Arch Biochem Biophys* 2000;**374**:334–8.

73. Panichi V, Migliori M, Taccola D, et al. Effects of 1,25(OH)2D3 in experimental mesangial proliferative nephritis in rats. *Kidney Int* 2001;**60**:87–95.

74. Makibayashi K, Tatematsu M, Hirata M, et al. A vitamin D analog ameliorates glomerular injury on rat glomerulonephritis. *Am J Pathol* 2001;**158**:1733–41.

75. Mizobuchi M, Morrissey J, Finch JL, et al. Combination therapy with an Angiotensin-converting enzyme inhibitor and a vitamin d analog suppresses the progression of renal insufficiency in uremic rats. *J Am Soc Nephrol* 2007;**18**:1796–806.

76. Migliori M, Giovannini L, Panichi V, et al. Treatment with 1,25-dihydroxyvitamin D3 preserves glomerular slit diaphragm-associated protein expression in experimental glomerulonephritis. *Int J Immunopathol Pharmacol* 2005;**18**:779–90.

77. Dong X, Craig T, Xing N, et al. Direct transcriptional regulation of RelB by 1alpha, 25-dihydroxyvitamin D3 and its analogs: physiologic and therapeutic implications for dendritic cell function. *J Biol Chem* 2003;**278**:49378–85.

78. Macconi D, Chiabrando C, Schiarea S, et al. Proteasomal processing of albumin by renal dendritic cells generates antigenic peptides. *J Am Soc Nephrol* 2009;**20**:123–30.

79. Repo JM, Rantala IS, Honkanen TT, et al. Paricalcitol aggravates perivascular fibrosis in rats with renal insufficiency and low calcitriol. *Kidney Int* 2007;**72**:977–84.

80. Tougaard L, Sorensen E, Brochner-Mortensen J, et al. Controlled trial of 1alpha-hydroxycholecalciferol in chronic renal failure. *Lancet* 1976;**1**:1044–7.

81. Christiansen C, Rodbro P, Christensen MS, et al. Deterioration of renal function during treatment of chronic renal failure with 1,25-dihydroxycholecalciferol. *Lancet* 1978;**2**:700–3.

82. Ritz E, Kuster S, Schmidt-Gayk H, et al. Low-dose calcitriol prevents the rise in 1,84-iPTH without affecting serum calcium and phosphate in patients with moderate renal failure (prospective placebo-controlled multicentre trial). *Nephrol Dial Transplant* 1995;**10**:2228–34.

83. Rix M, Eskildsen P, Olgaard K. Effect of 18 months of treatment with alfacalcidol on bone in patients with mild to moderate chronic renal failure. *Nephrol Dial Transplant* 2004;**19**:870–6.

84. Agarwal R, Acharya M, Tian J, et al. Antiproteinuric effect of oral paricalcitol in chronic kidney disease. *Kidney Int* 2005;**68**:2823–8.

85. Sezer S, Uyar M, Arat Z, et al. Potential effects of 1,25-dihydroxyvitamin D3 in renal transplant recipients. *Transplant Proc* 2005;**37**:3109–11.

86. Watson KE, Abrolat ML, Malone LL, et al. Active serum vitamin D levels are inversely correlated with coronary calcification. *Circulation* 1997;**96**:1755–60.

87. Park CW, Oh YS, Shin YS, et al. Intravenous calcitriol regresses myocardial hypertrophy in hemodialysis patients with secondary hyperparathyroidism. *Am J Kidney Dis* 1999;**33**:73–81.

88. Zittermann A, Schleithoff SS, Tenderich G, et al. Low vitamin D status: a contributing factor in the pathogenesis of congestive heart failure? *J Am Coll Cardiol* 2003;**41**:105–12.

89. Wu J, Garami M, Cheng T, et al. 1,25(OH)2 vitamin D3, and retinoic acid antagonise endothelin-stimulated hypertrophy of neonatal rat cardiac myocytes. *J Clin Invest* 1996;**97**:1577–88.

90. Alborzi P, Patel NA, Peterson C, et al. Paricalcitol reduces albuminuria and inflammation in chronic kidney disease: a randomised double-blind pilot trial. *Hypertension* 2008;**52**:249–55.

91. Mizobuchi M, Finch JL, Martin DR, et al. Differential effects of vitamin D receptor activators on vascular calcification in uremic rats. *Kidney Int* 2007;**72**:709–15.

92. Zhou C, Lu F, Cao K, et al. Calcium-independent and 1,25(OH)2D3-dependent regulation of the renin-angiotensin system in 1alpha-hydroxylase knockout mice. *Kidney Int* 2008;**74**:170–9.

93. Mancuso P, Rahman A, Hershey SD, et al. 1,25-Dihydroxyvitamin-D3 treatment reduces cardiac hypertrophy and left ventricular diameter in spontaneously hypertensive heart failure-prone (cp/+) rats independent of changes in serum leptin. *J Cardiovasc Pharmacol* 2008;**51**:559–64.

94. Bodyak N, Ayus JC, Achinger S, et al. Activated vitamin D attenuates left ventricular abnormalities induced by dietary sodium in Dahl salt-sensitive animals. *Proc Natl Acad Sci USA* 2007;**104**:16810–15.

95. Husain K, Ferder L, Mizobuchi M, et al. Combination therapy with paricalcitol and enalapril ameliorates cardiac oxidative injury in uremic rats. *Am J Nephrol* 2009;**29**:465–72.

96. Al-Aly Z. Arterial calcification: a tumor necrosis factor-alpha mediated vascular Wnt-opathy. *Transl Res* 2008;**151**:233–9.

97. Mathew S, Lund RJ, Chaudhary LR, et al. Vitamin D receptor activators can protect against vascular calcification. *J Am Soc Nephrol* 2008;**19**:1509–19.

98. Aihara K, Azuma H, Akaike M, et al. Disruption of nuclear vitamin D receptor gene causes enhanced thrombogenicity in mice. *J Biol Chem* 2004;**279**:35798–802.

99. Doherty TM, Tang W, Dascalos S, et al. Ethnic origin and serum levels of 1alpha, 25-dihydroxyvitamin D3 are independent predictors of coronary calcium mass measured by electron-beam computed tomography. *Circulation* 1997;**96**:1477–81.

100. London GM, Guerin AP, Verbeke FH, et al. Mineral metabolism and arterial functions in end-stage renal disease: potential role of 25-hydroxyvitamin D deficiency. *J Am Soc Nephrol* 2007;**18**:613–20.

101. Wolf M, Shah A, Gutierrez O, et al. Vitamin D levels and early mortality among incident hemodialysis patients. *Kidney Int* 2007;**72**:1004–13.

102. Barreto DV, Barreto FC, Liabeuf S, et al. Vitamin D affects survival independently of vascular calcification in chronic kidney disease. *Clin J Am Soc Nephrol* 2009;**4**:1128–35.

Chapter 26

Calcimimetics and calcilytics in the treatment of chronic kidney disease-mineral and bone disorder

Edward F. Nemeth

Introduction

Chronic kidney disease-mineral and bone disorder (CKD-MBD) is an umbrella term covering a number of distinct yet interrelated pathologies associated with terminal loss of kidney function.[1] One of the more common disorders of systemic mineral metabolism is secondary hyperparathyroidism (HPT), which is often accompanied by one of the various kinds of bone abnormalities of renal osteodystrophy and/or extraskeletal calcification. Secondary HPT (2HPT) is present to some degree in nearly all patients on renal replacement therapy. In many respects, 2HPT is a physiological response of the parathyroid glands to a loss of kidney function—it is an attempt to normalize lowered levels of $1,25\text{-}(OH)_2$vitamin D_3 and calcium, and elevated levels of phosphate by increasing the output of parathyroid hormone (PTH). Increased output of PTH is achieved by increasing the proliferation of parathyroid cells resulting in hyperplasia of all four glands. Increased glandular mass is accompanied by increased synthesis and secretion of PTH resulting in chronically elevated levels of plasma PTH. Prolonged 2HPT often leads to a high turnover form of renal osteodystrophy with marrow fibrosis, bone pain, and increased susceptibility to fracture. Additionally, 2HPT is often associated with increased vascular calcification that, in turn, predicts cardiovascular morbidity and mortality. Indeed, abnormalities in mineral metabolism are independent risk factors for all-cause and cardiovascular mortality in dialysis patients.

Recognizing this seemingly fundamental relationship between abnormal mineral metabolism and clinical outcomes prompted the National Kidney Foundation/Kidney Disease Outcomes Quality Initiative (KDOQI) to issue guidelines for circulating levels of PTH (150–300pg/mL), calcium (8.4–9.5mg/dL), phosphate (3.5–5.5mg/dL), and the calcium-phosphate product ($<55mg^2/dL^2$). These target ranges for blood chemistries can be used to define efficacy endpoints for the head-to-head comparative evaluation of therapies for 2HPT in patients with CKD.[2]

A skeletal resistance to the effects of PTH develops in patients with CKD and this underlies the KDOQI recommendation for maintaining PTH levels at about three-fold higher than normal.[3] A relative hypoparathyroidism can therefore develop in

CKD leading to low turnover bone abnormalities, such as osteomalacia and adynamic bone disease (ABD).[4,5] As the use of aluminum-based phosphate-binders has waned, the prevalence of osteomalacia has decreased, but that of ABD has increased. ABD is characterized by a lack of osteoblasts, and a corresponding low rate of bone formation and volume. Patients with ABD are less able to buffer a calcium load and are at increased risk for developing vascular calcification. Although plasma PTH levels within the KDOQI range are, by themselves, not often a good predictor of bone disease, very high or relatively low levels of PTH are generally prognostic of high or low turnover bone abnormalities. Bringing excessively high or low plasma PTH levels into the KDOQI range is therefore one goal in treating CKD-MBD.

Traditional treatments for 2HPT attempt to reduce circulating levels of PTH by increasing serum levels of calcium and/or 1,25-$(OH)_2$vitamin D_3. These approaches have met with limited success in achieving the recommended KDOQI targets for PTH, calcium, phosphate, and the calcium-phosphate (Ca × P) product. A recent study, for example, reported that only about half of the patients on conventional therapy were within target values for calcium and phosphate and less than a third were within those for PTH; only 9% of patients met the guidelines for all four parameters.[6] There is, therefore, room for improvement in the medical management of 2HPT.

A relatively new approach to treating CKD-MBD is the use of drugs that target the cell surface calcium receptor on parathyroid cells. The calcium receptor is a G protein-coupled receptor and the primary regulator of a number of distinct cellular functions including the synthesis and secretion of PTH and parathyroid cell proliferation.[7] Compounds that activate the calcium receptor are termed calcimimetics and they inhibit the secretion of PTH. Antagonists of the calcium receptor are termed calcilytics and they stimulate PTH secretion. Calcilytics might be useful in treating low turnover forms of renal osteodystrophy like adynamic bone disease. Orally administered calcimimetic and calcilytic compounds are a way to rapidly alter circulating levels of PTH independently of calcium, phosphate or vitamin D levels. Recent in-depth reviews of calcimimetic and calcilytic compounds have been published.[8,9]

Calcimimetic and calcilytic compounds

Calcimimetics

Calcimimetics are inorganic ions or organic compounds that mimic or potentiate the action of extracellular ionized calcium (Ca^{2+}) at the calcium receptor; they are classified as either *type I* or *type II* calcimimetics. The former activate the calcium receptor in the absence of extracellular Ca^{2+} and are agonists, whereas type II ligands act as positive allosteric modulators and require the presence of extracellular Ca^{2+} (or some other type I calcimimetic) to activate the calcium receptor. All the known type I calcimimetics are inorganic or organic polycations. Type II calcimimetics include the naturally occurring L-amino acids and several synthetic chemotypes of which the most therapeutically relevant are the phenylalkylamines. Phenylalkylamine compounds like NPS R-568 and cinacalcet are stereoselective and the R-enantiomers are 10–100-fold more potent than the corresponding S-enantiomers. As positive allosteric modulators, these calcimimetics shift the concentration-response curve for extracellular Ca^{2+} to the left. Type II calcimimetics thus increase the sensitivity of the calcium receptor to activation by extracellular Ca^{2+}.[8]

In normal rats or in rat models of 2HPT, the oral administration of NPS R-568 or cinacalcet causes a rapid fall in plasma levels of PTH, which reaches a nadir 2–4h following oral administration. The fall in plasma levels of PTH is dose-dependent and precedes that of serum Ca^{2+}; the longer PTH levels are depressed, the greater is the duration and magnitude of the decrease in serum levels of Ca^{2+}. The effect of NPS R-568 on levels of plasma PTH in normal rats parallels that seen *in vitro*: the concentration-response curve for plasma Ca^{2+} and PTH is shifted to the left, thereby reducing the set-point for extracellular Ca^{2+}.

In addition to these rapid effects on the secretion of PTH, calcimimetics additionally inhibit the synthesis of PTH and the proliferation of parathyroid cells in animal models of 2HPT. Both these likely contribute to the maintained lowering of plasma PTH levels following repeat dosing.

Both NPS R-568 and cinacalcet are relatively selective and do not affect the activity of a number of other G protein-coupled receptors at concentrations that maximally activate the calcium receptor. Moreover, these compounds can preferentially affect parathyroid cell gland functions even though the calcium receptor is expressed in many other cells in the body, particularly those involved in systemic mineral metabolism (C-cells, renal epithelial cells, certain bone cells). Thus, NPS R-568 and cinacalcet depress plasma levels of PTH at doses 30–40-fold lower than those that increase plasma levels of calcitonin. The hypocalcemic response following administration of either compound persists following an acute, total nephrectomy. The effects of these two calcimimetics on serum levels of calcium and phosphate in rats are largely, if not exclusively, due to their ability to lower circulating levels of PTH.

The pharmacodynamic properties of NPS R-568 and cinacalcet are essentially identical; they differ mostly in their pharmacokinetic properties with cinacalcet having a greater bioavailability and somewhat longer half-life following oral administration. The pharmacokinetics of cinacalcet has been assessed in rodents, monkeys, normal humans and in patients receiving hemodialysis or continuous ambulatory peritoneal dialysis. The pharmacokinetic profile of cinacalcet is essentially the same in normal humans and in those receiving either form of dialysis. Maximal plasma concentrations (C_{max}) of cinacalcet occur within 2–3h after a single oral dose. There is a dose-proportional increase in C_{max} and area under the plasma concentration-time curve (AUC) with cinacalcet doses up to 200mg once daily. These pharmacokinetic parameters and the plasma half-life of cinacalcet were similar when estimated on days with and without dialysis. Moreover, the degree of renal impairment did not affect the pharmacokinetic profile of cinacalcet. The dose-proportional increase in exposure to cinacalcet correlates inversely with plasma levels of PTH. The plasma concentration of cinacalcet that results in a 50% decrease in serum levels of PTH is 6.2ng/mL (about 15nM), a concentration similar to that causing a 50% decrease in PTH secretion *in vitro*.

Cinacalcet is metabolized by several hepatic cytochrome P_{450} enzymes, primarily CYP3A4, CYP2D6 and CYP1A2; none of the metabolites are biologically active on the calcium receptor and most (80%) are eliminated by renal excretion. Moderate to severe degrees of hepatic impairment will impede metabolism of cinacalcet and increase plasma exposure. Cinacalcet inhibits CYP2D6 *in vitro* and can therefore retard the metabolism of drugs that are metabolized by this enzyme, such as tricyclic antidepressants.

The expression of the calcium receptor, like that of the vitamin D receptor, is generally lower in pathological parathyroid cells from patients with primary or 2HPT when compared with normal tissue.[8] No mutations, however, have yet been detected in the coding region of the calcium receptor gene in either adenomatous or hyperplastic parathyroid glands. There is a correlation between the level of calcium receptor expression and the PTH-Ca^{2+} set-point; the set-point is higher in those patients with glands having the lowest expression levels. Like the receptor for vitamin D, expression of the calcium receptor appears to be lower in nodular, compared with diffuse areas of hyperplastic glands. Decreases in calcium receptor expression also occur in animal models of 2HPT. In these animal models, treatment with a calcimimetic increases the levels of expression of the calcium receptor and the vitamin D receptor.[10] These effects might contribute to the long-term clinical efficacy of calcimimetic compounds in patients with 2HPT.

Cinacalcet HCl has been approved for treating 2HPT in patients on dialysis and in patients with parathyroid cancer. In some European countries, it is additionally approved for treating primary HPT. It is marketed as Sensipar®, Mimpara® (Amgen), and Regpara® (Kyowa Kirin).

Calcilytics

Calcilytics are calcium receptor antagonists and several distinct small molecule chemotypes have been reported.[9] All these calcilytic compounds block calcium receptor-mediated increases in cytoplasmic concentrations of Ca^{2+} or inositol phosphates in heterologous expression systems, and shift the concentration-response curve for extracellular Ca^{2+} to the right, thus eliciting an apparent decrease in the sensitivity of the calcium receptor to activation by extracellular Ca^{2+}. This shift in the concentration-response curve does not, however, necessarily imply that these calcilytics act as negative allosteric modulators because such shifts would also be produced by a competitive antagonist. So at present there is no data that distinguishes the mechanism of action of different calcilytic compounds as there is for calcimimetic compounds.

As expected, the effects of calcilytics on parathyroid gland functions are generally the converse of those of calcimimetics. Several different calcilytics have been shown to stimulate secretion of PTH *in vitro* and to rapidly increase circulating levels of PTH following oral or systemic administration. Moreover, calcilytics stimulate the synthesis of PTH as assessed by increased levels of PTH mRNA levels in dissociated bovine parathyroid cells *in vitro*. However, calcilytics do not stimulate the proliferation of parathyroid cells, at least in ovariectomized (OVX) rats. While this might seem at odds with the profound inhibitory effect of calcimimetics on parathyroid cell proliferation, it is not necessarily so. Parathyroid cells have a very low mitotic index that increases rapidly and profoundly in animal models of renal failure and it is this *induced* proliferation that is so effectively blocked by calcimimetics. The effects of calcilytics on parathyroid cell proliferation in animal models of renal failure have not been examined.

Similarly, it is not known if calcilytics will decrease expression of the parathyroid calcium receptor in CKD.

Both long- and short-acting calcilytic compounds have been studied for effects on bone turnover in OVX rats.[9] The long-acting calcilytic NPS 2143 causes a sustained (>8h) increase in plasma levels of PTH in OVX rats and increases both bone formation and resorption; there is no net increase in volumetric bone mineral density (BMD). In contrast, a short-acting calcilytic (SB-423557) causes a transient (< 2h) increase in plasma levels of PTH and increases bone formation more so than resorption, thus resulting in a net increase in BMD. Neither the long- nor short acting calcilytic caused parathyroid gland hyperplasia when administered daily for 5 or 12 weeks to OVX rats.

In contrast to agonists and allosteric activators, antagonists of G protein-coupled receptors are typically not tissue selective. Cellular functions in cells that express the calcium receptor, but are not affected by therapeutic doses of a calcimimetic might very well be affected by a calcilytic. There is now compelling evidence that calcium receptors are functionally expressed in osteoblasts and chondrocytes and contribute significantly to skeletal development.[11] Effects of calcilytics on the osteoblast calcium receptor might negate any beneficial effects on low turnover forms of renal osteodystrophy achieved by intermittent increases in endogenous levels of plasma PTH. Similarly, calcilytics might affect the function of calcium receptors on smooth muscle cells and promote vascular calcification independent of any beneficial effect on the skeleton. Calcilytics have not been tested for effects on skeletal or vascular parameters in animal models of CKD with low turnover bone abnormalities.

Short-acting calcilytic compounds are currently in clinical development for the treatment of postmenopausal osteoporosis.

Calcimimetics and secondary hyperparathyroidism

Therapies for 2HPT should attempt to achieve both immediate and long-term goals. The immediate goals are to normalize serum levels of calcium and phosphate, correct the vitamin D deficiency, and control levels of PTH within the target range, typically <300pg/mL. The long-term goals of therapy would be to prevent parathyroid gland hyperplasia, maintain normal bone turnover, and reduce cardiovascular morbidity and mortality. Cinacalcet has been shown to improve the short-term biochemical parameters and there is emerging evidence that it might improve long-term clinical outcomes.

Biochemical parameters

There were three Phase 3 trials that formed the basis for regulatory approval of cinacalcet (Table 26.1).[12–14] These registration trials enrolled patients on hemodialysis or peritoneal dialysis and with plasma levels of intact PTH ≥300pg/mL. There was a 12- or 16-week dose titration phase, and a 10- or 14-week efficacy-assessment phase and the primary endpoint was the percentage of patients who achieved PTH levels ≤250pg/mL or a ≥30% reduction from baseline levels. A 30mg dose of cinacalcet was administered once daily and could be increased to 180mg during the dose-titration phase.

Table 26.1 Selected clinical studies with cinacalcet and vitamin D sterols in patients on dialysis.

Study	Baseline; iPTH pg/ml	Design and use of vitamin D	Percentage of patients achieving K/DOQI target (baseline → end of study)		
			PTH	Ca × P	Both
Phase 3 trials[12–14]	≥300	Double-blind, placebo-controlled; 26 weeks. Vitamin D held constant; could be reduced or increased only for safety reasons.(*Upper values are placebo; combined data from 3 separate studies[4]*)	<1 → 10 <1 → 56	34 → 36 37 → 65	0 → 6 0 → 41
TARGET[20]	>300–800 (biPTH >160–430)	Open-label; 16 weeks. 51% decrease in paricalcitol dose equivalents* by end of study	6 → 62	56 → 83	3 → 54
CONTROL[20]	150–300 (biPTH 80–160)	Open-label; 16 weeks. 49% decrease in paricalcitol dose equivalents* by end of study. 21% of patients completely stopped taking vitamin D sterols	91 → 85	21 → 72	17 → 47
OPTIMA[20]	> 300–800	Open-label; 23 weeks. 3% increase in paricalcitol dose equivalents* using conventional care algorithm (*upper values*); 22% decrease in dose using cinacalcet algorithm (*lower values*)	2 → 22 <1 → 71	59 → 58 60 → 77	0 → 16 0 → 59

*biPTH refers to PTH measured by the biointact assay as described in the text. Paricalcitol equivalents are defined as 2μg paricalcitol = 1.0μg doxercalciferol = 0.5μg calcitriol.

Treatment with cinacalcet for a total of 26 weeks significantly lowered plasma levels of PTH compared with baseline levels whereas PTH levels in the placebo-treated group tended to increase; the results in hemodialysis patients were similar to those in peritoneal dialysis patients. Treatment with cinacalcet significantly lowered levels of serum calcium and phosphate compared with those treated with placebo. The Ca × P product decreased by 14% in the cinacalcet group but remained unchanged in the placebo group and 89% of those who reached the primary endpoint had a reduction in the Ca × P product.

The data from all the Phase 3 studies were combined to assess the overall efficacy of cinacalcet relative to the KDOQI guidelines.[12] At baseline, the median plasma PTH levels of cinacalcet-treated and control subjects were similar (596 and 564pg/mL, respectively). After treatment for 6 months with cinacalcet, 56% of the subjects achieved mean plasma PTH levels at or below the upper limit of the KDOQI target (≤300pg/mL) compared with 10% of control subjects. Serum levels of calcium and phosphate were within the KDOQI target range in 49 and 46% of cinacalcet-treated subjects compared with 24 and 33%, respectively, in placebo-treated subjects. The target value for the Ca × P product was achieved in 65% of patients treated with cinacalcet compared with 36% of those treated with placebo. All these between group differences were highly significant. Perhaps the most striking index of efficacy is the percentage of patients achieving the targets for *both* serum PTH levels and Ca × P product, which none of the subjects met at baseline. After 6 months, this endpoint was achieved in 41% of cinacalcet-treated subjects but only 6% of placebo-treated subjects. In a long-term, open-label study, treatment with cinacalcet for 3 years caused a ≥30% reduction in plasma levels of PTH in 70% of the patients.[15]

Consistent with its mechanism of action as a positive allosteric modulator of the calcium receptor, treatment of dialysis patients with cinacalcet shifts the serum Ca^{2+}-PTH dose response curve to the left, thereby reducing the set-point for extracellular calcium.[16]

The reductions in plasma PTH levels reported in these studies mostly reflect changes in the level of the intact hormone. A head-to-head comparison of plasma PTH levels using a first-generation ('intact-PTH') and a second-generation immunometric assay ('bio-intact-PTH') showed that treatment with cinacalcet for 26 weeks lowered plasma levels of PTH in the same percentage of subjects (56%) and by the same magnitude (38%) using either assay.[17] In the control group, plasma PTH levels increased compared with baseline and the percentage increase was significantly greater (23%) with the second-generation than with the first-generation assay. The bioactive PTH/intact PTH ratio remained constant at 56% throughout the study. Thus, the absolute level of plasma PTH is assay-dependent, but the magnitude of the decrease from baseline and the proportion of patients responding to cinacalcet is independent of the assay used to measure PTH.

The most common adverse events in patients treated with cinacalcet are nausea and vomiting. The frequency of nausea is unrelated to the dose of cinacalcet, whereas that of vomiting is. These adverse events are mild to moderate in severity and resolve spontaneously in about one-third of patients. The incidence of nausea and vomiting can be reduced by administering cinacalcet with the first meal after dialysis rather than during dialysis. Calcium receptors are present in both the peripheral and central nervous systems, as well as in epithelial cells of the gastrointestinal tract and actions of cinacalcet at some or all these sites might contribute to untoward effects. The dose-dependent increases in vomiting, for example, might result from an action of cinacalcet in the area postrema, a region of the brain that expresses high levels of the calcium receptor. At doses that are used therapeutically to manage 2HPT, cinacalcet has little or no effect on serum levels of a number of different gastrointestinal hormones when measured at two or four hours after dosing.

Transient episodes of hypocalcemia (<7.5mg/mL) occur significantly more often in cinacalcet-treated patients; lowered calcium levels are an expected pharmacodynamic response of cinacalcet resulting from lowered levels of plasma PTH. Episodes of hypocalcemia are rarely associated with clinical symptoms and can be managed by adjusting the dialysate calcium concentration and/or changing the doses of calcium-containing phosphate binders and/or vitamin D sterols, as discussed below.

The collective results of these various prospective clinical trials demonstrate the efficacy and safety of cinacalcet in the treatment of 2HPT in patients on dialysis. A meta-analysis of the Phase 2 and 3 data confirms that treatment with cinacalcet improves mineral metabolism and the proportion of patients that achieve the KDOQI targets.[18]

A number of points deserve mention when considering the clinical results described so far. First, in all these studies, plasma PTH levels were measured 24h after the last dose of drug but prior to the dose on the following day. Yet the maximal decrease in plasma levels of PTH occurs 2–4h after dosing with cinacalcet. Thus, the levels of PTH reported in all these studies are an underestimate of the average levels over a 24h period. A much higher percentage of patients would have achieved the primary end-point if plasma PTH levels were measured at 2–4h after dosing. These studies thus provide a rather conservative estimate of efficacy. Secondly, although the decrease in plasma PTH level is transient, it does not return to baseline within 24h, a time when blood levels of cinacalcet are too low to affect PTH secretion. It is possible that this reflects the ability of calcimimetics to inhibit not only the secretion, but additionally the synthesis of PTH. Thirdly, more than 20% of all patients studied had severe HPT (>800pg/mL) yet most of those treated with cinacalcet achieved the KDOQI target for serum PTH and/or a ≤30% reduction from baseline levels. Thus, the degree of severity of 2HPT does not impact the efficacy of calcimimetics in lowering circulating levels of PTH. Fourthly, daily treatment with cinacalcet maintains plasma PTH at reduced levels for up to 3 years showing that tolerance to the effect of the drug does not develop. Finally, most of the patients studied were already receiving medications to manage 2HPT. For example, in the study of Block et al.,[12] sixty-seven per cent of the total patient population was already taking vitamin D sterols and 93% were taking phosphate binders. So nearly all the patients on 'placebo' were really receiving what was then standard of care. The fact that all these patients had plasma PTH levels >300pg/mL highlights the inadequacy of traditional therapies.

In all the Phase 3 trials, the dose of vitamin D sterol could be changed only for safety reasons; this was necessary to isolate the effect of cinacalcet independent of other medications. Vitamin D sterols can lower plasma levels of PTH, but often do so only at doses that increase serum levels of calcium and phosphate. Indeed, the increase in serum calcium levels likely contributes to the inhibitory effect of vitamin D on plasma levels of PTH. The more recent clinical studies with cinacalcet have therefore examined the combination of this calcimimetic with lower doses of vitamin D sterols.[19–21] In all these studies, it was found that the addition of cinacalcet to conventional therapy (vitamin D sterols plus phosphate binders) was significantly better in lowering plasma levels of PTH and the Ca × P product than was conventional therapy alone (Table 26.1; for reviews see references 22–24). Treatment with cinacalcet increased the percentage of patients achieving KDOQI targets and allowed doses of vitamin D sterols to be reduced by about 50%. Typically, there was an increase in the use of calcium-containing phosphate binders. The OPTIMA study[21] is a head-to-head comparison of best standard of care with cinacalcet, using an algorithm to optimize treatment with phosphate binders and vitamin D sterols, and the combination of these two therapies with cinacalcet. While optimal use of conventional therapy does improve the control of PTH, it does so less effectively than does treatment with cinacalcet combined with phosphate binders and low doses of vitamin D (Table 26.1).

The CONTROL study[20] is noteworthy because plasma levels of PTH were within the KDOQI target, but 79% of these patients had an elevated Ca × P product, perhaps resulting from the use of high doses of vitamin D sterols. Lowering the dose of vitamin D sterols and including cinacalcet permitted better control of the Ca × P product without sacrificing control of PTH levels. In particular, it was possible to lower the dose of vitamin D sterols (by about 20%) and still obtain improvements in KDOQI targets when cinacalcet was added to conventional therapy.

Long-term clinical outcomes

There remains the issue of whether the improvements in biochemical parameters of mineral metabolism obtained with cinacalcet will translate into clinically meaningful outcomes. A retrospective analysis of four similarly designed clinical trials (1184 subjects; 697 cinacalcet-treated subjects) revealed that randomization to cinacalcet significantly reduced the relative risk of parathyroidectomy, fracture, and cardiovascular hospitalization compared with conventional standard of care.[2] There are some small, observational studies with cinacalcet that hint at an improvement in clinical outcomes, but the trials that assess clinical endpoints are still underway. Until these results become available, it is mostly the preclinical results in animal models of 2HPT that offer some optimism for improved clinical outcomes by treating with cinacalcet.

Renal osteodystrophy

Table 26.2 lists the studies that have assessed the effects of cinacalcet on various skeletal parameters in patients with 2HPT. About half of the studies are case reports or include too few subjects to arrive at firm conclusions,[25–29] but significant effects of cinacalcet on markers of bone turnover have been reported in larger, randomized trials.[12,30–32] In general, treatment with cinacalcet decreased plasma levels of the bone formation markers bone-specific alkaline phosphatase (BSAP) and osteocalcin, and the resorption markers tartrate-resistant acid phosphatase (TRAP) and N-terminal telopeptide of type I collagen (NTx). In contrast, these bone turnover markers did not change or increased following treatment with placebo. As mentioned above, placebo in these studies refers to standard of care, and often includes treatment with phosphate-binders and vitamin D sterols.

A couple of studies have reported increases in BMD following treatment with cinacalcet but there are no prospective, appropriately designed studies to assess whether treatment with cinacalcet will increase BMD and/or decrease the risk of fracture. The study of Lien et al.[25] was randomized and placebo-controlled, but included pre-dialysis patients and different treatment regimens with cinacalcet. Nonetheless, when analyzed collectively, treatment with cinacalcet significantly increased BMD and improved the T-score of the proximal femur, but did not affect either parameter in the lumbar spine. There was a positive correlation between femur BMD and absolute decrease in plasma levels of PTH. In the subset of dialysis patients, treatment with cinacalcet resulted in a 2.2% increase in proximal femur BMD, whereas BMD decreased by 1.9% in patients treated with placebo.

Table 26.2 Clinical studies examining the effect of cinacalcet on skeletal parameters. The results are relative to baseline values

Study	Subjects and treatment duration	Results
Block et al. (2004)[12]	HD: 371 cinacalcet, 370 placebo; 26 weeks	Cinacalcet: ↓ BSAPPlacebo: ne on BSAP
Lien et al. (2005)[25]	HD: 6 cinacalcet, 4 placebo; 26 weeks CKD4:2 cinacalcet, 2 placebo; 6 weeks	Cinacalcet: ↑ BMD at proximal femur; ne at L2–L4Placebo: ↓ BMD at femur; ne at L2–L4
Messa et al. (2007)[26]	24 HD; 6 months	↑ OPG, ↓ fetuin-A
Bahner et al. (2008)[27]	HD case study; 13 months	↓ Bone pain
Bergua et al. (2008)[28]	9 renal transplant; 1 year	↑ BMD at radius
Eriguchi et al. (2008)[29]	HD case study; 68 weeks	↓ BSAP and NTx; ↑ BMD at distal radius
Fukagawa et al. (2008)[30]	HD: 72 cinacalcet, 71 placebo; 14 weeks	Cinacalcet: ↓ TRAP and osteocalcin; ne BSAPPlacebo: ne on TRAP, osteocalcin or BSAP
Malluche et al. (2008)[31]	HD: 19 cinacalcet, 13 placebo; 1 year	Cinacalcet: ↓ BSAP and NTx Placebo: ↑ BSAP and NTx
Shigematsu et al. (2009)[32]	199 HD; 1 year	↓ TRAP and NTx; ↑ BSAP at 4 weeks, ↓ at 1 year)

HD, hemodialysis; CKD4, stage 4 chronic kidney disease; OPG, osteoprotegerin; ne, no effect. Other abbreviations are defined in the text.

In only one study were bone biopsy samples collected (iliac crest).[31] At baseline, 84% of patients in each group had high bone turnover as assessed by the numbers of osteoblasts and osteoclasts and the activation frequency. After 1 year of treatment with cinacalcet, there were reductions in activation frequency and bone cell numbers; these parameters were also reduced in the placebo group but to a lesser extent. Treatment with cinacalcet did improve marrow fibrosis compared with the placebo-treated group. Three patients treated with cinacalcet developed adynamic bone disease, but in two of these, plasma levels of PTH were suppressed below 100pg/mL.

The limited clinical data, together with the diverse histologies that comprise renal osteodystrophy in this patient population, do not permit any conclusions to be made concerning the effects of cinacalcet on bone density or quality. Treatment with a calcimimetic, however, causes very striking improvements in bone quality in animal models of 2HPT.[8] Six weeks following a partial nephrectomy, rats developed a mild to moderate 2HPT with profound peritrabecular fibrosis; static and dynamic histomorphometry reveals a high turnover bone lesion. The daily oral administration of

NPS R-568 during the last 5 weeks completely prevented the development of osteitis fibrosa and tended to normalize histomorphometric parameters. Daily treatment with NPS R-568 additionally restored the decreases in volumetric cortical BMD and in cortical bone stiffness at the femoral mid-shaft, which was observed in vehicle-treated animals. Similar improvements in bone quality were observed when rats were treated with cinacalcet.

It has been suggested that daily, transient decreases in plasma levels of PTH caused by the administration of a calcimimetic might achieve qualitatively different effects on bone than sustained decreases in PTH levels.[33] Relevant to this hypothesis are data from a study comparing the effects of intermittent versus continuous administration of NPS R-568 in a rat model of mild 2HPT with a low turnover bone lesion accompanied by osteopenia and osteomalacia.[34] Daily, transient decreases in plasma levels of PTH, achieved by the oral administration of NPS R-568, increased femoral BMD whereas a sustained decrease in PTH, achieved by subcutaneous infusion of the calcimimetic, did not. Thus, intermittent decreases in plasma levels of PTH have markedly different effects on bone than do sustained decreases and, at least in this animal model, have an 'anabolic-like' effect on bone.

An ongoing clinical trial will determine whether any of the beneficial effects of calcimimetics on skeletal parameters noted in animal models will occur in patients on dialysis. The Bone Histomorphometry Assessment for Dialysis Patients with Secondary Hyperparathyroidism of End Stage Renal Disease (BONAFIDE) study will have a primary endpoint of change from baseline in bone formation rate, but it is not powered sufficiently to detect changes in the risk for fracture.

Parathyroid gland hyperplasia

In addition to their inhibitory effects on the synthesis and secretion of PTH, calcimimetics also inhibit parathyroid cell proliferation in animal models of 2HPT.[35,36] The inhibitory effect of calcimimetics on cellular proliferation is specific for parathyroid cells and is not observed in other cells that express the calcium receptor like C-cells or intestinal epithelial cells. Calcimimetics can completely prevent parathyroid gland hyperplasia when treatment is initiated at the time of kidney impairment and can halt the progression of hyperplasia in animals with established 2HPT. Moreover, calcimimetics inhibit parathyroid cell proliferation independently of the level of plasma phosphate and vitamin D. There are some recent clinical findings suggesting that cinacalcet might be able to reduce parathyroid gland hyperplasia in dialysis patients.

High-resolution color Doppler sonography was used to measure parathyroid gland volume in nine dialysis patients with severe 2HPT at baseline and after 24 to 30 months of daily dosing with cinacalcet.[37] Treatment with cinacalcet caused a significant, 68% reduction in the volume of parathyroid glands that had baseline volumes <500mm^3. Parathyroid glands that were larger at baseline ($\geq$500mm^3) were also reduced in size, but not significantly so. Larger glands might contain extensive regions of nodular hyperplasia and there is evidence to suggest that nodular parathyroid cells are less sensitive to regulation by calcimimetic compounds than are cells in areas of diffuse hyperplasia.[38]

Calcific uremic arteriolopathy (calciphylaxis)

This rare, but serious condition is characterized by cutaneous ischemia and necrosis, vascular calcification, and refractory infections; it is typically fatal. There have been three case reports of renal dialysis patients who developed calciphylaxis and who were successfully treated with cinacalcet (the most recent is reference 39). In all cases, treatment with cinacalcet lowered plasma levels of PTH, and normalized serum levels of calcium and phosphate; skin ulcerations healed following several months of treatment.

Vascular calcification and cardiovascular function

Vascular calcification, particularly of the coronary and aortic arteries, is highly predictive of cardiovascular morbidity and mortality in patients with CKD.[40,41] Vascular calcification is a regulated process involving the deposition of calcium and phosphate in atherosclerotic plaques and is associated with increased circulating levels of PTH, calcium and phosphate. Both NPS R-568[42] and cinacalcet[43] have been shown to prevent vascular calcification in animal models of 2HPT. Daily dosing with cinacalcet prevented calcification of the aortic arch and heart as indexed by histological staining with alizarin red or analysis of tissues for elemental calcium and phosphorous. The remodeling of the vasculature, characterized by a shift of smooth muscle cells to an osteoblastic phenotype, was also prevented by treatment with calcimimetics. While a direct action of calcimimetics on vascular calcium receptors might contribute to the prevention of calcification, it does not appear to be a necessary action because parathyroidectomy also prevents vascular calcification in animal models of 2HPT. Thus, the ability of calcimimetics to lower circulating levels of PTH and normalize mineral metabolism appear to be sufficient to prevent vascular calcification in preclinical models of 2HPT.

Improvements in systolic blood pressure, serum cholesterol levels, and cardiac remodeling following treatment with calcimimetics have also been reported in animal models of 2HPT (see reference 8). It is not yet known whether any of these beneficial effects on cardiovascular parameters will occur in dialysis patients treated with cinacalcet. Two prospective studies designed to assess the effects of cinacalcet on clinical outcomes are currently underway.[2] The first (a randomised vascular calcification study to evaluate the effects of cinacalcet; ADVANCE) will assess the ability of cinacalcet to reduce coronary artery calcification in patients on dialysis. The second (evaluation of cinacalcet therapy to lower cardiovascular events; EVOLVE) will determine the ability of cinacalcet to reduce all-cause mortality or first non-fatal cardiovascular event. In both studies, cinacalcet will be combined with lose-dose vitamin D and phosphate binders, and the outcome compared with that obtained by treatment with these conventional therapies alone.

Pediatric patients on dialysis

The effects of cinacalcet in children with 2HPT and on dialysis have been reported.[24] These were observational studies and involved a small number of subjects (total $n = 13$), but in both studies, treatment with cinacalcet caused a significant decrease in plasma levels of PTH compared with baseline.

A concern with the use of cinacalcet in pediatric patients is adverse effects of cinacalcet on growth, particularly because hypertrophic chondrocytes express the calcium receptor. In this respect, it is noteworthy that treatment with cinacalcet did not affect longitudinal bone growth and, in fact, increased body weight gain in a rat model of 2HPT.[44]

Pre-dialysis patients

Cinacalcet has been studied in patients with CKD and 2HPT, but not yet on dialysis.[22] In one study, the baseline level of plasma PTH was 240pg/mL, and 28 and 43% of the patients were on vitamin D sterols and phosphate binders, respectively. In cinacalcet-treated subjects, plasma levels of PTH fell by 33% after 2 weeks and remained at 30–40% of baseline throughout the study, whereas patients receiving placebo maintained PTH levels around baseline. Most patients treated with cinacalcet (56%) reached the primary endpoint ($\geq$30% decline from baseline in levels of PTH). There was a decrease in serum levels of calcium, and an increase in those of phosphate that occurred within 1 week and persisted throughout the study. Twenty-four-hour urinary calcium increased, whereas that of phosphate decreased. All these changes in serum and urine parameters can be explained by a decrease in plasma levels of PTH in the setting of a mostly functional kidney. It is difficult to determine if any of these effects results from actions of cinacalcet on calcium receptors in the kidney because such actions would result in effects very similar to those achieved by lowering plasma levels of PTH. Cinacalcet has not been approved for use in patients with Stage 3 or 4 CKD and its use in this patient population remains controversial.[45,46]

Renal transplant patients.

Kidney transplant in ESRD patients is typically successful and over time the 2HPT spontaneously resolves. However, the time taken to achieve normal bone and mineral metabolism takes several months, and there remain a variable percentage of patients (anywhere from 2 to 20%) that present with persistent 2HPT long after kidney transplantation.[47] Nine independent studies, comprising a total of 83 renal allograft recipients with persistent HPT and treated with cinacalcet for 10 weeks to 6 months, have been summarized by Chonchol and Wüthrich.[48] Treatment with cinacalcet lowered circulating levels of PTH and calcium in most of the patients. Serum phosphate levels did not change in five of the studies and slightly increased in the other three; there was no change in the Ca $\times$ P product. At present, there are no placebo-controlled, prospective studies using cinacalcet in renal transplant patients and cinacalcet is not approved for use in this patient population.

Calcilytics and low turnover renal osteodystrophy

PTH stimulates bone turnover and its net effect on BMD and fracture risk are dependent largely on pharmacokinetics: large, sustained increases in plasma levels of PTH decrease BMD and increase the risk of fracture whereas daily, intermittent increases in PTH increase BMD and decrease fractures. The relationship between circulating levels of PTH and the various skeletal abnormalities that comprise renal osteodystrophy is a long-standing and controversial issue.[49,50] It might well remain so until this pharmacokinetic aspect of PTH physiology is taken into account. In general, however, high levels of plasma PTH, above those recommended by the KDOQI guidelines are associated with a high turnover bone abnormality and osteitis fibrosa, whereas low levels are associated with a low turnover state. In patients with CKD, low bone turnover is almost always associated with decreased bone volume; mineralization can be normal (ABD) or impaired (osteomalacia). Because PTH is such an effective stimulator of bone turnover, the systemic administration of PTH, teriparatide or other related peptides that activate the PTH type 1 receptor might be useful in treating CKD patients with low-turnover forms of renal osteodystrophy. Alternatively, orally administered calcilytics could be used to increase endogenous levels of PTH in CKD patients with these sorts of bone abnormalities.

Two case reports using teriparatide to treat low turnover bone abnormalities have now been published.[51,52] The patients were receiving hemodialysis and had quite distinct disease natural histories, but both had low levels of PTH due to prior parathyroidectomy and both had a low turnover bone lesion. Daily treatment with teriparatide ($20\mu g$, s.c.) for 13 weeks or 18 months increased biochemical markers, and histomorphometric parameters of bone turnover in both patients. Significantly, clinical symptoms (necrosis due to calciphylaxis) improved in one of the patients.[51] The pharmacokinetics of teriparatide in patients receiving hemodialysis is not known, and these preliminary findings could be explained by a continuous or intermittent increase in plasma peptide levels. A decrease in glomerular filtration rate by itself does not impair the ability of teriparatide to increase BMD and decrease fracture incidence in postmenopausal women with osteoporosis.[53] In partially nephrectomized rats, daily subcutaneously administered PTH(1–37), but not continuously infused peptide, increased BMD of both cortical and trabecular bone in the proximal tibia metaphysis.[54] Longitudinal growth was also increased by intermittent, but not continuous administration of peptide. The evidence is thus fragmentary, but given what is known about PTH physiology, and the proven efficacy of PTH and teriparatide in treating osteoporosis, clinical studies of PTH peptides in CKD patients with low turnover renal osteodystrophy and relative hypoparathyroidism are warranted.

Endogenous levels of PTH can be elevated in patients receiving renal replacement therapy by lowering the concentration of calcium in the dialysate. Doing so in patients with ABD increases plasma markers of bone turnover;[55,56] bone formation rate in iliac crest biopsies also increases although the response of individual patients is variable.[57] Increasing plasma levels of PTH by lowering dialysate calcium is functionally equivalent to blocking the parathyroid cell calcium receptor so treatment with a calcilytic might increase bone turnover in patients with CKD and low turnover forms of renal osteodystrophy. Such an approach might be particularly useful in those CKD patients with ABD, but not yet on dialysis. However, and in contrast to exogenously administered peptides, the use of low concentrations of dialysate calcium or treatment with a calcilytic engenders the risk of developing or augmenting parathyroid gland hyperplasia. Indeed, prolonged (2 years) treatment with dialysate containing 1.0mM calcium increased the incidence of severe 2HPT by 2-fold compared with dialysate containing 1.75mM.[58] Although daily administration of a calcilytic for up to 3 months did not stimulate parathyroid cell proliferation in ovariectomized rats, CKD creates a different systemic background and concomitant increases in plasma levels of phosphate and/or decreases in vitamin D might unveil a proliferative effect of calcilytics on parathyroid cells.[8] A short-acting calcilytic that elicits a transient increase in plasma levels of PTH might be sufficient to increase bone turnover without stimulating parathyroid cell proliferation.

Summary

The introduction of calcimimetics into clinical practice has improved the management of 2HPT in patients receiving dialysis. The results obtained so far show that treatment with cinacalcet in combination with phosphate binders and low doses of vitamin D sterols can achieve KDOQI guidelines to an extent not possible with traditional therapy alone and in patients where these therapies fail to lower PTH levels. The unique feature of cinacalcet in comparison to traditional therapies is the inhibition of hormone secretion that results in a rapid lowering of plasma PTH levels. These rapid decreases in PTH levels occur independently of those of phosphate and 1,25-$(OH)_2$vitamin D_3 and reflect the dominant role of the calcium receptor in parathyroid physiology. Targeting this key receptor enables calcimimetics to inhibit several distinct functions including the synthesis and secretion of PTH and parathyroid cell proliferation. It has been suggested that in patients on dialysis, calcimimetics should be a first line therapy; levels of phosphate and calcium can then be managed with phosphate binders and active vitamin D sterols.[60]

Although optimal treatment with cinacalcet and traditional therapies clearly improves the biochemical abnormalities of 2HPT in dialysis patients, it is still uncertain if such effects will translate into clinically meaningful outcomes. The clinical usefulness of cinacalcet in managing 2HPT in patients not on dialysis is likewise uncertain. In these patients the question is not efficacy: cinacalcet is quite effective in lowering plasma levels of PTH in predialysis patients, and it appears to be generally effective in lowering PTH and calcium in renal transplant patients with persistent HPT. Rather, the concern is safety, specifically the mild, but sustained increases in levels of serum phosphate and urinary calcium. As mentioned earlier, these are the expected outcomes of lowering plasma levels of PTH in patients with some degree of kidney function. Additionally, actions of cinacalcet on renal calcium receptors might augment the effect of lowered plasma PTH levels. Fortunately, the pharmacology of the calcium receptor and G protein-coupled receptors in general, allows signaling-specific, activating ligands. It is quite possible to imagine calcimimetic chemotypes that inhibit parathyroid cell proliferation yet have minimal effects on synthesis and/or secretion of PTH and totally lack actions at renal calcium receptors. Therefore, there is reason to suppose that calcimimetics might achieve therapeutic benefits in patients with preserved kidney function. Continued research with cinacalcet in the clinic and with novel calcimimetic chemotypes in animal models of 2HPT is warranted.

Considerably more problematic is the use of calcilytics in low turnover forms of renal osteodystrophy. While the success of exogenously administered PTH peptides in treating osteoporosis provides a solid justification for studying calcilytics in the same indication, such vanguard data are not yet available for CKD patients with low turnover renal osteodystrophy. There are also a number of safety issues inherent in the use of a calcilytic compound that would not apply to exogenously administered PTH peptides. These include the possibility of triggering parathyroid cell proliferation and actions on calcium receptors in other tissues, particularly the skeleton and vascular smooth muscle. Nonetheless, both long and short-acting calcilytics are very effective in stimulating bone turnover and they could prove useful in treating ABD in patients with relative hypoparathyroidism.

References

1. Moe S, Drüeke T, Cunningham J, et al. Definition, evaluation, and classification of renal osteodystrophy: a position statement from Kidney Disease: Improving Global Outcomes (KDIGO). *Kidney Int* 2006;**69**:1945–53.

2. Cunningham J, Floege J, London G, et al. Clinical outcomes in secondary hyperparathyroidism and the potential role of calcimimetics. *NDT Plus* 2008;**1**(Suppl 1):i29–35.

3. Martin KJ, González EA. Metabolic bone disease in chronic kidney disease. *J Am Soc Nephrol* 2007;**18**:875–85.

4. Mucsi I, Hercz G. Relative hypoparathyroidism and adynamic bone disease. *Am J Med Sci* 1999;**317**:405–9.

5. Andress DL. Adynamic bone in patients with chronic kidney disease. *Kidney Int* 2008;**73**:1345–54.

6. Cannata-Andia JB, Carrera F. The pathophysiology of secondary hyperparathyroidism and the consequences of uncontrolled mineral metabolism in chronic kidney disease: the role of COSMOS. *NDT Plus* 2008;**1**(Suppl 1):i2–6.

7. Goodman WG, Quarles LD. Development and progression of secondary hyperparathyroidism in chronic kidney disease: lessons from molecular genetics. *Kidney Int* 2007;**74**:276–88.

8. Nemeth EF. Drugs acting on the calcium receptor: calcimimetics and calcilytics. In: J. P. Bilezikian, L. G. Raisz, & T. J. Martin (eds) *Principles of Bone Biology*, 3rd edn. New York: Academic Press, 2008a:1711–35.

9. Nemeth EF. Anabolic therapy for osteoporosis: calcilytics. *IBMS BoneKEy* 2008b;**5**:196–208.

10. Mendoza FJ, Lopez I, Canalejo R, et al. Direct upregulation of parathyroid calcium-sensing receptor and vitamin D receptor by calcimimetics in uremic rats. *Am J Physiol Renal Physiol* 2008;**296**:F605–13.

11. Chang W, Tu C, Chen T-H, et al. The extracellular calcium-sensing receptor (CaSR) is a critical modulator of skeletal development. *Sciencesignaling* 2008;**1**:1–13.

12. Block GA, Martin KJ, de Francisco ALM, et al. Cinacalcet for secondary hyperparathyroidism in patients receiving hemodialysis. *N Engl J Med* 2004;**350**:1516–67.

13. Lindberg JS, Culleton B, Wong G, et al. Cinacalcet HCl, an oral calcimimetic agent for the treatment of secondary hyperparathyroidism in hemodialysis and peritoneal dialysis: a randomised, double-blind, multicenter study. *J Am Soc Nephrol* 2005;**16**:800–7.

14. Moe SM, Chertow GM, Coburn, JW, et al. Achieving NKF-K/DOQI TM bone metabolism and disease treatment goals with cinacalcet HCl. *Kidney Int* 2005;**67**:760–71.

15. Moe SM, Cunningham J, Bommer J, et al. Long-term treatment of secondary hyperparathyroidism with the calcimimetic cinacalcet HCl. *Nephrol Dial Transplant* 2005;**20**:2186–93.

16. Valle C, Rodriguez M, Santamaria R, et al. Cinacalcet reduces the set point of the PTH-calcium curve. *J Am Soc Nephrol* 2008;**19**:2430–6.

17. Martin KJ, Jüppner H, Sherrard DJ, et al. First-and second-generation immunometric PTH assays during treatment of hyperparathyroidism with cinacalcet HCl. *Kidney Int.* 2005;**68**:1236–43.

18. Strippoli GFM, Palmer S, Tong A, et al. Meta-analysis of biochemical and patient-level effects of calcimimetic therapy. *Am J Kidney Dis* 2006;**47**:715–26.

19. Block GA, Zeig S, Sugihara J et al. Combined therapy with cinacalcet and low doses of vitamin D sterols in patients with moderate to severe secondary hyperparathyroidism. *Nephrol Dial Transplant* 2008;**23**:2311–18.

20. Chertow GM, Blumenthal S, Turner S, et al. Cinacalcet hydrochloride (Sensipar) in hemodialysis patients on active vitamin D derivatives with controlled PTH and elevated calcium x phosphate. *Clin J Am Soc Nephrol* 2006;**1**:305–12.

21. Messa P, Macário F, Yaqoob M et al. The OPTIMA study: assessing a new cinacalcet (Sensipar/Mimpara) treatment algorithm for secondary hyperparathyroidism. *Clin J Am Soc Nephrol* 2008;**3**:36–45.

22. Evenepoel P. Calcimimetics in chronic kidney disease: evidence, opportunities and challenges. *Kidney Intl* 2008;**74**:265–75.

23. Bushinsky DA, Piergiorgio M. Efficacy of early treatment with calcimimetics in combination with reduced doses of vitamin D sterols in dialysis patients. *NDT Plus* 2008;**1**(Suppl 1):i18–23.

24. Schlieper G, Floege J. Calcimimetics in CKD—results from recent clinical studies. *Pediatr Nephrol* 2008;**23**:1721–8.

25. Lien Y-HH, Silva AL, Whittman D. Effects of cinacalcet on bone mineral density in patients with secondary hyperparathyroidism. *Nephrol Dial Transplant* 2005;**20**:1232–7.

26. Messa P, Alerti L, Como G, et al. Calcimimetic increases osteoprotegerin and decreases fetuin-A levels in dialysis patients. *Nephrol Dial Transplant* 2007;**22**:2724–5.

27. Bahner U, Brandl M, Nies C, et al. Use of cinacalcet HCl to achieve the recommended targets of bone metabolism in a patient with therapy-resistant renal hyperparathyroidism. *J Renal Nutr* 2008;**18**:383–8.

28. Bergua C, Torregrosa J-V, Fuster D, et al. Effect of cinacalcet on hypercalcemia and bone mineral density in renal transplanted patients with secondary hyperparathyroidism. *Transplant* 2008;**86**:413–17.

29. Eriguchi R, Umakoshi J, Tominaga Y, et al. Successful treatment of inoperable recurrent secondary hyperparathyroidism with cinacalcet HCl. *NDT Plus* 2008;**4**:218–20.

30. Fukagawa M, Yumita S, Akizawa T, et al. Cinacalcet (KRN1493) effectively decreases the serum intact PTH level with favorable control of the serum phosphorous and calcium levels in Japanese dialysis patients. *Nephrol Dial Transplant* 2008;**23**:328–35.

31. Malluche HH, Monier-Faugere MC, Wang G, et al. An assessment of cinacalcet HCl effects on bone histology in dialysis patients with secondary hyperparathyroidism. *Clin Nephrol* 2008;**69**:269–77.

32. Shigematsu T, Akizawa T, Uchida E, et al. Long-term cinacalcet HCl treatment improved bone metabolism in Japanese hemodialysis patients with secondary hyperparathyroidism. *Am J Nephrol* 2009;**29**:230–6.

33. Nemeth EF, Bennett SA. Tricking the parathyroid gland with novel calcimimetic agents. *Nephrol Dial Trans* 1998;**13**:1923–5.

34. Ishii H, Wada M, Furuya Y, et al. Daily intermittent decreases in serum levels of parathyroid hormone have an anabolic-like action on the bones of uremic rats with low-turnover bone and osteomalacia. *Bone* 2000;**26**:175–82.

35. Wada M, Nagano N. Control of parathyroid cell growth by calcimimetics. *Nephrol Dial Transplant* 2003;**18**(Suppl):iii13–17.

36. Drüeke TB, Martin D, Rodriguez M. Can calcimimetics inhibit parathyroid hyperplasia? Evidence from preclinical studies. *Nephrol Dial Transplant* 2007;**22**:1828–39.

37. Meola M, Petrucci B, Barsotti G. Long-term treatment with cinacalcet and conventional therapy reduces parathyroid hyperplasia in severe secondary hyperparathyroidism. *Nephrol Dial Transplant* 2009;**24**:982–9.

38. Komaba H, Fukagawa M. Regression of parathyroid hyperplasia by calcimimetics—fact or illusion? *Nephrol Dial Transplant* 2009;**24**:707–9.

39. Mohammed IA, Sekar V, Bubtana AJ, et al. Proximal calciphylaxis treated with calcimimetic 'cinacalcet'. *Nephrol Dial Transplant* 2008;**23**:387–9.

40. AUaggi P, Kleerekoper M. Contribution of bone and mineral abnormalities to cardiovascular disease in patients with chronic kidney disease. *Clin J Am Soc Nephrol* 2008;**3**:836–43.

41. London GM. Bone-vascular axis in chronic kidney disease: a reality? *Clin J Am Soc Nephrol* 2009;**4**:254–7.

42. Koleganova N, Piecha G, Ritz E, et al. A calcimimetic (R-568), but not calcitriol, prevents vascular remodeling in uremia. *Kidney Int* 2009;**75**:60–71.

43. Kawata, T, Nagano N, Obi M, et al. Cinacalcet suppresses calcification of the aorta and heart in uremic rats. *Kidney Int* 2008;**74**:1270–7.

44. Nakagawa K, Pérez EC, Oh J, et al. Cinacalcet does not affect longitudinal growth but increases body weight gain in experimental uremia. *Nephrol Dial Transplant* 2008;**23**:2761–7.

45. Coyne DW. Cinacalcet should not be used to treat secondary hyperparathyroidism in stage 3–4 chronic kidney disease. *Nature Clin Prac Nephrol* 2008;**4**:364–5.

46. de Francisco ALM, Piñera C, Palomar R. Cinacalcet should be used to treat secondary hyperparathyroidism in stage 3–4 chronic kidney disease. *Nature Clin Pract Nephrol* 2008;**4**:366–7.

47. Sprague SM, Belozeroff V, Danese MD, et al. Abnormal bone and mineral metabolism in kidney transplant patients—a review. *Am J Nephrol* 2008;**28**:246–53.

48. Chonchol M, Wüthrich RP. Potential future uses of calcimimetics in patients with chronic kidney disease. *NDT Plus* 2008;**1**(Suppl 1):i36–41.

49. Goodman WG. Comments on plasma parathyroid hormone levels and their relationship to bone histopathology among patients undergoing dialysis. *Sem Dialysis* 2007;**20**:1–4.

50. Drüeke TB. Is parathyroid hormone measurement useful for the diagnosis of renal bone disease? *Kidney Int* 2008;**73**:674–6.

51. Elder G, Kumar KS. Calciphylaxis associated with chronic kidney disease and low bone turnover: management with recombinant human PTH-(1–34). *NDT Plus* 2008;**2**:97–9.

52. Lehmann G, Ott U, Maiwald J, et al. Bone histomorphometry after treatment with teriparatide (PTH 1-34) in a patient with adynamic bone disease subsequent to parathyroidectomy. *NDT Plus* 2008;**2**:49–51.

53. Miller PD, Schwartz EN, Chen P, et al. Teriparatide in postmenopausal women with osteoporosis and mild or moderate renal impairment. *Osteoporosis Int* 2007;**18**:59–68.

54. Schmitt CP, Hessing S, Oh J, et al. Intermittent administration of parathyroid hormone (1-37) improves growth and bone mineral density in uremic rats. *Kidney Int* 2000;**57:**1484–92.

55. Hamano T, Oseto S, Fujii N, et al. Impact of lowering dialysate calcium concentration on serum bone turnover markers in hemodialysis patients. *Bone* 2005;**36:**909–16.

56. Spasovski G, Gelev S, Masin-Spasovska J, et al. Improvement of bone and mineral parameters related to a dynamic bone disease by diminishing dialysate calcium. *Bone* 2007;**41:**698–703.

57. Haris A, Sherrard DJ, Hercz G. Reversal of a dynamic bone disease by lowering dialysate calcium. *Kidney Int* 2006;**70:**931–7.

58. Weinreich T, Ritz E, Passlick-Deetjen J. Long term dialysis with low-calcium solution (1.0mmol/l) in CAPD: Effects on bone mineral metabolism. *Periton Dial Int* 1996;**16:**260–8.

59. Wetmore JB, Quarles LD. Calcimimetics or vitamin D analogs for suppressing parathyroid hormone in end-stage renal disease: time for a paradigm shift? *Nature Clin Prac Nephrol* 2009;**5:**24–33.

Chapter 27

Medical therapy in chronic kidney disease

John Cunningham, Ewa Lewin, and
Justin Silver

Introduction

Management of mineral metabolism in the CKD patient aims to deal effectively with the complex interrelated series of perturbations that accompany progressive reduction of GFR. In this context, it is important not to lose sight of the two principle clinical endpoints that really matter to patients, namely loss of skeletal integrity and accelerated cardiovascular disease. Both of these are associated with serious morbidity and mortality. Some of these pathologies are difficult or impossible to reverse, leaving the patient with an indelible disease imprint. Current treatment strategies have evolved largely from an improved understanding of underlying pathophysiology and the belief, in some cases amounting to little more than hope (sometimes forlorn), that interventions that ameliorate or correct these abnormalities will translate to improved outcomes for patients. Unfortunately, this is by no means always the case and there is a conspicuous lack of robust evidence to support the utility of the majority of interventions that are made, particularly in the context of clinically relevant outcomes.

The perturbations that arise during the development of progressive CKD can be considered as primary or adaptive. Examples of the former are the failure of the diseased kidney to bioactivate vitamin D and a resulting deficiency of hormonal calcitriol. Similarly, a progressive failure to excrete phosphate can also be seen as a primary abnormality, and both this and the vitamin D disturbance can be detected quite early in the development of CKD. In the case of calcitriol generation, studies have shown significant reduction of mean plasma calcitriol when as little as 25% of GFR has been lost. Although plasma phosphate is well compensated until quite advanced CKD, adaptive responses to both the fall in calcitriol and the tendency of phosphate to rise, are detectable much earlier—PTH rises can be seen in an increasing number of patients as the GFR falls below 70% of normal, as can changes to the renal tubular handling of phosphate.[1] Further adaptive changes take place in the parathyroid glands with structural alterations to allow increased synthesis and release of PTH—changes that carry both benefits and drawbacks.[2] These changes are also associated with parallel abnormalities of the vasculature with a pronounced tendency towards medial calcification and the functional disturbances that go with this.

Specific treatment aspects in CKD stages 2–4

It is important to recognize that many of these patients remain 'under the radar' in respect of any medical attention at all, let alone from specialist nephrologists. In some ways this reflects the effectiveness of some of the adaptive responses and underlying redundancy, although increasingly a price is paid by patients in whom appropriate interventions are delayed.

Secondary hyperparathyroidism (2HPT) develops in the majority of untreated patients at this stage of CKD. Evidence that it is driven by a combination of inadequate synthesis of calcitriol by the kidney and impairment of normal renal phosphate handling encourages the notion that treatment should comprise replacement of deficient calcitriol and attempts to correct the abnormal renal phosphate handling. Deficiency of native vitamin D is endemic in this patient group and associates with 2HPT and other metabolic and vascular disturbances.[3] The significance, identification and treatment of vitamin D deficiency are discussed later in the chapter.

Replacement of deficient calcitriol using 'active' vitamin D compounds

This is generally straightforward. Any of the naturally occurring or semi synthetic vitamin D compounds can be used—calcitriol, paricalcitol and 22-oxacalcitriol all bind directly to the nuclear vitamin D receptor and are capable of substituting for the deficient hormone in any tissue in which it is expressed. Alfacalcidol (1α-hydroxyvitamin D_3) and doxercalciferol (1α-hydroxyvitamin D_2) are prodrugs that require hepatic 25-hydroxylation (unimpaired in CKD) for activation. All effectively obviate the need for renal 1α-hydroxylation and are highly effective in this setting. There is little evidence for a clinically significant advantage of any one of these metabolites over the others in this patient group,[4] although limited data have suggested that paricalcitol may be less calcemic and calciuric than some of the others.[5] Implementation of active vitamin D therapies at this stage has potentially beneficial effects to retard developing hyperparathyroidism and improves the abnormal bone histology associated with hyperparathyroidism.[6] Whether or not this translates to an improvement in the mechanical integrity of the skeleton is less clear, however.

Phosphate restriction

The failure of the diseased kidney to excrete phosphate properly is compensated in early and moderate CKD by progressive decreases in the tubular reabsorption of phosphate (TRP), driven by a combination of increasing hyperparathyroidism and increasing circulating levels of the phosphatonin, FGF23. These hormones serve to maintain serum phosphate within the normal range in the face of marked reduction of GFR until the final decompensation that inevitably occurs in advanced CKD. Predictably, the maintenance of normal serum phosphate in the face of increasing CKD can be sabotaged by measures that decrease PTH by targeting the parathyroids directly. Because these measures include therapeutic administration of active vitamin D compounds, we have the dilemma whereby the appropriate correction of the disturbance to the vitamin D endocrine system is likely to exacerbate the disturbed phosphate metabolism. Additional difficulties arise because active vitamin D metabolites used to treat hypocalcemia or hyperparathyroidism also up regulate intestinal phosphate absorption. A logical way around this is to implement dietary phosphate restriction, and/or oral phosphate binders, early in the genesis of CKD, perhaps even before serum phosphate has risen above the normal range. Experimentally such maneuvers are extremely effective in ameliorating the development of hyperparathyroidism and hyperparathyroid bone disease,[7] although evidence for this is less strong in clinical studies. Some work, particularly in children, does suggest that improvements to phosphate metabolism, hyperparathyroidism, and vitamin D metabolism may be generated by appropriate dietary phosphate restriction.[8] Benefits at the level of clinical outcomes have been harder to establish, though growth rate improved in children with CKD treated with aluminium hydroxide or calcium carbonate.[9]

Calcimimetics

Preliminary studies with calcimimetics have yielded disappointing results. Useful reduction of PTH has been accompanied by significant and problematic increases in serum phosphate, which would probably increase the need for phosphate binders in early CKD.

Despite these uncertainties, a logical way to proceed at this level is to use PTH as the initial trigger for intervention and not to wait for overt elevation of plasma phosphate, which arises later. Based on the known pathophysiology, it makes sense to construct the initial therapy with a combination of dietary phosphate restriction (or a phosphate binder), and a physiological dose of calcitriol or one of the other active vitamin D compounds discussed above. This implies giving calcitriol at a low dose—0.125μg daily, or equivalent for the other compounds, for example, with a phosphate binder given at modest dose. No therapies that specifically target the FGF23 disturbance are available.

Specific treatment aspects in CKD stages 5 and 5D

In these patients the adaptive responses to a fall in GFR are more extreme, but increasingly futile. Overt decompensation is evident. Untreated patients almost all manifest increasingly severe 2HPT at this stage, although those who have been vigorously, and perhaps over vigorously, treated during early stages of CKD will generally avoid hyperparathyroidism and might even fall to the other pathological extreme, namely adynamic bone disease. The vast majority of these patients will be significantly hyperphosphatemic and calcitriol concentration, if measured, is profoundly reduced. Standard treatment centers around prevention of hyperphosphatemia and therapies directly aimed at the overactive parathyroid gland, namely active vitamin D compounds and/or calcimimetic compounds. Adynamic bone disease is an increasingly important issue in these patients.[10] A reasonably well established collection of risk factors predispose to this, of which one of the most important is over zealous treatment of HPT in earlier stages of the CKD. There is considerable debate as to why this should be the case—the pathogenesis of adynamic bone disease is discussed in detail elsewhere, but the association between low PTH and adynamic bone disease has led to the view that the target for PTH should be set substantially above the upper limit of normal, and increasingly so as CKD progresses.[11] As in patients at earlier stages of CKD, there are potentially important conflicts between some of the available therapies. Thus, active vitamin D metabolites used to treat hypocalcemia or hyperparathyroidism almost invariably exacerbate problems with hyperphosphatemia—calcitriol is a potent up regulator of intestinal phosphate absorption. Furthermore, in some patients active vitamin D compounds given to treat hyperparathyroidism only do so at the expense of unacceptable rises of serum calcium. In this group of patients calcimimetics have a useful role in that they exert downward pressure on both PTH and calcium, and to a lesser extent on phosphate as well.[12]

In CKD 5D patients, manipulation of dialysis is also a potentially useful lever. Most striking are the beneficial effects that follow from a substantial increase in dialysis dose by using daily dialysis regimes.[13] These patients experience dramatic improvements in phosphate control, in many cases obviating the need for phosphate binders and occasionally even requiring phosphate supplementation. There is some evidence also that daily dialysis attenuates the underlying state of vitamin D deficiency seen in many dialysis patients.[14] Using more conventional dialysis regimens, worsening hyperphosphatemia is one of many unwanted consequences of under-dialysis of any cause. Choice of dialysate calcium concentration is also important when it comes to achieving satisfactory biochemical outcomes, although to what extent this translates to improved clinical outcomes is unclear. For example, the use of calcium-based phosphate binders is frequently associated with unwanted hypercalcemic episodes, the frequency of which can be reduced substantially by reducing the dialysate calcium concentration.[15]

In patients with adynamic bone disease, PTH may be increased by stimulating the patient's own parathyroids using a low calcium dialysate that gives the patient a burst of mild hypocalcemia at the time of each dialysis. Data exist to show that PTH increases significantly under such regimens and that there is an improvement in bone metabolism as judged by histological examinations and bone markers.[16] Patient level outcomes, such as fracture rate in response to these therapies are unknown.

Preventative measures

When considering these, it is sensible to pay attention to pathological developments that are potentially irreversible. It is here that prevention is particularly important. Three separate areas may be considered.

Parathyroid hyperplasia

Persisting stimulation of the parathyroid glands is associated with parathyroid cell hypertrophy and also increased proliferative activity. The former is largely reversible when down-regulatory inputs are applied to the parathyroids, but the latter appears to be essentially irreversible.[2] Parathyroid hyperplasia is, therefore, an entity that it is well worth avoiding because the only well established therapies for dealing with it revolve around surgery or other destructive measures. Vitamin D therapies become increasingly ineffective or are not tolerated as nodular hyperplasia progresses and, although calcimimetics remain effective in some of these patients, this is by no means always the case. Avoidance of parathyroid hyperplasia implies control of the principle stimulatory inputs, namely hypocalcemia, hyperphosphatemia, and failure of adequate suppressive input via the parathyroid vitamin D receptor. Achieving these objectives is not always easy in practice.

Skeletal integrity

Derangements to skeletal metabolism can fall within a wide spectrum in patients with advanced CKD, ranging from extremely low turnover adynamic bone disease to greatly accelerated high turnover hyperparathyroid disease. At both these extremes there is very marked impairment of mechanical integrity with increased fracture rate, bone pain, and in children failure of growth. Severe hyperparathyroid bone disease appears to respond well to measures that successfully reduce circulating PTH.[6] Less clear, however, is the extent to which the disturbed mechanical integrity reverts to premorbid levels—no studies have systematically examined this issue. At the other extreme, adynamic bone disease may be symptomatic and is a much more intractable lesion for which the only measures that have proved effective thus far are those designed to increase PTH—nearly all these patients have relatively low circulating PTH concentration.

Vascular calcification

This complication of CKD-MBD has important implications for cardiovascular health and mortality. No clinical evidence exists for useful reversibility although certain measures have been shown to retard further progression of established vascular calcification. The use of calcium free, rather than calcium based phosphate binders[17] has been shown to slow the progression of vascular calcification and an ongoing study using calcimimetics (ADVANCE) will also probe the possibility that calcimimetic treatment has a useful impact on the development of vascular calcification.

Management of advanced hyperparathyroidism

Many patients with CKD develop hyperparathyroidism despite the strict encouragement of adherence to preventative measures as outlined in this chapter. However, it requires a disciplined patient to adhere to a demanding medical regime when the only benefits are biochemical and complications that seem so distant, and this in addition to the other endless intrusions of being a dialysis patient. Many patients end up with hyperparathyroidism that often becomes remarkably advanced with serious skeletal and cardiovascular complications. The standard therapy of dietary advice, oral phosphorus binders, increased dialysis times, vitamin D analogues, where the serum phosphorus allows it, and calcimimetic drugs become ineffective and the patient requires parathyroidectomy. There is anecdotal evidence that calcimimetics in high doses for a prolonged period may be effective in some of these patients.

The indications for parathyroidectomy are:

◆ Persistent hypercalcemia despite stopping all calcium containing phosphorus binders.

- Persistent severe hyperphosphatemia despite intensive use of non-calcium containing phosphorus binders proportional to the food ingested at meals and increased dialysis time.
- Progressive and symptomatic soft tissue calcification with high bone turnover, including calcific uremic arteriolopathy (calciphylaxis).
- Severe progressive and symptomatic hyperparathyroidism despite intensive vitamin D analogue and calcimimetic therapy.
- Refractory pruritus.

The surgical approaches are either subtotal parathyroidectomy or total parathyroidectomy with parathyroid autotransplantation. There is no trial that prescribes the superiority of one approach over the other. There is successful experience, mainly in Japan, of parathyroid ablation by direct injection of the parathyroids with ethanol or active vitamin D compounds under sensitive ultrasound guidance.

Treatment of hyperphosphatemia

CKD is associated with development of hyperphosphatemia. The main causes are renal phosphate retention and disturbed bone formation. In early CKD renal excretion of phosphate is stimulated by enhanced levels of the phosphaturic hormones, FGF23 and PTH. Furthermore, the intestinal phosphate absorption is mildly impaired due to disturbed vitamin D metabolism and serum phosphate levels might therefore be normal or even slightly lower than normal in the early stages of renal failure. During the progression of CKD, phosphate retention eventually occurs, when GFR is reduced to below 25–20mL/min.

Control of hyperphosphatemia is a key therapeutic target in the management of CKD patients. Hyperphosphatemia is a cardiovascular risk factor in CKD. It was shown in epidemiological studies that serum phosphate is an independent risk factor for cardiovascular events and mortality in uremia. The pathogenesis is linked to the phosphate mediated induction of vascular calcification. In *in vitro* studies phosphate induced transformation of the phenotype of vascular smooth muscle cells from a contractile cell to a secretory cell expressing markers of osteoblastic lineage cell. Expression of these markers, osteopontin, osteocalcin, alkaline phosphatase, bone morphogenic proteins and the osteoblast specific transcription factors, RUNX2 and osterix was also demonstrated in the calcified vasculature of uremic patients. Recently, it was demonstrated in an *in vivo* model of atherosclerotic LDL receptor deficient mice with CKD, that hyperphosphatemia is a direct cause of vascular calcifications and that the skeleton is a significant contributor to hyperphosphatemia along with phosphate retention.[18]

Maintenance of normal skeletal remodeling

In experimental CKD, it has been shown that stimulation of bone formation and correction of adynamic bone disease by bone morphogenic protein 7 (BMP 7) treatment, resulted in correction of hyperphosphatemia, due to BMP7-driven stimulation of skeletal phosphate deposition.[18] This points toward a role of the skeleton in phosphate homeostasis and in the control of the levels of serum phosphate. Both low and elevated rates of skeletal remodeling contribute to hyperphosphatemia in CKD, due to excess bone resorption uncoupled to formation. Proper management of hyperphosphatemia would include the maintenance of normal skeletal remodeling. In uremia, the physiological levels of PTII are insufficient to maintain skeletal remodeling due to the complex phenomenon of skeletal resistance to the action of PTH. Therefore, PTH levels should be slightly elevated, as recommended in the published guidelines.[11]

Hopefully, new anabolic agents will be developed to treat the impaired skeletal remodeling in CKD. BMP 7 is a promising candidate.

Dietary phosphate restriction

Dietary phosphate restriction is the first step in the control of hyperphosphatemia. Food high in proteins such as meat and dairy products contribute with the largest amounts to the total dietary phosphate intake. Whole grain bread, nuts, fish and poultry are also high in this mineral. A significant increase in the daily intake of phosphate is due to the increasing use of industrial food processing practices, employing addition of phosphate. The usual intake of phosphate by normal adults is 1–1.8g per day. The phosphate-containing food additives contribute an estimated 470mg/day to an adult's daily phosphate intake in the United States.[19] Sixty per cent of dietary phosphate intake is absorbed. The bioavailability of phosphate varies in the different food sources. (See review by Uribarri J, *Semin Dial,* 2007). About 75% of phosphate from plants is in the form of phytate and is not bioavailable in the human intestine as the phytase enzyme is not secreted in humans. Phosphate from meat is easily digestible and well absorbed. Phosphate added in food processing is mostly in the form of inorganic salts and is almost completely absorbed.[19] Dietary phosphate restriction therefore requires prescription of a moderate protein intake and restricted consumption of highly processed food. This is only possible under supervision of a specialized renal dietician. Dietary restriction of phosphate intake to below 800mg/day is not recommended, since this will have a negative effect on the protein intake.

Adequate protein intake in dialysis patients of a minimum of 1g/kg/day is necessary to maintain a near neutral nitrogen balance, but will also increase the intake of phosphate. In patients on long-term dialysis, urinary excretion of phosphate is usually minimal. Therefore, phosphate balance is primarily determined by the net amount absorbed by the bowel and the quantity removed during dialysis therapy. Conventional dialysis regimes provide inadequate removal of phosphate from the circulation. Administration of compounds that bind phosphate in the bowel are necessary in dialysis patients and in advanced renal failure.

Oral phosphate binding agents

Oral phosphate binding agents (P-binders) lower the intestinal phosphate absorption by creating poorly soluble complexes in the intestinal tract. No interventional randomized controlled trials have examined the impact on survival of the reduction of serum phosphate by phosphate binder treatment. A recent epidemiological study by Isakova et al.,[20] based on a large cohort of incident hemodialysis patients tested the hypothesis that therapy with any P-binder versus none would be associated with survival benefit, and it was demonstrated that treatment with phosphate binder was independently associated with an improved survival. Phosphate binders, which are currently used in the clinical practice, include calcium-based agents, such as calcium carbonate and calcium acetate, and the non-calcium containing agents, sevelamer hydrochloride and lanthanum carbonate. All are effective at reducing serum phosphate levels. Calcium carbonate is widely used and is inexpensive. It contains, however, a high amount of elemental calcium and large doses are often necessary to attain sufficient control of serum phosphate. This may lead to hypercalcemia. Compared with calcium carbonate, calcium acetate has twice the binding capacity for phosphate per calcium absorbed. Whether use of calcium acetate might decrease the incidence of hypercalcemia is unknown. Hypercalcemia is the major side effect, associated with long-term use of calcium salts, either with or without concomitant vitamin D therapy. The case against the calcium-based P-binders has been accumulating for years, and their potential to contribute to total body calcium overload in CKD patients is an important clinical concern. However, no strong evidence is available to answer this question.

Results from observational studies indicate that exposure to calcium overload from P-binders is associated with increased aortic stiffness, measured by pulse wave velocity, and increased aorta calcification score in hemodialysis patients. Furthermore, a significant interaction was found between dosage of calcium containing P-binders and bone activity, indicating that a calcium load had a significantly greater impact on aorta calcifications in the presence of an adynamic bone disease.[21]

The major concern regarding the impact of the high calcium load, associated with the use of calcium-based P-binders, has lead to research towards development of non-calcium containing P-binders. The drug best examined in the clinical situation and, as such, the most promising is at present sevelamer hydrochloride. It is a synthetic non-absorbed polymer, which besides having phosphate binding capacity is a bile acid sequestrant, lowering cholesterol levels.

In a small study 129 patients, new to hemodialysis, were randomized to receive either calcium containing P-binders or sevelamer, and the effect on the development of coronary calcifications was evaluated.[22] At baseline, one-third of patients had no evidence of coronary artery calcifications. These subjects with zero calcification score did not develop significant calcifications for the next 18 months, despite calcium loading. Patients, who had significant calcifications at baseline showed progressive increases in the calcification score in both treatment arms. Use of calcium containing P-binders was combined with a more rapid progression of coronary calcifications than sevelamer. It is currently a matter of discussion, whether this potentially beneficial effect of sevelamer was due to a diminished calcium load. The sevelamer treated patients had significantly lower levels of LDL cholesterol. Thus, a reduction of cholesterol levels and not necessarily the reduced calcium load may provide an explanation for the reduced rate of cardiovascular calcifications. As such, in another small study on 203 prevalent hemodialysis patients, where statins were used to control the levels of

LDL cholesterol and the patients were treated either with calcium acetate or sevelamer, a similar progression of calcification was experienced.[23] A recent investigation on 101 hemodialysis patients tested the hypothesis that calcium containing P-binders might have a negative impact on bone remodeling, and thus might contribute to the progression of cardiovascular calcifications.[24] Bone biopsis were obtained at the entry and after 12 months of treatment with sevelamer or calcium acetate. There was no difference in the progression of calcifications or in the changes in bone remodeling. Similar results were obtained when the effect on bone of sevelamer was compared with that of calcium carbonate in 119 hemodialysis patients.[25] Treatment for 12 months with sevelamer resulted in no statistically significant changes in bone turnover or mineralization as compared with calcium carbonate.

Finally, in a large trial on prevalent hemodialysis patients, a total of 2103 patients were randomized to treatment with either calcium based P-binder or sevelamer. Surprisingly, all-cause mortality rate and cause-specific mortality (cardiovascular, infection, and others) rates were not significantly different in the two groups.[26] As such, lack of solid outcome data makes it difficult to justify the widespread utilization of sevelamer as first-line of therapy. The choice of agents should be individualized, depending upon the clinical circumstances. Sevelamer is currently the only agent that in prospective studies has demonstrated reduced progression of vascular calcifications, as compared with calcium-containing products. Patient groups with already established vascular calcifications are more likely to benefit from this therapy. As such, sevelamer hydrochloride might be considered as first-line of therapy in patients having extraskeletal and vascular calcifications. The mechanism and the relative importance of avoiding a calcium load versus a specific effect of sevelamer hydrochloride, awaits further elucidation. It remains also to be shown whether this effect might be shared by the other compounds, capable of reducing serum phosphate without increasing the calcium load.

The use of sevelamer hydrochloride in pre-dialysis stages of CKD is limited by its potential for aggravating the metabolic acidosis. Sevelamer carbonate has recently been tested in CKD patients not on dialysis. The compound was well-tolerated and effective in controlling plasma phosphate and plasma bicarbonate levels.

Lanthanum carbonate is a powerful P-binder which has the potential to reduce the pill burden and increase the patient compliance, as compared with other P-binders. It is well tolerated. Compared with calcium-based P-binders, lanthanum carbonate treatment was associated with a reduced incidence of hypercalcemia. However, to date, there are no data suggesting an advantage on morbidity and mortality with lanthanum carbonate, compared with other P-binders. An extremely low bioavailability and negligible renal clearance following oral administration has been documented in normal subjects. However, there is theoretical concern about the deposition of lanthanum, a rare earth element, in bone and liver. The rate of absorption of lanthanum is enhanced in chronic renal failure. Although no evidence of bone toxicity was found in dialysis patients after 1 year of treatment with lanthanum carbonate, a significant deposition of lanthanum was shown in bones. Once lanthanum enters bone tissue, its release is very slow, as lanthanum levels in bone remained detectable during the following two year of washout. In a cross-sectional study performed in 11 patients, who had been receiving lanthanum carbonate for 4–5 years, bone lanthanum concentrations were higher compared with patients, who had received lanthanum for 1 or 2 years, suggesting a progressive accumulation of lanthanum in bone.[6] These observations might have clinical implications for the long-term therapeutic use of lanthanum carbonate.[27] Although lanthanum carbonate is believed to be non-toxic, as compared with other forms of lanthanum, the long-term accumulation and long-term residence time in the body after stopping the administration requires detailed monitoring of the potential long term effects. In this respect, a recent report on its use for 6 years was without evidence of harmful side effects.

Use of P-binders containing aluminum leads to aluminum accumulation and its sequelae, such as osteomalacia, dementia, myopathy, and anemia. No safe dose of aluminum has been identified and aluminum salts should not be used in CKD patients. When there is a need for a short-term rescue therapy to achieve acute control of high phosphate levels lanthanum carbonate might be used instead.

The use of P-binders containing magnesium in conjunction with a dialysate low in magnesium may be efficacious. Recently, interest in magnesium salts has been revived due to the potential beneficial effect of magnesium on cardiovascular health. Whether administration of magnesium containing P-binders may reduce cardiac arrhythmias and vascular calcifications in dialysis patients needs to be evaluated in prospective studies. Large doses of magnesium will cause diarrhea and thus limit its use.

Recently, addition of salivary P-binding to the traditional treatment with P-binders has been proposed. An increase in salivary phosphate excretion, independent from food intake, was observed in CKD patients. Use of chitosan-loaded chewing gum in fasting periods significantly reduced serum phosphate levels.[28]

Dialysis treatment

An important cause of hyperphosphatemia is poor compliance, related both to dietary phosphate restriction and P-binder therapy. The effect of standard dialysis treatment on serum phosphate is relatively limited, due to the high volume of distribution of phosphate. There is a rapid rebound of serum phosphate after dialysis. Phosphate removal may be significantly improved by use of longer or more frequent dialysis. Daily or noctural hemodialyses are more efficient in controlling the serum phosphate levels. Noctural hemodialysis six nights weekly resulted in normalization of serum phosphate, despite an increase in dietary phosphate intake by 50% and discontinuation of P-binders.[29]

Future approaches

The characterization of molecular mechanisms involved in phosphate homeostasis is rapidly evolving. NaPi-2b on the intestinal brush border has been identified as being of importance for intestinal phosphate absorption. Inhibition of the intestinal transcellular phosphate transport is a potential new approach in the treatment of hyperphosphatemia in CKD patients. Experimentally, nicotinamide prevented development of hyperphosphatemia and significantly inhibited the intestinal phosphate absorption in adenine induced renal failure in rats, as assessed by influx of orally administered radiolabeled phosphate into the circulation. This effect was accompanied by a decrease in NaPi-2b expression in jejunum brush border membranes.[30] Recently, a randomized, double-blind, placebo-controlled, cross-over trial demonstrated that niacinamide was effective in controlling serum phosphate, when co-administered with P-binders in patients on hemodialysis.[31] Moreover, niacinamide increased serum HDL levels. The combination of phosphate reduction and a beneficial change in the lipid profile makes niacinamide a potentially attractive agent for further investigation, although side effects, such as thrombocytopenia might limit the clinical use of nicotinamide.

Several new factors- -the phosphatonins—which regulate the Na-Pi cotransporter abundance in the brush border membrane of the proximal tubule and thereby renal phosphate handling have recently been discovered.[32] As such in the future enhancing urinary excretion may be possible in CKD patients with some preserved tubular function. The most extensively studied phosphatonin is FGF23. Beside producing phosphaturia, the protein has additional effects on parathyroid function, depressing biosynthesis and secretion of PTH.[33]

Another phosphatonin, MEPE, is phosphaturic and has also been shown directly to reduce the intestinal phosphate absorption.[34] Recently, intestinal phosphate sensing has been demonstrated. An increase in luminal phosphate concentration was followed by release of an 'intestinal phosphatonin' and increase in the fractional excretion of phosphate by the kidney. Modulation of the phosphatonin system might have the potential to differentiate the regulation of the deranged phosphate homeostasis in uremia. In addition, the flux of phosphate from the extracellular fluid into bone and soft tissue is controlled by numerous factors as well and serum phosphate concentrations can be altered without changes in the intestinal absorption or in renal excretion.[32]

The maintenance of normal bone biology will probably become the most important target in the management of hyperphosphatemia in CKD patients. In this respect BMP 7 has been shown experimentally to ameliorate the skeletal lesions in uremic models of both adynamic bone disease and sec. HPT.[18]

Ergocalciferol and cholecalciferol prescription in CKD

Nutritional vitamin D deficiency is endemic in all populations and particularly in those who live in northern latitudes where there is a limited amount of ultraviolet light, those with a high content of melanin in their skin, and many others who either because of the constraints of time or modesty do not expose their bodies to the sun. We also obtain limited amounts of vitamin D in food such as fatty fish or food fortified with vitamin D. Plankton, which evolved 500 million years ago, are the lowest level of the food chain and they biosynthesize vitamin D using the energy of ultraviolet light and they are eaten by fish and hence to man. The proud place that vitamin D has in such lowly organisms illustrates its pivotal role in metabolism. Nutritional vitamin D status is best assessed by measuring serum 25(OH) vitamin D [25(OH)D] levels.

Considering that vitamin D deficiency is associated with adverse clinical outcomes in patients with normal kidney function (falls, fracture, mortality, and cancer) the adverse effects in CKD patients may very well be far worse. The KDIGO guidelines suggest that vitamin D be repleted aggressively in patients with CKD prior to the institution of dialysis, in an effort to provide substrate for hydroxylation to the active form of this vitamin and reduce secondary hyperparathyroidism.[11] The guidelines do not specify that dialysis patients should be repleted with nutritional vitamin D. It would seem wise to replete 25(OH)D in dialysis patients as for the general population.

In the normal population (Table 27.1) some facts on the relative relationship between 25(OH)D and 1,25(OH)$_2$D are presented. In normal subjects, the total plasma concentration of 25(OH)D is approximately 10^3 times higher than that of 1,25(OH)$_2$D. The binding affinity of 25(OH)D to vitamin D binding globulin is also about 10^3 times higher than that of 1,25(OH)$_2$D, leaving the free plasma concentrations of 25(OH)D and 1,25(OH)$_2$D at about the same level. The relative toxicity of 25(OH)D and 1,25(OH)$_2$D is therefore determined by their affinity to the vitamin D receptor (VDR), which is 500–1000 higher for 1,25(OH)$_2$D. The half-life for 25(OH)D is 25–30 days or longer, as compared with only 4–8h for 1,25(OH)$_2$D.

Levels of 25(OH)D below 32ng/mL are associated with increased PTH levels, reduced bone mineral density (BMD), and increased rates of hip fractures.[35] Such levels are therefore considered to represent insufficient vitamin D storage; levels between 15 and 30ng/mL are defined as vitamin D 'insufficiency', levels between 5 and 15ng/mL are characterized as vitamin D 'deficiency' and levels less than 5ng/mL as 'severe deficiency'.[36] Interestingly, 25(OH)D levels in the vast majority of the general population meet the definition of vitamin D insufficiency and a large percentage have serum levels less than 15ng/mL, thus qualifying as vitamin D deficient. Patients with CKD have long been known to suffer from vitamin D deficiency that was an integral component in the pathogenesis of the renal bone disease.[37] Lower serum 25(OH)D concentrations are found in those with lower vitamin D intake and in patients with renal failure. As always the role of vitamin D status on survival has been difficult to pinpoint. A retrospective, nested case-control study did evaluate 90-day survival in patients initiating hemodialysis. In this report,[38] patients who died within 90 days were more likely to be severely vitamin D deficient (defined as a serum 25(OH)D level < 10pg/mL). Patients who died within 90 days were also more likely to have serum 25(OH)D< 30pg/mL and not to have received vitamin D therapy with calcitriol or its analogs. In this report there was a significant relationship between the serum levels of 25(OH)D and those of calcium (direct relationship) and PTH (inverse relationship).

Table 27.1 Estimated levels in normal subjects

	25(OH)D	1,25(OH)$_2$D
Total plasma concentration—recommended values	32–50 ng/mL	32–50 pg/mL
	75–125 nmol/L	75–125 pmol/L
Total plasma concentration - relative levels	1000	1
Binding affinity to vitamin D binding globulin	1000	1
Free concentration—relative levels	1	1
Half life	25–30 days	4–8 h
Vitamin D receptor (VDR) affinity—relative values	1	500–1000
Relative toxicity—acute	1	500–1000
Relative toxicity—long term	100–200	1

Furthermore, a prospective study on chronic peritoneal dialysis patients followed for three years showed that serum 25(OH)D concentration (<30ng/mL) was associated with an increased risk of cardiovascular events.[39] In the Study for the Evaluation of Early Kidney disease (SEEK) hyperparathyroidism was evident at a GFR of 45mL/min, which correlated with the low serum 1,25(OH)$_2$D levels.[1] 25(OH)D levels correlated with serum 1,25(OH)$_2$D levels, but not in those with CKD stage 3 and later. It would be reasonable to ensure that patients with CKD at all stages have levels of 25(OH)D>30ng/mL. This is particularly so when one considers that vitamin D exerts a vast array of biological effects. The decrease in 1,25(OH)$_2$D may be a consequence of increased serum FGF23 levels, which have been shown to increase early in CKD before the development of serum mineral abnormalities and are independently associated with serum phosphate and 1,25(OH)$_2$D deficiency.[40] Increased FGF23 may contribute to maintaining normal serum phosphate levels in the face of advancing CKD, but may worsen 1,25(OH)$_2$D deficiency and thus may be a central factor in the early pathogenesis of 2HPT. So maintenance of a normal serum phosphate is of importance to prevent the decrease in 1,25(OH)$_2$D.

After renal transplantation a low serum 25(OH)D concentration is frequent, but few studies have evaluated the effects of normalizing serum 25-OHD concentration on serum PTH and calcium concentration, and on urinary calcium excretion in these patients. The replacement doses needed in transplanted patients who usually have 25(OH)D concentration <30ng/mL is in the order of 100,000U cholecalciferol every 2 weeks for 2 months (intensive phase) then every other month (maintenance phase).[41]

There is substantive scientific data showing that the biological actions of vitamin D are not only due to the action of the circulating 1,25(OH)$_2$D, but rather represent autocrine and paracrine actions.[42] It has been shown that 25(OH)D is taken up by many tissues where it is converted locally into 1,25(OH)$_2$D. This locally synthesized 1,25(OH)$_2$D is biologically active in an autocrine and paracrine manner. It has marked effects to decrease cell proliferation and hence perhaps prevent cancerous growth, stimulate the immune system, as well as the ability of macrophages to kill bacteria. To support these biological effects there is considerable epidemiological evidence.[35]

It therefore seems prudent to ensure that all of us have adequate levels of 25(OH)D and certainly patients with CKD. Thus, repletion of nutritional vitamin D appears important and doses of greater than the recommended 400–600IU for adults seem wise. The toxicity of larger doses in the range of 1000IU/day appears very low in that the toxic daily dose has been estimated as in excess of 10,000IU/day. Given that oral repletion of vitamin D is quite inexpensive and devoid of any appreciable risk, as opposed to the known risks of increased sunlight exposure, many will choose the oral route, although there is every reason to encourage exposure to sunlight that does not cause sunburn.

Active vitamin D analogs

1,25(OH)$_2$D is synthesized in the kidney, and is therefore deficient in CKD and is associated with the development of 2HPT. 1,25(OH)$_2$D actively increases intestinal calcium absorption and together with the higher serum calcium level would act to decrease serum PTH levels. It is now accepted therapy that CKD patients should receive $1,25(OH)_2D$ or an analogue to control their 2HPT. 2HPT begins to occur at eGFR levels of approximately $45mL/min/1.73m^2$, similar to the point where the median value of $1,25(OH)_2D$ begins to approach values deemed 'deficient' (22pg/mL) when using the values in the lowest tertile for this population.[1] Intravenous 1,25D analogs soon became the routine treatment in many countries aimed at ensuring patient compliance and higher blood levels. The costs to the health system soared. However, it has been questioned whether these extra costs have been of benefit to the patient. Palmer et al. performed a meta-analysis of all the published studies up to 2007 on vitamin D and CKD, and came to the conclusion that vitamin D compounds do not consistently reduce PTH levels, and that beneficial effects on patient-level outcomes are unproven.[43] The validity of the conclusions of this meta-analysis have, however, been severely questioned.[44] No evidence of superiority of newer vitamin D analogues over established vitamin D compounds for any outcome could be provided when these agents were compared directly in RCTs (e.g. paracalcitol against calcitriol resulted in a similar number of hyperphosphatemic episodes in patients on hemodialysis).[45] The lack of direct head-to-head trials comparing most of the newer with established agents makes it difficult to assess whether newer vitamin D agents have similar or different effects, even on biochemical outcomes, than established compounds. Similarly, no study exists showing that intravenous vitamin D compounds had any advantage over oral compounds.[43] The conclusions of Palmer et al. are in conflict with KDOQI opinion-based recommendations, but are in agreement with recommendations from other countries, such as the Australian recommendations, which concluded that there was insufficient evidence to recommend the use of newer vitamin D analogues over calcitriol.[46] The recommendations for the use of active vitamin D analogs have been accepted as 'cast in stone'. In the same way as higher hemoglobin targets and more intensive dialysis had strong support from seemingly unassailable biological and epidemiological evidence, suggesting that they would improve clinically relevant outcomes. However, subsequent randomized trials demonstrated that these interventions were not beneficial or actually caused harm. So, RCTs are eagerly awaited, but there are none in the offing as the pay-off would be limited for the drug companies that would normally finance such a study. Such trials should ideally not use biochemical markers as proxies for bone and cardiovascular end points in CKD. Modifications of PTH, calcium, or phosphorus by vitamin D, calcimimetics, and phosphate binders have as yet not been shown to improve patient-level bone and cardiovascular outcomes. The challenges are daunting.

Contraindications for the use of vitamin D analogs[47]

1) Hypercalcemia is the main symptom of vitamin D intoxication as vitamin D treatment enhances enteral calcium absorption and induces calcium release from bone. Hypercalcemia must therefore be considered an absolute contraindication for treatment with vitamin D analogs. It is not possible to monitor the active vitamin D treatment by plasma concentration (calcitriol, alphacalcidiol, paricalcitriol, and doxercalciferol) making hypercalcemia the main indicator of intoxication, as well as its degree. In the case of ergo/cholecalciferol treatment it is

possible to adjust the dose according to the plasma levels of 25(OH)D, however the laboratory results take time, and the evaluation and adjustment of treatment will therefore still depend mainly upon the calcium levels. It is also a question as to whether the generally accepted high normal range of calcium is, in fact, too high, and at what level of plasma calcium extra vitamin D (calcitriol, alphacalcidiol, paricalcitriol, and doxercalciferol or ergo/cholecalciferol) might result in extraskeletal calcifications.

2) In parallel with calcium vitamin D treatment enhances phosphorus absorption from the intestine and induces phosphorus release from bone. 1,25(OH)$_2$D does further stimulate the phosphatonin, FGF23, which normally (but not in dialysis patients) causes phosphaturia. Severe hyperphosphatemia might, as such, also be considered an absolute contraindication to vitamin D treatment. However, the more commonly encountered moderate hyperphosphatemia in dialysis patients often benefits from suppression of the secondary hyperparathyroidism by active vitamin D treatment.

3) Low PTH levels in non-parathyroidectomized (PTX) patients might result in adynamic bone disease. In such patients is treatment with active vitamin D analogs, in doses that further suppress PTH, contraindicated. However, it remains to be established whether these patients might, nevertheless, profit from a small dose of active vitamin (ineffective to suppress PTH further)—a dose which is sufficient to induce VDR activation in various tissues. In any case, the contraindication relates only to treatment with active vitamin D analogs, and patients who are not treated with active vitamin D should be provided with ergo/cholecalciferol in this setting. In PTX patients active vitamin D treatment is necessary in order to provide the patients with a calcitropic hormone.

4) The diagnosis of an adynamic bone disease in the case of higher PTH levels is difficult to establish without a bone biopsy. In biopsy proven adynamic bone disease is treatment with active vitamin D contraindicated.

5) In dialysis patients with significant vascular calcifications treatment with active vitamin D analogs should be restrictive due to the risk of further aggravation of the calcium/phosphorus burden and, as such, resulting in a worsening of the vascular calcifications. Increasing the level of concern is the observation that active vitamin D might have an independent adverse effect on the vasculature. This question remains unanswered as a beneficial effect of active vitamin D has also been shown.

6) Calciphylaxis represents a condition with severe obliterating calcifications of the small arterioles. Based upon the clinical experience from many casuistic reports aggressive attempts to reduce the calcium/phosphate burden should be initiated. Therefore, treatment with vitamin D analogs most be considered contraindicated in patients with calciphylaxis.

Useful rules of thumb

1) Provide sufficient erogocalciferol or cholecalciferol to maintain serum 25(OH) vitamin D levels > 30ng/mL. For patients with vitamin D deficiency, arbitrarily

defined as < 15ng/mL 25(OH)D, the equivalent of at least 2000 units per day given as a daily dose or the equivalent given weekly or every fortnight should prescribed. Once 25(OH)D levels are > 30ng/mL, which should be measured after three months of therapy, then the equivalent of 1000U/day is recommended. Cholecalciferol and ergocalciferol probably are both equally as effective treatments.[48]

2) For patients with a serum phosphorus in the target range and a serum calcium that is not high, if the serum PTH is increased then an active vitamin D analog should be prescribed. Calcitriol or 1α(OH) vitamin D_3 should be given at a dose of about 0.25µg/day and increased if the serum PTH is higher than about 2.5-fold the upper limit of the normal range for the assay used.

Calcimimetics

Calcimimetic agents provide an important additional therapeutic lever available to the nephrologist. These agents bind to the transmembrane domain of the calcium sensing receptor (CaSR) on parathyroid cells, and also on the same receptor in other tissues where it is expressed. The effect on the receptor is to augment its sensitivity to its principle directly acting ligands, calcium, and other polyvalent ions. The predictable effect of this on the parathyroid gland is to reduce the drive that the parathyroid gland receives from extracellular calcium with the result that in clinical practice both PTH and serum calcium fall simultaneously, in contrast to the effect of vitamin D metabolites in which PTH falls and calcium rises. This therapeutic profile is extremely useful in some patients with advanced CKD, particularly those in whom parathyroid dysregulation with underlying nodular hyperplasia makes active vitamin D compounds difficult or impossible to use. There is no doubt from a number of large well performed studies that calcimimetic agents when added to standard treatment greatly improve the biochemical control of hyperparathyroidism in CKD stage 5 patients.[49]

A number of studies have explored ways of identifying suitable patients and also how to integrate the use of calcimimetics with active vitamin D compounds.[50] Complex algorithms have been developed, but in essence the principle issue is determined by the relationship between PTH and the prevailing serum calcium concentration in any given patient. Table 27.2 illustrates this, defining the patients as either

Table 27.2 Vitamin D, calcimimetic, or both?

Vitamin D phenotype	Calcimimetic phenotype
PTH ↑	PTH ↑
Ca ↓	Ca ↑
Pi ↓	Pi ↑

In the 'vitamin D phenotype' serum calcium is in the mid- or lower part of the normal range. Active vitamin D compounds reduce PTH and any rise in serum calcium remains within the pre-existing headroom. The 'calcimimetic phenotype' has high or high/normal serum calcium. An active vitamin D compound reduces PTH, but exacerbates the hypercalcemia leading to treatment failure, whereas calcimimetics simultaneously reduce PTH and calcium, improving the biochemical profile. Combinations of vitamin D compounds and calcimimetics are frequently used—the effects on PTH are additive.

having a phenotype that invites treatment with vitamin D compounds or one that invites treatment with calcimimetics. The 'vitamin D phenotype' typically has hyperparathyroidism with serum calcium in the mid- or lower part of the normal range—here the deployment of active vitamin D compounds is likely to reduce PTH and any rise in serum calcium is likely to be acceptable in the context of the pre-existing headroom. Conversely, the 'calcimimetic phenotype' has elevated PTH with serum calcium in the upper part of the normal range or frankly above normal. Here, the use of an active vitamin D compound, while reducing PTH, exacerbates the hypercalcemia leading to treatment failure as a result of lack of efficacy or intolerance. It is in this patient group that calcimimetics have a particular appeal—simultaneous reduction of PTH and calcium serves to improve the biochemical profile dramatically. Combinations of vitamin D compounds and calcimimetics are frequently used—the effects on PTH are additive and a small dose of a calcimimetic renders patients more tolerant of active vitamin D and conversely active vitamin D compounds help to protect against potentially troublesome hypocalcemia in some calcimimetic treated patients.

The striking biochemical improvement seen with calcimimetic treatments raises the possibility that favorable responses to those biomarkers known to associate with poor skeletal and cardiovascular outcomes might result in calcimimetic induced improvements to both the skeleton and the cardiovascular system. A major study (evaluation of cinacalcet HCl therapy to lower CV events; EVOLVE) is underway to examine these possibilities—this study has recruited several thousand patients with hyperparathyroidism. Randomization is to continuation of standard therapy plus a placebo or to standard therapy plus a calcimimetic agent. The composite endpoint is a combination of mortality and various cardiovascular events. A *post hoc* analysis of four similar and large studies comparing standard treatment plus calcimimetic with standard treatment alone showed a 54% reduction of fracture rate and a 93% reduction of parathyroidectomy rate in the calcimimetic treated patients. Much less convincing changes were seen to some cardiovascular parameters.[51]

Acid-base control

Significant metabolic acidosis has long been appreciated as an important contributor to metabolic bone disease.[52] This causal relationship is most apparent in patients with reasonably good kidney function in whom renal tubular disorders, or other causes of chronic metabolic acidosis, such as urinary diversion or chronic diarrhea, have clearly been associated with the development of rickets in children and osteomalacia in adults. That this happens is not at all surprising given the important contribution that the skeleton makes to buffering in chronic metabolic acidosis and also the effect of acidosis to increase levels of calciuria. The similarity between the bone lesions of vitamin D deficiency and those of chronic metabolic acidosis prompted a series of experiments in the 1980s to examine the possibility that chronic metabolic acidosis affected the skeleton by impairing the bioactivation of vitamin D. The picture that emerged was a mixed one—at the level of the kidney there is experimental evidence for impairment of calcitriol production in circumstances where the synthetic apparatus has already been up-regulated by calcium deficiency.[53,54] Further support for a role of acidosis *per se* comes from clinical studies in which effective treatment of chronic metabolic acidosis with alkali alone has been associated with demonstrable healing of the underlying skeletal lesions.[55] In these studies, measurement of vitamin D metabolites showed no significant change. Overall, the available evidence strongly supports the use of regular oral alkali therapy to correct underlying chronic metabolic acidosis in the expectation that skeletal morbidity will be avoided and also that nutritional status will be protected.

Much less clear is the importance of metabolic acidosis seen in patients with advanced uremia. In CKD stage 5D, the acidosis is largely titrated by bicarbonate ingress during dialysis. Nevertheless, the propensity of patients to manifest chronic mild or even moderate metabolic acidosis in this setting varies considerably and some work points to benefits from rigorous correction of acidosis in dialysis patients.[56] There are clear practical difficulties with this—sodium bicarbonate at anything above small doses is poorly tolerated in ECF expanded dialysis patients and other difficulties are associated with exuberant bicarbonate replacement during dialysis. The potential advantages of daily dialysis in this context are substantial, although the patient level improvements documented with these treatments have not convincingly been linked to correction of acidosis *per se*.

Summary

The management of the bone and mineral disorders in patients with CKD is challenging. As outlined in this chapter the management differs according to the stage of CKD, as well as the particular changes in serum biochemical and skeletal parameters. However, careful attention at an early stage of CKD to the pathophysiological principles presented here and the use of simple available therapy together with a disciplined patient will very often prevent unnecessary suffering for the patient.

References

1. Levin A, Bakris GL, Molitch M, et al. Prevalence of abnormal serum vitamin D, PTH, calcium, and phosphorus in patients with chronic kidney disease: results of the study to evaluate early kidney disease. *Kidney Int* 2007;**71**:31–8.

2. Goodman WG, Quarles LD. Development and progression of secondary hyperparathyroidism in chronic kidney disease: lessons from molecular genetics. *Kidney Int* 2008;**74**:276–88.

3. London GM, Guerin AP, Verbeke FH, et al. Mineral metabolism and arterial functions in end-stage renal disease: potential role of 25-hydroxyvitamin D deficiency. *J Am Soc Nephrol* 2007;**18**:613–20.

4. Cunningham J. New vitamin D analogues for osteodystrophy in chronic kidney disease. *Pediatr Nephrol* 2004;**19**:705–8.

5. Andress DL, Coyne DW, Kalantar-Zadeh K, et al. Management of secondary hyperparathyroidism in stages 3 and 4 chronic kidney disease. *Endocr Pract* 2008;**14**:18–27.

6. Malluche HH, Mawad H, Monier-Faugere MC. Effects of treatment of renal osteodystrophy on bone histology. *Clin J Am Soc Nephrol* 2008;**3**(Suppl 3):S157–63.

7. Slatopolsky E, Caglar S, Pennell JP, et al. On the pathogenesis of hyperparathyroidism in chronic experimental renal insufficiency in the dog. *J Clin Invest* 1971;**50**:492–9.

8. Portale AA, Booth BE, Halloran BP, Morris RCJ. Effect of dietary phosphorus on circulating concentrations of 1,25-dihydroxyvitamin D and immunoreactive parathyroid hormone in children with moderate renal insufficiency. *J Clin Invest* 1984;**73**:1580–9.

9. Mak RH, Turner C, Thompson T, et al. Suppression of secondary hyperparathyroidism in children with chronic renal failure by high dose phosphate binders: calcium carbonate versus aluminium hydroxide. *Br Med J (Clin Res Ed)* 1985;**291**:623–7.

10. Mucsi I, Hercz G. Adynamic bone disease: pathogenesis, diagnosis and clinical relevance. *Curr Opin Nephrol Hypertens* 1997;**6**:356–61.

11. KDIGO clinical practice guideline for the diagnosis, evaluation, prevention, and treatment of Chronic Kidney Disease-Mineral and Bone Disorder (CKD-MBD). *Kidney Int* 2009;Suppl:S1–130.

12. Block GA, Martin KJ, de Francisco AL, et al. Cinacalcet for secondary hyperparathyroidism in patients receiving hemodialysis. *N Engl J Med* 2004;**350**:1516–25.

13. Kooienga L. Phosphorus balance with daily dialysis. *Semin Dial* 2007;**20**:342–5.

14. Nessim SJ, Jassal SV, Fung SV, Chan CT. Conversion from conventional to nocturnal hemodialysis improves vitamin D levels. *Kidney Int* 2007;**71**:1172–6.

15. Sawyer N, Noonan K, Altmann P, Marsh F, Cunningham J. High-dose calcium carbonate with stepwise reduction in dialysate calcium concentration: effective phosphate control and aluminium avoidance in hemodialysis patients. *NephrolDial Transplant* 1989;**4**: 105–9.

16. Haris A, Sherrard DJ, Hercz G. Reversal of adynamic bone disease by lowering of dialysate calcium. *Kidney Int* 2006;**70**:931–7.

17. Chertow GM, Burke SK, Raggi P. Sevelamer attenuates the progression of coronary and aortic calcification in hemodialysis patients. *Kidney Int* 2002;**62**:245–52.

18. Mathew S, Tustison KS, Sugatani T, et al. The mechanism of phosphorus as a cardiovascular risk factor in CKD. *J Am Soc Nephrol* 2008;**19**:1092–105.

19. Uribarri J. Phosphorus homeostasis in normal health and in chronic kidney disease patients with special emphasis on dietary phosphorus intake. *Semin Dial* 2007;**20**:295–301.

20. Isakova T, Gutierrez OM, Chang Y, et al. Phosphorus binders and survival on hemodialysis. *J Am Soc Nephrol* 2009;**20**:388–96.

21. London GM, Marchais SJ, Guerin AP, et al. Association of bone activity, calcium load, aortic stiffness, and calcifications in ESRD. *J Am Soc Nephrol* 2008;**19**:1827–35.

22. Block GA, Spiegel DM, Ehrlich J, et al. Effects of sevelamer and calcium on coronary artery calcification in patients new to hemodialysis. *Kidney Int* 2005;**68**:1815–24.

23. Qunibi W, Moustafa M, Muenz LR, et al. A 1-year randomised trial of calcium acetate versus sevelamer on progression of coronary artery calcification in hemodialysis patients with comparable lipid control: the Calcium Acetate Renagel Evaluation-2 (CARE-2) study. *Am J Kidney Dis* 2008;**51**:952–65.

24. Barreto DV, Barreto FC, de Carvalho AB, et al. Phosphate binder impact on bone remodeling and coronary calcification—results from the BRiC study. *Nephron Clin Pract* 2008;**110**:c273–83.

25. Ferreira A, Frazao JM, Monier-Faugere MC, et al. Effects of sevelamer hydrochloride and calcium carbonate on renal osteodystrophy in hemodialysis patients. *J Am.Soc.Nephrol.* 2008;**19**:405–12.

26. Suki WN, Zabaneh R, Cangiano JL, et al. Effects of sevelamer and calcium-based phosphate binders on mortality in hemodialysis patients. *Kidney Int* 2007;**72**:1130–7.

27. Drueke TB. Lanthanum carbonate as a first-line phosphate binder: the 'cons'. *Semin Dial* 2007;**20**:329–32.

28. Savica V, Calo LA, Monardo P, et al. Salivary phosphate-binding chewing gum reduces hyperphosphatemia in dialysis patients. *J Am Soc Nephrol* 2009;**20**:639–44.

29. Mucsi I, Hercz G, Uldall R, et al. Control of serum phosphate without any phosphate binders in patients treated with nocturnal hemodialysis. *Kidney Int* 1998;**53**:1399–404.

30. Eto N, Miyata Y, Ohno H, Yamashita T. Nicotinamide prevents the development of hyperphosphatemia by suppressing intestinal sodium-dependent phosphate transporter in rats with adenine-induced renal failure. *Nephrol Dial Transplant* 2005;**20**:1378–84.

31. Cheng SC, Young DO, Huang Y, Delmez JA, Coyne DW. A randomised, double-blind, placebo-controlled trial of niacinamide for reduction of phosphorus in hemodialysis patients. *Clin J Am Soc Nephrol* 2008;**3**:1131–8.

32. Berndt T, Thomas LF, Craig TA, et al. Evidence for a signaling axis by which intestinal phosphate rapidly modulates renal phosphate reabsorption. *Proc Natl Acad Sci USA* 2007;**104**:11085–90.

33. Ben Dov IZ, Galitzer H, Lavi-Moshayoff V, et al. The parathyroid is a target organ for FGF23 in rats. *J Clin Invest* 2007;**117**:4003–8.

34. Berndt T, Kumar R. Phosphatonins and the regulation of phosphate homeostasis. *Ann Rev Physiol* 2007;**69**:341–59.

35. Holick MF. Resurrection of vitamin D deficiency and rickets. *J Clin Invest* 2006;**116**:2062–72.

36. Vieth R, Bischoff-Ferrari H, Boucher BJ, et al. The urgent need to recommend an intake of vitamin D that is effective. *Am J Clin Nutr* 2007;**85**:649–50.

37. Eastwood JB, Stamp TC, Harris E, De Wardener HE. Vitamin-D deficiency in the osteomalacia of chronic renal failure. *Lancet* 1976;**2**:1209–11.

38. Wolf M, Shah A, Gutierrez O, et al. Vitamin D levels and early mortality among incident hemodialysis patients. *Kidney Int* 2007;**72**:1004–13.

39. Wang AY-M, Lam CW-K, Sanderson JE, et al. Serum 25-hydroxyvitamin D status and cardiovascular outcomes in chronic peritoneal dialysis patients: a 3-y prospective cohort study. *Am J Clin Nutr* 2008;**87**:1631–8.

40. Gutierrez O, Isakova T, Rhee E, et al. Fibroblast growth factor-23 mitigates hyperphosphatemia but accentuates calcitriol deficiency in chronic kidney disease. *J Am Soc Nephrol* 2005;**16**:2205–15.

41. Courbebaisse M, Thervet E, Souberbielle JC, et al. Effects of vitamin D supplementation on the calcium-phosphate balance in renal transplant patients. *Kidney Int* 2009;**75**:646–51.

42. Bikle D. Nonclassic Actions of Vitamin D. *J Clin Endocrinol Metab* 2009;**94**:26–34.

43. Palmer SC, McGregor DO, Macaskill P, et al. Meta-analysis: vitamin D compounds in chronic kidney disease. *Ann Intern Med* 2007;**147**:840–53.

44. Olgaard K, Lewin E. Use (or misuse) of vitamin D treatment in CKD and dialysis patients. *Nephrol Dial Transplant* 2008;**23**:1786–9.

45. Sprague SM, Llach F, Amdahl M, Taccetta C, Batlle D. Paricalcitol versus calcitriol in the treatment of secondary hyperparathyroidism. *Kidney Int* 2003;**63**:1483–90.

46. Elder G, Faull R, Branley P, Hawley C. The CARI guidelines. Management of bone disease, calcium, phosphate and parathyroid hormone. *Nephrol (Carlton)* 2006;**11**(Suppl. 1):S230–61.

47. Lewin E, Olgaard K. When is vitamin D contraindicated in dialysis patients? *Semin Dial* 2009;**22**:240–2.

48. Holick MF, Biancuzzo RM, Chen TC, et al. Vitamin D2 is as effective as vitamin D3 in maintaining circulating concentrations of 25-hydroxyvitamin D. *J Clin Endocrinol Metab* 2008;**93**:677–81.

49. Moe SM, Cunningham J, Bommer J, et al. Long-term treatment of secondary hyperparathyroidism with the calcimimetic cinacalcet HCl. *Nephrol Dial Transplant* 2005;**20**:2186–93.

50. Schlieper G, Floege J. Calcimimetics in CKD-results from recent clinical studies. *Pediatr. Nephrol.* 2008; **23**:1721–8.

51. Cunningham J, Danese M, Olson K, Klassen P, Chertow GM. Effects of the calcimimetic cinacalcet HCl on cardiovascular disease, fracture, and health-related quality of life in secondary hyperparathyroidism. *Kidney Int* 2005;**68**:1793–800.

52. Richards P, Chamberlain MJ, Wrong OM. Treatment of osteomalacia of renal tubular acidosis by sodium bicarbonate alone. *Lancet* 1972;**2**:994–7.

53. Bushinsky DA, Favus MJ, Schneider AB, et al. Effects of metabolic acidosis on PTH and 1,25(OH)2D3 response to low calcium diet. *Am J Physiol* 1982;**243**:F570–5.

54. Cunningham J, Bikle DD, Avioli LV. Acute, but not chronic, metabolic acidosis disturbs 25-hydroxyvitamin D3 metabolism. *Kidney Int* 1984;**25**:47–52.

55. Cunningham J, Fraher LJ, Clemens TL, Revell PA, Papapoulos SE. Chronic acidosis with metabolic bone disease. Effect of alkali on bone morphology and vitamin D metabolism. *Am J Med* 1982;**73**:199–204.

56. Chiu YW, Kopple JD, Mehrotra R. Correction of metabolic acidosis to ameliorate wasting in chronic kidney disease: goals and strategies. *Semin Nephrol* 2009;**29**:67–74.

Chapter 28

Chronic kidney disease-mineral and bone disorder (CKD-MBD) in children

Sevcan A. Bakkaloglu, Katherine Wesseling-Perry, and Isidro B. Salusky

Introduction

Abnormalities in mineral metabolism and bone structure are an almost universal finding in chronic kidney disease (CKD) in childhood,[1] and result in significant complications. Many are similar to those seen in adults with CKD (e.g. fractures, bone pain, and avascular necrosis), but others are unique to children (e.g. growth failure and skeletal deformities), which may result in significant physical disability when left untreated. Such skeletal changes reflect disturbances in endochondral bone formation at the level of the epiphyseal growth plate as well as the alterations in bone turnover, mineralization and volume common to the adult population.[2]

Accordingly, treatment and prevention of renal bone diseases is of critical importance in managing the alterations in bone and growth plate that occur early in the course of CKD and are accompanied by the development of cardiovascular complications. A growing body of evidence demonstrates that cardiovascular disease is the leading cause of morbidity and mortality in adult and pediatric patients with CKD, and that therapies designed to treat the skeletal consequences of CKD affect the progression of vascular pathology. Such findings led to a reclassification of the biochemical, skeletal, and vascular complications associated with progressive kidney disease. Together, these alterations are termed 'CKD mineral and bone disorder' ('CKD-MBD'),[2] while the term 'renal osteodystrophy' exclusively defines bone morphology and is therefore one aspect of the CKD-MBD.[2] This chapter summarizes the specific aspects related to normal skeletal development, and the major aspects of the pathogenesis, clinical manifestations, histological features, and therapeutic interventions currently used in the management of CKD-MBD. Particular emphasis has been placed on the clinical manifestations and treatment strategies that distinguish pediatric patients from their adult counterparts, and on the differences in the management of CKD-MBD across the spectrum of CKD.

Normal growth and development of the skeleton

Most bones are first formed as a cartilage model or anlage. Subsequently, around the eighth week of gestation, endochondral ossification begins. The central anlage degrades and mineralizes, allowing for the ingrowth of blood vessels and the osteoprogenitor cells that are precursors of bone-forming cells. Concurrently, osteoblasts arise in the periosteum in the anlage midshaft, depositing the beginnings of the cortex and establishing the diaphyseal primary ossification centre followed by an epiphyseal secondary ossification centre.[3] The growth plate, the essential structure for longitudinal bone growth, is located between these two sites of ossification. Chondrocytes within the growth plate undergo proliferation, growth, maturation, and necrosis, regulated by the Indian hedgehog gene and parathyroid hormone (PTH)-related protein (PTHrP), among others.[4] During this highly regulated process, three distinct chondrocyte zones develop: the reserve zone, proliferative zone, and hypertrophic zone, corresponding to different stages of chondrocyte differentiation.

Vascular endothelial growth factor (VEGF) signaling is critical for the conversion of a vascular cartilage to highly vascular bone. Angiogenesis is a key feature in endochondral ossification and longitudinal bone growth. Blood vessels migrate into the epiphysis via cartilage canals that form a discrete network that gives rise to the marrow space. Development of the mature bone marrow requires the excavation of the provisional cartilaginous matrix, mainly through the actions of matrix metalloproteases and tartrate resistant acid phosphatase.[5] After excavation of provisional cartilaginous matrix and following angiogenesis, mesenchymal cells of the cartilage canals transform into osteocytes, establishing a permanent bone matrix. Thus, remodeling of the cartilage matrix and modeling of the bone matrix are fine-tuned events that eventually result in progressive elongation of bone.[5]

In children, skeletal growth occurs by processes of bone modeling and remodeling. Modeling, defined as simultaneous bone formation and resorption on different bone surfaces, is the basis for large increases in bone size during growth. Remodeling, in which resorption and formation occur sequentially at the same location because of local coupling, allows for maintenance and repair of the skeleton.[6] Although several hormones (parathyroidhormone (PTH), calcitonin, insulin, growth hormone (GH), thyroid hormone, 1,25-dihydroxyvitamin D_3 (1,25$(OH)_2D_3$), glucocorticoids and sex steroids), and growth factors (insulin-like growth factor-1 (IGF-1), fibroblast growth factor-23 (FGF23), transforming growth factor-β superfamily of cytokines), interleukins, and prostaglandins are known to regulate bone formation; three tumor necrosis factor (TNF) family molecules, the receptor activator of NF-kappaB (RANK), its ligand RANKL, and the decoy receptor of RANKL, osteoprotegerin (OPG), (RANK Ligand/RANK/OPG system) are now recognized as the dominant pathway regulating bone remodeling.[7]

Longitudinal bone growth is driven by the growth plate, whereas the periosteum drives bone growth in width. Bone elongates as the growth plate and bone front move progressively away from the centre of the bone. This process continues until the end of puberty, when the growth plate completes fusion. Appositional modeling at the periosteum, on the other hand, results in the growth of the diameter or width of the long bone.[6] During puberty and early adult life, endosteal apposition, and trabecular thickening provide maximum skeletal mass and strength (peak bone mass).

Disturbances in bone modeling, remodeling, and growth in CKD

Growth retardation is the hallmark of CKD in children. Multiple factors contribute to suboptimal growth including protein and calorie malnutrition, metabolic acidosis, alterations in mineral and bone metabolism, and end-organ growth hormone resistance.[8] Despite correction of acidosis and anemia, normalization of serum calcium and phosphorus levels, and vitamin D sterol therapy replacement, the majority of children with CKD continue to grow poorly. Growth failure worsens as renal function declines; the average height of children with even mild CKD (GFR 50–70mL/min/1.73m^2) is 1 SD (SDS) below the average for healthy children. CKD stage 3 and 4 (GFR 25–49 mL/min/1.73m^2) are associated with a height SDS of –1.5, and, at the time of initiation of dialysis, the mean height SDS is –1.8. Along with the psychosocial disadvantages associated to growth failure, uremic children with growth deficits have been demonstrated to have an increased risk of death.[9]

Chronic metabolic acidosis has been linked to delayed linear growth in patients with renal tubular acidosis and normal renal function, and correction of metabolic acidosis often leads to acceleration in growth velocity. Growth hormone (GH) secretion, serum IGF-1, and hepatic IGF-1 mRNA, along with GH receptor and IGF-1 receptor expression are reduced in acidotic rats, while the expression of IGF binding protein 2 (IGFBP-2) and IGFBP-4, which serve as negative modulators of IGF-I, are increased. Moreover, the stimulatory effect of IGF-I on chondrocytic proliferation and differentiation are markedly attenuated under acidic conditions.[8,10,11]

Despite correction of acidosis, growth retardation persists in children with CKD. Secondary hyperparathyroidism (2HPT), the most common skeletal lesion of pediatric renal osteodystophy, and calcitriol deficiency have also been shown to contribute to growth failure. Treatment of 2HPT with small doses of daily oral calcitriol improves growth velocity. However, over suppression of serum PTH levels with large doses of vitamin D sterols in conjunction with calcium-based phosphate binders may result in the adynamic renal osteodystrophy, growth failure, and progressive vascular calcification.[8,10] Indeed, vitamin D analogues suppress osteoblastic activity and inhibit chondrocyte proliferation in a dose-dependent fashion *in vitro*, while vitamin D sterols increase expression of a number of IGFBPs which sequester IGF-1.[11] Unfortunately, specific PTH target values in children in all stages of CKD remain controversial; some data suggest that normal growth velocity in moderate stages of CKD (stages 3 and 4) is associated with PTH levels in the normal range, while others demonstrate a linear correlation between growth velocity and PTH levels in the same patient population.[10] According to current recommendations PTH levels should be maintained within the upper limit of the normal range in early CKD (stages 1–3); while values between 3–5 times the upper limit of normal in stage 5 CKD to attain normal rates of bone turnover.[1,10]

GH resistance also contributes to impaired linear growth in renal failure. In CKD, poor growth develops despite normal or increased serum GH levels. Serum levels of IGF-I are normal or slightly low in children with CKD while levels of inhibitory circulating IGF binding proteins 1, 2, and 3 are increased; these changes may explain, in part, the resistance to GH therapy.[11] Improved growth velocity during recombinant human GH (rhGH) therapy has been ascribed to increased bioavailability of IGF-1 to target tissues. Children who are treated with maintenance dialysis respond less well to rhGH therapy than children with less severe CKD, possibly due, in part, to the inhibitory effects of calcitiol therapy—required for the control of 2HPT in the majority of pediatric dialysis patients—on chondrocyte proliferation. Indeed, therapy with calcitriol blunts the stimulatory effect of recombinant human growth hormone in animals with renal failure.[12] Studies in uremic animals have demonstrated comparable growth during IGF-I treatment as with GH therapy. However, combined therapy with GH and IGF-I have little added benefit and complications such as hypoglycemia, along with the need for twice daily administration of IGF-I limits the potential use of such anabolic agent in pediatric patients. Newer treatment modalities targeting the GH resistance with recombinant human IGFBP3 (rhIGFBP3) and IGFBP displacers are under investigation and may prove to be more effective in treating growth failure in CKD.[11]

Bony deformities are also common in pediatric patients with CKD, and disturbances in endochondral bone formation have been demonstrated on autopsy material obtained from children with CKD.[13] Marked chondroclastic erosion and abnormal vascularization of the growth plate cartilage contribute to the pathogenesis of growth retardation and slipped capital epiphyses in children with renal bone disease. Downregulation of PTH/PTHrP mRNA expression is evident in growth plate sections from pediatric patients with end-stage renal disease. Furthermore, the growth plate characteristics are different in experimental models of adynamic bone and 2HPT in rats with renal failure.[14] These disturbances may contribute to the skeletal resistance to PTH in renal failure, marked growth retardation, and the alterations in growth plate ossification found in patients with CKD.[10,15]

Renal bone diseases across the spectrum of CKD

Subtle signs of renal osteodystrophy begin when the GFR decreases to 50 percent of normal (stage 3 disease),[16] and these children should be monitored for evidence of bone disease by physical examination and laboratory evaluation. Physical findings may include muscle pain, weakness, and bony changes, such as varus and valgus deformities of the long bones. Serum FGF23 levels increase early in the course of CKD while PTH and $1,25(OH)_2D_3$ levels are within the normal range, as well as calcium phosphorus levels. FGF23 enhances phosphate excretion by the kidney and inhibit 1α-hydroxylase activity and leading to reductions in $1,25(OH)_2D_3$ levels.[10] Abnormalities in bone histology are common in stage 3 and 4 diseases and these were associated with elevated serum PTH carboxyl-terminal levels.[8–10,15] Serum PTH levels are inversely correlated with GFR, and the majority of patients with GFR less than 50 mL/min have increased serum PTH levels and high turnover bone disease.

Bone lesions of high bone turnover, due to 2HPT remain the most common skeletal lesion of renal osteodystrophy in children treated with maintenance dialysis.[15] Defects in skeletal mineralization are also prevalent in patients with CKD[17] and may contribute to such outcomes as bony deformities, bone pain, and growth retardation.[8,10]

Thus, the KDIGO guidelines recommend the evaluation of three bone histological key variables: bone turnover, mineralization, and volume, in all patients with CKD.[2]

Bone turnover

The most common lesion of renal osteodystrophy in pediatric patients treated with dialysis is high bone turnover associated with 2HPT. In this form of bone lesion, increased numbers of osteoblasts and osteoclasts and variable degrees of peritrabecular fibrosis are present (Fig. 28.1A,B). Activation of osteoclasts is mediated through PTH; the result is increased resorption of both mineral and matrix along the trabecular surface and within the haversian canals of cortical bone. Different factors are involved in the development of such cellular activity and among them: insulin-like growth factor-1 (IGF-1), cytokines, microfractures, elevated thyroxine or PTH levels. Increased quantities of woven osteoid, exhibiting haphazard arrangement of collagen fibers in contrast to the usual lamellar pattern of osteoid in normal bone, are present.[8,10]

At the other end of the spectrum of bone turnover, adynamic bone disease is characterized by a reduced bone formation rate, decreased numbers of osteoblasts and osteoclasts, an absence of fibrosis, lack of osteoid accumulation (Fig. 28.1C,D). Adynamic bone is extremely rare in early stages of CKD. The prevalence in pediatric dialysis patients is between 15 and 20%, although it may occur in up to 33% of subjects after receiving large intermittent doses of calcitriol and calcium-based binders for the treatment of 2HPT.[18] Adynamic bone is associated with relatively low PTH levels, low alkaline phosphatase levels, higher levels of serum calcium with an increased tendency for hypercalcemic episodes and higher risk for vascular calcification.[18] The long-term consequences of adynamic renal osteodystrophy include increased risks of skeletal fractures, delayed fracture healing, and the development of soft tissue and vascular calcifications. In pre-pubertal children, adynamic renal osteodystrophy has been associated with a reduction in linear growth.[9,10,18]

Mineralization

Although renal osteodystrophy has traditionally been defined according to the type of bone turnover, alterations in skeletal mineralization are also prevalent in CKD.[19] Defective mineralization that is associated with low to normal bone turnover termed 'osteomalacia',[2] while 'mixed lesion' defines the skeletal histology of high bone turnover combined with defective mineralization. The histomorphometric characteristics of osteomalacia include the presence of wide osteoid seams, an increased number of osteoid lamellae, an increase in the trabecular surface covered with osteoid, and diminished rates of mineralization and bone formation. Fibrosis is often absent (Fig. 28.1E). In long-term dialysis patients, osteomalacia that is refractory to vitamin D therapy is most commonly a result of aluminum intoxication, but currently the mineralization abnormalities are highly prevalent in the absence of aluminum intoxication.[8] The mixed lesion is characterized by increased osteoid seams, fibrosis, and high bone turnover (Fig. 28.1F).

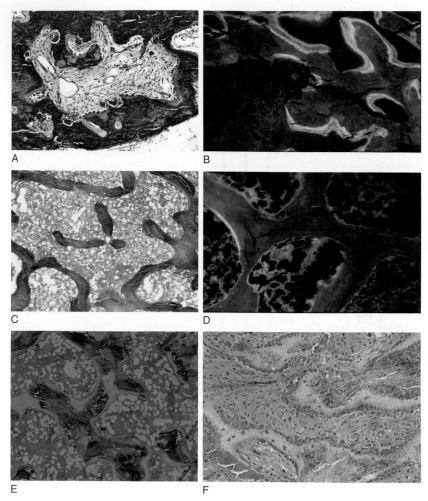

Fig. 28.1 Bone histology slides. **(A,B)** Osteitis fibrosa. (A) Under light microscopy, an increase in cellular activity, osteoid accumulation, erosion, and fibrosis are visible. (B) An increase in double tetracycline labeling signifies an increase in bone turnover rate. (C,D) Adynamic bone. (C) Under light microscopy, decreased cellular activity with minimal osteoid accumulation. (D) A decrease in double tetracycline labeling signifies a decrease in bone turnover rate. (E) Osteomalacia characterized by heavy osteoid accumulation. (F) Mixed renal osteodystrophy: Increased cellular activity, marrow fibrosis, and increased osteoid.

Although the mechanisms of skeletal mineralization are incompletely understood, factors such as 25 hydroxy vitamin D_3 ($25(OH)D_3$) deficiency and altered FGF23 metabolism have been implicated in their pathogenesis. In the general population, nutritional $25(OH)D_3$ deficiency results in osteomalacia and a similar phenotypic expression may occur in pediatric patients with CKD. FGF23 may also contribute to

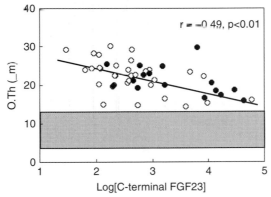

Fig. 28.2 Relationship between log [C-terminal FGF23] and osteoid thickness (O.Th) in pediatric dialysis patients. Open circles depict patients with residual renal function; closed circles depict aneuric patients. The shaded area represents the normal range for osteoid thickness in children with normal kidney function.

this defect; indeed, both over expression and ablation of FGF23 in mice are associated with abnormal mineralization of osteoid, although by different mechanisms. The phosphaturic effect of increased FGF23 may cause rickets and osteomalacia through an insufficiency of mineral substrate. The mechanisms leading to impaired mineralization in FGF23-null animals, which have severe hyperphosphatemia and normal or elevated serum calcium levels, remain uncertain; however, osteomalacia in these animals suggests that FGF23 may play a direct role in skeletal mineral deposition.[10] In pediatric dialysis patients higher FGF23 concentrations may be associated with decreases in osteoid thickness and shorter osteoid maturation times; i.e. with improvements in skeletal mineralization (Fig. 28.2).[20]

Extraskeletal and vascular calcification

Extraskeletal calcification, including vascular calcification, has long been associated with uremia in the adult population. Less appreciated is its occurrence in a substantial proportion of pediatric patients with renal failure. Milliner et al. found post-mortem evidence of soft tissue and vascular calcification in 72 of 120 (60%) children with end-stage renal disease, 43 (36%) of whom had systemic calcinosis.[21] The most common sites of calcification were blood vessels, lungs, kidneys, heart, and coronary arteries, central nervous system, and stomach.[21] Structural and functional abnormalities and calcification in the large vessels begin as early as the first decade of life in patients with CKD. Hypercalcemia, hyperphosphatemia, elevated calcium × phosphorus ion product, high doses of vitamin D sterols, and hyperparathyroidism have all been implicated in the progression of the burden of extraskeletal calcification in pediatric CKD patients. Additionally, the time on dialysis is a strong independent predictor of vascular damage and calcification.[22–24]

In-vivo and *in-vitro* studies have demonstrated that vascular calcification is an active, highly regulated, cell-mediated process that involves a balance between inducers and inhibitors of calcification, as described in Chapter 17. In CKD, hyperphosphatemia, hypercalcemia, and a myriad of promineralization factors are enhanced, while inhibitors of calcification, including fetuin-A and klotho are reduced. Pediatric patients on maintenance dialysis with calcification had lower fetuin-A and higher OPG than those without calcification, which were associated with increased vascular stiffness and calcification.[25,26] Levels of circulating FGF23 may also contribute; indeed, increased levels have been associated with increased mortality in incident dialysis patients in the adult population.[27] Klotho, phosphatonins, and mainly FGF23 in renal failure are discussed in detail in Chapters 21, 23, and 24, respectively.

Biochemical determinations

The development of 2HPT

The kidneys regulate intestinal calcium and phosphorus absorption by converting 25-hydroxy vitamin D_3 [25(OH)D_3], the storage form of vitamin D, to 1,25(OH)$_2D_3$ (calcitriol), the active form of vitamin D, by means of the enzyme 1-α-hydroxylase. In the early stages of CKD, reduced renal phosphate excretion is the primary stimulus for a cascade of events, in which FGF23-dependent suppression of renal 1,25(OH)$_2D_3$ production is a necessary adaptive response to limit the gastrointestinal absorption of phosphate. Along with preventing the stimulation of gastrointestinal phosphate absorption by 1,25(OH)$_2D_3$, the phosphaturic action of FGF23 represents a mechanism to maintain neutral phosphate balance.[28] Thus, increased FGF23 and subsequent suppression of calcitriol synthesis occur early in CKD, before alterations in calcium, phosphorus, or PTH can be detected. Low circulating levels of calcitriol, due to a combination of rising FGF23 values and declining renal mass, stimulate a release of PTH. Elevation of circulating PTH ensues from FGF23-mediated reductions in 1,25(OH)$_2D_3$ production and from impaired gastrointestinal calcium absorption.[28] In the early stages of CKD, elevated circulating PTH may result in normal calcium with normal or even low serum phosphate levels. In advanced CKD stages, very low circulating calcitriol levels result in hypocalcemia due to decreased intestinal calcium absorption. Concurrently, impaired glomerular filtration limits phosphorus excretion and hyperphosphatemia ensues. Both hypocalcemia and hyperphosphatemia occur late in the stage of CKD and stimulate PTH release, resulting in dramatically elevated circulating PTH levels (Fig. 28.3).[8,10,28]

Over time, chronic hypocalcemia, hyperphosphatemia, and low circulating calcitriol levels by different mechanisms lead to parathyroid gland hyperplasia. Since the half-life of parathyroid cells is long—on the order of 30 years—hyperplasia is difficult to reverse once established. PTH secretion from enlarged parathyroid glands may become uncontrollable due to the non-suppressible basal activity of a large number of parathyroid cells. Chronic stimulation of parathyroid glands may also lead to chromosomal changes that result in autonomous, unregulated growth and hormone release.[8,10]

Calcium and phosphorus

Due to rising PTH levels, serum calcium levels are within the normal range until late in the course of CKD.[10] Likewise, serum phosphorus levels are usually maintained in

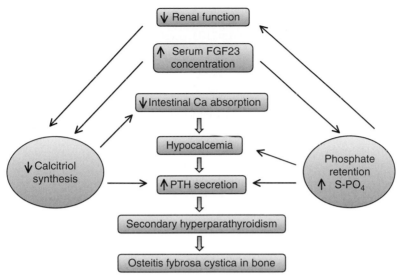

Fig. 28.3 Pathogenesis of 2HPT.

the normal range throughout mild to moderate CKD. Elevated serum PTH and FGF23 levels increase renal phosphate excretion, thus maintaining overall phosphate balance until GFR declines to 25–30% of normal. In late (stage 4) CKD, hyperphosphatemia ensues and contributes to 2HPT.[10,28]

Fibroblast growth factor 23

Although declining values of $1,25(OH)_2D_3$ have been traditionally implicated as the initial event of the altered mineral and bone metabolism associated with CKD, recent data suggest that an increase in circulating levels of FGF23 may precede declining $1,25(OH)_2D_3$ levels and thus may be the initial trigger in the development of 2HPT.[28] Indeed, serum FGF23 levels increase early in the course of CKD prior to any changes in serum calcium, phosphorus, PTH or $1,25(OH)_2D_3$ levels. FGF23 is a phosphaturic hormone, made in bone, that was first identified in patients with tumor-induced osteomalacia, autosomal dominant hypophosphatemic rickets, and X-linked hypophosphatemic rickets. In these conditions, elevated circulating levels of FGF23 result in renal phosphate wasting and suppression of $1,25(OH)_2D_3$ production. FGF23 levels may be regulated by phosphorus intake and serum values increase as CKD progresses, becoming markedly elevated in individuals with end-stage kidney disease. In patients with CKD, $1,25(OH)_2D_3$ levels are inversely related to levels of circulating FGF23, suggesting that the hormone may play a significant role in mineral metabolism-in declining active vitamin D levels in CKD, specifically.[29] FGF23 levels have been implicated in parathyroid gland regulation; higher levels of FGF23 have been shown to suppress PTH release,[30] but other investigators did not confirm such original observations.[31] FGF23 has also been shown to act directly on PTH secretion *in vitro*, through a mechanism independent of its actions on vitamin D metabolism (FGF23 in CKD is reviewed in Chapter 24).[10]

Vitamin D

In patients with CKD, serum $1,25(OH)_2D_3$ levels decline via an FGF23-mediated mechanism early in the course of kidney dysfunction, before any changes in serum calcium or phosphorus concentrations occur and prior to any rise in serum PTH levels. The decline in calcitriol levels seems to be adaptive response in CKD to limit the toxic effects of hyperphosphatemia. In late stages of CKD, phosphate retention and increased serum phosphorus levels directly suppress 1α-hydroxylase activity.[1,8,10,28]

Low circulating levels of $1,25(OH)_2D_3$ have consequences for many tissues. Aside from its effect on intestinal calcium absorption, $1,25(OH)_2D_3$ plays a direct role in the suppression of PTH gene transcription (*vide infra*). Animal studies also indicate that $1,25(OH)_2D_3$ is essential for normal skeletal physiology—particularly in growing animals—and that this effect may not be mediated by the vitamin D receptor (VDR). Mice that lack the VDR [i.e. mice unable to respond to the actions of $1,25(OH)_2D_3$ through its classical receptor] are phenotypically similar to those lacking the 1α-hydroxylase gene itself (i.e. mice unable to generate $1,25(OH)_2D_3$); both sets of mice are hypocalcemic with markedly elevated serum PTH levels, parathyroid gland hyperplasia, and rickets.[8] However, a diet replete in calcium, phosphorus, and lactate is sufficient to normalize the serum calcium, phosphorus, and PTH levels, and to prevent the development of rickets in VDR deficient animals. By contrast, this 'rescue diet' is unable to completely reverse growth plate abnormalities in 1α-hydroxylase deficient mice, suggesting that $1,25(OH)_2D_3$, acting through a receptor other than the classical VDR, may be essential for proper growth plate development.[32] $1,25(OH)_2D_3$ has also been shown to regulate the renin-angiotensin system; 1α-hydroxylase deficient mice demonstrate cardiac hypertrophy and dysfunction, which are reversed with angiotensin converting enzyme blockade. Thus, $1,25(OH)_2D_3$ may be essential for cardiac health, a finding that may explain observational data suggesting that active vitamin D sterol therapy improves survival in patients treated with maintenance dialysis.[8]

Native $25(OH)D_3$ deficiency is prevalent in patients with CKD, and low levels of this form of $25(OH)D$ also contribute to altered mineral metabolism. Although conversion of $25(OH)D_3$ to $1,25(OH)_2D_3$, in individuals with normal renal function, is a substrate-independent process, it becomes a substrate-dependent process in patients with CKD. Several studies have also documented a high prevalence of $25(OH)D_3$ deficiency in adult and pediatric patients with CKD; this prevalence increases as renal function declines and the vast majority of patients treated with maintenance dialysis have insufficient vitamin D storage.[1,33] Patients with CKD are at increased risk of vitamin D deficiency for several reasons:

+ many are chronically ill with little outdoor (sunlight) exposure;
+ CKD dietary restrictions, particularly of dairy products, curtail the intake of vitamin D rich food and lead to decreased dietary calcium intake, resulting in greater conversion of $25(OH)D_3$ to $1,25(OH)_2D_3$, thus necessitating higher vitamin D intake and/or production. Skin synthesis of vitamin D in response to sunlight is reduced in individuals with CKD.[33]

Since levels of $25(OH)D_3$ below 32ng/mL are associated with increased PTH levels, reduced bone mineral density (BMD), and increased rates of hip fractures in the general population, such levels are therefore considered to represent insufficient vitamin D storage. Apart from its conversion to $1,25(OH)_2D_3$, $25(OH)D_3$ may have its own effect on tissues. Indeed, supplementation with ergocalciferol has been shown to decrease serum PTH levels in patients with CKD. Recent evidence demonstrates that 1α-hydroxylase is present in the parathyroid glands; thus, $25(OH)D_3$ is converted inside the gland to $1,25(OH)_2D_3$, suppressing PTH.[34] Furthermore, $25(OH)D_3$ administration suppresses PTH synthesis even when parathyroid gland 1α-hydroxylase is inhibited, indicating that $25(OH)D_3$ may contribute to PTH suppression, independent of its conversion to $1,25(OH)_2D_3$.[33] In addition to the parathyroid gland and bone, arterial smooth muscle cells, pancreatic islet cells, macrophages, T and B cells, hepatocytes, lung alveolar cells, dermal keratinocytes, and renal parenchymal cells have been shown to respond to vitamin D.[35] Many of the effects on these organ systems appear to be due to the immune-regulatory role of vitamin D. Recent investigations suggest that $25(OH)D_3$ has a direct effect on macrophage function that cannot be reproduced by active $1,25(OH)_2D$ administration. Indeed, macrophages have their own 1α-hydroxylase and require sufficient ambient levels of $25(OH)D_3$ substrate in order to produce internal $1,25(OH)_2D_3$. Serum from patients who are vitamin D deficient induce a lower bactericidal response than serum from vitamin D replete individuals, suggesting decreased macrophage function under conditions of vitamin D deficiency.[36]

Parathyroid hormone

Serum PTH levels are widely used as non-invasive markers in distinguishing low-turnover lesions from osteitis fibrosa.[19] During the past 25 years, this first-generation PTH immunometric assay (1st PTH-IRMA) has proven to be a reasonable predictor of the different subtypes of renal osteodystrophy. It has also performed well in assessing the therapeutic response to active vitamin D sterols in patients with renal failure. Since the first generation (1st) assays measure both full-length molecule and amino-terminally truncated fragments, second generation (2nd) PTH assays have been developed which measure, exclusively, the full-length molecule ('PTH(1–84)'). Second generation PTH-IRMA and, mainly, the ratio between PTH(1–84)/amino-truncated PTH fragment (calculated from the differences in PTH levels determined between 1st and 2nd PTH-IRMAs) was suggested a better predictor of bone turnover than 1st PTH-IRMA.[8–10]; however, these findings were not confirmed by subsequent investigations.[37,38] Taking into consideration the crucial role of serum PTH concentrations in the diagnosis and treatment of renal osteodystrophy, 2nd PTH-IRMA may provide important new insights into the physiology of parathyroid gland function. At present, however, measurements of PTH using either 1st or 2nd PTH-IRMAs have shown similar accuracy for predicting bone turnover in patients undergoing maintenance dialysis. The current available data do not yet support the claim that 2nd PTH-IRMAs provide an advantage over 1st PTH-IRMAs for the diagnosis of the different subtypes of renal bone diseases in adult and pediatric patients treated with dialysis.[1,8,10]

Table 28.1 Target PTH levels by the stage of chronic kidney disease (CKD)

CKD stage	GFR range (mL/min/1.73m²)	Target intact PTH (pg/mL)
3	30–59	*35–70 **10–65
4	15–29	*70–110 **10–65
5	<15 or dialysis	*200–300 **130–195

*NKF-KDOQI 2005.[1]
**Klaus G, et al. European PD Group, 2006.[39]

Therefore, current recommendations for target PTH levels are based on measurements obtained by the 1st generation PTH assay based on cross-sectional studies with bone biopsy data from children treated with maintenance dialysis and receiving either low dose oral calcitriol or no vitamin D sterol therapy.[1]

Increasing skeletal resistance to the actions of PTH requires that PTH be maintained at higher levels in advanced stages of CKD (Table 28.1). Down regulation of the PTH receptor, decreased expression of osteoblast differentiation factor, and increased levels of osteoclastogenesis inhibitory factors occur with decreased renal function, contributing to the skeletal resistance to PTH. In patients with CKD stage 3, PTH levels within the normal range generally correspond to normal rates of bone formation, while mildly increased levels above the upper limit of normal suggest the presence of 2HPT. In patients undergoing maintenance dialysis who are either untreated or are receiving small daily oral doses of calcitriol, PTH(7–84) levels of approximately two to five times the upper limit of normal generally correspond to normal bone formation rates (1,10,39). Over suppression of PTH in patients on dialysis has also been shown to result in growth failure, hypercalcemia, and adynamic bone. In summary, PTH levels should be maintained in the range appropriate to the stage of CKD; levels appropriate for early stages of CKD would indicate low-turnover disease in patients treated with dialysis, while appropriate levels for stage 4 CKD represent osteitis fibrosa in stage 3 CKD.[9,10]

Radiographic features of renal osteodystrophy

Radiographs are the most widely used imaging technique to detect and monitor bone disease in patients with renal failure. Subperiosteal erosion is the most common radiographic finding in 2HPT, and its severity can correlate with serum PTH and alkaline phosphatase levels, but radiographs can be normal in patients with moderate to severe histological features of osteitis fibrosa cystica on bone biopsy.[8]

In pediatric patients, metaphyseal changes (i.e. growth zone lesions that are termed 'rickets-like lesions') are common. In severe 2HPT, the growth plate cartilage may appear widened and poorly mineralized.[40] The radiographic changes arising from

2HPT may be difficult to differentiate from true rachitic abnormalities. However, the radiographic features of slipped epiphyses resulting from osteitis fibrosa are present in uremic children, but absent in rickets resulting from vitamin D deficiency. These findings are best detected by hand radiographs and several techniques, including the use of fine-grain films and magnification with a hand lens, are used to enhance sensitivity. Subperiosteal erosions can occur at any site, but they are typically found along the radial margins of the middle phalanges of the second and third digits in adults. In contrast, phalangeal involvement may not be present in young children, but rather involve the lateral aspect of the distal radius and ulna, and medial side of the proximal tibia. Subperiosteal erosions also occur in the distal ends of clavicles, on the surface of the ischium and pubis, at the sacroiliac joints, and at the junction of the metaphysis and diaphysis of long bones.[8,15]

Other findings include brown tumors, which are intra-osseous soft tissue masses that appear as well-defined lytic lesions in the metaphyses of long bones, jaws, ribs, and ilium. In addition, periosteal neostosis (new bone formation), intracortical resorption, erosion of the terminal phalanges (acro-osteolysis), and absence of the lamina dura on dental films are also evident in 2HPT. Radiographic abnormalities of the skull in 2HPT can include:

* a diffuse 'ground-glass' appearance;
* a generalized mottled or granular appearance;
* focal radiolucencies;
* focal sclerosis.[8]

Although radiographic findings of osteomalacia are less specific than those of 2HPT, the presence of Looser's zones and fractures in bones, such as vertebrae, ribs, and hips, are more common in patients with osteomalacia.

X-rays may also be helpful in the detection of extraskeletal calcifications (Fig. 28.4A–D).

New generation high-resolution CT and MRI scanners may also be used to evaluate bone microarchitecture in metabolic bone disease and to estimate fracture risk. Although promising initial reports in uremic animals, clinical utility of these techniques remains to be defined.[41] One such technique, peripheral quantitative computed tomography (pQCT) selectively measures volumatic densities of cortical and trabecular bone in the appendicular skeleton. Trabecular bone density appears higher and cortical bone density lower in pediatric dialysis patients with high turnover disease compared to adynamic bone;[8,15] however, a recent study emphasizes the limitations of pQCT, including a large intra and intersubject variability in the bone density measurements by CT scan (imaging of renal osteodystrophy is reviewed in Chapter 12).[42]

Treatment of CKD-MBD in children

The goal of treatment is to maintain bone remodeling within the normal according to the stage of CKD and prevent the development of vascular calcifications.

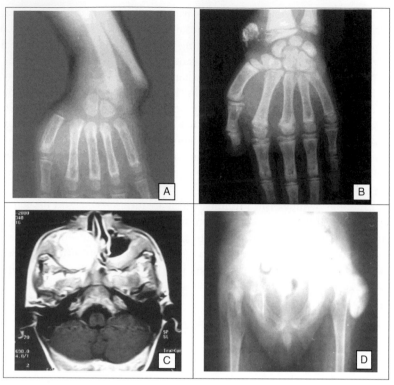

Fig. 28.4 Radiological findings of renal osteodystrophy. (A) Wrist dislocation, irregular distal epiphyseal contours of radius and ulna and severe osteopenia. (B) Acro-osteolysis in the distal phalanx of the thumb and intravascular calcification in arteriovenous fistula of a 15-year-old boy. (C) A solid mass due to 2HPT in the maxillar sinus resulting in proptosis. (D) Bone X-ray revealed osteopenia and soft tissue calcification next to the left femoral proximal metaphysis.

Dietary modifications

The average phosphorus intake of both adults and children in the US population is approximately 1500–2000mg/day and 60–70% of the dietary intake is absorbed. Thus, dietary phosphorus restriction is often necessary to prevent the development and progression of 2HPT, and extraskeletal calcifications in patients with advanced renal failure. Treatment goals include maintaining serum phosphorus levels within normal limits for age and avoiding calcium-phosphorus ion product above $55mg^2/dL^2$.[29] In the early stages of CKD, dietary phosphate restriction alone is sufficient in preventing hyperphosphatemia because serum phosphorus levels are within the normal range in the vast majority of patients. However, strict adherence to dietary phosphate restriction is often difficult because low phosphate diets are unpalatable, especially to older children and adults, and because phosphorus intake is directly linked with protein intake with 10–12 mg of phosphorus accompanying each gram of protein. Adequate protein intake is necessary for growth in children and for maintenance of lean body mass in adults. Current dietary recommendations suggest that adults with CKD ingest between 0.8 and 1 g/kg/day of protein and that children, depending on age, ingest anywhere from 1 to 2.5 g/kg/day.[1,29] This translates to a minimum phosphate ingestion of approximately 800 mg/day of phosphate. Since serum FGF23 are elevated early in the course of CKD, it would be interesting in the future to assess the effects of therapy targeted to normalize FGF23 levels prevents the development of 2HPT and vascular calcifications.

Standard prescription peritoneal dialysis and hemodialysis remove insufficient phosphate (300–400 mg/day for peritoneal dialysis and 800 mg/treatment for hemodialysis) to maintain normal serum phosphorus levels. Thus, phosphate binders are often required in these patients. It is essential to monitor serum phosphorus levels regularly to prevent hypophosphatemia, which may result from aggressive dietary restriction and the use of large doses of phosphate-binding agents. Infants are particularly at risk for hypophosphatemia due to low phosphorus intake, large doses of phosphate binders, higher phosphate removal by peritoneal dialysis due to larger peritoneal surface area, and possibly nutritional repletion.[8,10,15]

Phosphate-binding agents

Phosphate-binding agents reduce intestinal phosphate absorption by forming poorly soluble complexes with phosphorus in the intestinal tract. Aluminum-containing phosphate binders were frequently used in the past, but long-term treatment led to bone disease, encephalopathy, and anemia. The use of aluminum-containing phosphate binders should therefore be restricted to the treatment of severe hyperphosphatemia (>7mg/dL) associated with hypercalcemia or an elevated calcium-phosphorus ion product, since both conditions will be aggravated by calcium-containing compounds. In such cases, the dose of aluminum hydroxide should not exceed 30 mg/kg/day and the lowest possible dose should be given only for a limited period of approximately 4–6 weeks. Plasma aluminum levels should be monitored regularly. Concomitant intake of citrate-containing compounds should be avoided since citrate increases intestinal aluminum absorption and increases the risk of acute aluminum intoxication. Constipation is a common side effect and can be relieved by stool softeners.[8,15,43]

Calcium-containing salts are recommended as the mainstay in phosphorus binding therapy in CKD stages 3 through 5 and also serve as a source of supplemental calcium. Doses should be taken with meals if the calcium salt is used as a phosphate binder and taken between meals if given for hypocalcemia. The recommended dose is proportional to the phosphorus content of the meal, and adjusted to achieve acceptable serum levels of calcium and phosphorus. Several calcium salts are commercially available, including calcium carbonate, calcium acetate, and calcium citrate. Calcium carbonate is the primarily used compound, and studies in adults and children have shown its efficacy in controlling serum phosphorus levels.[1,8–10] The required doses of calcium carbonate ranged widely, from 64–1,578 mg/kg/day in one study, to

21–228 mg/kg/day in another. One study provided data on the absolute dose of elemental calcium required to control PTH: 240–6000 mg elemental calcium per day.[1] In general, starting doses for calcium carbonate and calcium acetate are 600–1500 mg and 375–750 mg of elemental calcium per day, respectively. Raising the dose 2–4 fold may be necessary, especially in younger children. However, the use of large doses of calcium-based binders has been linked to the development of vascular calcifications in adult and pediatric patients treated with maintenance dialysis as well as in adults with stage 4 CKD.[22,24,25,44,45] Total calcium intake from calcium-based phosphate binders should not exceed twice the daily recommended intake for dietary calcium (maximum to not exceed 2.5 g/day). Hypercalcemia (serum calcium values greater than 10.2 mg/dL) should first be treated by switching to calcium-free phosphate binder therapy and reduction in dialysate calcium concentration. If persistent, discontinuation of active vitamin D sterols may be required.[1]

To limit the vascular calcification risks associated with the use of calcium salts, alternative phosphate binders have been developed. Sevelamer hydrochloride (RenaGel[R]), a calcium- and metal-free hydrogel of cross-linked poly-allylamine, has been shown to lower serum phosphorus, the calcium-phosphorus ion product, and PTH without inducing hypercalcemia in adult patients treated with hemodialysis. It is now increasingly utilized as the primary phosphate binder in children with renal failure and has been shown in prospective trials to lower serum phosphorus levels effectively and control the skeletal lesions of 2HPT without increasing serum calcium levels in children treated with dialysis.[9,10,17,43] Sevelamer has allowed the use of higher doses of active vitamin D sterols without inducing increments in serum calcium and thus, enhancing the margin of safety of therapy with active vitamin D analogues. Sevelamer also halts the progression of vascular calcification, while such lesions increase during calcium-containing binder therapy in adult hemodialysis patients. In addition to its effects on serum phosphorus levels, sevelamer has been shown to decrease concentrations of total serum cholesterol and low-density lipoprotein cholesterol, but to increase high-density lipoprotein levels. These effects may offer additional benefits in reducing cardiovascular complications in patients with end-stage renal disease. Mild acidosis may occur in patients treated with sevelamer HCL, thus, a modified form, sevelamer carbonate, has recently been introduced. This new compound is an effective phosphate binder as sevelamer HCl, but serum bicarbonate levels are higher and chloride concentrations are lower.[9,10,43]

Clinical trials have demonstrated that lanthanum carbonate, a calcium-free phosphate binder, also effectively controls serum phosphorus and PTH levels without inducing changes in serum calcium levels. However, lanthanum is a heavy metal absorbed in the intestine and accumulates in body tissues, especially in the liver and other organs in the different experimental models. Lanthanum also accumulates in the growth plate of animals with normal renal function, and, in dialysis patients, lanthanum also accumulates in bone where it persists for as long as 2 years despite discontinuation of the drug.[9,10,43,46] Further long-term studies are therefore needed to confirm the safety of such compound before widespread use is recommended in children.

Vitamin D therapy

Treatment with vitamin D is aimed at controlling serum PTH levels and the resultant high turnover bone disease. Current evidence indicates that treatment of $25(OH)D_3$ deficiency and therapy with active vitamin D sterols reduce PTH values and have beneficial effects beyond bone and mineral metabolism.

Assessment and treatment of 25(OH) vitamin D deficiency

Treatment with $25(OH)D_3$, in the form of ergocalciferol or cholecalciferol, reduces PTH values in patients with CKD stages 2–4. Thus, the KDOQI recommendations include measurement of $25(OH)D_3$ levels in pediatric patients with CKD and treatment with either ergocalciferol or cholecalciferol if serum levels are below 30 ng/mL.[1] Treatment of $25(OH)D_3$ deficiency should be based on $25(OH)D_3$ levels, as recommended by current guidelines (Table 28.1). Although current recommendations do not mention $25(OH)D_3$ repletion in individuals treated with maintenance dialysis, recent data from several centers suggest that $25(OH)D_3$ deficiency increases the risk for mortality in the dialysis population[47], likely through pleotrophic effects on the cardiovascular and immune systems[31,32]. Thus, $25(OH)D_3$ therapy should be considered in patients with all stages of CKD who display values below 30 ng/mL.[1,9] The potential role of treatment with ergocalciferol or cholecalciferol on the control of 2HPT and the mineralization defect remains to be determined, as well as the efficacy of combined therapy with active vitamin D sterols.

Treatment with active vitamin D sterols

Several studies have documented the efficacy of intermittent and daily oral calcitriol therapy for management of 2HPT both in children and in adults with advanced renal failure.[8–10,16] Bone pain diminishes, muscle strength, and gait-posture improve, and osteitis fibrosa frequently resolves either partially or completely. Active vitamin D sterol doses should be titrated based on serum PTH, calcium, and phosphorus values. Since higher PTH levels are required to maintain normal bone remodeling with progression of CKD, titration of therapy with vitamin D should be performed according to the specific stage of CKD. In early CKD, if PTH levels are above the upper limit of normal, the first step is to replete $25(OH)D_3$ deficiency; if values are still elevated therapy with active vitamin D sterols should be initiated. PTH levels slightly above the normal range are desirable in later (stage 4) CKD, 1 while, in dialysis patients, PTH concentrations between three to five times the upper limit of normal generally correspond to normal bone formation rates (Table 28.1).[1,9,10,16]

Daily doses of oral calcitriol and alfacalcidol ranging from 0.25 to 1.5 µg/day are effective in controlling PTH levels in the majority of patients with CKD stages 2–4. In dialysis patients, $1,25(OH)_2D_3$ doses given thrice weekly either by IV injection or by oral pulse therapy are effective in reducing serum PTH levels and allow for the administration of higher weekly calcitriol doses before the development of hypercalcemia when used with calcium-free phosphate binders. Dosage regimens range from 0.5–1.0 to 3.5–4.0 µg

Table 28.2 Recommended supplementation for vitamin D deficiency/insufficiency in children with CKD stages 3–4[1]

Serum 25(OH)D (ng/mL)	Definition	Ergocalciferol dose (vitamin D₂)	Duration (months)	Comment
<5	Severe vitamin D deficiency	8000IU/day orally × 4 weeks (50000IU/week × 4 weeks); then 4000IU/day × 2 months (50000IU 2 × per month for 2 months)	3 months	Measure 25 (OH) vitamin D levels after 3 months
5–15	Mild vitamin D deficiency	4000IU/day orally × 12 weeks (50000IU every other week, for 12 weeks	3 months	Measure 25 (OH) vitamin D levels after 3 months
16–30	Vitamin D deficiency	2000IU/day orally (50000IU every 4 weeks)	3 months	Measure 25 (OH) vitamin D levels after 3 months

three times weekly or 2.0–5.0 µg twice weekly. In all patients, doses should be adjusted according to target values for serum calcium, phosphorus and PTH and stage of CKD. The doses should be adjusted at frequent intervals.[8] This approach will prevent the development of adynamic bone disease and possibly vascular calcifications.[13,16]

In order to minimize the side effects associated with calcitriol therapy, mainly hypercalcemia, new vitamin D sterols, such as 22-oxacalcitrol (maxicalcitol, available in Japan) and 19-nor-1,25 dihydroxyvitamin D₂ (paricalcitol) and 1-alpha-hydroxyvitamin D₂ (doxercalciferol; available in the United States) have been approved for clinical use.[9,10] Over the past decade, these new therapies have become integral to the management of renal osteodystrophy. Indeed, studies have demonstrated the effectiveness of paricalcitol and doxercalciferol in decreasing serum PTH in patients with 2HPT accompanied by stable calcium and phosphorus values in adults and in children.[9,25] However, despite their common usage and higher survival rates in adult dialysed patients,[45] there is very limited information on the specific effects of these new vitamin D analogues on bone histology in patients with CKD. However, current evidence demonstrated that when such compounds are utilized with calcium-free phosphate binders, there is a substantial reduction in the development of hypercalcemic episodes.

Calcimimetics

Cinacalcet HCl, an allosteric activator of the calcium sensing receptor, is used for treatment of 2HPT. This small organic molecule reduces serum PTH levels and decreases the calcium-phosphorous ion product in adult patients treated with maintenance dialysis, regardless of the specific phosphate-binding agent. There is very limited information on the value of cinacalcet in a small cohorts of pediatric patients and such studies have shown that cinacalcet is an effective additional drug for the treatment of 2HPT in children. Studies in animals also suggest that the use of calcimimetic agents may play a role in reversing the process of vascular calcification. Clinical studies in adult patients have also shown that treatment with cinacalcet may prevent the need for parathyroidectomy, lower the risk of fracture and reduce vascular calcification in patients with chronic renal failure.[9,10] Due to the presence of the calcium sensing receptor on the growth plate, these agents should be used with caution in growing children. Studies are required to carefully evaluate the specific effects of such therapy in pediatric patients treated with dialysis.

Growth hormone therapy

Recombinant growth hormone (rhGH) should be considered in children with growth failure that does not respond to optimization of nutrition, correction of acidosis and control of renal osteodystrophy. Serum phosphorus and PTH levels should be within target values prior to the initiation of rhGH. Serum phosphorus levels should be less than 1.5 times the upper limit for age and 1st PTH-IRMA levels less than 1.5 times the upper target values for the CKD stage prior to rhGH therapy.[1] GH therapy will increase serum PTH levels during the initial first months of therapy; therefore, serum PTH levels should be monitored monthly. GH therapy should be temporarily discontinued if PTH levels exceed three times the upper target value for the CKD stage.[1]

Bone disease after successful renal transplantation

Successful kidney transplantation corrects many of the metabolic abnormalities associated with the development of renal osteodystrophy. Despite a well-functioning graft, however, osteopenia, growth failure, spontaneous fractures, and avascular necrosis remain prevalent in adult and pediatric kidney recipients. Significant bone loss has been shown to occur as early as 3–6 months after kidney transplantation. Several factors are implicated in the development of bone disease after transplantation, including persistent alterations in mineral metabolism, prolonged immobilization, and the use of immunosuppressive agents required to maintain graft function.[48,49]

In both adult and pediatric kidney recipients, bone histological changes associated with 2HPT have been shown to resolve within 6-12 months after kidney transplantation. However, some patients have persistently elevated rates of bone turnover, while others develop adynamic lesions, despite moderately elevated serum PTH levels.[49] Bone biopsy data from pediatric kidney recipients indicate that 67% of patients with stable graft function have indices of bone formation rate within the normal range, while 10% have adynamic bone lesion, and 23% have bone lesions characteristic of 2HPT.[50] Bone resorption is typically increased, leading to a net loss of bone mass over time. Serum PTH levels are unable to discriminate between adynamic, normal, and increased bone turnover in the pediatric transplant population.[50] The use of maintenance corticosteroids have been implicated in these alterations; steroids decrease intestinal calcium absorption, enhance urinary calcium excretion, inhibit osteoblastic activity, decrease bone formation, and increase osteoclastic activity and bone resorption.[49] Likewise, cyclosporine has been reported to increase both bone formation and bone resorption, and reduce cancellous bone volume in the rat.[49] By contrast, azathioprine has been shown to have minimal impact on skeletal remodeling. The role of other immunosuppressive agents, such as mycophenolate mofetil, as potential modifiers of bone formation and bone resorption has not been evaluated.

While bone turnover may return to normal, defective skeletal mineralization is present in the majority of pediatric transplant recipients.[50] Osteoid volume is increased while mineral apposition rate is markedly reduced.[50] Although the factors responsible for the persistent increase in osteoid formation remain to be fully explained, corticosteroid use may contribute, as may persistent imbalances in PTH, vitamin D, and FGF23 metabolism.[51]

After successful kidney transplantation with standard immunosuppressive regimens (daily corticosteroids, calcineurin inhibitor, and anti-metabolite), growth may be accelerated by an improvement in kidney function, but catch-up growth may not be observed even in children who undergo transplantation very early in life. Moreover, height deceleration occurs in approximately 75% of patients who undergo transplantation before the age of 15 years.[52] The etiology of persistent growth retardation is not completely understood, but immunosuppressive agents, persistent 2HPT, altered vitamin D and FGF23 metabolism, and the persistence of defective skeletal mineralization may all contribute. Children receiving steroid-free immunosuppressive regimens, those treated with alternate day steroids and those with better height SDS at the time of transplant attain the greatest final adult height.[52] Recombinant human growth hormone (rhGH) has been used in children with significant height deficit after kidney transplantation. A substantial increase in linear growth occurs within the first year of rhGH therapy, but the magnitude of growth response may decline thereafter.[53]

Cardiovascular disease continues to be prevalent after renal transplantation. The presence of hypertension is strongly linked to increased carotid artery intima-media thickness and poor vessel distensibility in children.[24] Electron beam computed tomography data also indicate that vascular calcifications, present in young adults on dialysis, do not regress post-transplantation and may contribute to the burden of cardiovascular disease in this population.[54]

References

1. K/DOQI clinical practice guidelines for bone metabolism and disease in children with chronic kidney disease. *Am J Kidney Dis* 2005;**46**(4 Suppl 1):S1–121.

2. Moe S, Drueke T, Cunningham J, et al. Definition, evaluation, and classification of renal osteodystrophy: a position statement from Kidney Disease: Improving Global Outcomes (KDIGO). *Kidney Int* 2006;**69**:1945–53.

3. Olsen BR, Reginato AM, Wang W. Bone development. *Annu Rev Cell Dev Biol* 2000;**16**: 191–220.

4. Wagner EF, Karsenty G. Genetic control of skeletal development. *Curr Opin Genet Dev* 2001;**11**:527–32.

5. Blumer MJ, Longato S, Fritsch H. Structure, formation and role of cartilage canals in the developing bone. *Ann Anat* 2008;**190**:305–15.

6. Rauch F. Bone accrual in children: adding substance to surfaces. *Pediatrics* 2007;**119**: S137–40.

7. Boyce BF, Xing L. Functions of RANKL/RANK/OPG in bone modeling and remodeling. *Arch Biochem Biophys* 2008;**473(2)**:139–46.

8. Kuizon BD, Salusky IB. Renal osteodystrophy. In: E. D. Avner, W. E. Harmon, & P. Niaudet (eds), *Pediatric Nephrology* (5th edn). Philadelphia: Lippincott Williams & Wilkins, 2004:1347–73.

9. Sanchez CP. Mineral metabolism and bone abnormalities in children with chronic renal failure. *Rev Endocr Metab Disord* 2008;**9**:131–7.

10. Wesseling K, Bakkaloglu S, Salusky I. Chronic kidney disease mineral and bone disorder in children. *Pediatr Nephrol* 2008;**23**:195–207.

11. Tönshoff B, Kiepe D, Ciarmatori S. Growth hormone/insulin-like growth factor system in children with chronic renal failure. *Pediatr Nephrol* 2005;**20**:279–89.

12. Sanchez CP, He YZ. Daily or intermittent calcitriol administration during growth hormone therapy in rats with renal failure and advanced 2HPT. *J Am Soc Nephrol* 2005;**16**:929–38.

13. Krempien B, Mehls O, Ritz E. Morphological studies on pathogenesis of epiphyseal slipping in uremic children. *Virchows Arch A Pathol Anat Histol* 1974;**362**:129–43.

14. Salusky IB, Kuizon BG, Jüppner H. Special aspects of renal osteodystrophy in children. *Semin Nephrol* 2004;**24**:69–77.

15. Kuizon BD, Salusky IB. Bone diseases in children with chronic renal failure In: T. Drueke & I. B. Salusky (eds) *The Spectrum of Renal Osteodystropy*. Oxford: Oxford University Press, 2001:309–33.

16. National Kidney Foundation. K/DOQI clinical practice guidelines for chronic kidney disease: evaluation, classification and stratification. *Am J Kidney Dis* 2002;**39**(Suppl 1): S1–266.

17. Salusky IB, Goodman WG, Sahney S, et al. Sevelamer controls parathyroid hormone-induced bone disease as efficiently as calcium carbonate without increasing serum calcium levels during therapy with active vitamin D sterols. *J Am Soc Nephrol* 2005;**16**:2501–8.

18. Sanchez CP. Adynamic bone revisited: is there progress? *Perit Dial Int* 2006;**26**:43–8.

19. Salusky IB, Ramirez JA, Oppenheim W, Gales B, Segre GV, Goodman WG. Biochemical markers of renal osteodystrophy in pediatric patients undergoing CAPD/CCPD. *Kidney Int* 1994;**45**:253–8

20. Wesseling-Perry K, Pereira RC, Wang H, et al. Relationship between plasma fibroblast growth factor-23 concentration and bone mineralization in children with renal failure on peritoneal dialysis. *J Clin Endocrinol Metab* 2009;**94**:511–17

21. Milliner DS, Zinsmeister AR, Lieberman E, Landing B. Soft tissue calcification in pediatric patients with end-stage renal disease. *Kidney Int* 1990;**38**:931–6

22. Mitsnefes MM, Kimball TR, Kartal J, et al. Cardiac and vascular adaptation in pediatric patients with chronic kidney disease: role of calcium-phosphorus metabolism. *J Am Soc Nephrol* 2005;**16**:2796–803

23. Shroff RC, Donald AE, Hiorns MP, et al. Mineral metabolism and vascular damage in children on dialysis. *J Am Soc Nephrol* 2007;**18**:2996–3003

24. Mitsnefes MM. Cardiovascular complications of pediatric chronic kidney disease. *Pediatr Nephrol* 2008;**23**:27–39

25. Schoppet M, Shroff RC, Hofbauer LC, Shanahan CM. Exploring the biology of vascular calcification in chronic kidney disease: what's circulating? *Kidney Int* 2008;**73**:384–90.

26. Shroff RC, Shah V, Hiorns MP, et al. The circulating calcification inhibitors, fetuin-A and osteoprotegerin, but not matrix Gla protein, are associated with vascular stiffness and calcification in children on dialysis. *Nephrol Dial Transplant* 2008;**23**:3263–71.

27. Gutierrez OM, Mannstadt M, Isokava T et al. Fibroblast growth factor 23 and mortality among patients undergoing hemodialysis. *N Engl J Med* 2008;**359**:584–92.

28. Wetmore JB, Quarles LD. Calcimimetics or vitamin D analogs for suppressing parathyroid hormone in end-stage renal disease: time for a paradigm shift? *Nat Clin Pract Nephrol* 2009;**5**:24–33.

29. Gutierrez O, Isakova T, Rhee E, et al. Fibroblast growth factor-23 mitigates hyperphosphatemia but accentuates calcitriol deficiency in chronic kidney disease. *J Am Soc Nephrol* 2005;**16**:2205–15.

30. Ben-Dov IZ, Galitzer H, Lavi-Moshayoff V, et al. The parathyroid is a target organ for FGF23 in rats. *J Clin Invest* 2007;**117**:4003–8.

31. Imanishi Y, Inaba M, Nakatsuka K, et al. FGF23 in patients with end-stage renal disease on hemodialysis. *Kidney Int* 2004;**65**:1943–6.

32. Demay MB. Mechanisms of vitamin D receptor action. *Ann NY Acad Sci* 2006;**1068**:204–13.

33. National Kidney Foundation. K/DOQI clinical practice guidelines for bone metabolism and disease in chronic kidney disease. *Am J Kidney Dis* 2003;**42**(4 Suppl 3):S1–201.

34. Ghazali A, Fardellone P, Pruna A, et al. Is low plasma 25-(OH) vitamin D a major risk factor for hyperparathyroidism and Looser's zones independent of calcitriol? *Kidney Int* 1999;**55**:2169–77.

35. Adorini L. Intervention in autoimmunity: the potential of vitamin D receptor agonists. *Cell Immunol* 2005;**233**:115–24.

36. Liu PT, Stenger S, Li H, et al. Toll-like receptor triggering of a vitamin D-mediated human antimicrobial response. *Science* 2006;**311**:1770–3.

37. Salusky IB, Goodman WG, Kuizon BD, et al. Similar predictive value of bone turnover using first- and second-generation immunometric PTH assays in pediatric patients treated with peritoneal dialysis. *Kidney Int* 2003;**63**:1801–8.

38. Coen G, Bonucci E, Ballanti P, et al. PTH 1–84 and PTH '7–84' in the noninvasive diagnosis of renal bone disease. *Am J Kidney Dis* 2002;**40**:348–54.

39. Klaus G, Watson A, Edefonti A, et al. Prevention and treatment of renal osteodystrophy in children on chronic renal failure: European guidelines. *Pediatr Nephrol* 2006;**21**:151–9.

40. Mehls O. Renal osteodystrophy in children: Etiology and clinical aspects. In: R. N. Fine & A. Gruskin (eds), *Endstage Renal Disease in Children*. Philadelphia: Saunders, 1984:227–50.

41. Leonard MB. A structural approach to the assessment of fracture risk in children and adolescents with chronic kidney disease. *Pediatr Nephrol* 2007;**22**:1815–24.

42. Lee DC, Gilsanz V, Wren TA. Limitations of peripheral quantitative computed tomography metaphyseal bone density measurements. *J Clin Endocrinol Metab* 2007;**92**:4248–53.

43. Salusky IB. A new era in phosphate binder therapy: what are the options? *Kidney Int* 2006;**105**(Suppl.):S10–15.

44. Goodman WG, Goldin J, Kuizon BD, et al. Coronary-artery calcification in young adults with end-stage renal disease who are undergoing dialysis. *N Engl J Med* 2000;**342**:1478–83.

45. Block GA, Hulbert-Shearon TE, Levin NW, Port FK. Association of serum phosphorus and calcium × phosphate product with mortality risk in chronic hemodialysis patients: a national study. *Am J Kidney Dis* 1998;**31**:607–17.

46. Drüeke TB. Lanthanum carbonate as a first-line phosphate binder: the 'cons'. *Semin Dial* 2007;**20**:329–32.

47. Wolf M, Shah A, Gutierrez O, et al. Vitamin D levels and early mortality among incident hemodialysis patients. *Kidney Int* 2007;**72**:1004–13.

48. Julian BA, Laskow DA, Dubovsky J, Dubovsky EV, Curtis JJ, Quarles LD. Rapid loss of vertebral mineral density after renal transplantation. *N Engl J Med* 1991;**325**:544–50.

49. Mitterbauer C, Oberbauer R. Bone disease after kidney transplantation. *Transpl Int* 2008;**21**:615–24.

50. Sanchez CP, Salusky IB, Kuizon BD, et al. Bone disease in children and adolescents undergoing successful renal transplantation. *Kidney Int* 1998;**53**:1358–64.

51. Evenepoel P, Naesens M, Claes K, Kuypers D, Vanrenterghem Y. Tertiary 'hyperphosphatoninism' accentuates hypophosphatemia and suppresses calcitriol levels in renal transplant recipients. *Am J Transplant* 2007;**7**:1193–200.

52. Hokken-Koelega AC, van Zaal MA, van BW, et al. Final height and its predictive factors after renal transplantation in childhood. *Pediatr Res* 1994;**36**:323–8.

53. Fine RN, Yadin O, Nelson PA, et al. Recombinant human growth hormone treatment of children following renal transplantation. *Pediatr Nephrol* 1991;**5**:147–51.

54. Ishitani MB, Milliner DS, Kim DY, et al. Early subclinical coronary artery calcification in young adults who were pediatric kidney transplant recipients. *Am J Transplant* 2005;**5**:1689–93.

Chapter 29

Bone disease in renal transplant recipients

Stuart M. Sprague and Klaus Olgaard

Introduction

The incidence of chronic kidney disease (CKD) and end-stage kidney disease (ESKD) is increasing worldwide. With newer immunosuppressant drugs and treatment protocols, post-kidney transplant prognosis is improving, with the current 1-year survival rate greater than 90%. Despite these advances, not all sequelae of CKD and ESKD are, however, reversed after transplantation. As a result of CKD and co-morbid conditions, many patients have underlying bone disorders (Table 29.1) that can persist after kidney transplantation. Furthermore, metabolic changes after transplantation, as well as medications used to manage the transplant patient may contribute to disorders in bone and mineral metabolism. This chapter addresses some of the causes and types of bone disorders observed following kidney transplantation, and the associated changes in bone and mineral metabolism as well as a summary of current therapeutic options.

Changes in mineral metabolism following kidney transplantation

Ideally, successful kidney transplantation corrects the abnormalities of mineral metabolism leading to secondary hyperparathyroidism (2HPT) and renal osteodystrophy during uremia. This includes reversal of uremia, abolition of hypocalcemia, hyperphosphatemia, and acidosis, restoration of calcitriol production, and reversal of skeletal resistance to PTH and vitamin D.[1] The scope and magnitude of the biochemical abnormalities of CKD-MBD fluctuate dramatically in the early post-transplant period compared with the late post-transplant period, the latter depending on the level of kidney function.

The incidence of hypercalcemia after kidney transplantation is non-negligible, and varies between 8.5 and 65%. The natural evolution of hypercalcemia after successful kidney transplantation is, in most cases, a spontaneous resolution.[2,3] The pathogenesis of post-transplant hypercalcemia is not necessarily due to persistent 2HPT. Several factors, such as resolution of soft tissue calcifications, immobilization, high doses of corticosteroid treatment, and hypophosphatemia might all contribute.

Table 29.1 Pre-transplant risk factors for development of post-transplant bone disease

---

1. **A history of previous bone disease**
   Renal osteodystrophy:
   (a) Secondary HPT
   (b) Osteomalacia
   (c) Mixed bone disease
   (d) Adynamic bone disease
   (e) Aluminum intoxication

2. **Previous drug treatment with**
   (a) Active vitamin D analogs and calcium
   (b) Previous steroid treatment
   (c) Treatment with other immunosuppressive drugs
   (d) Anticonvulsant therapy

3. **Other factors:**
   (a) Immobilization
   (b) Malnutrition
   (c) Gonadal insufficiency
   (d) History of fractures
   (e) History of musculoskeletal symptoms

4. **Low BMD**

5. **Renal diagnosis**

6. **Type and duration of dialysis**

Chronic hyperparathyroidism plays a major role in bone loss both before and post transplantation.[4] 2HPT is very common post-transplant and some studies demonstrate that greater than 50% of transplanted patients have elevated PTH levels even after two years.[5] Elevations in PTH are invariably a consequence of the patient's pre-transplant physiology. Both duration of dialysis and degree of 2HPT pre-transplant predict higher post-transplant PTH values.[6] Between 1.3 and 20% will later have to undergo parathyroidectomy (PTX).[2,7] The criteria for PTX after kidney transplantation are in most centers symptomatic hypercalcemia or asymptomatic hypercalcemia with inappropriately elevated levels of PTH one or more years after the successful kidney transplantation with normal kidney function.[2,3] The risk of developing post-transplant HPT increases with the duration of dialysis[2,8] and with the severity of the pre-transplant 2HPT.[8,9] Thus, the degree of parathyroid hyperplasia is believed to determine the ability of the parathyroid glands to involute after transplantation.[10] One would expect patients requiring PTX to have the most severe changes of the parathyroid glands, such as monoclonal nodular hyperplasia and formation of adenomas. Histological examination of parathyroid glands that were removed due to severe persistent post-transplant 2HPT revealed diffuse hyperplasia in most cases and only rarely adenomas.[11] This is in contrast to the findings in glands removed from uremic patients, where nodular hyperplasia was the most prevalent.[12,13] The reason for this rather surprising finding is not quite clear. However, molecular studies are probably required to detect for monoclonality.[14]

In the clinical situation, the majority of patients with 2HPT will, despite previous long-term uremia, demonstrate a significant decrease in plasma PTH after kidney transplantation. Some proportion of this decrease in measured plasma PTH might be due to better clearance of C-terminal PTH fragments as a result of the improvement in GFR, as most of the assays that have been used until recently co-measure some long C-terminal fragments.[15,16] In most cases plasma PTH return to near normal with time[5] as PTH levels are consistently below pre-transplant values by 6 months post-transplant.[5] After 6 months, a median decrease of 54% in PTH has been observed. However, in some patients PTH concentrations may remain elevated for many years.[5] Furthermore, normalization of GFR is necessary for the normalization of the PTH levels.[17] However, in transplanted patients with reduced GFR, elevated PTH levels are to be expected due to the degree of kidney dysfunction and independently of whether the patients are transplanted or not. In addition to the degree to which kidney function is restored, correction of 2HPT is also influenced by vitamin D status,[18] phosphorus metabolism, and persistent hypocalcemia caused by hypercalciuria and/or poor intestinal absorption secondary to steroids and/or vitamin D deficiency.

Hypophosphatemia is a common problem following successful kidney transplantation. Hypophosphatemia can be exacerbated by immunosuppressant medications, diuretics, persistent hyperparathyroidism, and tubular dysfunction.[19] The role of phosphatonins, such as FGF23, in perpetuating hypophosphatemia following kidney transplantation is of particular interest.[20] The majority of patients have moderate to severe hyperphosphatemia at the time of transplantation and phosphorus concentrations tend to decrease dramatically immediately following transplantation, however this decrease can be transient.[5] In some patients hypophosphatemia persists as 2–40% of patients can have hypophosphatemia at 6 months following transplantation.[5,21] It appears that the degree of hypophosphatemia is not associated with the GFR.[22]

Disorders of *vitamin D* metabolism play a major role in bone and mineral disorders in CKD prior to transplantation, which may continue into the post transplant period. Vitamin D deficiency is essentially endemic in CKD patients,[23] which persists post transplantation with mean vitamin D levels being reported as low as 10 ng/mL (95% CI 8.2–14.3).[24]

Metabolic acidosis also contributes to bone loss as many transplant patients may have metabolic acidosis from persistent CKD, medication-induced diarrhea, and renal tubular acidosis. The association of metabolic acidosis with bone loss has been demonstrated in the general population. Whether extrapolating these findings to the transplant population is appropriate is unknown. There are limited studies in transplant patients with some of the studies unable to demonstrate an association of between bone loss and acidosis.[25]

Impact of renal transplantation on bone

Several factors impact bone following transplantation, which include ongoing kidney disease with biochemical abnormalities and immunosuppressive medications (Table 29.2). Loss of bone mass after kidney transplantation occurs primarily in the first 12 months, predominantly in cortical bone. The main alteration is an uncoupling of bone remodeling, resulting in a decrease of bone formation; with persistent bone resorption, net

Table 29.2 Post-transplant risk factors for the development of post-transplant bone disease

1.	Low GFR
2.	Persistent HPT
3.	Severe hypercalcuria
4.	Severe hypophosphatemia
5.	Low plasma 1,25-dihydroxyvitamin D levels,
6.	Gonadal insufficiency
7.	Drug therapy (a) Glucocorticoids (b) Calcineurin inhibitors (c) Loop diuretics
8.	Persistently low BMD after transplantation

bone loss results. Rojas et al.[26] examined the early alterations in osteoblast number and surfaces immediately following kidney transplantation in a cohort of prospectively evaluated patients. Osteoid volume, osteoid thickness, osteoid resorption surface, and osteoclast surface were above the normal range before transplant and remained increased approximately 35 days after transplantation, while osteoid and osteoblast number and surfaces were significantly decreased, together with an inhibition of bone formation and mineralization. An important observation was that although none of the pre-transplant biopsy specimens showed evidence of apoptosis, 45% of post-transplant biopsy specimens showed significant apoptosis after only an average of 35 days. The degree of apoptosis was associated with the total glucocorticoid dose. Thus, early post-transplant apoptosis, and a decrease in osteoblast number and osteoblast surface play a contributory role in the pathogenesis of post-transplant bone disease that may be related directly to the use of glucocorticoids.

A retrospective bone biopsy study of 57 patients after kidney transplantation was performed by Lehmann et al.[27] The mean time between transplantation and bone biopsy was 53.5 months. Seven histological subgroups were identified: normal, osteitis fibrosa cystica, mild osteitis fibrosa, mixed uremic bone disease, osteomalacia, adynamic renal bone disease, and non-renal osteodystrophy, which included osteoporosis. Patients with osteitis fibrosa cystica and osteoporosis had received the highest doses of prednisolone. In all the subgroups, the mean values for creatinine, alkaline phosphatase, and PTH were increased. Patients with osteitis fibrosa cystica and mild osteitis fibrosa (as well as those with normal histology) showed the highest values for PTH and increased alkaline phosphatase levels. Given the limited number of patients in the study, no significant correlations were observed. However, a variable degree of histological abnormalities were observed following transplantation that could not have been predicted by biochemical testing, confirming that pre-existing bone disease persists in the post-transplant period.

Cueto-Manzano et al.[28] evaluated 45 bone biopsies of post–kidney transplant patients whose treatment included cyclosporine monotherapy, azathioprine and prednisone, or triple therapy. Compared with age- and sex-matched controls, none of the groups showed a significant reduction in bone mineral density (BMD) in the lumbar spine or femoral neck. However, when compared with young normal controls, osteopenia was detected in the femoral neck, except in premenopausal women. There was no significant difference in BMD related to immunosuppressant regimen, sex, or menopausal status. The histopathological diagnosis also did not differ among the immunosuppressant regimens. A subgroup analysis of 21 patients with normal PTH levels showed that cyclosporine monotherapy was associated with a more pronounced decrease in bone thickness compared with the other regimens.[28] In addition, there was a reduction in trabecular appositional rate compared with the azathioprine and prednisone group. Multiple regression analysis showed that gender and time after transplantation were the most significant factors predicting bone volume and mineralizing surface. Predictive factors for eroded bone surface and osteoclast number included age and time on dialysis before transplantation.

Role of immunosuppression

During the early perioperative period; medications, inflammation, and immobilization can contribute to bone loss. Inflammatory cytokines contribute to bone loss by affecting RANKL and osteoprotegerin influencing osteoclastogenesis.[29] The largest influence on early post-transplant bone loss appears to be the use of corticosteroids. Steroids can induce bone loss in multiple different ways such as impairing bone formation, accelerating breakdown, and causing a negative calcium balance. Steroids promote a negative calcium balance by decreasing gastrointestinal absorption and increasing urinary excretion. Steroids also impair gonadal hormone production. Steroids can induce apoptosis of osteoblasts and osteocytes, and inhibit osteoblast replication, and differentiation resulting in an imbalance of osteoclast, and osteoblast number and function causing bone loss.[30] Long-term steroid use tends to produce a low turnover state, which may play a critical role in subsequent fracture development. The induction phase of immunosuppression generally utilizes high doses of steroids and even small doses of steroids have been correlated with bone loss.[31]

Another potential serious adverse effect of steroids is avascular necrosis (AVN).[32] The mechanism of AVN is not entirely clear, but may be due to steroid's effect on the endothelial and smooth muscle cells, damaging veins resulting in venous stasis and poor drainage. AVN can affect anywhere from 3 to 41% of patients.[33] AVN tends to occur early after transplantation, usually within the first 12 months and there appears to be a higher risk in patients under the age of 40.[34] High dose steroids (over 4g) given intravenously are also associated with an increased risk of AVN.[35,36] With the decrease in steroid use over the years, the incidence of bilateral AVN has decreased from 79% in 1991 to 14% in 2002 correlating with decreased steroid usage.[34,37] Despite decreased dependence on high doses of steroids in modern immunosuppressant protocols, AVN still occurs. While there are no proven effective means to salvage an affected joint, steroid minimization may help to limit disease progression, and prevent disease in the contra-lateral hip.

Calcineurin inhibitors such as cyclosporine and tacrolimus affect bone as well. However, apparently contradictory results have been observed between *in vivo* and *in vitro* studies. In *in vivo* animal studies cyclosporine produces high turnover associated bone loss.[38] Cyclosporine is thought to affect bone metabolism by increasing osteoclast number and bone turnover as evidenced by increased osteocalcin. Although not as well studied it appears that tacrolimus has a similar effect on bone.[39] In contrast, *in vitro* studies have suggested that both cyclosporine and tacrolimus inhibit osteoclastic bone resorption.[40]

Clinical observations have been unable to clarify the effect of calcineurin inhibitor's on bone metabolism.[41] However, one study demonstrated that cyclosporine resulted in bone loss, as measured by serial BMDs, independent of steroid exposure,[42] while another study was not able to detect a difference between tacrolimus and cyclosporine.[43] Some studies have found cyclosporine to be more toxic to bones than tacrolimus,[44,45] but they are confounded by the use of lower doses of steroids in the tacrolimus arm.[45] The physiological effect of calcineurin inhibitors is thought to be opposite that of steroids and hypothetically they should offset each other. It has also been suggested that calcineurin inhibitors actually cause an uncoupling of bone processes and though their direct effect on bone cells is to inhibit bone resorption, they actually stimulate circulating bone resorptive cytokines resulting in net bone loss.[46] Although there are limited available data regarding MMF, sirolimus, and azathioprine, an effect on bone has not been identified.

Fractures, bone density, and histology post-transplant

Fracture risk is increased in patients with CKD and the risk of suffering a fracture increases further following kidney transplantation. This elevated risk continues for the life of the transplant[47] and increases with time.[48] By 5 years post-transplant up to 50% of patients experience at least one fracture. Reported fracture incidences in transplant recipients range anywhere from 5% to greater than 60%.[47,49] This wide range of reported fracture rates is a consequence of the varied methodology used in obtaining these data. Whether determining fracture rates by questionnaire, patient encounters, or documented radiographic evidence dramatically affects the result. The relative risk of fracture depends on the populations being used for comparison. Male kidney transplant recipients have an overall 5-fold increased fracture risk compared with the general population, whereas female kidney transplant recipients age 25–44 have an 18-fold increased risk and the 45–64-year-old female cohort has a 34-fold increased risk.[50] Dialysis patients have an increased incidence of both hip and spinal fractures relative to the general population but a decreased incidence compared with transplant recipients.[51] Using kidney failure patients as the comparison group for transplant patients will dampen the magnitude of relative risk of fracture, although the difference remains noteworthy. Studies using USRDS data from over 100,000 patients reveal a 34% increased risk of hip fracture in transplant recipients compared with those with kidney failure.[51]

A study of transplant patients hospitalized for fracture showed that renal transplant recipients had an adjusted risk of fracture of 4.59 (95% CI of 3.59–6.31) compared with the general population and an increased risk of mortality of 1.6 (95% CI 1.13–2.26).[52] With aging of the transplant population and with the acceptance of transplanting older individuals, this problem is poised to become even larger.

Fractures result from a decrease in bone mass and quality which results in decreased bone strength.[53] In addition, conditions such as peripheral neuropathy and an increased likelihood of falls contribute to fracture risk. Bone strength is determined by impaired bone quality and bone quantity. Bone quality is a function of its turnover and level of mineralization. Bone quantity is difficult to assess in patients with kidney failure, particularly those on dialysis. In the general public, bone density serves as a surrogate for bone quantity; however, it cannot assess bone quality. It is unlikely that it is as robust a surrogate in patients with kidney disease or in the transplant population.

When evaluated by BMD, osteoporosis is very common in kidney transplant patients, affecting anywhere from 27 to 57%.[54] This decrease in bone density can be associated with an increased fracture risk in transplant patients,[55] although the risk of diminished BMDs is better characterized in non-kidney patients.[56] Most studies have not found BMDs to have the same predictive value for fracture as noted in the general population. Nevertheless, many physicians obtain BMD studies in transplant recipients. How BMD findings should be used to direct therapy remains to be determined.

Bone biopsies reveal an array of qualitative abnormalities both early and late after transplant including, but not limited to, low bone turnover, osteomalacia, and high turnover disease. Low turnover or adynamic bone disease is characterized by decreased osteoblast and osteoclast function resulting in decreased deposition of new mineralized bone, and decreased removal of old and possibly microfractured bone. Osteomalacia or defective mineralization may also be present. Adynamic bone disease and osteomalacia may occur simultaneously. High turnover bone disease is a consequence of overactive osteoblasts and osteoclasts. New osteoid and mineralized bone is laid down rapidly and old bone is quickly removed. Similarly, both high turnover and osteomalacia may occur simultaneously. When the osteoclast activity outpaces the osteoblast activity, decreased bone mass ensues. High turnover bone disease is frequently, but not universally associated with hyperparathyroidism. It is difficult to accurately estimate the prevalence of different bone lesions as a limited number of studies have included post-transplant bone biopsies. As well, the relative contribution of the different bone pathologies changes with modifications in CKD-MBD management. To that end, adynamic bone disease may be more common now than previously appreciated.[57]

Although documenting the type or cause of bone disease in a transplant recipient may sound academic it can be clinically useful. Aside from providing a practical guide for treatment decisions it may help predict which bones are most at risk for fracture. Steroids tend to affect the cancellous bone and cause adynamic bone disease, whereas hyperparathyroidism primarily affects cortical bone and causes increased bone turnover.[58] Cancellous bone involvement affects the spine. Although spinal compression fractures can be asymptomatic they may also result in profound back pain, decreased mobility, respiratory compromise, and a decreased quality of life. Cortical bone is found predominantly in long bones of the appendicular skeleton. Several studies have found a propensity for fractures in the appendicular skeleton, especially the feet, in kidney transplant recipients.[50] Evaluating 432 kidney transplant recipients Ramsey-Goldman et al. observed 33 fractures of which 28 where appendicular and 5 were axial. Hip fractures are also debilitating cortical fractures and their occurrence is increased in both dialysis and transplant patients.[49,52,59]

Evaluation of bone disease post-transplantation

Given the prevalence of bone disease in kidney transplant recipients, they should be monitored regularly for changes in bone and mineral metabolism. BMD may be measured using dual energy X-ray absorptiometry scans at the time of transplant. Recommendations are that they should be repeated at least once, 1–2 years after transplant, but such scans are not diagnostic of bone loss or bone disease. In contrast to the Caucasian female population, the utility of BMD has not been well defined in patients with CKD or following transplantation population.[60] BMD estimates the amount of mineralized bone, but does not reflect the degree of bone turnover. BMD cannot reveal subperiosteal resorption in patients with severe osteitis fibrosa or looser zones in those with severe osteomalacia. Thus, it is not surprising that BMD has not been proven to provide good fracture risk prediction in kidney transplant recipients. Newer imaging modalities such as Micro-CT may help to assess bone quality in the future.[61] Further work is needed to clarify the utility of these newer techniques.

The utility of bone biomarkers in transplant recipients is questionable. Although changes in biomarkers provide a sense of underlying changes in bone formation and dissolution, the values may not be discriminating enough to diagnose the underlying pathology for any given patient. Cruz et al.[62] performed bone biopsies at the time of transplant and 5 months later. Biomarkers normalized before changes in bone histomorphometry were observed indicating that there may be a time lag between improvements in markers and underlying bone pathology. Biomarker concentrations change after transplant. Generally osteocalcin and PTH change in parallel and decrease with time post transplantation. Urinary collagen cross-links remain stable or decrease post-transplantation, while alkaline phosphatase tends to have a more unpredictable course.[48,63] Similar contradictory data exist for osteocalcin and urinary collagen breakdown products.

Bone mineralization, strength, and fracture rate are determined mostly by the three-dimensional architecture of the bone matrix, which can only be determined on bone biopsy, the gold standard for identification and classification of post-transplant bone disease. Abnormalities of bone are nearly uniformly observed, but the etiology and pathology are widely variable. The etiology of transplant bone lesion is multifactorial. Patients come to transplantation with pre-existing bone lesions of CKD-MBD, which are not always improved by transplantation. In addition, new insults to bone occur, including the potentially deleterious effects of various immunosuppressive agents, the impaired kidney function frequently observed in kidney transplant patients, and other factors particular to each patient, such as post-menopausal status, presence of diabetes, smoking, physical activity, and duration of dialysis and transplantation.[64–66] Based on a few bone biopsy studies in transplant patients, glucocorticoids appear to be the primary determinant of subsequent bone volume and turnover. Thus, the cumulative and mean prednisone dose correlated negatively with bone turnover, whereas there was no correlation with cyclosporine cumulative dose or serum PTH.[57] The possible role of calcineurin inhibitors such as cyclosporine or tacrolimus remains incompletely studied, with contradictory reports on their effects on bone turnover.[57]

Intuitively, it would seem that bone biopsies for transplant patients with worsening BMD or with multiple fractures would be useful. However few centers perform bone biopsies on transplant patients. This is likely because performing a bone biopsy is costly, may be uncomfortable for the patient and there are few centers with the expertise to appropriately interpret the pathology. Consequently, whether or not the increased use of bone biopsies would aid clinicians in providing more appropriate treatment and lead to better outcomes for patients with reduction in post-transplant fractures is unknown. Furthermore, a quantitative analysis and definition of bone histology and clinical consequences following transplantation has not been performed. Clearly a detailed study of bone histology following transplantation is warranted.

Treatment options for post-transplant bone disease

The goal for treatment of post–kidney transplant bone disease should be the prevention of fractures. Although BMD is used as a surrogate for identifying bone disease, whether BMD can predict fracture risk and whether improvement in BMD is associated with reduction in fracture risk in the kidney transplant population are unknown. How to approach or treat patients once a diagnosis is made can be even more problematic than making an appropriate diagnosis because of the limited number of studies addressing treatment of bone disorders in transplant patients. Several treatment regimens have been utilized; including steroid withdrawal, vitamin D, bisphosphonates, cinacalcet, parathyroidectomy, and teriparatide (Tables 29.3 and 29.4). These treatments are generally associated with an improvement in BMD; however, no studies have been shown to demonstrate a reduction in fracture risk.

Rapid tapering of *corticosteroids* is recommended, if possible, to minimize bone loss. If there is evidence of osteopenia or osteoporosis before transplant, steroid-free protocols may be considered. Early steroid withdrawal has been shown to result in improvement in BMD in the lumbar spine and femoral neck 1 year after transplantation.[67] Unfortunately, this was an uncontrolled study with a very small number of patients. Thus, there are very few data showing a beneficial effect of steroid withdrawal on the prevention of fractures or improvement in BMD.

Treatment for *hypophosphatemia* is phosphorus supplementation, either through foods or oral supplements. If the phosphorus is low enough to cause muscle weakness, intravenous phosphorous supplementation may be indicated. The net effect of low phosphorus levels on bone density, strength, and risk for fracture is not well known; however, prolonged and severe hypophosphatemia could lead to osteomalacia.

Both CKD and transplant patients have a high incidence of *vitamin D* deficiency. Vitamin D deficiency and insufficiency are associated with CVD, autoimmune disorders, malignancies, bone disease and musculoskeletal weakness, and insulin resistance.[68] Unfortunately, there are no RCTs of vitamin D supplementation in patients following kidney transplantation. However, given the magnitude of vitamin D deficiency, and the high prevalence of many of the disorders associated with vitamin D deficiency in the general population, it appears reasonable to treat deficiency.[69] Thus, supplementation with either ergocalciferol or cholecalciferol is suggested, but the optimal treatment regimen is not known,[70] nor is the sufficient level of calcidiol well defined. It is also important to point out that the primary source of vitamin D is sunlight, and the increased risk of skin cancer in kidney transplant patients mandates use of appropriate sun-screen protection, further increasing the need for oral intake of vitamin D.

Table 29.3 Prophylaxis and/or treatment of post-transplant bone disease

1.	Vitamin D—calcitriol 0.25–0.5µg/day or 600–1000U of cholecalcifereol/day
2.	Calcium intake of 1000mg/day—post-menopausal women 1500mg/day
3.	Avoid loop diuretics, if possible—use thiazides
4.	Restore normal gonadal function
5.	Restore normal thyroid function
6.	Treat persistent severe hypophosphatemia
7.	Treat persistent hypomagnesemia
8.	Treat persistent hyperparathyroidism, secondary as well as tertiary HPT
9.	Use the least possible dose of glucocorticoids, consider alternate day therapy
10.	Use of 'bone sparing steroids' might be considered
11.	Use of bisphosphonates might be considered in some patients.
	(a) Patients with severe secondary and tertiary HPT and osteomalacia might have to be excluded.
	(b) Bisphosphonates should probably be avoided when GFR< 30mL/min

Few studies have evaluated the effects of active vitamin D therapy in kidney transplant patients. A positive change in BMD was observed in subjects who where treated with either calcitriol or alfacalcidol compared with subjects who were assigned to 'no treatment' or placebo groups. In a controlled, blinded study,[42] it was demonstrated that kidney transplant recipients who were given calcium and calcitriol had significantly less bone loss in the lumbar spine and increased BMD in the distal radius and femoral neck compared with transplant patients given calcium alone or placebo (Table 29.4). The patients given calcium and calcitriol did not develop significant hypercalcemia or deterioration of kidney function during the 2 years of the study.

One study on long-term kidney transplant patients (> 12 months from transplant) evaluated the effect of calcitriol plus calcium carbonate vs. no treatment by bone biopsies in addition to BMD as an endpoint.[71] Although significant improvement in BMD was observed after 1 year in the treatment group, no differences were observed between the treatment and non-treatment groups. After 1 year of treatment, patients in the treatment group had a suppression of PTH, together with an increase in serum calcium (within normal limits), as compared with the non-treatment group. The bone biopsy results showed that bone turnover was better in 43% of the control biopsies and 12% of the calcitriol biopsies, but worse in 28% of the control biopsies and 50% of the calcitriol biopsies. Therefore, it appears as though there was development of low turnover in the treatment group. Unfortunately, no important clinical outcomes, such as mortality, hospitalizations, or fractures were evaluated in any of these studies.

Thus, if the patient does not have hypercalcemia, vitamin D, and calcium supplements could be used to prevent steroid-related osteopenia. If the GFR is less than 30mL/min and the patient has hyperparathyroidism, active vitamin D sterols could be used in addition to dietary vitamin D supplements. Serum calcium, phosphorus, and PTH levels need to be monitored closely, and used to adjust the doses of therapy,

Table 29.4 Treatment options for post-kidney transplant bone disease

Study	No. of subjects	Intervention	Results
Vitamin D			
Josephson et al.[42]	64	Ca carb Ca carb + calcitriol placebo	Ca carb: no effect on BMD Ca carb + calcitriol: increased BMD in distal radius and femoral neck
Cueto-Manzano[71]	45	Ca carb + calcitriol non-treatment	Non-significant improvement in BMD Tendency for low turnover bone disease
Bisphosphonates			
Fan et al.[72]	25	Pam placebo	Preserved BMD in lumbar spine and femoral neck at 1 year
Fan et al.[73]	17	Pam Placebo	Preserved BMD in femoral neck at 4 years
Torregrosa et al.[75]	84	Risen, Ca + Vit D Ca + Vit D	Increased BMD in lumbar spine at 1 year
Jeffrey et al.[77]	117	Alen + Ca Calcitriol + Ca	Increased BMD in lumbar spine in both groups Increased BMD in femur in Alen group
Coco et al.[80]	59	Pam, Vit D + Ca Vit D + Ca	Preserved BMD in vertebral spine at 6 and 12 months Increased risk of adynamic bone disease
Walsh et al.[79]	93	Pam, Vit D + Ca Vit D + Ca	Preserved BMD in vertebral spine at 12 month Fracture rate 3.3% versus 6.4%/year in Pam verse control
Nowacka-Cieciura etal.[90]	66	Alen or Risen non-treatment	Increased BMD in femoral neck
Grotz et al.[76]	80	Iban Non-treatment	Less decrease in BMD in lumbar spine, femur and less spinal deformities
Calcimimetics			
Serra et al.[81]	11	Cinacal 30mg/day PTH decreased 21.8%	Ca decreased 11.4%
Kruse et al.[82]	14	Cinacal 30mg/day	Ca decreased by 11.8%; PTH decreased, but not significantly
Bergua et al.[83]	9	Cincal 30mg/day, titrated at 6 months to Ca	Ca decreased 14.4%; PTH decreased 30.5%; increased BMD
Leca et al.[86]	10	Cinacal 30–60mg/day	Ca decreased 12.7%; PTH decreased 40–50%
Srinivas et al.[85]	11	Cinacal 30mg/day	Ca decreased 17.9%; PTH decreased, but not significantly
Szwarc et al.[84]	9	Cinacal 30mg/day	Ca decreased 12%; PTH decreased 22%
Teriparatide			
Cejka et al.[89]	24	Teriparatide Ca + Vit D Ca + Vit D	No change in BMD at femoral neck

Abbreviations: Ca, calcium; Ca carb, calcium carbonate; Alen, alendronate; Risen, risendronate; Pam, pamidronate; Iban, ibandronate; Cinacal, cinacalcet; Vit D, vitamin D; PTH, parathyroid hormone; BMD, bone mineral density.

Bisphosphonates act via inhibition of osteoclasts, thereby inhibiting bone resorption. Several studies (Table 29.4) have evaluated the role of bisphosphonates and suggest that bisphosphonate therapy may be useful in preventing or treating bone loss after kidney transplantation. Protocols between the studies were different, making overall comparisons nearly impossible. Fan et al. demonstrated that intravenous pamidronate administered at transplant and 1 month post-transplantation improved BMD in the lumbar spine and femoral neck at 12[72] and 48[73] months post-transplantation compared with controls. Increased BMD in the femoral neck was observed following 12 months in a group of patients who were administered either oral alendronate or residronate within the first month following transplantation compared with no specific therapy.[74] Torregrosa et al.[75] showed that patients who received risendronate had increased BMD in the lumbar spine up to 1 year after transplant compared with patients who received only calcium and vitamin D. Loss of trabecular and cortical bone assessed by BMD was prevented by parenteral ibandronate at when administered at baseline and 3, 6, and 9 months after transplantation.[76] Fewer vertebral deformities by X-ray were also observed in the ibandronate group compared with the controls.

The effect of bisphosphonates in prevalent kidney transplant patients with established osteopenia or osteoporosis was evaluated in 117 patients with reduced BMD. Patients were randomized to daily oral alendronate and calcium vs. calcitriol and calcium.[77] There was no untreated control group in this study. After 1 year of therapy both treatments showed significant increases in lumbar spine and femur BMD. However, no differences between groups were demonstrated. In another non-randomized, controlled study by Conley et al., the use of bisphosphonates was retrospectively evaluated in 554 kidney transplant patients who had at least two BMD analyses. Patients who received bisphosphonates after the first year of transplantation showed improved BMD, but did not have reduced fracture rate when compared with those who did not receive the anti-resorptive agents.[78] A randomized controlled study by Walsh et al.[79] demonstrated that pamidronate treatment resulted in improvement in BMD in lumbar spine, and tended to have decreased fractures compared with therapy with vitamin D and calcium. Unfortunately, the study was not powered to detect differences in fracture rates.

There was one study which evaluated bone histomorphometry as an end point. Coco et al.,[80] also treated patients with parenteral pamidronate at baseline, 1, 2, 3, and 6 months after transplantation. Rapid decrease of lumbar spine BMD was prevented in the pamidronate group, however, no changes in hip BMD were observed. There were no differences in the number of fractures between the groups after 1 year. Bone biopsies were performed at the time of transplant in 21 patients and in 14 patients after 6 months—six in the pamidronate group and eight in the control group. The mean activation frequency, a measure of bone turnover, after 6 months was significantly lower in the pamidronate-treated patients than in the controls. All of the pamidronate patients had adynamic bone disease on the 6-month biopsy; four patients with initial HPT and one with mixed uremic osteodystrophy developed adynamic disease. In the control group, three of eight patients had adynamic bone disease and the rest were mixed. The bone turnover improved in five of eight (62%) among the control biopsies and in none of the pamidronate biopsies. It worsened in one control biopsy (12%) and five of six (83%) pamidronate biopsies. In the second biopsy, three subjects had prolonged mineralization lag time (MLT), indicating either osteomalacia or very little tetracycline uptake. In the control group, none of the biopsies had increased osteoid thickness, although several had elevated MLT. The data provided do not allow a clear interpretation of mineralization. Mean bone volume was normal in both groups. In the pamidronate group, there was no change from baseline. Overall, bone histomorphometry revealed development of adynamic bone disease in the pamidronate treated patients, but the results are limited by a small number of subjects with a short follow-up time. It also is not clear if the potential benefit from preserving bone volume and fracture reduction outweighs the potential harm of decreased bone formation and/or prolonged mineralization. These studies should raise caution about the indiscriminate use of bisphosphonates in kidney transplant patients, especially since bisphosphonates are not recommended in patients with reduced GFR.

The *calcimimetic*, cinacalcet (Sensipar in the US and Mimpara in Europe), increases the sensitivity of the calcium-sensing receptor of the parathyroid cells to extracellular calcium, and has been shown to normalize serum calcium and PTH levels in patients with primary or secondary hyperparathyroidism. Studies by Serra et al.[81] and Kruse et al.[82] were the first to show an improvement in serum calcium and PTH concentrations in patients with persistent post-transplant hyperparathyroidism, hypercalcemia, and normal allograft function without detectable changes in fractional calcium excretion. More recently, Bergua et al.[83] also demonstrated that cinacalcet decreased serum calcium and PTH levels, as well as increased BMD, in post–kidney transplant patients with persistent hyperparathyroidism. Studies showing the beneficial effects of cinacalcet are listed in Table 29.4. In more than 50 kidney transplant patients with persistent hypercalcemia and hyperparathyroidism, cinacalcet led to an overall reduction in serum calcium and PTH levels.[81–86] In several of the studies improvement in hypophosphatemia was also noted, and kidney function did not appear to be affected adversely by cinacalcet. Thus, cinacalcet may be indicated in the setting of persistent hyperparathyroidism and hypercalcemia. An appropriately designed prospective study on the use of cinacalcet in post-transplant hypercalcemia and hyperparathyroidism would provide valuable information.

Surgical *parathyroidectomy* (PTX) has also been shown to increase bone mass after kidney transplantation.[87] One retrospective study of 14 patients demonstrated that PTX post-transplantation resulted in a 10% increase in bone mass after a median follow up of 26 months. The gain in bone density was greatest for those with osteoporosis and osteopenia; however, this study is difficult to interpret due to the inclusion of nine patients (64%) on steroid free regimens.[88] Indications for PTX include symptomatic or severe hypercalcemia, symptomatic bone disease or fracture, vascular calcification, or calciphylaxis with persistent hyperparathyroidism for more than 1 year after transplantation. Care should also be focused upon the GFR after PTX, as some small studies have found a decline. When considering cinacalcet or PTX, it is important to understand that optimal target ranges for post-transplant PTH levels have not been established.

Teriparatide is a recombinant amino-terminal parathyroid hormone with full physiological activity that has been shown to increase BMD and decrease fracture risk in large cohorts of post-menopausal women. Cejka et al.[89] demonstrated that teriparatide administered to kidney transplant patients for 6 months was safe, but did not alter

BMD in the lumbar spine or distal radius compared with the placebo group. However, BMD at the femoral neck remained stable in those given teriparatide, compared with a decrease in the placebo group. In addition, after 6 months, no significant differences between the two groups were detected in fractures, bone histology, vitamin D levels, PTH levels, kidney function, or serological bone markers. Future studies are needed in the renal transplant population.

Summary

Even after a successful kidney transplantation with good kidney function, many patients suffer from disabling skeletal symptoms. Ten to 60% of patients may develop a fracture, mainly of the cancellous bones, but also of the vertebrae. Incidence of fractures is greater in female patients and much higher in diabetic kidney transplanted recipients. Furthermore, more than half of kidney transplant recipients develop a significant reduction of the bone mineral content (BMC/BMD), which is mainly manifested in the vertebrae and the hips.

The etiology of the post-transplant bone disease is multifactorial, depending upon the pre-transplant skeletal condition of the patient, upon the immunosuppressive therapy administered after transplantation, upon post-transplant hormonal disturbances and upon the GFR obtained after transplantation. Bone biopsy studies have revealed alterations of bone remodeling that are reflecting a decrease in bone formation despite continuing bone resorption. Prophylaxis and treatment of the post-transplant bone disease should take into consideration the numerous pathogenic factors involved, which might vary significantly from patient to patient. As such, a 'simple' and easy to manage protocol to be provided to all post-transplant patients has yet to be developed.

References

1. Lewin E, Wang W, Olgaard K. Reversibility of experimental secondary hyperparathyroidism. *Kidney Int* 1997;**52**(5):1232–41.
2. D'Alessandro AM, Melzer JS, Pirsch JD, et al. Tertiary hyperparathyroidism after renal transplantation: operative indications. *Surgery* 1989;**106**:1049–55; discussion 1055–6.
3. Parfitt AM. Hypercalcemic hyperparathyroidism following renal transplantation: differential diagnosis, management, and implications for cell population control in the parathyroid gland. *Min Electrolyte Metab* 1982;**8**(2):92–112.
4. Cruz DN, Wysolmerski JJ, Brickel HM, et al. Parameters of high bone-turnover predict bone loss in renal transplant patients: a longitudinal study. *Transplantation* 2001;**72**:83–8.
5. Sprague SM, Belozeroff V, Danese M, Martin L, Olgaard K. Abnormal bone and mineral metabolism in kidney transplant patients—a review. *Am J Nephrol* 2008;**28**:246–53.
6. Edwards RM, Contino LC, Gellai M, Brooks DP, et al. Parathyroid hormone-1 receptor downregulation in kidneys from rats with chronic renal failure. *Pharmacology* 2001;**62**(4):243–7.
7. Schmid T, Muller P, Spelsberg F. Parathyroidectomy after renal transplantation: a retrospective analysis of long-term outcome. *Nephrol Dial Transplant* 1997;**12**:2393–6.
8. Messa P, Sindici C, Cannella G, et al. Persistent secondary hyperparathyroidism after renal transplantation. *Kidney Int* 1998;**54**:1704–13.
9. Torres A, Lorenzo V, Salido E. Calcium metabolism and skeletal problems after transplantation. *J Am Soc Nephrol* 2002;**13**:551–8.

10. McCarron DA, Muther RS, Lenfesty B, Bennett WM. Parathyroid function in persistent hyperparathyroidism: relationship to gland size. *Kidney Int* 1982;**22**:662–70.

11. Kilgo MS, Pirsch JD, Warner TF, Starling JR. Tertiary hyperparathyroidism after renal transplantation: surgical strategy. *Surgery* 1998;**124**:677–83; discussion 683–4.

12. Valimaki S, Farnebo F, Forsberg L, Larsson C, Farnebo LO. Heterogeneous expression of receptor mRNAs in parathyroid glands of secondary hyperparathyroidism. *Kidney Int* 2001;**60**:1666–75.

13. Matsushita H, Hara M, Endo Y, et al. Proliferation of parathyroid cells negatively correlates with expression of parathyroid hormone-related protein in secondary parathyroid hyperplasia. *Kidney Int* 1999;**55**:130–8.

14. Drueke TB. Cell biology of parathyroid gland hyperplasia in chronic renal failure. *J Am Soc Nephrol* 2000;**11**:1141–52.

15. Brossard JH, Cloutier M, Roy L, Lepage R, Gascon-Barré M, D'Amour P. Accumulation of a non-(1-84) molecular form of parathyroid hormone (PTH) detected by intact PTH assay in renal failure: importance in the interpretation of PTH values. *J Clin Endocrinol Metab* 1996;**81**:3923–9.

16. Martin KJ, Akhtar I, Gonzalez EA. Parathyroid hormone: new assays, new receptors. *Semin Nephrol* 2004;**24**:3–9.

17. Claesson K, Frodin L, Rastad J. Calcium homeostasis after kidney transplantation: a prospective study. *Transplant Proc* 1995;**27**:3465.

18. Reinhardt W, Bartelworth H, Jockenhövel F, et al. Sequential changes of biochemical bone parameters after kidney transplantation. *Nephrol Dial Transplant* 1998;**13**:436–42.

19. Ghanekar H, Welch BJ, Moe OW, Sakhaee K. Post-renal transplantation hypophosphatemia: a review and novel insights. *Curr Opin Nephrol Hypertens* 2006;**15**(2):97–104.

20. Pande S, Ritter CS, Rothstein M, et al. FGF23 and sFRP-4 in chronic kidney disease and post-renal transplantation. *Nephron Physiol* 2006;**104**:23–32.

21. Saha HH, Salmela KT, Ahonen PJ, et al. Sequential changes in vitamin D and calcium metabolism after successful renal transplantation. *Scand J Urol Nephrol* 1994;**28**:21–7.

22. Ozdemir FN, Afsar B, Akgul A, Usluoğullari C, Akçay A, Haberal M. Persistent hypercalcemia is a significant risk factor for graft dysfunction in renal transplantation recipients. *Transplant Proc* 2006;**38**:480–2.

23. LaClair RE, Hellman RN, Kraus M, et al. Prevalence of calcidiol deficiency in CKD: a cross-sectional study across latitudes in the United States. *Am J Kidney Dis* 2005;**45**:1026–33.

24. Querings K, Girndt M, Geisel J, Georg T, Tilgen W, Reichrath J. 25-hydroxyvitamin D deficiency in renal transplant recipients. *J Clin Endocrinol Metab* 2006;**91**:526–9.

25. Welch AA, Bingham SA, Reeve J, Khaw KT. More acidic dietary acid-base load is associated with reduced calcaneal broadband ultrasound attenuation in women but not in men: results from the EPICNorfolk cohort study. *Am J Clin Nutr* 2007;**85**:1134–41.

26. Rojas E, Carlini RG, Clesca P, et al. The pathogenesis of osteodystrophy after renal transplantation as detected by early alterations in bone remodeling. *Kidney Int* 2003;**63**:1915–23.

27. Lehmann G, Ott U, Stein G, Steiner T, Wolf G. Renal osteodystrophy after successful renal transplantation: a histomorphometric analysis in 57 patients. *Transplant Proc* 2007;**39**:3153–8.

28. Cueto-Manzano AM, Konel S, Hutchison AJ, et al. Bone loss in long-term renal transplantation: histopathology and densitometry analysis. *Kidney Int* 1999;**55**:2021–9.

29. Cunningham J. Pathogenesis and prevention of bone loss in patients who have kidney disease and receive long-term immunosuppression. *J Am Soc Nephrol* 2007;**18**:223–34.

30. Weinstein RS, Jilka RL, Parfitt AM, Manolagas SC. Inhibition of osteoblastogenesis and promotion of apoptosis of osteoblasts and osteocytes by glucocorticoids. Potential mechanisms of their deleterious effects on bone. *J Clin Invest* 1998;**102**:274–82.

31. Mikuls TR, Julian BA, Bartolucci A, Saag KG. Bone mineral density changes within six months of renal transplantation. *Transplantation* 2003;**75**:49–54.

32. Heerfordt J, Olgaard K, Madsen S. Osteoscintigraphic changes in kidney-transplanted patients. *Nephron* 1978;**21**:86–94.

33. Meakin CJ, Hopson CN, First MR. Avascular (aseptic) necrosis of bone following renal transplantation. *Int J Artif Organs* 1985;**8**:19–20.

34. Marston SB, Gillingham K, Bailey RF, Cheng EY. Osteonecrosis of the femoral head after solid organ transplantation: a prospective study. *J Bone Jt Surg Am* 2002;**84-A**:2145–51.

35. Lausten GS, Egfjord M, Olgaard K. Metabolism of prednisone in kidney transplanted patients with necrosis of the femoral head. *Pharmacol Toxicol* 1993;**72**(2):78–83.

36. Kubo T, Fujioka M, Yamazoe S, et al. Relationship between steroid dosage and osteonecrosis of the femoral head after renal transplantation as measured by magnetic resonance imaging. *Transplant Proc* 1998;**30**:3039–40.

37. Kopecky KK, Braunstein EM, Brandt KD, et al. Apparent avascular necrosis of the hip: appearance and spontaneous resolution of MR findings in renal allograft recipients. *Radiology* 1991;**179**:523–7.

38. Epstein S, Dissanayake IR, Goodman GR, et al. Effect of the interaction of parathyroid hormone and cyclosporine a on bone mineral metabolism in the rat. *Calcif Tissue Int* 2001;**68**(4):240–7.

39. El Haggan W, Barthe N, Vendrely B, et al. One year evolution of bone mineral density in kidney transplant recipients receiving tacrolimus versus cyclosporine. *Transplant Proc* 2002;**34**:1817–18.

40. Stern PH. The calcineurin-NFAT pathway and bone: intriguing new findings. *Mol Interv* 2006;**6**(4):193–6.

41. Brandenburg VM, Westenfeld R, Ketteler M. The fate of bone after renal transplantation. *J Nephrol* 2004;**17**:190–204.

42. Josephson MA, Schumm LP, Chiu MY, Marshall C, Thistlethwaite JR, Sprague SM. Calcium and calcitriol prophylaxis attenuates posttransplant bone loss. *Transplantation* 2004;**78**:1233–6.

43. Albano L, Casez JP, Bekri S, et al. Effects of tacrolimus vs cyclosporin-A on bone metabolism after kidney transplantation: a cross-sectional study in 28 patients. *Nephrol Ther* 2005;**1**(2):115–20.

44. Monegal A, Navasa M, Guanabens N, et al. Bone mass and mineral metabolism in liver transplant patients treated with FK506 or cyclosporine A. *Calcif Tissue Int* 2001;**68**(2): 83–6.

45. Goffin E, Devogelaer JP, Lalaoui A, et al. Tacrolimus and low-dose steroid immuno-suppression preserves bone mass after renal transplantation. *Transpl Int* 2002;**15**(2–3):73–80.

46. Gal-Moscovici A, Popovtzer MM. New worldwide trends in presentation of renal osteodystrophy and its relationship to parathyroid hormone levels. *Clin Nephrol* 2005;**63**(4):284–9.

47. Vautour LM, Melton LJ, Clarke BL, Achenbach SJ, Oberg AL, McCarthy JT. Long-term fracture risk following renal transplantation: a population-based study. *Osteoporos Int* 2004;**15**(2):160–7.

48. Sprague SM, Josephson MA. Bone disease after kidney transplantation. *Semin Nephrol* 2004;**24**:82–90.

49. Ball AM, Gillen DL, Sherrard D, et al. Risk of hip fracture among dialysis and renal transplant recipients. *J Am Med Ass* 2002;**288**:3014–18.

50. Ramsey-Goldman R, Dunn JE, Dunlop DD, et al. Increased risk of fracture in patients receiving solid organ transplants. *J Bone Miner Res* 1999 **14**:456–63.

51. Stehman-Breen CO, Sherrard DJ, Alem AM, et al. Risk factors for hip fracture among patients with end-stage renal disease. *Kidney Int* 2000;**58**:2200–5.

52. Abbott KC, Oglesby RJ, Hypolite IO, et al. Hospitalisations for fractures after renal transplantation in the United States. *Ann Epidemiol* 2001;**11**(7):450–7.

53. Borah B, Gross GJ, Dufresne TE, et al. Three-dimensional microimaging (MRmicroI and microCT), finite element modeling, and rapid prototyping provide unique insights into bone architecture in osteoporosis. *Anat Rec* 2001;**265**(2):101–10.

54. Marcen R, Caballero C, Uriol O, et al. Prevalence of osteoporosis, osteopenia, and vertebral fractures in long-term renal transplant recipients. *Transplant Proc* 2007;**39**:2256–8.

55. Durieux S, Mercadal L, Orcel P, et al. Bone mineral density and fracture prevalence in long-term kidney graft recipients. *Transplantation* 2002;**74**:496–500.

56. Marshall D, Johnell O, Wedel H. Meta-analysis of how well measures of bone mineral density predict occurrence of osteoporotic fractures. *Br Med J* 1996;**312**(7041):1254–9.

57. Monier-Faugere MC, Mawad H, Qi Q, Friedler RM, Malluche HH. High prevalence of low bone turnover and occurrence of osteomalacia after kidney transplantation. *J Am Soc Nephrol* 2000;**11**:1093–9.

58. Parker CR, Freemont AJ, Blackwell PJ, Grainge MJ, Hosking DJ. Cross-sectional analysis of renal transplantation osteoporosis. *J BoneMiner Res* 1999;**14**:1943–51.

59. Dooley AC, Weiss NS, Kestenbaum B. Increased risk of hip fracture among men with CKD. *Am J Kidney Dis* 2008;**51**:38–44.

60. Jamal SA, Hayden JA, Beyene J. Low bone mineral density and fractures in long-term hemodialysis patients: a meta-analysis. *Am J Kidney Dis* 2007;**49**:674–81.

61. Nickolas TL, Leonard MB, Shane E. Chronic kidney disease and bone fracture: a growing concern. *Kidney Int* 2008;**74**:721–31.

62. Cruz EA, Lugon JR, Jorgetti V, Draibe SA, Carvalho AB. Histological evolution of bone disease 6 months after successful kidney transplantation. *A m J Kidney Dis* 2004;**44**:747–56.

63. D'Angelo A, Calò L, Giannini S, et al. Parathyroid hormone and bone metabolism in kidney-transplanted patients. *Clin Nephrol* 2000;**53**(Suppl.):19–22.

64. Weisinger JR, Carlini RG, Rojas E, Bellorin-Font. Bone disease after renal transplantation. *Clin J Am Soc Nephrol* 2006;**1**:1300–13.

65. Rix M, Lewin E, Olgaard K. Post-transplant bone disease. *Transpl Rev* 2003;**17**:176–86.

66. Olgaard K, Sprague SM. Post-transplant bone disease. In: K. Olgaard, (ed.) C linical Guideto Bone and Mineral Metabolism in CKD. New York: National Kidney Foundation 2006:141–52.

67. Zhang R, Alper B, Simon E, Florman S, Slakey D. Management of metabolic bone disease in kidney transplant recipients. *Am J Med Sci* 2008;**335**:120–5.

68. Holick MF. Vitamin D deficiency. *N Engl J Med* 2007;**357**:266–81.

69. Olgaard K, Lewin E. Use (or misuse) of vitamin D treatment in CKD and dialysis patients. *Nephrol Dial Transplant* 2008;**23**:1786–9.

70. Cannell JJ, Hollis BW, Zasloff M, Heaney RP. Diagnosis and treatment of vitamin D deficiency. *Expert Opin Pharmacother* 2008;**9**:107–18.

71. Cueto-Manzano AM, Konel S, Freemont AJ, et al. Effect of 1,25-dihydroxyvitamin D3 and calcium carbonate on bone loss associated with long-term renal transplantation. *Am J Kidney Dis* 2000;**35**:227–36.

72. Fan SL, Almond MK, Ball E, Evans K, Cunningham J. Pamidronate therapy as prevention of bone loss following renal transplantation. *Kidney Int* 2000;**57**:684–90.

73. Fan SL, Kumar S, Cunningham J. Long-term effects on bone mineral density of pamidronate given at the time of renal transplantation. *Kidney Int* 2003;**63**:2275–9.

74. Nowacka-Cieciura E, Cieciura T, Baczkowska T, et al. Bisphosphonates are effective prophylactic of early bone loss after renal transplantation. *Transplant Proc* 2006;**38**:165–7.

75. Torregrosa JV, Fuster D, Pedroso S, et al. Weekly risedronate in kidney transplant patients with osteopenia. *Transpl Int* 2007;**20**(8):708–11.

76. Grotz W, Nagel C, Poeschel D, et al. Effect of ibandronate on bone loss and renal function after kidney transplantation. *J Am Soc Nephrol* 2001;**12**:1530–7.

77. Jeffery JR, Leslie WD, Karpinski ME, Nickerson PW, Rush DN. Prevalence and treatment of decreased bone density in renal transplant recipients: a randomised prospective trial of calcitriol versus alendronate. *Transplantation* 2003;**76**:1498–502.

78. Conley E, Muth B, Samaniego M, et al. Bisphosphonates and bone fractures in long-term kidney transplant recipients. *Transplantation* 2008;**86**:231–7.

79. Walsh SB, Altmann P, Pattison J, et al. Effect of pamidronate on bone loss after kidney transplantation: a randomised trial. *J Am Kidney Dis* 2009;**53**:856–65.

80. Coco M, Glicklich D, Faugere MC, et al. Prevention of bone loss in renal transplant recipients: a prospective, randomised trial of intravenous pamidronate. *J Am Soc Nephrol* 2003;**14**:2669–76.

81. Serra AL, Schwarz AA, Wick FH, Marti HP, Wüthrich RP. Successful treatment of hypercalcemia with cinacalcet in renal transplant recipients with persistent hyperparathyroidism. *Nephrol Dial Transplant* 2005;**20**:1315–19.

82. Kruse AE, Eisenberger U, Frey FJ, Mohaupt MG. The calcimimetic cinacalcet normalises serum calcium in renal transplant patients with persistent hyperparathyroidism. *Nephrol Dial Transplant* 2005;**20**:1311–14.

83. Bergua C, Torregrosa JV, Fuster D, Gutierrez-Dalmau A, Oppenheimer F, Campistol JM. Effect of cinacalcet on hypercalcemia and bone mineral density in renal transplanted patients with secondary hyperparathyroidism. *Transplantation* 2008;**86**:413–17.

84. Szwarc I, Argilés A, Garrigue V, et al. Cinacalcet chloride is efficient and safe in renal transplant recipients with posttransplant hyperparathyroidism. *Transplantation* 2006;**82**:675–80.

85. Srinivas TR, Schold JD, Womer KL, et al. Improvement in hypercalcemia with cinacalcet after kidney transplantation. *Clin J Am Soc Nephrol* 2006;**1**:323–6.

86. Leca N, Laftavi M, Gundroo A, et al. Early and severe hyperparathyroidism associated with hypercalcemia after renal transplant treated with cinacalcet. *Am J Transplant* 2006;**6**:2391–5.

87. Chou FF, Hsieh KC, Chen YT, Lee CT. Parathyroidectomy followed by kidney transplantation can improve bone mineral density in patients with secondary hyperparathyroidism. *Transplantation* 2008;**86**:554–7.

88. Collaud S, Staub-Zahner T, Trombetto A, et al. Increase in bone mineral density after successful parathyroidectomy for tertiary hyperparathyroidism after renal transplantation. *World J Surg* 2008;**32**:1795–801.

89. Cejka D, Benesch T, Krestan C, et al. Effect of teriparatide on early bone loss after kidney transplantation. *Am J Transplant* 2008;**8**:1864–70.

90. Nowacka-Cieciura E, Durlik M, Cieciura T, et al. Positive effect of steroid withdrawal on bone mineral density in renal allograft recipients. *Transplant Proc* 2001;**33**:1273–7.

Chapter 30

Imaging and intervention of parathyroid hyperplasia

Hirotaka Komaba, Motoko Tanaka, and Masafumi Fukagawa

Introduction

Parathyroid hyperplasia is one of the characteristic features of secondary hyperparathyroidism (2HPT) in patients with chronic kidney disease (CKD).[1] Development of marked parathyroid hyperplasia is associated with diminished responsiveness to medical therapies including active vitamin D therapy. Such refractory patients with marked parathyroid hyperplasia often require intervention therapy, i.e. surgical parathyroidectomy and percutaneous ethanol injection therapy (PEIT).[2] Thus, the evaluation of parathyroid hyperplasia is an essential step for the management of HPT in CKD patients.

Until recently, imaging of the parathyroid glands has been mainly aimed at the preoperative identification and localization of abnormal parathyroid glands. However, recently developed imaging methods provide additional quantitative and qualitative information on various types and stages of parathyroid hyperplasia. These kinds of information are not only useful for preoperative diagnosis, but also for the selection of medical or surgical therapeutic approaches. In this chapter, we would like to summarize the recent advances of parathyroid imaging for the evaluation of 2HPT.

Detection and localization of abnormal parathyroid glands

Available methods of parathyroid imaging

Many options of imaging methods are currently available for the detection of abnormal parathyroid glands. Non-invasive methods such as ultrasonography, computed tomography (CT), magnetic resonance imaging (MRI), and ^{99m}Tc-methoxyisobutyl isonitrile (MIBI) scintigraphy are widely used in clinical practice. Use of such imaging methods have been deliberately tested and compared for their sensitivity and specificity mainly in patients with primary HPT. In these patients, it is well accepted that accurate preoperative imaging is useful to identify uncommon or ectopic lesions and to determine if minimally invasive surgery can be appropriately performed.[3–5]

However, in CKD patients with 2HPT, use of imaging procedures as preoperative examination still remains controversial.[6] This is attributable to the fact that multiglandular hyperplastic disease is the most common finding in these patients and all glands need to be localized before surgery to perform total parathyroidectomy with autotransplantation.[7] This is in sharp contrast to patients with primary HPT, where solitary adenoma is responsible for 89% of primary HPT,[8] which can be intensively sought at surgery.

Another characteristic of parathyroid hyperplasia in 2HPT is that the size of parathyroid gland can be an indicator for the severity of parathyroid hyperplasia.[2] Thus, evaluation of parathyroid hyperplasia by imaging procedures provides useful information. For this purpose, ultrasonography is the method of choice because it is non-invasive, repeatable, and easily accessible, while application of other imaging methods, i.e. MIBI scintigraphy, CT, or MRI, should be considered in case of suspected ectopic and unidentified glands.

Variations in number and localization of parathyroid

The number and location of parathyroid glands are highly variable. Such variations should be carefully considered in the interpretation of parathyroid imaging. About 80–90% of people have four glands, while 5–10% have five glands, and 5% have three glands. Less than 5% of people have five or more glands, up to 12 has been reported in one case.[9]

The development of parathyroid glands during embryogenesis is a complex process and takes place in the 8–10mm embryo. Interestingly, the third branchial pouch gives rise to the 'lower' parathyroid glands together with thymus, while the fourth branchial pouch, which is caudal to the third branchial pouch, gives rise to the 'upper' parathyroid glands.[10]

Because of their migration process, the location of lower parathyroid glands is more variable than that of upper parathyroid glands, resulting in a variety of ectopic glands such as mediastinal, intrathyroidal, and undescended glands. Such glands may be overlooked readily during parathyroidectomy and can be responsible for persistent or recurrent HPT.[11]

Size of parathyroid as a useful marker

Parathyroid hyperplasia can be divided into two types with different morphological features, i.e. diffuse and nodular hyperplasia.[12] Nodular hyperplasia is considered to be a more advanced type of hyperplasia, and is associated with a lower density of both calcium-sensing receptors (CaSR)[13] and vitamin D receptors (VDR)[14] than diffuse hyperplasia. These altered qualities are considered to be the central feature responsible for resistance to active vitamin D treatment. It is, therefore, quite important to distinguish diffuse from nodular hyperplasia when treating 2HPT in CKD patients.

For this purpose, the most informative approach is to determine the size of the parathyroid glands which can be estimated by three-dimensional measurement ($\pi/6 \times a \times b \times c$, where a, b, c represent the diameters of the gland in three-dimensions).

According to our clinical experience, patients with one or more enlarged glands larger than 0.5 cm^3 or 1cm in diameter are usually refractory to calcitriol therapy in the long term.[15] Other researchers also reported that patients with enlarged parathyroid glands larger than 11mm in diameter[16] or 300mm^3 in diameter [17] were less responsive to maxacalcitol therapy than those with smaller glands. Histological studies reported that glands heavier than 0.5g[19] were composed of nodular hyperplasia in most cases.

Together, these data indicate that the critical size is 0.5 cm^3 or 1cm in diameter for the treatment of 2HPT. Parathyroid glands larger than this size may well be composed of nodular hyperplasia, and therefore are in general refractory to medical therapies including active vitamin D therapy.[2] However, it should be noted here that whether calcimimetics alone or in combination with active vitamin D sterols are capable of controlling HPT in patients with nodular hyperplasia has not yet fully been proven. Thus, in the era of calcimimetics, the utility of measuring parathyroid gland size as a marker of disease severity should be re-examined by future studies.

High resolution ultrasonography

High resolution ultrasonography is an established imaging method used most frequently in the evaluation of parathyroid hyperplasia.[18–20] To provide optimal images, ultrasonography should be performed with linear array transducers at 7.5MHz or higher and the beam should be focused at 1.5–3.0cm from the body surface. The threshold of ultrasonography depends on the operator experience and the state-of-the-art device, wich explains the wide range of reported sensitivity from 24 to 90% in patients with 2HPT.[20–33]

Image of parathyroid hyperplasia usually represents as a low echoic lesion behind middle or lower thyroid (Fig. 30.1A). Normal parathyroid gland measures 6 × 5 × 2mm and this size is generally within the detection limits of such probes. However, abnormal parathyroid glands with less fat cell tissue can be detected even if they have the size of normal glands.[18]

Parathyroid hyperplasia in CKD patients is usually larger than primary adenoma and varies in shape. The ultrasonographic pattern of glands is frequently associated with severity of parathyroid hyperplasia; when the glands show a heterogeneous pattern associated with several daughter nodules, as shown in Fig. 30.1B, the histologic findings often indicate nodular hyperplasia.[18,19]

Evaluation of blood supply to the parathyroid glands by power Doppler ultrasonography is another useful tool for the diagnosis of parathyroid hyperplasia in CKD patients (Fig. 30.1C).[18–20] Positive blood supply excludes cystic lesions and nodular lesions within thyroid, which is very useful to distinguish intrathyroidal parathyroid glands from nodular thyroid lesions (Fig. 30.1D). Furthermore, ample blood supply may suggest vigorous cell growth and nodule formation,[19,20] as discussed below.

The major weak point of ultrasonography is that glands located behind the esophagus, trachea, sternum, and those in caudal part of thymus can not be detected, although upper mediastinum can be accessible by ultrasonography. For these ectopic glands, the combination of other imaging method such as CT, MRI, and MIBI scintigraphy should be used.[3–6]

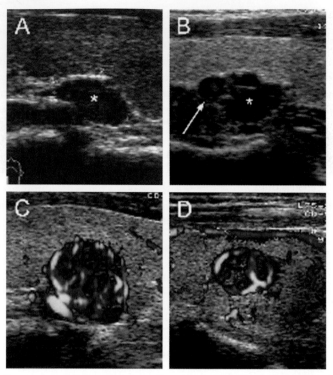

Fig. 30.1 Ultrasonographic images of parathyroid gland. (A) Typical parathyroid hyperplasia with uniform low echogenicity (asterisk) located posterior to the inferior aspect of the right thyroid lobe. (B) Heterogeneous parathyroid hyperplasia (asterisk) associated with a daughter nodule (arrow). (C) Power Doppler ultrasonography shows abundant vascularity within markedly hyperplastic parathyroid gland. (D) Parathyroid hyperplasia located wholly within the thyroid, which can be distinguished from nodular thyroid lesions by use of power Doppler ultrasonography. Courtesy of Dr. Jeongsoo Shin and Mr. Yasushi Shimizu (Motomachi HD Clinic, Kobe, Japan).

CT and MRI

CT can provide precise anatomical information on cervical and ectopic parathyroid glands. Examination of neck and mediastinum is the primary advantage of CT. In most institutions, CT is used as adjuvant imaging to search for ectopic parathyroid glands.[4]

The radiographic density of parathyroid tissue by plain CT is about the same as that of muscle and lower than that of thyroid tissue (Fig. 30.2); however, it is sometimes difficult to detect parathyroid glands close to or within the thyroid gland. By enhancement, density of parathyroid becomes greater than muscle and lower than thyroid, thus making it more easily recognizable. Artefacts caused by adjacent bones, in particular shoulder bones and sternum, and metallic clips from previous surgery. False positive results may result from tortuous vessels, lymph nodes and thyroid nodules.[6]

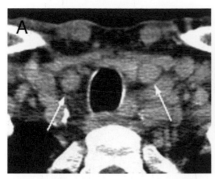
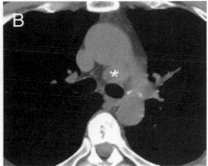

Fig. 30.2 CT images of parathyroid gland. (A) There are two hyperplastic parathyroid glands located inferior to both lobes of the thyroid gland (arrows). (B) Mediastinum ectopic parathyroid hyperplasia located posterior to the ascending aorta (asterisk).

The overall sensitivity of CT for preoperative localization of primary adenoma ranges between 46 and 80%,[3] while little data have been reported in 2HPT. By using technique with 0.5cm slices, this imaging modality would become more sensitive. Recently, the use of four-dimensional CT (4D-CT) has been proposed as a new tool for precise localization of hyperfunctioning parathyroid glands.[34,35] This new technique combines three-dimensional anatomic imaging with functional assessment that derives from changes in perfusion of contrast over time. Despite several disadvantages, such as radiation exposure, availability, and high cost, the use of 4D-CT appears promising in 2HPT.

MRI has also been shown to be useful for the detection of abnormal parathyroid glands in CKD patients with 2HPT.[6] Parathyroid hyperplasia is typically low signal intensity in T1-weighed images and high signal intensity in T2-weighed images; however, it is sometimes isotense or hyperintense on both T1- and T2-weighed sequences (Fig. 30.3A,B). Several studies suggest that MRI is more sensitive than CT, and the reported sensitivity of MRI in 2HPT ranges between 42 and 80%.[23,25, 36–38]

Until recently, gadolinium-enhanced MRI has been frequently performed to provide better sensitivity for the localization of parathyroid glands even in dialysis patients. However, due to the recently identified serious relevance to the development of nephrogenic systemic fibrosis, its routine use is currently not recommended in advanced CKD patients.[39]

Scintigraphy

The classic subtraction scan with ^{201}Tl and $^{99m}TcO_4^-$ has been recently replaced by MIBI scintigraphy. MIBI was originally developed as a cardiac imaging agent, and its uptake by abnormal parathyroid tissue was incidentally noted in 1989.[40] Because MIBI is retained in parathyroid glands for longer time of periods than in the thyroid, single isotope, double phase technique can be performed. Typically, it is performed at 10–15 min (early phase) and 2–3h (late phase) after tracer administration

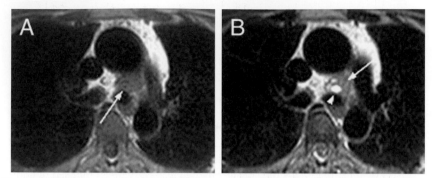

Fig. 30.3 MR images of parathyroid gland. Same case as Fig. 30.2B. (A) T1-weighted image shows a low-signal mass (arrow) located in the superior mediastinum. (B) Corresponding T2-weighted image shows a high-signal spot (arrowhead) within an isotense mass (arrow). Parathyroidectomy was performed via transthoracic approach, and histological analysis revealed parathyroid hyperplasia associated with cystic degeneration.

(Fig. 30.4A,B). Imaging can be performed using planar, single photon emission computed tomography (SPECT), or hybrid SPECT/CT.[41]

The superiority of MIBI scintigraphy has been repeatedly confirmed in patients with primary adenoma.[5] However, in CKD patients, MIBI uptake by parathyroid hyperplasia is lower than that by adenoma and its sensitivity for localization of parathyroid hyperplasia has been reported to be 35–89%.[21–31,42–52] Thus, several clinicians are against routine preoperative scintigraphy before initial surgery for 2HPT,[29,47,51] while others emphasize the need of this procedure to prevent persistent or

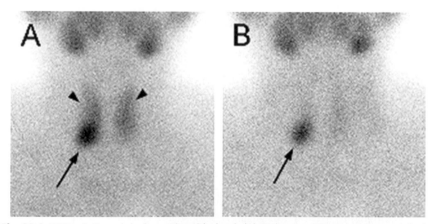

Fig. 30.4 MIBI scintigraphy of parathyroid gland. (A) Early scan (10min) shows uptake in the parathyroid hyperplasia (arrow) and physiological uptake in the thyroid gland (arrowheads). (B) Delayed scan (2h) shows retention of radiotracer in the parathyroid hyperplasia (arrow), with washout of radiotracer in the thyroid gland.

recurrent HPT[7,11] that accounts for as high as 10–30%.[68–70] Given that MIBI-positive parathyroid glands may suggest histological subtype of nodular hyperplasia,[38,49] parathyroid scintigraphy may help detect hyperfunctional ectopic glands that may cause persistent or recurrent HPT. The addition of ^{123}I subtraction,[25,33] SPECT,[26,48] SPECT/CT,[56] or low-dose dobutamine infusion[57] may improve the sensitivity of MIBI scintigraphy, although further research is needed to confirm the practical utility.

Evaluation of parathyroid cell function by imaging

Parathyroid size and weight

As discussed, parathyroid glands heavier than 0.5g are usually composed of nodular hyperplasia.[12] In patients treated by total parathyroidectomy with autotransplantation, relapse of transplanted glands often develops if the fragments were taken from a gland heavier than 0.5g.[12] The size detected by ultrasonography correlates well with the actual gland weight,[12,58] so it is suggested that the parathyroid gland size can be an indicator of the stage of parathyroid hyperplasia, i.e. diffuse or nodular hyperplasia.[2]

In dialysis patients with 2HPT, the total size or weight of parathyroid glands usually exhibits significant correlation with basal PTH levels.[58,59] The correlation is much better with stimulated, peak plasma PTH.[60] A recent study also reported that the weight of a resected parathyroid gland is significantly correlated with the corresponding PTH reduction after the removal of each parathyroid gland.[58]

Interestingly, the size of parathyroid glands may be modified during medical therapies such as active vitamin D sterols[61] and calcimimetic agents.[62] Based on several clinical data, reduction of parathyroid size may occur more frequently in small glands than in markedly enlarged glands associated with nodular hyperplasia. It is possible, although not proven, that such regression of hyperplasia may lead to a long-term controllability of the patient's 2HPT.[15] Ultrasonography may be the best tool to follow-up on such parathyroid gland changes during medical treatment, because it is less costly and easily accessible.

Blood supply to parathyroid hyperplasia

It is well known that parathyroid adenoma in patients with primary HPT usually exhibit increased blood supply on power Doppler imaging. Similarly, parathyroid hyperplasia in CKD patients also frequently demonstrate increased vascularity, especially in enlarged parathyroid glands.[18–20]

Several clinical studies have reported that high blood flow signals evaluated by power Doppler ultrasonography were associated with pathological features of nodular hyperplasia.[19,20] Furthermore, suppression of parathyroid cell activity by medical therapies, such as active vitamin D sterols[63] and calcimimetics,[62] can be assessed by the decrease or disappearance of detectable blood flow, which is sometimes associated with anechoic areas of cystic degeneration.[62] Evaluation of blood supply by this method is also helpful to make diagnosis of autoinfarction of parathyroid glands.[64]

Thus, evaluation of parathyroid vascularity by power Doppler ultrasonography is highly useful in clinical practice; however, detection of blood supply still depends on the device performance and there is no standardized scoring system. For quantitative evaluation of parathyroid vascularity, these issues should be resolved in near future.

Cell activity assessment by scintigraphy

Parathyroid tissue uptake of MIBI depends on the number and the activity of mitochondria,[65] and therefore may be an indicator of metabolic activity of the cells. Furthermore, recent studies have shown that MIBI uptake is associated not only with cell cycle,[66] cell proliferation, and weight,[44] but also with histology of parathyroid glands. i.e. diffuse or nodular hyperplasia.[38,49] In addition, diminished MIBI uptake has been reported in association with spontaneous remission of HPT due to autoinfarction of the glands.[87] Thus, parathyroid scintigraphy can be an indicator of severely advanced parathyroid hyperplasia in patients with 2HPT, although other factors such as expression of P-glycoprotein or the multidrug resistance-related protein may also influence the radiotracer uptake.[68–70]

Several studies reported that parathyroid scintigraphy can reflect the suppression of parathyroid cell activity by calcitriol pulse therapy.[71] A recent preliminary report also suggested that calcimimetics suppress MIBI uptake in 2HPT.[72] In these studies, the presence of severe parathyroid hyperplasia, reflected by high MIBI uptake, has been shown to predict the responsiveness to medical therapies, as has been shown in the studies of ultrasonography.

Reduction of parathyroid function under ultrasonographic guidance

Patients with severe 2HPT that is refractory to medical treatment should be treated with interventional therapy, i.e. parathyroidectomy and PEIT.[2] PEIT of parathyroid glands was originally developed as an alternative to conventional surgical parathyroidectomy by Italian pioneers during the 1980s[73] and has become widespread as a procedure for the treatment of refractory HPT.[74–77]

Based on the accumulated clinical data, the first guidelines for PEIT were established by the Japanese Society for Parathyroid Intervention in 2003[78] and they have recently been updated in 2008.[79] These guidelines reinforced the concept of 'selective PEIT', where an enlarged gland with nodular hyperplasia is selectively destroyed by ethanol injection and the remaining glands with diffuse hyperplasia are controlled by medical therapy, such as active vitamin D analogues.[80] This policy is partly in contrast to that of surgical parathyroidectomy, which does not usually require postoperative medical treatment to manage parathyroid function (Fig. 30.5).[7] In this regard, it is noteworthy that recent clinical observations suggest that patients who have one enlarged gland are best suited to selective PEIT.[81] It is very important to recognize the number and location of parathyroid glands when selecting the optimal method of intervention.

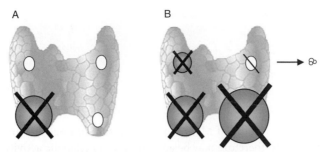

Fig. 30.5 Schematic representation of parathyroid intervention. (A) Selective PFIT. An enlarged parathyroid gland with nodular hyperplasia (grey gland) is destroyed selectively by ethanol injection and other glands with diffuse hyperplasia (white glands) are managed by medical therapy. (B) Total parathyroidectomy with autotransplantation. All glands are surgically removed and fragments from the smallest gland (white gland) are transplanted in the forearm muscle.

With the advances in equipment and imaging techniques, we can perform PEIT more efficiently and safely than ever. The sensitivity of ultrasonography has become high enough to detect smaller glands and to identify the tip of the needle. The injection of each 0.1mL of ethanol into parathyroid glands can be performed by monitoring Doppler blood flow mapping. To confirm the destruction of parathyroid tissue by ethanol injection, routinely use of Doppler color imaging is recommended.[79]

Figure 30.6 illustrates a representative procedure of selective PEIT. In Fig. 30.6A, an enlarged gland with abundant blood supply is detected with power Doppler mode. Then under B mode (Fig. 30.6B), a 22g PEIT needle (arrowheads) is inserted into the centre of the selected parathyroid gland (arrow) and a mixture of 90% ethanol with 0.1% lidocaine is injected slowly. The amount of ethanol at the initial injection should be less than 80% of the estimated volume of the parathyroid gland. It is very important to prevent the leak of ethanol to the surrounding tissue. After the ethanol injection, the echo-density of the parathyroid becomes higher (arrow) (Fig. 30.6C). Finally, disappearance of blood supply is confirmed by power Doppler imaging. As shown in Fig. 30.6D, successful PEIT usually results in a reduction in the volume and vascularity after a long-term follow-up.

PEIT can cause pain, hematomas or paralysis of the recurrent laryngeal nerve, so it should be performed with care. If the PTH concentration does not decrease even after five sessions of PEIT, clinicians should discontinue PEIT to avoid tissue adhesion due to the injected alcohol, a condition which may lead to difficulty in subsequent parathyroidectomy.[79]

Direct calcitriol injection and other procedures for parathyroid intervention

The direct injection route can be used not only for ethanol, but also for other agents such as calcitriol or its analogues (percutaneous vitamin D injection therapy; PDIT).[82,83] Clinical studies of PDIT for dialysis patients have shown that these

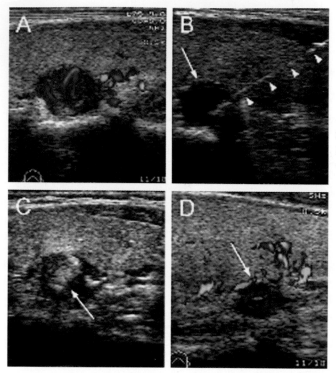

Fig. 30.6 Procedure of selective PEIT. (A) Enlarged parathyroid gland (11.8×10.1×8.7mm) with hypervascularity is detected with power Doppler mode. (B) PEIT needle (arrowheads) is inserted into the parathyroid gland (arrow). (C) Post-procedure ultrasonography shows echogenic changes related to ethanol injection (arrow). (D) The same gland after 12 months, showing a reduced volume (7.5×5.5×4.8mm) with minimal residual vascularity (arrow). Courtesy of Dr. Jeongsoo Shin and Mr. Yasushi Shimizu (Motomachi HD Clinic, Kobe, Japan). See text for details.

procedures effectively suppress PTH secretion, regress parathyroid hyperplasia, and thereby restore the responsiveness to conventional medical therapy.[82,83] The potential mechanism of these effects is suggested to be through the direct effect on PTH secretion, upregulation of both VDR and CaSR, and induction of apoptosis of parathyroid cells.[84,85] Because calcitriol and its analogues are not as toxic to parathyroid cells as ethanol, the risk of recurrent nerve palsy in PDIT is lower than that in PEIT, while at least two or three times of injections are usually needed to suppress PTH secretion.

By using the method of direct injection procedure, it has recently become possible to transfer functional genes into parathyroid cells and thereby modulate parathyroid function. A recent preliminary study reported that direct injection of CaSR- and VDR- inducted adenovirus into parathyroid glands resulted in upregulation of CaSR and VDR expression, respectively.[86] Although not applicable to humans at present, this technique is promising as it may clarify various signaling pathways related to cell function and proliferation activity in 2HPT.

Summary

Evaluation of parathyroid hyperplasia by various imaging methods provides useful information in CKD patients. Routine examination of parathyroid by high resolution ultrasonography is recommended in CKD patients with increased PTH levels. Evaluation of parathyroid size and blood supply by power Doppler ultrasonography is highly useful for the differentiation between diffuse and nodular hyperplasia. With such advances in ultrasound imaging, interventional therapies such as PEIT became a practical therapeutic modality to control severe HPT, especially in patients with one enlarged gland. For preoperative localization, scintigraphy in combination with either MRI or CT adds more information especially on ectopic glands, although routine use of these modalities at initial surgery still remains controversial. When these modalities are inconclusive or negative despite the presence of severe HPT, other procedures such as selective venous sampling and positron emission tomography with ^{11}C-methionin[48,51] may be indicated. Further progress of parathyroid imaging techniques would provide more accurate localization and quantitative evaluation of parathyroid hyperplasia and would open new approaches to rational treatment strategies for 2HPT.

References

1. Drueke TB. Cell biology of parathyroid gland hyperplasia in chronic renal failure. *J Am Soc Nephrol* 2000;**11**:1141–52.

2. Fukagawa M, Nakanishi S, Kazama JJ. Basic and clinical aspects of parathyroid hyperplasia in chronic kidney disease. *Kidney Int* 2006;**70**(Suppl 102):S3–7.

3. Mariani G, Gulec SA, Rubello D, et al. Preoperative localisation and radioguided parathyroid surgery. *J Nucl Med* 2003;**44**:1443–58.

4. Fakhran S, Branstetter BF 4th, Pryma DA. Parathyroid imaging. *Neuroimag Clin N Am* 2008;**18**:537–49.

5. Palestro CJ, Tomas MB, Tronco GG. Radionuclide imaging of the parathyroid glands. *Semin Nucl Med* 2005;**35**:266–76.

6. Fuster D, Torregrosa JV, Setoain X, et al. Localising imaging in secondary HPT. *Minerva Endocrinol* 2008;**33**:203–12.

7. Tominaga Y. Surgical management of secondary HPT in uremia. *Am J Med Sci* 1999;**317**:390–7.

8. Ruda, JM, Hollenbeak, CS, Stack, BC Jr. A systematic review of the diagnosis and treatment of primary HPT from (1995) to (2003). *Otolaryngol Head Neck Surg* 2005;**132**:359–72.

9. Grimelius L, Akerström G, Johansson H, Bergström R. Anatomy and histopathology of human parathyroid glands. *Pathol Annu* 1981;**16**:1–24.

10. Mansberger AR Jr, Wei JP. Surgical embryology and anatomy of the thyroid and parathyroid glands. *Surg Clin North Am* 1993;**73**:727–46.

11. Tominaga Y, Katayama A, Sato T, et al. Re-operation is frequently required when parathyroid glands remain after initial parathyroidectomy for advanced secondary HPT in uremic patients. *Nephrol Dial Transplant* 2003;**18**(Suppl 3): iii65–70.

12. Tominaga Y, Tanaka Y, Sato K, Nagasaka T, Takagi H. Histopathology, pathophysiology, and indications for surgical treatment of renal HPT. *Semin Surg Oncol* 1997;**13**:78–86.

13. Gogusev J, Duchambon P, Hory B, et al. Depressed expression of calcium receptor in parathyroid gland tissue of patients with HPT. *Kidney Int* 1997;**51**:328–36.

14. Fukuda N, Tanaka H, Tominaga Y, Fukagawa M, Kurokawa K, Seino Y. Decreased 1,25-dihydroxyvitamin D3 receptor density is associated with a more severe form of parathyroid hyperplasia in chronic uremic patients. *J Clin Invest* 1993;**92**:1436–42.

15. Fukagawa M, Kitaoka M, Yi H, et al. Serial evaluation of parathyroid size by ultrasonography is another useful marker for the long-term prognosis of calcitriol pulse therapy in chronic dialysis patients. *Nephron* 1994;**68**:221–8.

16. Okuno S, Ishimura E, Kitatani K, et al. Relationship between parathyroid gland size and responsiveness to maxacalcitol therapy in patients with secondary HPT. *Nephrol Dial Transplant* 2003;**18**:2613–21.

17. Tominaga Y, Inaguma D, Matsuoka S, et al. Is the volume of the parathyroid gland a predictor of Maxacalcitol response in advanced secondary HPT? *Ther Apher Dial* 2006;**10**:198–204.

18. Kitaoka M. Ultrasonographic diagnosis of parathyroid glands and percutaneous ethanol injection therapy. *Nephrol Dial Transplant* 2003;**18**(Suppl 3):ii27–30.

19. Vulpio C, Bossola M, De Gaetano A, et al. Ultrasound patterns of parathyroid glands in chronic hemodialysis patients with secondary HPT. *Am J Nephrol* 2008;**28**:589–97.

20. Onoda N, Kurihara S, Sakurai Y, et al. Evaluation of blood supply to the parathyroid glands in secondary HPT compared with histopathology. *Nephrol Dial Transplant* 2003;**18**(Suppl 3):iii34–7.

21. Light VL, McHenry CR, Jarjoura D, Sodee DB, Miron SD. Prospective comparison of dual-phase technetium-99m-sestamibi scintigraphy and high resolution ultrasonography in the evaluation of abnormal parathyroid glands. *Am Surg* 1996;**62**:562–7.

22. Ishibashi M, Nishida H, Strauss HW et al. Localisation of parathyroid glands using technetium-99m-tetrofosmin imaging. *J Nucl Med* 1997;**38**:706–11.

23. Ishibashi M, Nishida H, Hiromatsu Y, Kojima K, Tabuchi E, Hayabuchi N. Comparison of technetium-99m-MIBI, technetium-99m-tetrofosmin, ultrasound and MRI for localisation of abnormal parathyroid glands. *J Nucl Med* 1998;**39**:320–4.

24. Torregrosa JV, Palomar MR, Pons F, et al. Has double-phase MIBI scintigraphy usefulness in the diagnosis of HPT? *Nephrol Dial Transplant* 1998;**13**(Suppl 3):37–40.

25. Wakamatsu H, Noguchi S, Yamashita H, et al. Parathyroid scintigraphy with 99mTc-MIBI and 123I subtraction: a comparison with magnetic resonance imaging and ultrasonography. *Nucl Med Commun* 2003;**24**:755–62.

26. Spanu A, Migaleddu V, Manca A, et al. The usefulness of single photon emission computerised tomography with pinhole collimator (P-SPECT) in preoperative localisation of hyperfunctioning parathyroid glands in patients with secondary HPT. *Radiol Med* 2003;**106**:399–412.

27. Takeyama H, Shioya H, Mori Y, et al. Usefulness of radio-guided surgery using technetium-99m methoxyisobutylisonitrile for primary and secondary HPT. *World J Surg* 2004;**28**:576–82.

28. Fuster D, Ybarra J, Ortin J, et al. Role of pre-operative imaging using 99mTc-MIBI and neck ultrasound in patients with secondary HPT who are candidates for subtotal parathyroidectomy. *Eur J Nucl Med Mol Imaging* 2006;**33**:467–73.

29. Lai EC, Ching AS, Leong HT. Secondary and tertiary HPT: role of preoperative localisation. *ANZ J Surg* 2007;**77**:880–2.

30. Kasai ET, da Silva JW, Mandarim de Lacerda CA, Boasquevisque E. Parathyroid glands: combination of sestamibi-(99m)Tc scintigraphy and ultrasonography for demonstration of hyperplasic parathyroid glands. *Rev Esp Med Nucl* 2008;**27**:8–12.

31. Sukan A, Reyhan M, Aydin M, et al. Preoperative evaluation of HPT: the role of dual-phase parathyroid scintigraphy and ultrasound imaging. *Ann Nucl Med* 2008;**22**:123–31.

32. Kawata R, Kotetsu L, Takamaki A, Yoshimura K, Takenaka H. Ultrasonography for preoperative localisation of enlarged parathyroid glands in secondary HPT. *Auris Nasus Larynx* 2009;**36**:461–5.

33. Périé S, Fessi H, Tassart M, et al. Usefulness of combination of high-resolution ultrasonography and dual-phase dual-isotope iodine 123/technetium Tc 99m sestamibi scintigraphy for the preoperative localisation of hyperplastic parathyroid glands in renal HPT. *Am J Kidney Dis* 2005;**45**:344–52.

34. Rodgers SE, Hunter GJ, Hamberg LM, et al. Improved preoperative planning for directed parathyroidectomy with 4-dimensional computed tomography. *Surgery* 2006;**140**: 932–40.

35. Mortenson MM, Evans DB, Lee JE, et al. Parathyroid exploration in the reoperative neck: improved preoperative localisation with 4D-computed tomography. *J Am Coll Surg* 2008;**206**:888–95.

36. Ishibashi M, Nishida H, Hiromatsu Y, Kojima K, Uchida M, Hayabuchi N. Localisation of ectopic parathyroid glands using technetium-99m sestamibi imaging: comparison with magnetic resonance and computed tomographic imaging. *Eur J Nucl Med* 1997;**24**: 197–201.

37. Ishibashi M, Nishida H, Strauss HW, et al. Localisation of parathyroid glands using technetium-99m-tetrofosmin imaging. *J Nucl Med* 1997;**38**:706–11.

38. Nishida H, Ishibashi M, Hiromatsu Y, et al. Comparison of histological findings and parathyroid scintigraphy in hemodialysis patients with secondary hyperparathyroid glands. *Endocr J* 2005;**52**:223–8.

39. Grobner T, Prischl FC. Gadolinium and nephrogenic systemic fibrosis. *Kidney Int* 2007;**72**:260–4.

40. Coakley AJ, Kettle AG, Wells CP, O'Doherty MJ, Collins RE. 99Tcm sestamibi—a new agent for parathyroid imaging. *Nucl Med Commun* 1989;**10**:791–4.

41. Lavely WC, Goetze S, Friedman KP et al. Comparison of SPECT/CT, SPECT, and planar imaging with single- and dual-phase (99m)Tc-sestamibi parathyroid scintigraphy. *J Nucl Med* 2007;**48**:1084–9.

42. McHenry CR, Lee K, Saadey J, Neumann DR, Esselstyn CB Jr. Parathyroid localisation with technetium-99m-sestamibi: a prospective evaluation. *J Am Coll Surg* 1996;**183**:25–30.

43. Wada A, Sugihara M, Sugimura K, Kuroda H. Magnetic resonance imaging (MRI) and technetium-99m-methoxyisonitrile (MIBI) scintigraphy to evaluate the abnormal parathyroid gland and PEIT efficacy for secondary HPT. *Radiat Med* 1999;**17**:275–82.

44. Takebayashi S, Hidai H, Chiba T, Takagi Y, Nagatani Y, Matsubara S. Hyperfunctional parathyroid glands with 99mTc-MIBI scan: semiquantitative analysis correlated with histologic findings. *J Nucl Med* 1999;**40**:1792–7.

45. Hung GU, Wang SJ, Lin WY. Tc-99m MIBI parathyroid scintigraphy and intact parathyroid hormone levels in HPT. *Clin Nucl Med* 2003;**28**:180–5.

46. Gotthardt M, Lohmann B, Behr TM, et al. Clinical value of parathyroid scintigraphy with technetium-99m methoxyisobutylisonitrile: discrepancies in clinical data and a systematic metaanalysis of the literature. *World J Surg* 2004;**28**:100–7.

47. Ogi S, Fukumitsu N, Uchiyama M, Mori Y, Takeyama H. The usefulness of radio-guided surgery in secondary HPT. *Ann Nucl Med* 2004;**18**:69–71.

48. Otto D, Boerner AR, Hofmann M, et al. Pre-operative localisation of hyperfunctional parathyroid tissue with 11C-methionine PET. *Eur J Nucl Med Mol Imaging* 2004;**31**: 1405–12.

49. Custódio MR, Montenegro F, Costa AF, et al. MIBI scintigraphy, indicators of cell proliferation and histology of parathyroid glands in uremic patients. *Nephrol Dial Transplant* 2005;**20**:1898–903.

50. Lomonte C, Buonvino N, Selvaggiolo M, et al. Sestamibi scintigraphy, topography, and histopathology of parathyroid glands in secondary HPT. *Am J Kidney Dis* 2006;**48**: 638–44.

51. Tang BN, Moreno-Reyes R, Blocklet D, et al. Accurate pre-operative localisation of pathological parathyroid glands using 11C-methionine PET/CT. *Contrast Media Mol Imaging* 2008;**3**:157–63.

52. Papanikolaou V, Vrochides D, Imvrios G, et al. Tc-99m sestamibi accuracy in detecting parathyroid tissue is increased when combined with preoperative laboratory values: a retrospective study in 453 greek patients with chronic renal failure who underwent parathyroidectomy. *Transplant Proc* 2008;**40**:3163–5.

53. Rothmund M, Wagner P. Reoperations for persistent and recurrent secondary HPT. *Ann Surg* 1988;**207**:310–14.

54. Kessler M, Avila JM, Renoult E, Mathieu P. Reoperation for secondary HPT in chronic renal failure. *Nephrol Dial Transplant* 1991;**6**:176–9.

55. Gagné ER, Ureña P, Leite-Silva S, et al. Short and long term efficacy of total parathyroidectomy with immediate autografting compared with subtotal parathyroidectomy in hemodialysis patients. *J Am Soc Nephrol* 1992;**3**:1008–17.

56. Serra A, Bolasco P, Satta L, Nicolosi A, Uccheddu A, Piga M. Role of SPECT/CT in the preoperative assessment of hyperparathyroid patients. *Radiol Med* 2006;**111**:999–1008.

57. Quagliata A, López JJ, Guissoli P, Gambini JP, Hermida JC, Alonso O. Dobutamine modulated Tc-99m MIBI scintigraphy in secondary HPT in uremic patients. *Clin Nucl Med* 2007;**32**:782–6.

58. Kakuta T, Tanaka R, Kanai G, et al. Relationship between the weight of parathyroid glands and their secretion of parathyroid hormone in hemodialysis patients with secondary HPT. *Ther Apher Dial* 2008;**12**:385–90.

59. Inaba M, Okuno S, Chou H, et al. Positive correlation of serum bio-intact PTH(1-84) but not intact PTH with parathyroid gland size in hemodialysis patients. *Biomed Pharmacother* 2006;**60**:62–5.

60. McCarron DA, Muther RS, Lenfesty B, Bennett WM. Parathyroid function in persistent HPT: Relationship to gland size. *Kidney Int* 1982;**22**:662–70.

61. Fukagawa M, Okazaki R, Takano K, et al. Regression of parathyroid hyperplasia by calcitriol-pulse therapy in patients on long-term dialysis. *N Engl J Med* 1990;**323**: 421–2.

62. Meola M, Petrucci I, Barsotti G. Long-term treatment with cinacalcet and conventional therapy reduces parathyroid hyperplasia in severe secondary HPT. *Nephrol Dial Transplant* 2009;**24**:982–9.

63. Pretolesi F, Silvestri E, Di Maio G, et al. US imaging and color Doppler in patients undergoing inhibitory therapy with calcitriol for secondary HPT. *Eur Radiol* 1997;**7**:721–5.

64. Tanaka M, Tominaga Y, Itoh K, et al. Autoinfarction of the parathyroid gland diagnosed by power Doppler ultrasonography in a patient with secondary HPT. *Nephrol Dial Transplant* 2006;**21**:1092–5.

65. Chiu ML, Kronauge JF, Piwnica-Worms D. Effect of mitochondrial and plasma membrane potentials on accumulation of hexakis (2-methoxyisobutylisonitrile) technetium(I) in cultured mouse fibroblasts. *J Nucl Med* 1990;**31**:1646–53.

66. Torregrosa JV, Fernández-Cruz L, Canalejo A, et al. (99m)Tc-sestamibi scintigraphy and cell cycle in parathyroid glands of secondary HPT. *World J Surg* 2000;**24**:1386–90.

67. Tanaka M, Tominaga Y, Sawatari E, et al. Infarction of mediastinal parathyroid gland causing spontaneous remission of secondary HPT. *Am J Kidney Dis* 2004;**44**:762–7.

68. Bhatnagar A, Vezza PR, Bryan JA, et al. Technetium-99m-sestamibi parathyroid scintigraphy: effect of P-glycoprotein, histology and tumor size on detectability. *J Nucl Med* 1998;**39**:1617–20.

69. Yamaguchi S, Yachiku S, Hashimoto H, et al. Relation between technetium 99m-methoxyisobutylisonitrile accumulation and multidrug resistance protein in the parathyroid glands. *World J Surg* 2002;**26**:29–34.

70. Shiau YC, Tsai SC, Wang JJ, Ho ST, Kao A. Detecting parathyroid adenoma using technetium-99m tetrofosmin: comparison with P-glycoprotein and multidrug resistance related protein expression–a preliminary report. *Nucl Med Biol* 2002;**29**:339–44.

71. Torregrosa JV, Fuster D, Ybarra J, Ortín J, Moreno A, Valveny N. Predicting the effect of intravenous calcitriol on parathyroid gland activity using double-phase technetium Tc 99m-sestamibi scintigraphy. *Am J Kidney Dis* 2004;**44**:476–80.

72. Torregosa JV, Fuster D, Martin G, Casellas J, Cruzado JM. MIBI scintigraphy can predict the effect of cinacalcet in patients on dialysis with secondary HPT. (Abstract.) *J Am Soc Nephrol* 2008;**19**:5A.

73. Solbiati L, Giangrande A, Pra LD, Belloti E, Cantu P, Ravetto C. Percutaneous ethanol injection of parathyroid tumor under US guidance: treatment for secondary HPT. *Radiology* 1985;**155**:607–10.

74. Giangrande A, Castiglioni A, Solbiati L, Allaria P. Ultrasound-guided percutaneous fine-needle ethanol injection into parathyroid glands in secondary HPT. *Nephrol Dial Transplant* 1992;**7**:412–21.

75. Kitaoka M, Fukagawa M, Ogata E, Kurokawa K. Reduction of functioning parathyroid cell mass by ethanol injection in chronic dialysis patients. *Kidney Int* 1994;**46**:1110–17.

76. Fletcher S, Kanagasundaram NS, Rayner HC, et al. Assessment of ultrasound guided percutaneous ethanol injection and parathyroidectomy in patients with tertiary HPT. *Nephrol Dial Transplant* 1998; **13**: 3111–17.

77. Kakuta T, Fukagawa M, Fujisaki T, et al. Prognosis of parathyroid function after successful percutaneous ethanol injection therapy guided by color Doppler flow mapping in chronic dialysis patients. *Am J Kidney Dis* 1999;**33**:1091–9.

78. Fukagawa M, Kitaoka M, Tominaga Y, et al. Guidelines for percutaneous ethanol injection therapy of the parathyroid glands in chronic dialysis patients. *Nephrol Dial Transplant* 2003;**18**(Suppl 3):iii31–3.

79. Onoda N, Fukagawa M, Tominaga Y, et al. New clinical guidelines for selective direct injection therapy of the parathyroid glands in chronic dialysis patients. *NDT Plus* 2008;**1**(Suppl 3):iii26–8.

80. Tanaka M, Fukagawa M. Medical management after parathyroid intervention. *NDT Plus* 2008;**1**(Suppl 3):iii18–20.

81. Koiwa F, Kakuta T, Tanaka R, Yumita D. Efficacy of percutaneous ethanol injection therapy (PEIT) is related to the number of parathyroid glands in hemodialysis patients with secondary HPT. *Nephrol Dial Transplant* 2007;**22**:522–8.

82. Kitaoka M, Onoda N, Kitamura H, Koiwa F, Tanaka M, Fukagawa M. Percutaneous calcitriol injection therapy (PCIT) for secondary HPT: multicentre trial. *Nephrol Dial Transplant* 2003;**18**(Suppl 3):38–41.

83. Shiizaki K, Hatamura I, Negi S, et al. Percutaneous maxacalcitol injection therapy regresses hyperplasia of parathyroid and induces apoptosis in uremia. *Kidney Int* 2003;**64**:992–1003.

84. Shiizaki K, Negi S, Hatamura I, et al. Biochemical and cellular effects of direct maxacalcitol injection into parathyroid gland in uremic rats. *J Am Soc Nephrol* 2005;**16**:97–108.

85. Shiizaki K, Negi S, Hatamura I, et al. Direct injection of calcitriol or its analog into hyperplastic parathyroid glands induces apoptosis of parathyroid cells. *Kidney Int* 2006;**70**(Suppl 102):S12–15.

86. Shiizaki K, Hatamura I, Nakazawa E, Fukagawa M, Akizawa T, Kusano E. Successful induction of target genes in parathyroid cell by direct injection technique. (Abstract.) *NDT Plus* 2008;**1**(Suppl 2):ii211.

Chapter 31

Surgical management of secondary hyperparathyroidism

Emile Sarfati and Tilman B. Drüeke

Anatomical and embryological aspects

The surgical treatment of secondary hyperparathyroidism is based on a perfect knowledge of parathyroid anatomy and embryology. Whatever the procedure chosen it is necessary to find and expose all parathyroid glands.

Embryology

The parathyroid glands arise as proliferation of endodermal cells at the lateral tip of the third and fourth pharyngeal pouches. The third pouch gives rise to the inferior parathyroid (PIII) glands and to the thymus. This common origin explains the tight anatomical links of both inferior parathyroids and thymus. The fourth pouch gives rise to the superior parathyroid (PIV) glands. The parathyroid bodies migrate in the 13–14mm embryonic stage. An important anatomic event occurs with the deflexion of the neck and the descent of the heart and the large vessels. The inferior parathyroid glands (PIII) dragged by the thymic sketch descend toward the upper mediastinum. They are abandoned more or less at the same height as the lower thyroid pole or within the thyro-thymic ligament. During their migration the inferior glands may be left very high above the upper thyroid pole (parathymus)[1] or very low into the anterior and upper mediastinum with the thymus. The migration of the superior glands (PIV) is short and these glands remain close to the posterior part of the middle thyroid lobe. The superior glands are never far from the lower thyroid artery. In 85% of cases they are located less than 2cm from the crossing between the lower thyroid artery and the inferior laryngeal nerve.[2,3] This crossing explains the more or less tight links of the superior and inferior glands near the lower thyroid artery.[4]

Of interest, evidence was found nearly 10 years ago for an essential role of two genes in the embryonic development of the parathyroids, namely GATA3[5] and Gcm2.[6] The latter is a transcription factor that is exclusively expressed in the parathyroid glands, at least in mice, since Gcm2-deficient mice lack parathyroid glands. Surprisingly, Gcm2-deficient mice have serum PTH levels identical to wild-type animals, at least under conditions of normal calcium intake, with PTH being secreted by the thymus, by still to be defined cells.[7] The existence of such an auxiliary source of PTH, at least in the mouse, provides one among several potential explanations for the long known capacity of the organism to regulate calcium and phosphate metabolism in a parathyroid independent way. Moreover, it is also in line with the high incidence of PTH-producing tumors in thymus. Our understanding of the precise mode of action of these genes requires further research. The significance of the observations made in *Gcm2*-deficient mice for human parathyroid gland development is unclear at present. However, its significance for PTH synthesis has been demonstrated in two case reports where *Gcm2* mutations were found respectively in a patient with isolated idiopathic hypoparathyroidism[8] and a highly consanguineous Pakistani family with autosomal recessive familial idiopathic hypoparathyroidism.[9]

Number of glands

The parathyroid glands are usually four. Gilmour[4] identified four glands in 87% of 428 autopsy cases. Åkerström et al.,[2] in their study of 203 autopsies, identified four glands in 84% of cases. When only three glands are found, one should consider that the fourth has been missed or wrongly considered as a bilobated gland what actually are two stack glands.

Supernumerary glands exist in more than 13% of cases reported in autopsy studies,[3] with mostly five glands, and exceptionally six glands or more. In chronic renal failure patients with secondary hyperparathyroidism the frequency of supernumerary glands is probably higher, small parathyroid rudiments left in various sites during embryologic migration becoming hyperplastic as the result of uremic stimulation. These supernumerary glands may be located anywhere in the embryological migration areas of parathyroid glands. They are mostly found in the thyro-thymic ligament and within the upper pole of the thymus.[3]

Location of glands

Parathyroid gland positions are mostly symmetric. Therefore, when the glands on one side have been found, this should facilitate the exploration of the other side.[2] This is valuable for the identification of eutopic and ectopic positions.

The superior parathyroid glands are most frequently located in contact with the posterior edge of the thyroid, just above the intersection between the recurrent laryngeal nerve and the inferior thyroid artery within a circumscribed area of 2cm in diameter (Fig. 31.1). High location of superior parathyroid glands at the level of the superior thyroid pole was found by Åkerström et al. in 2% and location above the upper thyroid pole in less than 1% of patients.[2] When not found in their usual position the superior parathyroid gland is often found in a medial position on the inferior constrictor of the pharynx, under the pharyngeal perimisium. True intrathyroidal parathyroid superior glands are rare; they are often located between the inferior thyroid artery branches or subcapsularly, in a protrusion of the thyroid. When superior glands are heavy and enlarged they may slip against the prevertebral plans, behind the inferior thyroid artery and the recurrent laryngeal nerve, pulled by the negative pressure of the chest into the posterior superior mediastinum.[7] Thus, they are found in the latero- or retro-esophageal space.

The inferior parathyroid glands are more widely located (Fig. 31.2). Their commonest location is close to the lower thyroid pole, on its posterolateral face, in front of the recurrent laryngeal nerve. The glands can be found in the thyro-thymic ligament or in

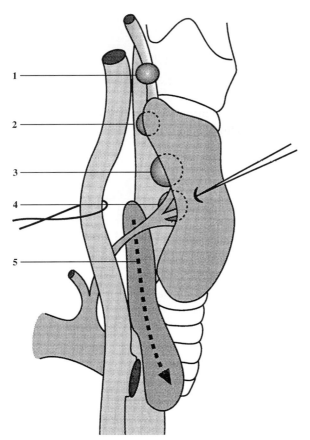

Fig. 31.1 Locations of the superior parathyroid glands. (1 and 2) Rare high ectopic position. (3 and 4) Common locations, representing over 80% of cases (Åkerström[2]). (5) Heavy and enlarged superior parathyroid glands, potentially slipped behind the inferior thyroid artery into the posterior superior mediastinum.

the upper thymus. Two per cent of inferior glands are in highly ectopic location by lack of embryological migration and 5% are in a really low intramediastinal position.[3]

Supernumerary glands may have exceptional ectopic locations (Fig. 31.3). Glands located within the thyroid are very rare,[10,11] and some greater, irregular, multilobated, and subcapsular glands appear to be intrathyroid glands, especially in uremic hyperparathyroidism. Hyperplastic glands have been described in the middle mediastinum,[12,13] outside the jugular carotid vessels,[11] and within the vagal nerve.[14]

Total parathyroidectomy with autotransplantation

In 1973, Geis et al. reported the first experience with total parathyroidectomy with autotransplantation (total PTX + AT) into the sternocleidomastoid muscle[15] and in 1978 Wells et al. described the technique of total PTX + AT into the forearm.[16]

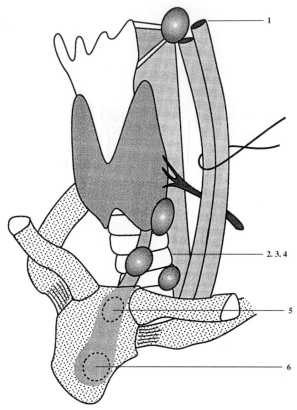

Fig. 31.2 Locations of the inferior parathyroid glands. (1) Undescended inferior gland. (2–4) Common locations, representing over 85% of cases (Åkerström[2]). (5 and 6) Mediastinal intrathymic glands.

This technique has become the procedure of choice for surgical management of uremic hyperparathyroidism in several institutions.[17,18]

All identified parathyroid glands are excised, placed in a 4°C Ringer solution and a biopsy specimen of each gland is performed for histological confirmation. The neck wound is then closed and the forearm, which is not bearing an arteriovenous fistula, is prepared for autotransplantation. The parathyroid tissue of the smallest gland is cut into cubes of about 1–2mm³. About 10 pieces of tissue weighing approximately 50–60mg are placed into separate muscle pockets of a forearm muscle. After having made certain that there is no bleeding into the muscle pockets to avoid widespread contamination with parathyroid tissue, the pockets are sutured and closed with non-absorbable material. As described by Wells et al.,[16] parathyroid tissue is cryopreserved for potential future re-implantation, in case hypoparathyroidism develops. In our experience of more than 400 cases cryopreserved tissue was never useful. One case of severe hypoparathyroidism after renal transplantation has been successfully treated with recombinant PTH.[19] Careful selection of tissue for autotransplantation is important to prevent early graft-dependent recurrence of hyperparathyroidism.[18,20]

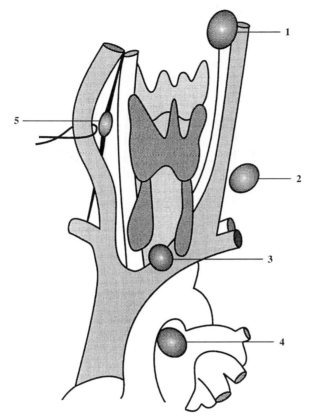

Fig. 31.3 Very rare locations of parathyroid glands. (1) Undescended inferior parathyroid gland. (2) Gland outside the cervical vessels, (3) Anterior mediastinal, extrathymic gland. (4) Gland in the middle mediastinum. (5) Intravagal parathyroid gland.

Tissue should be taken from a gland with no nodular formations or from non nodular parts of the smallest gland available. Welsh et al.[21] used the gland with the lowest density. Niederle et al.[22] proposed to separate monoclonal regions with high proliferative activity from polyclonal regions with low activity, before proceeding to autotransplantation, based on extemporaneous stereomicroscopy selection. The monoclonal tissue is characterized morphologically by the absence of fat cells and by an increased number of nucleoli and binuclear cells.

Other locations for autografting have been proposed. Diethelm et al.[23] performed autotransplantation in the sternocleidomastoid muscle and Kinnaert et al.[24] chose subcutaneous presternal autografting.

Subtotal parathyroidectomy

In 1960, Stanbury et al.[25] reported the first case of uremic hyperparathyroidism cured by subtotal parathyroidectomy and in 1964 Mac Phaul et al.[26] published efficacious, subtotal parathyroidectomy for tertiary hyperparathyroidism.

All the four parathyroid glands must be indentified and the two cervicomediastinal thymic tracts excised not to miss an possible supernumerary gland or rudiments of parathyroid tissue. One parathyroid gland, the smallest and less nodular one, should be subtotally resected after meticulous dissection, leaving in place a 50mg remnant before the other glands are resected. Care must be taken to leave a well vascularized fragment in place in order to avoid necrosis and permanent tetany. Subtotal resection can be repeated in a second gland if the first remnant does not appear to be adequately vascularized. The remnant is then marked with a non-absorbable suture for eventual re-operation. We usually choose the smallest and less nodular gland and, if possible, a gland which is localized far from the laryngeal nerve. Routine cryopreservation of parathyroid tissue may help to solve the problem of permanent hypoparathyroidism.

Total parathyroidectomy without autotransplantation

Complete removal of all parathyroid tissue was recommended by Ogg in 1967,[27] but since this first report only few authors reported their experience with such a treatment for uremic hyperparathyroidism.[28–30] Total parathyroidectomy has been abandoned by most centers since reports of severe osteomalacia attributed to hypoparathyroidism.[31,32] Moreover, the osteomalacia caused by aluminium accumulation could be worsened by hypoparathyroidism or transformed into adynamic bone disease. This being said, Kaye et al.[30] reported improvement of bone disease after total parathyroidectomy and Ljutic et al.[33] did not find evidence of low turnover bone disease in a follow-up period of up to 18 years in their patients. It must be pointed, however, out that parathyroidectomy was found to be really total in none of the patients in Kaye's series and in only 10% of Ljutic's series. In elderly patients, who are not eligible for renal transplantation, one may consider to perform total parathyroidectomy without immediate autotransplantation, but in such cases cryopreservation would be preferable. Secondary re-implantation with cryopreserved tissue is then possible, in case deleterious bony effects of hypoparathyroidism become manifest.

Advantages and disadvantages of total parathyroidectomy followed by immediate autotransplantation, compared with subtotal parathyroidectomy

Operative difficulties

There is no substantial difference in operative difficulties between these two procedures. The exploration of the neck, which takes most of the time with both procedures and consists to find and excise all parathyroid glands, is the same for total PTX + AT as for subtotal PTX. Total PTX + AT may be more of a time consuming procedure. Clearly, operative complications such as recurrent laryngeal nerve injury, would be expected to occur with equal frequency regardless of whether subtotal PTX or total PTX + AT is performed.[34]

Assessment of the parathyroid tissue left in place

With total PTX + AT there is a better guarantee of the quantity of tissue left in place (namely re-implanted tissue). Parathyroid tissue for transplantation should be chosen from non-nodular parts of one of the glands as this tissue should exhibit the least potential secretory dysregulation and display a lesser tendency for proliferation. Selection of such tissue may be easier when the glands are removed and sliced.[30] However, with subtotal PTX, a meticulous dissection of each gland allows in most cases to choose and quantify adequately the tissue remnant from the less severely diseased parathyroid gland. With total PTX + AT local monitoring of graft function is theoretically possible, but there are practical limitations. A clear-cut concentration gradient of plasma PTH between both arms will reflect graft tissue secretory function. However, it is not always easy to know whether the secretion of autografted tissue actually is insufficient or, on the contrary, excessive. In case of a very high PTH concentration in blood drawn from a vein of the grafted forearm side, but a normal or only slightly elevated systemic PTH level, one can conclude that the secretory activity of PTH by the autograft is satisfactory.

Persistent hyperparathyroidism

The incidence of persistent hyperparathyroidism is not dependent on the surgical procedure. It is due to a missed gland during cervical exploration and occurs with equal frequency regardless of the procedure. Kessler et al.[35] reported in their series of uremic hyperparathyroidism an incidence of persistent hyperparathyroidism of 8%. They further showed that a supernumerary gland was responsible in 2.7% of cases. Edis et al.[36] reported an incidence of persistent hyperparathyroidism of 16.4%, with a supernumerary gland being responsible in 5.5%. Meakins et al.[37] reported persistently high systemic PTH levels after successful parathyroidectomy in 25% of cases, suggestive of a missed supernumerary gland.

Hypoparathyroidism

Immediate post-operative hypocalcemia is more marked in response to total PTX + AT than in response to subtotal PTX. The prolonged period of postoperative hypoparathyroidism during which the grafted tissue is not yet vascularized, may span 3–6 months, and require the administration of large doses of calcium supplements and active vitamin D3 derivatives. However, we found that the long-term incidence of hypoparathyroidism was similar with either surgical procedure.[38]

Recurrent hyperparathyroidism

The main problem with both surgical procedures is that in the long run, despite an often excellent initial response, the evolution of the parathyroid status is mostly influenced by factors other than the type of surgery performed, in particular the subsequent control of metabolic and hormonal abnormalities.

Rothmund et al.[39] performed a randomized, prospective trial in 40 dialysis patients, comparing the technique of total PTX + AT with that of subtotal PTX. There were two cases of recurrence in the subtotal PTX group but none in the total PTX + AT group. Critical analysis of these results, however, demonstrates that there is no difference with either strategy for initial operation. We found that the long term frequency of recurrence was similar with these two procedures,[38] as did others.[40]

Comparing 23 patients having undergone total PTX without autotransplantation with 64 patients after subtotal PTX, Kerstin Lorenz[41] concluded that total versus subtotal PTX were equally safe and successful procedures with same frequency of hypocalcemic episodes, but total PTX was superior with regard to prevention of recurrence. As others,[42] we feel that total PTX without autotransplantation is a treatment option only for those patients who are not expected to receive a kidney transplant.

Difficulties with re-operation

In case of persistent hyperparathyroidism difficulties with re-operation would be expected to be identical with subtotal PTX and total PTX + AT. Persistence is due to a missed cervical or mediastinal gland and does not depend on the choice of the initial procedure. The main cause of unsuccessful operation is a missed supernumerary gland, which should be found in about 13% of cases and removed by routine cervical thymectomy.[2]

In our experience, recurrence after subtotal parathyroidectomy for uremic hyperparathyroidism occurs within an average time period of 7 years. It can be due to late hyperplasia of a remnant gland or a supernumerary gland. An association of these two causes is not uncommon and can be treated by same cervicotomy. Re-operation is not very difficult, in case the remnant gland has been marked with non-absorbable suture or with a titanium clip during the first operation. Explorative and localization procedures before re-operation, such as cervical echography and ^{99m}Tc-sestamibi scintigraphy, are generally very helpful.

Re-operation for recurrence after total PTX + AT has been considered to be easier than after subtotal PTX because re-operation on forearm autografts is felt to be simpler than re-operation in the neck.[43] Moreover, it can be performed under local anesthesia with no morbidity.[44] However, the management of graft-dependent hyperparathyroidism sometimes poses major problems and its most difficult aspect may be to substantiate the diagnosis. Even the proof of transplant function by a significant forearm/systemic venous PTH gradient does not exclude additional functioning parathyroid tissue in the neck or in the mediastinum as the cause of hyperparathyroidism.[45]

In our experience the forearm graft was the only cause of recurrence in less than 50% of cases. The hyperplastic tissue was often localized in the neck or mediastinum and many patients had concomitant hyperplastic autografts and cervical or mediastinal hyperplastic recurrence.[46] Palpation, cervical US, forearm US and ^{99m}Tc-sestamibi scintigraphy of both forearm and cervicomediastinal areas are helpful to localize the source of PTH excess. Measurement of peripheral serum intact PTH levels before and after a 10min complete ischemic blockade of the arm bearing the autograft often allows one to distinguish graft-dependent recurrence from cervical and mediastinal recurrence.[47] In case of confirmed graft-dependent hyperfunction, a conservative approach removing only enlarged fragments has been proposed.[48] In our experience such partial parathyroidectomy has been possible in several cases. The autografts are more or less deeply embedded in the muscle. Some of them are hypotrophic, whereas others are hypertrophic. However, the attempt to locate them precisely is rather difficult, even under general anesthesia. In some cases the growth of the transplanted fragments is dramatically increased, with widespread hyperplastic tissue sometimes simulating neoplastic transformation.[49] In case of graft-dependent recurrence, we prefer to remove all the transplanted tissue as completely as possible and perform cryopreservation for potential secondary, delayed autotransplantation.

Post-operative management

Immediately after surgery serum calcium levels must be monitored twice a day during 4 days and then every 2 days, before each dialysis session in case the patient is treated by intermittent hemodialysis. The extent to which the serum calcium decreases is related to the severity of ostetis fibrosa. In case of profound hypocalcemia the patient may require calcium gluconate infusions for several days or even weeks. Only a few patients present clinical signs of hypocalcemia with tetany, even in case of severe hypocalcemia.

Practically speaking, when serum calcium levels decrease to below 1.75mmol/L an IV infusion of high doses of calcium gluconate is administered to increase and maintain serum calcium at a level near 2.2mmol/l or higher. Subsequently, the doses are gradually reduced and replaced by oral calcium carbonate and/or alfacalcidol or calcitriol (1–2µg/day).

Interest of imaging techniques before surgery

The challenge for the surgeon in the treatment of uremic hyperparathyroidism is to find the four parathyroid glands and potential supernumerary glands. Persistence or recurrence of uremic hyperparathyroidism is a problem encountered by all surgeons, even when they have major experience with the treatment of this disease. We do not think that imaging techniques lead to a more complete localization of parathyroid glands and most experienced surgeons doubt the utility of imaging techniques at initial operation.[49,50] Takagi et al.[51] routinely combined preoperative localization procedures with US, CT, ^{201}Tl scanning and MRI. They found preoperative localization studies helpful with a 97% success rate of surgery. However, most ectopic parathyroid glands were small and found within the thymic tongue. They could not be detected by preoperative localization. Poor sensitivity of ^{99m}Tc-sestamibi scintigraphy has been reported in uremic patients,[51] emphasizing that imaging techniques should be reserved for persistent or recurrent uremic hyperparathyroidism [52]. Figure 31.4 shows the localization of hyperplastic parathyroid glands at various infrequent locations with MRI, CT scan, or even simple chest X-ray methods. Figure 31.5 demonstrates the value of ^{99m}Tc-sestamibi scintigraphy to locate ectopic glands before re-operation.

In case of re-operation the use of localization procedures has improved the ability to identify the site of abnormal parathyroid tissue.[53] Our present approach is to try, before re-operation, to visualize twice the same gland with non invasive procedures. We perform US and ^{99m}Tc-sestamibi scintigraphy with factor analysis of dynamic structures,[54,55] and if necessary cervicothoracic CT scan and MRI. Successful localization

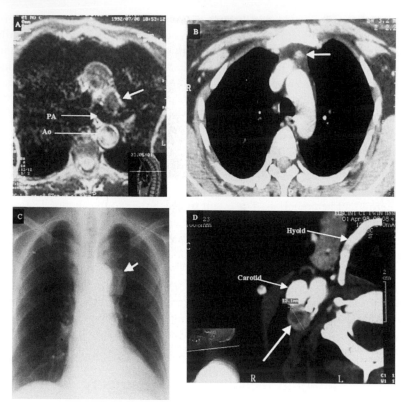

Fig. 31.4 Imaging procedures before re-operations. (A) Hyperplastic gland in the middle mediastinum (RMI). (B) Hyperplastic gland in the thymus (CT scan). (C) Hyperplastic gland in the anterior mediastinum (chest X-ray). (D) Intravagal hyperplastic gland (CT scan).

and a directed operation can result in a 95 % success rate.[56,57] High resolution sonography and ^{99m}Tc-sestamibi scintigraphy appear to be useful in the diagnosis of graft-dependent hyperparathyroidism. Intraoperative nuclear guidance has not improved the outcome of initial parathyroid surgery.[58–60] At present, we are in the process of evaluating the potential usefulness of the gamma detector for re-operations in case of graft-dependent recurrence, with encouraging initial results.

Current surgical treatment at our institution

From 1970 to 2008, we have operated 3057 patients for uremic hyperparathyroidism. At present, we prefer performing subtotal PTX, leaving in place a well vascularized remnant parathyroid tissue weighing 50–60mg. Routine thymectomy is performed. We have no longer done routine cryopreservation of parathyroid tissue in the last 8 years. In case of technical difficulties with necrosis of the four glands we perform total PTX + AT. In the few patients who are not candidates for renal transplantation total PTX without autotransplantation may be considered as an operative alternative.

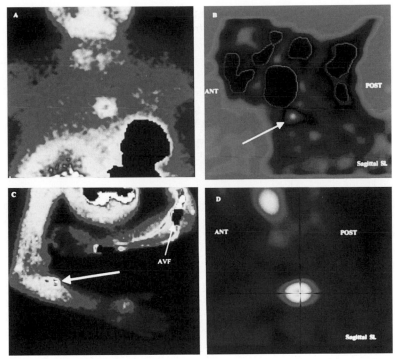

Fig. 31.5 Interest of ^{99m}Tc-sestamibi scintigraphy before re-operation. (A) Anterior intramediastinal supernumerary gland. (B) Undescended inferior parathyroid gland. (C) Autograft-dependent recurrence. (D) Fifth gland in the middle mediastinum.

In case of recurrent or persistent hyperparathyroidism we perform total PTX with cryopreservation of non-nodular parathyroid tissue which can be autotransplanted, if required.

Indications of surgical parathyroidectomy

Surgical removal of the parathyroid glands remains the final, symptomatic treatment of the most severe forms of secondary hyperparathyroidism in patients with CKD who fail to respond to or comply with medical treatment, including dietary phosphate restriction and optimal dialysis management in those with end-stage kidney disease, or who do not tolerate it because of major adverse events which are not infrequent,[55,56] as also recommended by the recent KDIGO guidelines (KDIGO, 2009[74]). Medical treatment failure is difficult to define. No randomized controlled trial on hard patient outcomes has ever been performed comparing surgical with medical treatment of severe secondary hyperparathyroidism. Therefore, there is no such thing as an absolute serum PTH threshold above which neck surgery becomes mandatory. The recent introduction of the calcimimetic cinacalcet, which represents a new class of PTH lowering drugs, has rendered the criteria for the indication of parathyroidectomy even more uncertain. Using this novel treatment approach it is possible to reduce high serum intact PTH levels, say above 800pg/mL, to a considerable extent, and even down to the range of normal in at least some patients.[61] It is impossible at present to predict in which patient full normalization of serum PTH will be possible, and in which other patient there will be partial or complete resistance to cinacalcet treatment. As a general rule, the higher the baseline PTH value, the higher is the probability that the correction of severe hyperparathyroidism will remain incomplete with medical treatment.

The presence of a severe form of parathyroid over function must be proved by clinical, biochemical and radiological evidence. If the serum calcium is low normal or low, medical treatment should always be attempted first. In general, surgical parathyroidectomy should only be done in cases where circulating intact PTH values are extremely elevated (> 1000–1500pg/mL), together with an increase in plasma total alkaline phosphatases (or better bone-specific alkaline phosphatase), and only after one or several medical treatment attempts have been unsuccessful in decreasing plasma iPTH using active vitamin D derivatives, cinacalcet, or both, in association with appropriate phosphate binders. Bone histomorphometry examination is rarely needed. Clinical symptoms and signs, such as pruritus and osteoarticular pain, are non-specific and, therefore, are not good criteria for operation by their own. Similarly, an isolated increase in plasma calcium and/or phosphorus, even in case of co-existing soft tissue calcifications, is not a sufficient criterion for surgical PTX. However, in the concomitant presence of a very high plasma PTH level the latter disturbances may contribute to favor the decision of parathyroid surgery. A concomitant aluminium overload should be excluded or treated, if present, before performing PTX.

Another criterion for the indication of surgical neck exploration is the ultrasonographic demonstration of one or several parathyroid glands with an estimated volume ≥ 1.0 cm^3 or a mass ≥ 1.0g.[62] In that case, the type of excessive parathyroid proliferation is considered to be nearly always monoclonal or multiclonal, that is made of one or several benign tumours.[63] This form of parathyroid hyperplasia is probably difficult to control by conservative means, at least in the long run. In keeping with this, it has been shown that the suppressibility of PTH secretion by calcium is negatively correlated with parathyroid tissue mass.[64] It must be pointed out, however, that the absence of ultrasonographic evidence of parathyroid gland enlargements is not a contraindication to surgery, in case severe hyperparathyroidism is present based on clinical and biochemical evidence.

Whether the frequency of surgical parathyroidectomy has changed during the past 10–20 years is a matter of debate. In the USA, both an increase[65] and a decrease[66] have been reported between the years 1990 and 2002. This discrepancy can probably be explained by differences in the hemodialysis cohorts studied, and in treatment and prevention strategies among centers. The introduction of cinacalcet into clinical practice has certainly allowed a reduction in frequency of parathyroidectomy further, as suggested by the *post-hoc* analysis of a prospective randomized controlled trial in chronic hemodialysis patients of cinacalcet treatment on top of optimal classical PTH lowering therapy.[67]

An interesting question is whether parathyroidectomy is associated with better patient outcome, as compared to no parathyroidectomy. A study with a large sample size in the US showed lower long-term mortality in dialysis patients who underwent parathyroidectomy compared with a matched cohort.[66] However, this was a retrospective, observational study. Short-term, postoperative mortality was high at 3.1% and the better long-term outcome after parathyroidectomy may be due to selection bias, as in the study by Trombetti et al.[68] In that study, patients undergoing parathyroidectomy were younger and had fewer comorbidities. However, when the authors proceeded toward a case–control analysis, this difference was no longer significant.

Contraindications of surgical parathyroidectomy

There are a number of local and general contraindications. Some anatomical variants in the neck region and several systemic diseases may render a cervicotomy procedure difficult, if not impossible. In particular, the co-existence of a severe, erosive cervical spondylarthropathy in association with dialysis amyloidosis must be looked for since in this instance cervical hyperextension may lead to spinal cord compression and quadriplegia.[69] In case such a pathology is suspected a NMR study must be done to excluded a severe lesion of the atlas/axis region. A previous cervicotomy renders re-operation more difficult and more dangerous, concerning the risk of recurrent nerve or phrenic nerve lesions. Only an endocrine surgeon with long-standing expertise should perform cervical re-interventions.

Severe cardiac or pulmonary failure may be a contraindication to general anesthesia as well. In such cases one can exceptionally remove under local anesthesia, through two successive lateral cervicotomies, the four hyperplastic glands or, if not technically possible, only the enlarged and easily found glands, similarly to what is occasionally done in debilitated patients with primary parathyroid adenoma. Finally, ultrasonographically-guided alcohol injection has also been successfully used as an alternative to surgery since its initial description in 1982.[70] This technique has been greatly developed in Japan and is currently in use in their dialysis patients (see Chapter 30).[70,71] However, our own experience with this technique has been disappointing, as has been that of other teams outside Japan.[72,73] Moreover, surgical removal after ethanol injection may become more difficult because of the local induction of fibrous tissue.

Summary

The surgical management of severe secondary hyperparathyroidism in patients with chronic kidney failure remains the ultimate solution in those who fail to respond to medical treatment or cannot comply with it. Among the various surgical techniques available, the most frequently used are subtotal parathyroidectomy, total parathyroidectomy with immediate autotransplantation of parathyroid tissue, total parathyroidectomy without autotransplantation, and total parathyroidectomy with delayed autotransplantation. At present, we prefer performing subtotal parathyroidectomy. Local and general contraindications to parathyroidectomy include erosive cervical spondylarthropathy and several systemic diseases. The presence of severe cardiac or pulmonary failure may be a contraindication to general anesthesia. In such cases, local anesthesia with two successive lateral cervictomies may be exceptionally used.

References

1. Edis AJ, Purnell DC, Heerden JAV. The undescendent 'parathymus'. An occasional cause of failed neck exploration for hyperparathyroidism. *Ann Surg* 1979;**190:**64–8.

2. Åkerström G, Malmaeus J, Bergström R. Surgical anatomy of human parathyroid glands. *Surgery* 1984;**95:**14–21.

3. Wang CA. The anatomic basis of parathyroid surgery. *Ann Surg* 1976;**183:**271–5.

4. Gilmour JR. The gross anatomy of the parathyroid glands. *J Pathol Bact* 1938;**46:**133–49.

5. van Esch H, Groene P, Nesbit MA, et al. GATA3 haplo-insufficiency causes human HDR syndrome. *Nature* 2000;**406:**419–22.

6. Gunther T, Chen ZF, Kim J, et al. Genetic ablation of parathyroid glands reveals another source of parathyroid hormone. *Nature* 2000;**406:**199–203.

7. Cope O. The story of hyperparathyroidism at the Massachusetts General Hospital. *N Engl J Med* 1966;**274:**1174.

8. Ding CL, Buckingham B, Levine MA. Familial isolated hypoparathyroidism caused by a mutation in the gene for the transcription factor GCMB. *J Clin Invest* 2001;**108:** 1215–20.

9. Baumber L, Tufarelli C, Patel S, et al. Identification of a novel mutation disrupting the DNA binding activity of GCM2 in autosomal recessive familial isolated hypoparathyroidism. *J Med Genet* 2005;**42:**443–8.

10. Sarfati E, Ferron Pd, Gossot D, Assens P, Dubost C. Adénomes parathyroïdiens de sièges inhabituels ectopiques ou non. *J Chir* 1987;**124:**24–9.

11. Thompson NW, Eckhauser FE, Harness JK. The anatomy of primary hyperparathyroidism. *Surgery* 1982;**92:**814–21.

12. McHenry C, Walsh M, Jarosz H, et al. Resection of parathyroid tumor in the aortopulmonary window without prior neck exploration. *Surgery* 1988;**104:**1090–4.

13. Sarfati E, Assens P, Charpentier YL, Lubetsky J, Dubost C. Un adénome parathyroïdien de localisation exceptionnelle au médiastin moyen. *J Chir* 1985;**122:**515–17.

14. Reiling RB, Cady B, Clerkin EP. Aberrant parathyroid adenoma within vagus nerve. *Lahey Clin Bull* 1972;**21:**158–62.

15. Geis WP, Popovtzer MM, Corman JL, Halgrimson CG, Groth CG, Starzl TE. The diagnosis and treatment of hyperparathyroidism after renal homotransplantation. *Surg Gynecol Obstet* 1973;**137:**997–1010.

16. Wells SA, Stirman JA, Bolman RM, Gunnels JC. Transplantation of the parathyroid glands. Clinical and experimental results. *Surg Clin N Am* 1978;**58:**391–402.

17. Niederle B, Roka R, Brennan MF. The transplantation of parathyroid tissue in man: Development, indication, technique and results. *Endocr Rev* 1982;**3:**245–79.

18. Rothmund M. Surgical treatment of secondary hyperparathyroidism: indication, operative management and results. *Prog Surg* 1986;**18:**186–205.

19. Mahajan A, Narayanan M, Jaffers G, Concepcion L. Hypoparathyroidism associated with severe mineral bone disease postrenal transplantation, treated successfully with recombinant PTH. *Hemodial Int* 2009;**13:**547–50.

20. Åkerström G, Rastad J, Ljunglall S, Ridefelt P, Juhilin C, Gylfe E. Cellular physiology and pathophysiology of parathyroid gland. *World J Surg.* 1991;**15:**672–80.

21. Welsh CL, Taylor GW, Cattel WR, Baker LRI. Parathyroid surgery in chronic renal failure: subtotal parathyroidectomy or autotransplantation? *Br J Surg* 1984;**71:**591–3.

22. Niederle B, Hörandner H, Roka R, Woloszczuk W. Morphological and functional studies to prevent graft-dependent recurrence in renal osteodystrophy. *Surgery* 1989;**106**:1043–8.

23. Diethelm AG, Adams PL, Murad TM, et al. Treatment of secondary hyperparathyroidism in patients with chronic renal failure by total parathyroidectomy and parathyroid autograft. *Ann Surg* 1981;**193**:777–93.

24. Kinnaert P, Salmon I, Decoster-Gervy C, et al. Total parathyroidectomy and presternal subcutaneous implantation of parathyroid tissue for renal hyperparathyroidism. *Surg Gynecol Obstet* 1993;**176**:135–9.

25. Stanbury SW, Lumb GA, Nicholson WF. Elective subtotal parathyroidectomy for renal hyperparathyroidism. *Lancet* 1960;**1**:793–7.

26. McPhaul JJ, McIntosh DA, Hammond WS, Park OK. Autonomons secondary renal parathyroid hyperplasia. *N Engl J Med* 1964;**271**:1342–5.

27. Ogg CS. Total parathyroidectomy in the treatment of secondary (renal) hyperparathyroidism. *Br Med J* 1967;**4**:331–4.

28. Hampl H, Steinmuller T, Frohling P, et al. Long-term results of total parathyroidectomy without autotransplantation in patients with and without renal failure. *Miner Electrolyte Metab* 1999;**25**:161–70.

29. Hampl H, Steinmuller T, Stabell U, Klingenberg HJ, Schnoy N, Neuhaus P. Recurrent hyperparathyroidism after total parathyroidectomy and autotransplantation in patients with long-term hemodialysis. *Miner Electrolyte Metab* 1991;**17**:256–60.

30. Kaye M, D'Amour P, Henderson J. Elective total parathyroidectomy without autotransplantation in end-stage renal disease. *Kidney Int* 1989;**35**:1390–9.

31. Drezner MK, Neelon FA, Jowsey J, Lebovitz HE. Hypoparathyroidism: a possible cause of osteomalacia. *J Clin Endocrinol Metab* 1977;**45**:114–22.

32. Felsenfeld AJ, Harrelson JM, Gutman RA, Wells SA, Jr., Drezner MK. Osteomalacia after parathyroidectomy in patients with uremia. *Ann Intern Med* 1982;**96**:34–9.

33. Ljutic D, Cameron JS, Ogg CS, Turner C, Hicks JA, Owen WJ. Long term follow up after total parathyroidectomy without parathyroid reimplantation in chronic renal failure. *Quarterly J Med* 1994;**87**:685–92.

34. Campbell DA, Dafoe DC, Swartz RD. Medical and surgical management of secondary hyperparathyroidism. In: NW Thompson (ed.) *Endocrine Surgery Update.* 1983:385–402.

35. Kessler M, Avila JM, Renout E, Mathieu P. Reoperation for secondary hyperparathyroidism in chronic renal failure. *Nephrol Dial Transplant* 1991;**6**:176–9.

36. Edis AJ, Levitt MD. Supernumerary parathyroid glands: implications for the surgical treatment of secondary hyperparathyroidism. *World J Surg* 1987;**11**:398–401.

37. Meakins JL, Milne CA, Hollomby DJ, Goltzman D. Total parathyroidectomy parathyroid hormone level and supernumerary glands in hemodialysis patients. *Clin Invest Med* 1984;**7**:21–5.

38. Gagné ER, Ureña P, Leite-Silva S, et al. Short and long-term efficacy of total parathyroidectomy with immediate autografting compared with subtotal parathyroidectomy in hemodialysis patients. *J Am Soc Nephrol* 1992;**3**:1008–17.

39. Rothmund M, Wagner PK, Schark C. Subtotal parathyroidectomy versus total parathyroidectomy and autotransplantation in secondary hyperparathyroidism: a randomised trial. *World J Surg* 1991;**15**:745–50.

40. Neonakis E, Wheeler MH, Krishnan H, Coles GA, Davies F, Woodhead S. Results of surgical treatment of renal hyperparathyroidism. *Arch Surg* 1995;**130**:643–8.

41. Lorenz K, Ukkat J, Sekulla C, Gimm O, Brauckhoff M, Dralle H. Total parathyroidectomy without autotransplantation for renal hyperparathyroidism: experience with a qPTH-controlled protocol. *World J Surg* 2006;**30**:743–51.

42. Shih ML, Duh QY, Hsieh CB, et al. Total parathyroidectomy without autotransplantation for secondary hyperparathyroidism. *World J Surg* 2009;**33**:248–54.

43. Skinner KA, Zuckerman L. Recurrent secondary hyperparathyroidism: an argument for total parathyroidectomy. *Arch Surg* 1996;**131**:724–7.

44. Takagi H, Tominaga Y, Uchida K. Subtotal versus total parathyroidectomy with forearm autograft for secondary hyperparathyroidism in chronic renal failure. *Ann Surg* 1984;**200**:18–23.

45. Saxe A. Parathyroid transplantation: a review. *Surgery* 1984;**95**:507–26.

46. Dubost C, Kracht M, Assens P, Sarfati E, Zingraff J, Drüeke T. Reoperation for secondary hyperparathyroidism in hemodialysis patients. *World J Surg* 1986;**10**:654–60.

47. Casanova D, Sarfati E, Francisco AD, Amado JA, Arias M, Dubost C. Secondary hyperparathyroidism: diagnosis of site of recurrence. *World J Surg* 1991;**15**:546–50.

48. Niederle B, Roka R, Hörandner H. Rezidivierender renaler Hyperparathyreoidismus: Reoperationen am Autotransplantat. *Wien Klin Wschr* 1988;**100**:369–72.

49. Klempa I, Steinan U, Frei U, Koch KM, Usadel KH, Röttger P. Morphologische Aspekte der Parathyreoideatransplantation: Beitrag zur klinischen Relevanz des induzierten, invasiven Gewebswachstums. *Chirurg* 1978;**49**:704–10.

50. Kaplan EL, Yashiro T, Salti G. Primary hyperparathyroidism in the (1990s). *Ann Surg* 1992;**216**:215–300.

51. Takagi H, Tominaga Y, Uchida K. Evaluation of image diagnosing methods of enlarged parathyroid glands in chronic renal failure. *World J Surg* 1986;**10**:605–9.

52. Piga M, Bolasco P, Satta L, et al. Double-phase parathyroid technetium-99m-MIBI scintigraphy to identify functional autonomy in secondary hyperparathyroidism. *J Nucl Med* 1996;**37**:565–9.

53. O' Doherty MJ. Radionuclide parathyroid imaging. *J Nucl Med* 1997;**38**:840–1.

54. Billotey C, Aurengo A, Najean Y, et al. Identifying abnormal parathyroid glands in the thyroid uptake area using technetium-99m-sestamibi and factor analysis of dynamic structures. *J Nucl Med* 1994;**35**:1631–6.

55. Miller DL, Doppman JL, 133- TSTLopaipwhusPINimR. Localisation of parathyroid adenomas in patients who have undergone surgery. Part I. Noninvasive imaging methods. *Radiology* 1987;**162**:133–9.

56. Brennan MF, Norton JA. Reoperation for persistent and recurrent hyperparathyroidism. *Ann Surg* 1985;**201**:40–8.

57. Zingraff J, Léger A, Skhiri H, Billotey C, Sarfati E, Drüeke T. Localisation of ectopic parathyroid tissue: usefulness of 99mTc sesta-mibi scanning in a dialysis patient with severe secondary hyperparathyroidism (Teaching Point). *Nephrol Dial Transplant* 1996;**11**:2504–6.

58. Bonjer HJ, Bruining HA, Pols HA, et al. Intraoperative nuclear guidance in benign hyperparathyroidism and parathyroid cancer. *Eur J Nucl Med* 1997;**24**:246–51.

59. Bonjer HJ, Bruining HA, Pols HA, et al. Methoxyisobutylisonitrile probe during parathyroid surgery: tool or gadget? *World J Surg* 1998;**22**:507–11.

60. Shen W, Duren M, Morita E, et al. Reoperation for persistent or recurrent primary hyperparthyroidism. *Arch Surg* 1996;**131**:861–7.

61. Moe SM, Chertow GM, Coburn JW, et al. Achieving NKF-K/DOQI(TM) bone metabolism and disease treatment goals with cinacalcet HCl. *Kidney Int* 2005;**67**:760–71.

62. Ritz E. II. Early parathyroidectomy should be considered as the first choice. *Nephrol Dial Transplant* 1994;**9**:1819–21.

63. Arnold A, Brown MF, Ureña P, Gaz RD, Sarfati E, Drüeke TB. Monoclonality of parathyroid tumors in chronic renal failure and in primary parathyroid hyperplasia. *J Clin Invest* 1995;**95**:2047–54.

64. Indridason OS, Pieper CF, Quarles LD. Predictors of short-term changes in serum intact parathyroid hormone levels in hemodialysis patients: role of phosphorus, calcium, and gender. *J Clin Endocrinol Metab* 1998;**83**:3860–6.

65. Foley RN, Li SY, Liu JN, Gilbertson DT, Chen SC, Collins AJ. The fall and rise of parathyroidectomy in US hemodialysis patients, (1992) to (2002). *J Am Soc Nephrol* 2005;**16**:210–18.

66. Kestenbaum B, Seliger SL, Gillen DL, et al. Parathyroidectomy rates among United States dialysis patients: 1990–1999. *Kidney Int* 2004;**65**:282–8.

67. Cunningham J, Danese M, Olson K, Klassen P, Chertow GM. Effects of the calcimimetic cinacalcet HCl on cardiovascular disease, fracture, and health-related quality of life in secondary hyperparathyroidism. *Kidney Int* 2005;**68**:1793–800.

68. Trombetti A, Stoermann C, Robert JH, et al. Survival after parathyroidectomy in patients with end-stage renal disease and severe hyperparathyroidism. *World J Surg* 2007;**31**:1014–21.

69. Rousselin B, Hélénon O, Zingraff J, et al. Pseudotumor of the craniocervical junction during long-term hemodialysis. *Arthr Rheum* 1990;**33**:1567–73.

70. Giangrande A, Castiglioni A, Solbiati L, Allaria P. Ultrasound-guided percutaneous fine-needle ethanol injection into parathyroid glands in secondary hyperparathyroidism. *Nephrol Dial Transplant* 1992;**7**:412–21.

71. Kitakoa M, Fukagawa M, Ogata E, Kurokawa K. Reduction of functioning parathyroid cell mass by ethanol injection in chronic dialysis patients. *Kidney Int* 1994;**46**:1110–17.

72. de Barros Gueiros JE, Chammas MC, Gerhard R, et al. Percutaneous ethanol (PEIT) and calcitrol (PCIT) injection therapy are ineffective in treating severe secondary hyperparathyroidism. *Nephrol Dial Transplant* 2004;**19**:657 63.

73. Fletcher S, Kanagasundaram NS, Rayner HC, et al. Assessment of ultrasound guided percutaneous ethanol injection and parathyroidectomy in patients with tertiary hyperparathyroidism. *Nephrol Dial Transplant* 1998;**13**:3111–17.

74. KDIGO clinical practice guidelines for the diagnosis, evaluation, prevention, and treatment of Chronic Kidney Disease-Mineral and Bone Disorder (CKD-MBD). *Kidney Int*; Supp. 2009;**113**:S1–130.

Chapter 32

Morbidity and mortality related to disturbances in mineral metabolism in CKD

Geoffrey A. Block, Jorge B. Cannata-Andia, and David Goldsmith

The chains of habit are too weak to be felt until they are too strong to be broken[1]

Introduction

The magnitude of the exaggerated morbidity and mortality experienced by patients with chronic kidney disease is truly remarkable and despite being described some time ago, remains largely unexplained. In a modern cohort of over 1.1 million patients, Go and colleagues demonstrated that compared with patients with an eGFR greater than 60mL/min, patients with an eGFR < 60 mL/min had a hazard ratio (HR) for death from any cause of 1.2–5.9 and a HR for any cardiovascular (CV) event of 1.4–3.4 despite extensive statistical adjustment for co-morbidity.[2] A similar situation exists for patients receiving dialysis who continue to experience mortality rates in excess of 225/1000 patient years, a rate nearly 6 times that of the general age matched population. Five-year survival of patients on hemodialysis remains only 31% and patients on dialysis greater than 5 years have a mortality rate in excess of 250/1000 patient years.[3] This is comparable with or worse than many major solid-organ malignancy and, unlike malignancy, there is no known 'cure' for end-stage kidney disease with the exception of organ transplantation. When successful, transplantation restores kidney function towards normal, and is associated with lower mortality than is seen in matched 'wait listed' dialysis patients.

It has been suggested that disturbances in mineral metabolism [specifically calcium (Ca), phosphorus (P), parathyroid hormone (PTH) and vitamin D] contribute to this exaggerated risk and there is substantial biological plausibility for this assertion. While much of the past literature in this area focused on overtly abnormal biochemical values in patients with end-stage renal disease, more recently a great deal of attention has been directed towards the adverse effects of disturbances in mineral metabolism at much earlier stages of chronic kidney disease. In a recent evaluation of 1800 community-based patients older than 40 years, hyperparathyroidism was present in 56% of those with eGFR < 60mL/min, thereby providing evidence of dysregulated calcium, phosphorus and vitamin D even with relatively mild reduction in kidney function.[4]

Since the early 1990s there have been numerous studies showing increased mortality with increased serum levels of Ca, P, and PTH in patients receiving hemodialysis. As a result, K/DOQI guidelines published in 2003, established target values for these parameters within narrow ranges (150–300pg/mL for PTH; 3.5–5.5mg/dL for P; and 8.4–9.5mg/dL for Ca).[5] However, as highlighted by the recently published and strictly evidence-based KDIGO guidelines, the K/DOQI guidelines were developed largely on the basis of observational reports rather than results from randomized clinical trials.[6] Rather surprisingly, fundamentally important questions about the role of treatment of disordered mineral metabolism have not been adequately addressed. To date, there have been no prospectively designed randomized clinical trials that have shown *any* patient level benefit with *any* treatment for abnormal Ca, P, PTH, or vitamin D level. Thus, it must be emphasized that, despite the consistent associations between abnormal levels of Ca, P, and PTH with morbidity and mortality in patients with CKD that are described below, there is no established evidence that there is a *causal* relationship between any of these minerals and the associated events. Notwithstanding these important limitations, in this chapter we describe the reported associations between disordered mineral metabolism and morbidity and mortality in patients with CKD. A recent systematic review of the English language literature describing these associations in patients with CKD describes considerable methodological issues with many of the papers cited here.[7] Of the 35 papers that met the inclusion criteria in this review, only nine were rated as 'good' for assessment for all-cause mortality and only one paper was rated as 'good' for assessment of cardiovascular mortality (Table 32.1). Readers are strongly encouraged to review this excellent systematic review in its entirety. The Dialysis Outcomes and Practice Patterns Study (DOPPS) has been collecting data prospectively related to laboratory values and clinical outcomes in a random sample patients on hemodialysis from 1996 to the current year and is currently in its fourth phase. Global trends in the serum levels of calcium, phosphorus and PTH are shown in Fig. 32.1.[8] Data from this multinational long-term observational study have been instrumental in further clarifying the often discrepant results from smaller, short-term, national, or regional reports.

Readers are also encouraged to read the 2009 KDIGO Workgroup Recommendations on the Evaluation, Prevention and Treatment of CKD-MBD which addresses these important issues and highlights the lack of randomized clinical trial data upon which to base clinical practice guidelines.[6] These guidelines discuss the importance of basing therapeutic decisions on trends in laboratory values, rather than on a single value and suggest taking into account all available CKD-MBD assessments (such as the presence or absence of vascular calcification). Finally, despite the common practice of utilizing the mathematical construct of the product of the serum calcium × serum phosphate, the KDIGO guidelines remind us that outcomes related to this construct are primarily driven by those related to phosphorus and recommend that individual values of serum calcium and phosphorus be used to guide therapy.

Phosphorus

There have been an abundance of observational reports describing an association between higher levels of serum P and adverse clinical outcomes in subjects with

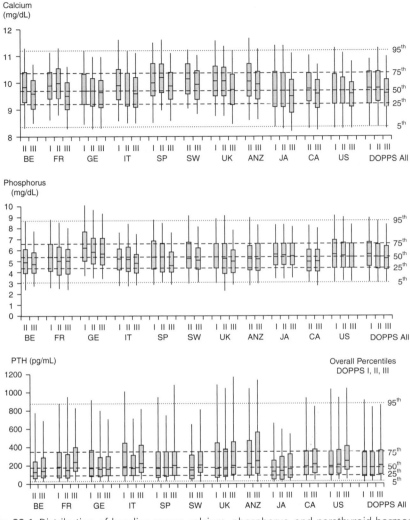

Fig. 32.1 Distribution of baseline serum calcium, phosphorus, and parathyroid hormone (PTH) levels by country and Dialysis Outcomes and Practice Patterns Study (DOPPS) phase. Box plots show weighted 25th to 75th percentiles (box) with median (line), and 5th and 95th percentiles (whiskers) for each country and phase of DOPPS. Horizontal lines indicate these percentiles for serum calcium (percentiles: 5th = 7.9, 25th = 8.7, 50th = 9.2, 75th = 9.8, and 95th = 10.7mg/dL), serum phosphorus (percentiles: 5th = 3.0, 25th = 4.3, 50th = 5.4, 75th = 6.5, and 95th = 8.7mg/dL), and PTH (percentiles: 5th = 28, 25th = 83, 50th = 177, 75th = 342, and 95th = 893pg/mL) for the overall DOPPS sample. To convert serum calcium or albumin-corrected calcium (calciumAlb) in mg/dL to mmol/L, multiply by 0.25; serum phosphorus in mg/dL to mmol/L, multiply by 0.323; PTH levels expressed in pg/mL and ng/L are equivalent. Abbreviations: BE, Belgium; FR, France; GE, Germany; IT, Italy; SP, Spain; SW, Sweden; UK, United Kingdom; ANZ, Australia-New Zealand; JA, Japan; CA, Canada; US, United States. (From:Tentori et al. *Am J Kidney Dis* 2008;**52**:519–30.)

Table 32.1 Assessment of the quality of observational studies assessing the risk of clinical outcomes with mineral abnormalities based upon the STROBE statement (22 items)

Reference	Introduction				Methods						
	Abstract	Rationale	Objective	Study design	Setting	Inclusion criteria	Variable	Data source	Bias	Study size	Quantitative variable
Block, 1998 [19]	•	•	•	•	•	•		•	•		•
Block, 2004 [20]	•	•	•	•	•	•		•	•		•
Chang, 2006 [21]	•	•	•	•	•	•		•	•		
Foley, 1996 [22]	•	•	•	•	•	•		•	•	•	•
Ganesh, 2001 [23]	•	•	•	•	•	•		•	•	•	•
Jassal, 1996 [24]		•	•	•	•			•	•	•	
Kalantar, 2006 [25]	•	•	•	•	•	•	•	•	•	•	•
Kato, 2006 [51]	•	•	•	•							
Kestenbaum, 2005 [26]	•	•	•	•	•	•	•	•	•	•	•
Kimata, 2007 [27]	•	•	•	•	•	•		•	•		
Leggat, 1998 [28]		•	•					•	•		
Lowrie, 1990 [29]	•		•	•	•			•	•		
Marco, 2003 [52]		•	•	•	•			•	•	•	•
Melamed, 2006 [30]	•	•	•	•	•	•		•	•		•
Menon, 2005 [31]		•	•	•		•			•		
Noordzij, 2005 [32]	•	•	•	•	•	•		•	•	•	•
Noordzij, 2006 [50]	•	•	•	•	•	•	•	•	•	•	

	Results					Discussion					
Statistic methods	Participant	Descriptive data	Outcome data	Result	Other analyses	Key result	Limitation	Interpretation	External validity	Funding	Total
•		•		•	•	•	•	•	•		17/22
•		•		•	•	•	•	•	•		17/22
•		•		•	•	•	•	•			15/22
•	•	•		•	•	•	•	•			18/22
•	•	•		•	•	•	•	•			18/22
•	•	•		•		•	•				13/22
•	•	•	•	•		•	•	•			19/22
		•		•		•	•	•	•		10/22
•	•	•		•		•	•	•	•		19/22
		•				•		•			11/22
		•				•		•			7/22
		•		•		•		•			10/22
		•				•	•	•	•		13/22
		•	•		•	•	•	•	•		16/22
•		•		•		•	•	•			11/22
•	•	•	•	•	•	•	•	•			19/22
	•	•	•			•	•	•			16/22

(Continued)

Table 32.1 (*Continued*) Assessment of the quality of observational studies assessing the risk of clinical outcomes with mineral abnormalities based upon the STROBE statement (22 items)

Reference	Introduction				Methods						
	Abstract	Rationale	Objective	Study design	Setting	Inclusion criteria	Variable	Data source	Bias	Study size	Quantitative variable
Port, 2004 [33]		•	•	•	•			•	•		
Rodriguez-Benot, 2005 [34]	•	•	•	•		•		•	•		
Saran, 2003 [35]	•	•	•	•	•			•			
Slinin, 2005 [36]	•	•	•	•	•		•	•	•		•
Stack, 2001 [56]		•	•	•			•	•	•	•	
Stevens, 2004 [37]	•	•	•	•	•	•	•	•	•	•	•
Tentori, 2007 [39]	•	•	•	•	•	•		•	•		•
Voormolen, 2007 [38]		•	•	•		•	•	•	•	•	•
Young, 2004 [40]			•		•			•	•		
Young, 2005 [54]			•		•			•	•		

	Results					Discussion					
Statistic methods	Participant	Descriptive data	Outcome data	Result	Other analyses	Key result	Limitation	Interpretation	External validity	Funding	Total
						•		•		•	9/22
	•			•	•	•		•			12/22
		•		•		•		•			10/22
		•				•	•		•		14/22
•	•	•			•	•	•	•			15/22
•	•	•				•	•	•	•		18/22
•		•			•	•	•	•	•	•	17/22
	•	•				•	•	•			14/22
						•		•			6/22
		•				•	•	•			8/22

Items that were of good quality are highlighted and added to achieve a total score out of 22.
The description of each item is as follows: (1) Title/abstract: reporting of study design and a balanced summary of the method and results; (2) Background/rationale: the scientific rationale behind the study has been reported; (3) Objectives: specific objectives and hypotheses have been reported; (4) Study design: key elements of the study design presented early in the paper; (5) Setting: location of the study, relevant dates including periods of enrolment, exposure, follow-up and data collection have been described; (6) Participants: eligibility criteria and source/method of selection of participants described;
(7) Variables: outcomes, exposure, predictors, potential confounders and effect modifiers have been clearly defined. The type of confounders and the reasons for its adjustment were reported; (8) Data sources/ measurement: for each variable of interest, data source and method of assessment described;
(9) Bias: efforts undertaken to address source of bias; (10) Study size: explanation of how the study size was arrived at; (11) quantitative variables: explanation of the handling of the quantitative variables in the analyses; (12) Statistical methods: description of methods used to control confounding, sensitivity analyses and how missing data and lost to follow-up was addressed; (13) Participants: number of individuals reported at each stage of study, e.g. numbers potentially eligible, examined for eligibility, confirmed eligible, included in the study, completed follow-up and analysed; (14) Descriptive data: characteristics of study participants including demographic, clinical and social; (15) Outcome data:
time-dependent information on outcomes; (16) Main results: unadjusted estimates and if applicable, confounder-adjusted estimates and their precision; (17) Other analyses: reporting of subgroup analysis or sensitivity analysis; (18) Key results: key results were summarized with respect to study objectives;
(19) Limitations: the study discussed key limitations taking into account the source of potential bias or imprecision; (20) Interpretation: a cautious overall interpretation was given considering the objectives, limitations and results from similar studies; (21) Generalizibility: the external validity of the results were discussed; (22) Funding: the source of funding and the role of funders was provided.

chronic kidney disease. Originally described as associated with mortality in 1990 in patients on hemodialysis, interest in phosphorus increased with the 1998 publication by USRDS investigators demonstrating a 6% increase in the relative risk (RR) of mortality per 1mg/dL increase in serum P among prevalent subjects on hemodialysis.[9] Subsequent reports utilizing independent, large datasets from various large US dialysis providers and from the DOPPS all confirmed a 4–8% increase in the RR of death per 1mg/dL increase in serum P in patients treated with hemodialysis.[10,11] Although many in the community attempt to use observational data to ascertain the precise threshold for serum P at which the RR of mortality increases, we strongly caution that this is both difficult and ill-advised. Generally, increases in the RR of all-cause mortality seem to cluster around 5–5.5mg/dL in these subjects, although this is by no means consistent across all observational reports. Among the references cited above, the threshold for mortality increased at 5mg/dL, 5.5mg/dL, >6mg/dL, and > 6.5mg/dL in subjects on hemodialysis. Because P is currently thought to contribute to vascular calcification as the primary mechanism accounting for its' adverse effects, the relationship between serum P and cardiovascular specific mortality and cardiovascular events has also been examined. Assessed as a continuous variable, four studies report a 9–13% increase in the RR of cardiovascular mortality associated with a 1mg/dL increase in serum P.[7] The threshold for increased RR of cardiovascular mortality seems to similarly cluster near 5.5mg/dL; however, data from the USRDS waves 1, 3, and 4 found a graded increase in the RR of any CV event beginning at serum P levels >4.5mg/dL.[12] As would be expected, it appears that hemodialysis patients with previous evidence of CV disease are at greatly exaggerated risk of CV death associated with elevations in serum P, particularly when it is associated with elevations in serum calcium as shown in Fig. 32.2. Lending substantial strength to the hypothesis that phosphorus, *per se*, is contributing directly to morbidity and mortality is recent data in subjects with chronic kidney disease not receiving dialysis and in the general population that similarly report a direct association between serum P levels and cardiovascular events, all-cause mortality, and cardiovascular mortality. Several independent investigators have shown that patients with CKD not on dialysis have a 23–62% increase in the RR of all-cause mortality associated with a 1mg/dL increase in serum P.[13] The threshold for this increased RR appears to cluster around 3.5mg/dL in subjects with CKD (RR 1.32–1.90) even after extensive statistical adjustment. This same threshold of 3.5mg/dL was also seen as an inflection point for increased RR (1.27) in an analysis of CV events and mortality in 4127 patients with pre-existing coronary artery disease.[14] In this *post-hoc* evaluation of the Cholesterol and Recurrent Events trial, higher levels of serum phosphate were associated with an increased risk of new heart failure and myocardial infarction. Sigrist et al. have reported that among subjects with stages 4 and 5 CKD, increases in serum P are associated with increases in vascular calcification, arterial stiffness and death.[15] Perhaps the most remarkable insights have recently come from subjects in the general population without CKD. The Framingham Offspring Study was the first to report that among subjects with no evidence of either CV disease or CKD and followed for 13 years, there was a 55% increase in the RR of a new cardiovascular event even after adjustment for eGFR and traditional CV risk factors.[16] The Atherosclerosis Risk in Communities Study (ARIC)

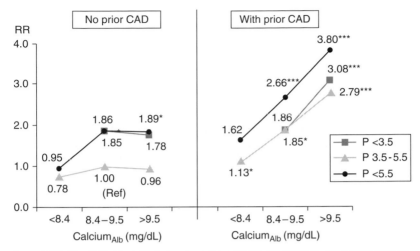

* p=0.01-0.05, *** p<0.001; Adjusted for factors shown above plus age, sex, black race, cause of CKD, years on dialysis, smoking (active), UFR, BMI, spKt/V, Hgb, albumin, iPTH, cholesterol, triglycerides, % lymphocytes and neutrophils, vascular access, and 14 summary comorbid conditions. Calcium-ALB = albumin-corrected calcium. Reprinted with permission of Dr. Fritz Port.

Fig. 32.2 Relative coronary mortality risk by calcium and phosphorus. (From Block GA, Cunningham J. *Clinical Guide to Bone and Mineral Metabolism in CKD*, K. Olgaard (ed.). National Kidney Foundation, 2006; Figure 1 from Chapter 4.) Used with permission from Arbor Research.

followed 15,732 adults prospectively for 13 years and reported that baseline serum P levels were associated with future stroke and death although not with coronary events.[17] Widely accepted surrogates of cardiovascular health including LVH and increased ankle-brachial index have also been associated with serum P levels above 3.5mg/dL (LVH) or 4.0mg/dL (ABI) in community-based studies of subjects without chronic kidney disease.[18,19]

In summary, although many of the published reports have significant methodological issues there are consistent data that find an independent, graded relationship between levels of serum P, and morbidity and mortality in patients with or without CKD. While the precise threshold for increased risk appears to cluster around 5.0–5.5mg/dL for patients with ESRD we do not endorse the use of this value as a target for therapeutic treatment nor as an indicator of quality of care. Several reports have demonstrated that the complex relationships that exist between serum levels of calcium, phosphorus and PTH, as well as their interaction with the treatment options that include calcium containing phosphate binders, vitamin D and calcimimetics, preclude the use of single values of any particular biochemical variable to determine 'optimal' or 'target' treatment values. In fact, work by Stevens et al. suggests that in addition to the inherent complexity described above, the nature of the RR conferred by combinations of these parameters varies with the duration of CKD.[20] Further confounders not yet identified are likely to be present. Furthermore, data from patients with non-dialysis dependent CKD and data from community living subjects without CKD demonstrating increased risk when serum P values rise progressively *within the normal range* above 3.5mg/dL suggest that, in fact, 'optimal' or 'target' P values are likely to be significantly lower than what has been reported for subjects with ESRD. The newly published KDIGO guidelines recognize this and suggest that when serum P values rise above normal, observational data suggest that it should be reduced *towards* normal. However, as emphasized earlier, there are *no* clinical trials conducted showing any patient level benefit of *any* treatment aimed specifically to lower serum P.

Calcium

Data regarding the relationship between levels of serum calcium and adverse events are less consistent than those with serum phosphorus. In part this may be a result of the fact that serum calcium values do not accurately reflect actual calcium balance and it is likely that many patients on hemodialysis are in long-term positive calcium balance due to the use of calcium containing phosphate binders, activated vitamin D and a moderate to high dialysate calcium concentration. A recent calculation of calcium balance in patients on dialysis suggests that 80% of patients on a 2.5 mEq/L calcium dialysate bath are in positive calcium balance.[21] Several reports describe an increased mortality associated with *lower* levels of serum calcium, while others report either a *lack of* a relationship or an increased mortality associated with *increased* serum calcium levels. Serum calcium levels tend to be at the low end of normal in patients with advanced CKD and increase during the first 6 months of dialysis and thereafter remain generally stable.[22] Over the decade that the DOPPS has been collecting data, mean serum calcium levels in patients on dialysis have had a significant decline (0.09mg/dL per phase). Nonetheless, nearly 25% of current prevalent patients on hemodialysis have serum calcium values greater than 10mg/dL while fewer than 5% of such patients have serum calcium <8.4mg/dL.[6]

Early reports described an increased risk of mortality associated with serum calcium below 8.8mg/dL; however, subsequent reports that adjusted for a wider range of potentially confounding variables found no such increased risk and, in fact, show a progressive decline in the RR of death with lower serum calcium levels. A possible explanation for this discrepancy is offered by data from DOPPS I–III which show an increased RR of all-cause and cardiovascular mortality associated with serum calcium <7.5mg/dL only in patients with an albumin greater than 3.8g/L and no such increase RR of death associated with low serum calcium values in patients with albumin less than 3.8g/L.[8] As described for PTH below, this highlights the complexity of interpretation of individual laboratory values in patients with multiple, simultaneous, and competing risk factors for adverse outcomes. Additionally, no data is available regarding the effect of calcimimetic therapy and its associated reduction in serum calcium values with clinical outcomes. Preliminary data suggest that prescription of cinacalcet increases the proportion of subjects with low serum calcium and yet is associated with an improvement in both all-cause and cardiovascular survival.[23] Conclusive data will be provided from the ongoing Evaluation of Cinacalcet HCL Therapy to Lower CardioVascular Events (EVOLVE; clinicaltrials.gov identifier NCT 00345839) clinical trial, which is a large, global randomized, prospective clinical trial evaluating whether the addition of cinacalcet to hemodialysis patients with secondary

HPT affects a composite endpoint including survival, myocardial infarction, heart failure, and peripheral vascular disease.

Data regarding the relationship between elevated serum calcium and adverse events are more consistent than those for low serum calcium. As detailed by Covic et al., nine studies have assessed the risk associated with increased serum calcium in dialysis patients and six find a significant relationship.[7] Each 1mg/dL increase in serum calcium is associated with approximately a 12–22% increase in RR of death. Categorical analysis suggests that, when serum calcium is at the high end of normal or overtly above normal there is an increase in the RR of all-cause and cardiovascular mortality. The precise threshold for this increase risk varies among reports but is generally in the range of >9.5–9.7mg/dL to as high as >10.2–10.5mg/dL. As mentioned earlier, 25% of prevalent patients on dialysis globally have serum calcium values above this range and the precise increase in risk almost certainly varies with underlying co-morbidity (Fig. 32.2), and with combinations of calcium, phosphorus and PTH. Observational data have thus far provided no clear evidence of increased risk of morbidity or mortality associated with serum calcium in patients with CKD not yet receiving dialysis nor in community dwelling patients without CKD. The Framingham Offspring Study ($n = 3368$) found no relationship between serum calcium and incident cardiovascular disease while the ARIC Study ($n = 15,732$) found no association between serum calcium and coronary heart disease or death in a 12-year follow-up period.[16,17]

Parathyroid hormone

Parathyroid hormone is secreted by the parathyroid glands as a polypeptide containing 84 amino acids. It acts to increase the concentration of calcium (Ca^{2+}) in the blood by acting upon the parathyroid hormone receptor in three parts of the body. PTH plasma half-life is approximately 2–4min. Caution is required, therefore, in trying to over-interpret the cross-sectional association between outcomes months to years later, with a single measurement of a hormone with a very short half-life.

Back in the very early days of nephrology Klahr, Massry, Slatopolsky, and others cited the possibility that PTH was one of many uremic toxins.[24] This idea is still relevant today, despite the proliferation of known uremic toxins, and the much greater evident complexity in pathomechanisms that are impacted by chronic kidney failure. PTH has been incriminated in not just hyperparathyroidism and high-turnover bone lesions, but also dyslipidemia, anemia, neuropathy, LVH (with chronotropic and inotropic actions) and encephalopathic complications. Thus, it can be imagined that, directly or indirectly, PTH might be associated with adverse clinical outcomes.

There are some useful analyses that have attempted to examine the relationship between low, normal (whatever definition is accepted for this), and raised plasma PTH levels and adverse outcomes. A recent report from the DOPPS reported on 25,588 patients with end-stage renal disease on hemodialysis therapy for longer than 180 days at 925 facilities in DOPPS I (1996–2001), DOPPS II (2002–2004), or DOPPS III (2005–2007).[8] Distributions of mineral metabolism markers differed across DOPPS countries and phases, as shown in Fig. 32.1. Survival models identified categories with the lowest mortality risk for calcium (8.6–10.0mg/dL), CaAlb (7.6–9.5mg/dL), phosphorus

(3.6–5.0mg/dL), and PTH (101–300pg/mL). The greatest risk of mortality was found for calcium or CaAlb levels greater than 10.0mg/dL, phosphorus levels greater than 7.0mg/dL, and PTH levels greater than 600pg/mL, and in patients with combinations of high-risk categories of calcium, phosphorus, and PTH.

The systematic literature review by Covic and co-workers identified 11 studies that analyzed the relationship between raised PTH levels and mortality.[7] Seven of these studies showed a significant association (see, reference 7 for full details). Two studies assessed mortality with every 100pg/mL increase in PTH and reported significant increases in the relative risk, by 1 and 4%, respectively. Categorical models revealed a significant increase in the mortality risk in only four of the seven studies. The categories of PTH levels at which the mortality risk increased significantly were >300pg/mL; >308pg/mL (HR, 1.68, reference: 160–308); >480pg/mL (HR: 1.17); 600–900pg/mL (RR: 1.08, reference: 150–300); 900–1200pg/mL (RR: 1.18, reference: 150–300) and >1200pg/mL (RR: 1.24, reference: 150–300). In general, the reports appear to support a uniform increase in the RR of death associated with PTH levels >600pg/mL in patients receiving dialysis, a level consistent with the recent DOPPS report suggesting that the lowest risk category is a PTH 101–600pg/mL.[8]

Four studies assessed the association between mortality risk and K/DOQI targets, but showed conflicting results depending upon the categorization choices. Categorical analysis identified a significant risk at PTH levels between 600 and 900pg/mL,[20] but not at >300pg/mL relative to the reference of 150–300pg/mL. Using a dichotomous PTH analysis, one study reported a significant decrease in risk by 11% in patients with levels within the target compared with those beyond it. No significant relationship was observed between low PTH levels and risk of mortality. This last feature seems at odds with the increasing feeling that adynamic or low-turnover bone disease is especially linked to soft-tissue deposition of excess calcium and phosphorus.

Some recent data regarding the relationship between PTH and outcome have been analyzed from the 4D study assessing atorvastatin use in type II diabetic dialysis patients.[25] Patients in the 4D study had a mean age of 66 ± 8 years, and 54% were male. Among patients without wasting (albumin >3.8g/dL, $n = 586$), the risks of death and cardiovascular events (CVE) during 4 years of follow-up significantly increased by 23 and 20% per unit increase in logPTH. Patients in the highest PTH tertile had a 74% higher risk of death [HR(adj) 1.74, 95% CI 1.27–2.40] and a 49% higher risk of CVE [HR(adj) 1.49, 95% CI 1.05–2.11] compared with patients in the lowest PTH tertile. In contrast, no effect was found in patients with wasting. Additional analyses in strata of BMI showed that PTH significantly impacted on death and CVE [HR(logPTH)(adj) 1.15 and 1.14, respectively] only in patients without, but not in patients with wasting. This is an important consideration given that most patients on dialysis have dozens of contemporaneous risk factors for death, which either co-exist or conspire by interaction. In the context of advanced loss of muscle, strength, more inflammation, and lower albumin, PTH is no longer the most important factor in driving mortality. If, however, patients were well nourished and stronger, and thus with a lower event rate and most events occurring later, the effect of PTH on mortality could be detected again as a signal. Wasting modifies the association of PTH with adverse outcomes in diabetic dialysis patients. Thus, the authors concluded that high PTH levels are of concern in the patients without wasting, while the effect of PTH on mortality is nullified in the patients with wasting. Whether similar confounders affect reported relationships for other biochemical markers of CKD-MBD (calcium and phosphorus) is unknown.

Data on mortality risk with PTH changes in pre-dialysis patients are seriously lacking and assertions about 'optimal' levels of PTH for patients with CKD not yet on dialysis cannot be supported with either observational or clinical trial data. For this reason the KDIGO guidelines state that the 'target' value for patients with CKD is unknown and recommend only that when PTH levels are elevated or raising that modifiable factors such as hyperphosphatemia, hypocalcemia and vitamin D deficiency be evaluated and treated.

Vitamin D

Vitamin D is a steroid hormone that has long been known for its key role in the regulation of calcium and phosphorus and bone metabolism, in addition it is an important nutrient with great implications in human health.[26] The vitamin D hormonal system comprises different metabolites derived from the precursor cholecalciferol (vitamin D_3), which is mainly generated under the influence of ultraviolet light in the skin, a minor proportion is of dietary origin. Endogenous vitamin D belongs to the vitamin D_3 series, while some vitamin D supplements extracted from plants, such as ergocalciferol, belong to the vitamin D_2 series.

Worldwide, nearly one billion people have inadequately low levels of calcidiol [25(OH)D_3], the main indicator of overall vitamin D nutritional status. In patients with CKD apart from the calcidiol deficiency (<15ng/mL) or insufficiency (<30ng/mL), there is an additional problem due to the reduction of renal mass and consequently of 1-alpha hydroxylase, which is followed by reduction in the serum levels of calcitriol, the natural physiological vitamin D receptor activator (VDRA).[4,27] In the past it was assumed that in CKD patients the calcidiol concentration was irrelevant, but now there is a body of evidence that demonstrate that calcidiol can activate the VDR and it can contributes to the overall vitamin D effect on target organs. This matter is important also in the dialysis population, as these mostly elderly patients have rather inactive life style and reduced exposure to sunshine, with a consequent reduction in the actinic synthesis of cholecalciferol.

Until recently, in patients with CKD, the VDRA has been mainly used in the treatment of SHPT, however, there is increasing evidence demonstrating that vitamin D exerts effects beyond parathyroid hormone and bone metabolism with important implications in morbidity and mortality. Nevertheless, the detrimental or beneficial effect of VDRAs use is still a controversial issue. The concern about the harmful effect of VDRAs is mainly based on the fact that in experimental models, high doses of calcitriol have shown to increase vascular calcification and some human data also support this notion.[28] On the other hand, experimental studies have shown that low and more physiological dose of VDRAs may have a cardioprotective effect. Observational studies carried out mainly in CKD 5 patients have shown overall mortality advantages with the use of VDRAs despite a demonstrable ability to increase serum levels of calcium and phosphorus.

One of the seminal contributions in this area was the study performed by Teng et al., who showed in a large observational study differences in survival in CKD 5 patients receiving two different VDRAs.[29] It was speculated that the potential survival advantage was mediated by the less calcemic and phosphatemic effects of the new VDRA, paricalcitol, but the survival benefit was sustained for almost all levels of phosphorus and calcium. While many efforts have concentrated on the likely effects of VDRAs on survival data, which suggests that while the beneficial effect of VDRAs may partly be due to different effects on calcium and phosphorus, potential explanations for the survival benefit being attributed to VDRA's include their differential effects on Ca and P, but may also be due to other important pleiotropic effects of the VDRAs. Disorders in cardiovascular function, inflammation, immune response, insulin resistance, and others, are all well documented clinical and experimental correlates associated with vitamin D metabolism.[30,31] Animals lacking the VDR show higher renin levels, hypertension, left ventricular hypertrophy, cardiomyocyte contractile abnormalities, and muscle dysfunction.[32] A differential effect of the VDRAs in the vasculature with different impact on vascular calcifications has been shown.[33] In addition, low VDRAs have been associated with inflammation and higher C Reactive protein levels, and physiological doses of active vitamin D have shown protective cardiovascular effects reducing the inflammatory response to cardiovascular injury, the myocardial cell hypertrophy and proliferation. As such, part of these paradoxical effects of vitamin D in the cardiovascular system can be explained by the different dose of VDRAs used. High pharmacological doses of VDRAs may favor vascular calcification, whereas more physiological doses may have protective effects.

VDRAs have also shown to be able to reduce fibrosis, inflammation and proteinuria with potential positive benefits on the progression of CKD.[30] Furthermore, low VDRA levels have been also associated to increased risk of cancer, infections, and immune disorders; accordingly, the use of different VDRA activators have been associated with better outcomes in all these disorders. A good example of this likely general beneficial effect is the important reduction in neoplastic and infectious mortality observed with the use of low dose of oral calcitriol.[34] A role of VDRAs deficiency in the life expectancy of CKD has been supported by a series of observational studies showing that calcidiol, calcitriol, alphacalcidol and paricalcitol treatment has been associated with better survival in CKD patients at all stages, but mainly in CKD 5.[8,29,34–36] Ravani et al. showed that serum calcidiol was an independent negative predictor of progression of CKD and death in CKD 2–5 patients, Teng et al. and Tentori et al. showed in different large scale studies that intravenous administration of different forms of VDRAs have been associated with a 15–26% improvement in survival in CKD 5 patients.[35,37] Recently, Naves et al. showed a 42–48% reduction in overall, cardiovascular, infectious, and neoplastic mortality associated to the use of oral forms of VDRA despite the potentially lower bioavailability of this via of administration.[34] They also found that the main survival benefit was seen in patients receiving mean daily doses of less than 1µg with the highest reduction associated with the lowest dose of 0.25µg/day.

However, it is necessary to reiterate that observational, experimental and mechanistic studies, no matter how well or rigorously conducted, still are an incomplete proof that VDRAs directly impact CKD outcomes. In particular, observational data regarding relationships between medication exposure and clinical outcome are susceptible to confounding by indication and there are several examples in the literature in which randomized clinical trials have not supported even strong beneficial relationships reported from observational data. Indeed, a recent re-evaluation of DOPPS data using sophisticated instrumental variable modeling techniques, failed to find a relationship between VDRA exposure and clinical outcome.[38]

Summary

It is reasonably clear that observational data support a significant relationship between biochemical markers of CKD-MBD (calcium, phosphorus, and PTH) and adverse clinical outcomes, and yet many fundamental questions remain unanswered. Do these observational data suggest or support a causal relationship between laboratory values and outcome? Should we establish clinical treatment target value guidelines based on observational data? What are the optimal values for these parameters? Does intervention to reduce elevated levels have an impact on clinical outcome? The answers to these questions are likely to be far more complex than can be answered by even well done observational studies.

While it is common to isolate single laboratory values when conducting such analyses in order to identify an independent relationship between the laboratory variable and a clinical outcome, the reality of clinical medicine is such that clinicians are faced with interpreting laboratory variables *in aggregrate*. Several reports have now attempted to replicate such complexity and consistently report that the RR is greatest among patients with simultaneously high calcium and phosphorus, often in association with overtly low (< 130pg/dL) or high (>600pg/dL) PTH.[20] Supporting the complex nature of these relationships and the importance of treating multiple abnormal laboratory values concurrently, Danese et al. have shown that patients who achieve combinations of K/DOQI targets for Ca, P, and PTH have a survival advantage compared with those who achieve only a single parameter in target.[39] These investigators further demonstrated the importance of *consistent* control of mineral metabolism as shown in Fig. 32.3

It is almost certain that there is no single threshold value for calcium, phosphorus or PTH that independent of the other variables is 'optimal'. Indeed, it appears that the 'target' value is a moving target that is likely to be modified by each patients unique underlying risk profile that changes over time. Data from Stevens et al. suggests that the optimal combination of calcium, phosphorus, and PTH varies with dialysis vintage,[20] while data from the 4D study suggests that it varies by concurrent illness. Thus, we urge providers to use restraint and caution when trying to establish universal and widely applied target values.

In general, it appears that elevations in phosphorus above the upper limit of normal can be demonstrably associated with adverse outcomes in patients with CKD on dialysis and that this threshold may be lower for patients with CKD not on dialysis or without CKD. Whether intervention to reduce the phosphate burden or reduce serum levels can modify this risk remains uncertain.

We agree with the recommendations of KDIGO that encourage the urgent conduct of randomized clinical trials to establish definitive evidence of the role of abnormal

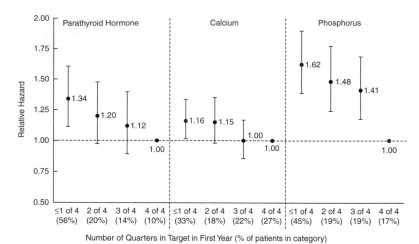

Fig. 32.3 Consistent control of mineral and bone disorder in incident hemodialysis patients. Time in target: relationship between quarters in target and risk for death. HR and 95% CI for number of quarters in target PTH, Ca, and P. Values in parentheses represent the proportion of patients in each category at baseline. (From: Danese MD, et al.. *Clin J Am Soc Nephrol* 2008;**3**:1423–9.

mineral metabolism in the exaggerated CV risk in patients with CKD and we caution against the rising tide of reliance upon observational data to define 'optimal' care. Nephrology is currently mired in the unenviable situation where observational data are used to generate clinical treatment 'guidelines', rather than being used to generate hypotheses to be tested with randomized controlled clinical trials. Unfortunately, such an approach has often proven to be erroneous when ultimately tested in properly conducted clinical trials. Remarkably, there are some in the community who go so far as to suggest that, on the basis of observational data alone, such randomized controlled trials are precluded from being conducted on ethical grounds. This intellectual nihilism must be resisted at all costs.

References

1. Haynes RB, Haynes GA. What does it take to put an ugly fact through the heart of a beautiful hypothesis? *Evid Based Med* 2009;**14**(3):68–9.
2. Go AS, Chertow GM, Fan D, McCulloch CE, Hsu CY. Chronic kidney disease and the risks of death, cardiovascular events, and hospitalization. *N Engl J Med* 2004;**351**(13):1296–305.
3. U.S. Renal Data System, USRDS 2008 Annual Data Report: *Atlas of Chronic Kidney Disease and End-Stage Renal Disease in the United States.* 2008, National Institutes of Health, National Institute of Diabetes and Digestive and Kidney Diseases: Bethesda, MD.
4. Levin A, Bakris GL, Molitch, M, et al. Prevalence of abnormal serum vitamin D, PTH, calcium, and phosphorus in patients with chronic kidney disease: results of the study to evaluate early kidney disease. *Kidney Int* 2007;**71**(1):31–8.
5. K/DOQI clinical practice guidelines for bone metabolism and disease in chronic kidney disease. *Am J Kidney Dis* 2003;**42**(4 Suppl 3):S1–201.

6. Group, K.D.I.G.O.K.C.-M.W., KDIGO clinical practice guideline for the diagnosis, evaluation, prevention, and treatment of chronic kidney disease-mineral and bone disorder (CKD-MBD). *Kidney International* 2009;**76**(Supp 113):S1–S130.

7. Covic A, Kothawala P, Bernal M, Robbins S, Chalian A, Goldsmith D. Systematic review of the evidence underlying the association between mineral metabolism disturbances and risk of all-cause mortality, cardiovascular mortality and cardiovascular events in chronic kidney disease. *Nephrol Dial Transplant* 2009;**24**:1506–23

8. Tentori F, Blayney MJ, Albert JM, et al. Mortality risk for dialysis patients with different levels of serum calcium, phosphorus, and PTH: the Dialysis Outcomes and Practice Patterns Study (DOPPS). *Am J Kidney Dis* 2008;**52**(3):519–30.

9. Block GA, Hulbert-Shearon TE, Levin NW, Port FK, Association of serum phosphorus and calcium x phosphate product with mortality risk in chronic hemodialysis patients: a national study. *Am J Kidney Dis* 1998;**31**(4):607–17.

10. Block GA, Klassen PS, Lazarus JM, Ofsthun, N, Lowrie EG, Chertow GM. Mineral metabolism, mortality, and morbidity in maintenance hemodialysis. *J Am Soc Nephrol* 2004;**15**(8):2208–18.

11. Young EW, Albert JM, Satayathum S, et al. Predictors and consequences of altered mineral metabolism: the Dialysis Outcomes and Practice Patterns Study. *Kidney Int* 2005;**67**(3):1179–87.

12. Foley RN, Collins AJ, Herzog CA, Ishani A, Kalra PA. Serum phosphorus levels associate with coronary atherosclerosis in young adults. *J Am Soc Nephrol* 2009;**20**(2): 397–404.

13. Kestenbaum B, Sampson, JN, Rudser, KD, et al. Serum phosphate levels and mortality risk among people with chronic kidney disease. *J Am Soc Nephrol* 2005;**16**(2):520–8.

14. Tonell M, Sacks F, Pfeffer M, Gao Z, Curhan G. Relation between serum phosphate level and cardiovascular event rate in people with coronary disease. *Circulation,* 2005;**112**(17):2627–33.

15. Sigrist MK, Taal MW, Bungay P, McIntyre, CW. Progressive vascular calcification over 2 years is associated with arterial stiffening and increased mortality in patients with stages 4 and 5 chronic kidney disease. *Clin J Am Soc Nephrol* 2007;**2**(6):1241–8.

16. Dhingra R, Sullivan, LM, Fox CS, et al. Relations of serum phosphorus and calcium levels to the incidence of cardiovascular disease in the community. *Arch Intern Med* 2007;**167**(9):879–85.

17. Foley RN, Collins AJ, Ishani, A, Kalra, PA. Calcium-phosphate levels and cardiovascular disease in community-dwelling adults: the Atherosclerosis Risk in Communities (ARIC) Study. *Am Heart J* 2008;**156**(3):556–63.

18. Foley RN. (2009) Phosphate Levels and Cardiovascular Disease in the General Population. *Clin J Am Soc Nephrol* 2009;**4**(6):1136–9.

19. Foley RN, Collins AJ, Herzog CA, Ishani A, Kalra PA. Serum phosphate and left ventricular hypertrophy in young adults: the coronary artery risk development in young adults study. *Kidney Blood Press Res* 2009;**32**(1):37–44.

20. Stevens LA, Djurdjev O, Cardew S, Cameron EC, Levin A. Calcium, phosphate, and parathyroid hormone levels in combination and as a function of dialysis duration predict mortality: evidence for the complexity of the association between mineral metabolism and outcomes. *J Am Soc Nephrol* 2004;**15**(3):770–9.

21. Gotch FA. Pro/Con debate: the calculation on calcium balance in dialysis lower the dialysate calcium concentrations (propart). *Nephrol Dial Transplant* 2009;**24**(10):2994–6.

22. Melamed ML, Eustace JA, Plantinga L, et al. Changes in serum calcium, phosphate, and PTH and the risk of death in incident dialysis patients: a longitudinal study. *Kidney Int* 2006;**70**(2):351–7.

23. St Peter WL, Li Q, Persky M, Nieman K, Arko C, Block GA. Cinacalcet Use Patterns and Effect on Laboratory Values and Other Medications in a Large Dialysis Organization, 2004 through 2006. *Clin J Am Soc Nephrol* 2009;**4**:354–360.

24. Slatopolsky E, Martin KJ, Hruska KA. Parathyroid hormone metabolism and its potential as a uremic toxin. *Am J Physiol Renal Physiol* 1980;**239**:F1–F12.

25. Drechsler C, Krane V, Grootendorst DC. The association between parathyroid hormone and mortality in dialysis patients is modified by wasting. *Nephrol Dial Transplant* 2009;**24**:3151–7.

26. Holick MF. Vitamin D: importance in the prevention of cancers, type 1 diabetes, heart disease, and osteoporosis. *Am J Clin Nutr* 2004;**79**(3):362–71.

27. Cannata-Andia JB and Gomez Alonso C. Vitamin D deficiency: a neglected aspect of disturbed calcium metabolism in renal failure. *Nephrol Dial Transplant* 2002;**17**(11):1875–8.

28. Valdivielso JM, Cannata-Andia J, Coll B, Fernandez E. A New Role for the Vitamin D Receptor Activation in Chronic Kidney Disease. *Am J Physiol Renal Physiol* 2009.

29. Teng M, Wolf M, Lowrie E, Ofsthun N, Lazarus JM, Thadhani R. Survival of patients undergoing hemodialysis with paricalcitol or calcitriol therapy. *N Engl J Med* 2003;**349**(5):446–56.

30. Alborzi P, Patel NA, Peterson C, et al. Paricalcitol reduces albuminuria and inflammation in chronic kidney disease: a randomized double-blind pilot trial. *Hypertension* 2008;**52**(2):249–55.

31. Timms PM, Mannan N, Hitman GA, et al. Circulating MMP9, vitamin D and variation in the TIMP-1 response with VDR genotype: mechanisms for inflammatory damage in chronic disorders? *QJM* 2002;**95**(12):787–96.

32. Bodyak N, Ayus JC, Achinger S, et al. Activated vitamin D attenuates left ventricular abnormalities induced by dietary sodium in Dahl salt-sensitive animals. *Proc Natl Acad Sci U S A* 2007;**104**(43):16810–5.

33. Cardus A, Panizo S, Parisi E, Fernandez E, Valdivielso JM, et al. Differential effects of vitamin D analogs on vascular calcification. *J Bone Miner Res* 2007;**22**(6):860–6.

34. Naves-Diaz M, Alvarez-Hernandez D, Passlick-Deetjen J, et al. Oral active vitamin D is associated with improved survival in hemodialysis patients. *Kidney Int* 2008;**74**(8):1070–8.

35. Ravani P, Malberti F, Tripepi G, et al. Vitamin D levels and patient outcome in chronic kidney disease. *Kidney Int* 2009;**75**(1):88–95.

36. Shoji T, Shinohara K, Kimoto E, et al. Lower risk for cardiovascular mortality in oral 1alpha-hydroxy vitamin D3 users in a haemodialysis population. *Nephrol Dial Transplant* 2004;**19**(1):179–84.

37. Teng M, Wolf M, Ofsthun MN, et al. Activated injectable vitamin D and hemodialysis survival: a historical cohort study. *J Am Soc Nephrol* 2005;**16**(4):1115–25.

38. Tentori F, Albert JM, Young EW, et al. The survival advantage for haemodialysis patients taking vitamin D is questioned: findings from the Dialysis Outcomes and Practice Patterns Study. *Nephrol Dial Transplant* 2009;**24**(3):963–72.

39. Danese MD, Belozeroff V, Smirnakis K, Rothman KJ. Consistent Control of Mineral and Bone Disorder in Incident Hemodialysis Patients. *Clin J Am Soc Nephrol* 2008;**3**:1423–29.

Index

Page numbers followed by "f" indicate figures, those followed by "t" indicate tables.